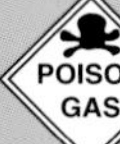

TOXIC BY INHALATION: Materials that have bee ... inhalation, and the shipping paper states: Poison-I ... marked: "Inhalation Hazard" and labeled "Poison." ... placarded "Poison" or "Poison Gas" as appropriate in addition to the primary hazard requirements. **Note:** 1000 lb exception does not apply to vehicles carrying these materials.

HAZARD CLASS/ DIVISION	LABEL	PLACARD	GUIDELINE
DIVISION 4.1	FLAMMABLE SOLID 4	FLAMMABLE SOLID 4	6
DIVISION 4.2	SPONTANEOUSLY COMBUSTIBLE 4	SPONTANEOUSLY COMBUSTIBLE 4	
DIVISION 4.3	DANGEROUS WHEN WET 4	DANGEROUS WHEN WET 4	6
DIVISION 5.1	OXYDIZER 5.1	OXYDIZER 5.1	7
DIVISION 5.2	ORGANIC PEROXIDE 5.2	ORGANIC PEROXIDE 5.2	8
DIVISION 6.1 (PG I & PG II)	POISON GAS 6	POISON GAS 6	10
DIVISION 6.1 (PG III)	HARMFUL STOW AWAY FROM FOODSTUFF 6	HARMFUL STOW AWAY FROM FOODSTUFF 6	10
CLASS 7 (YELLOW III)	RADIOACTIVE CONTENTS ACTIVITY 7	RADIOACTIVE 7	12
CLASS 8	CORROSIVE 8	CORROSIVE 8	13
CLASS 9	9	9	ii*

ii,* insufficient information; must identify specific substance

MIXED LOADS: When the total weight of two or more Table II materials is 1000 lbs (454 kg) or more, a DANGEROUS placard may be used. If 5000 lbs (2268 kg) or more of any Table II materials are loaded at one location, use its class placard.

EMERGENCY CARE FOR

HAZARDOUS MATERIALS EXPOSURE

EMERGENCY CARE FOR

HAZARDOUS MATERIALS EXPOSURE

PHILLIP L. CURRANCE, EMT-P, RHSP
Senior Paramedic Lakewood Fire Department (Ret)
Hazardous Materials Emergency Response Training Coordinator
Rocky Mountain Education Center/OSHA Training Institute
Red Rocks Community College Lakewood, Colorado;
Deputy Commander
Central U.S. National Medical Response Team—Weapons of Mass Destruction
Colorado 2 Disaster Medical Response Team
Denver, Colorado

Bruce Clements, MPH
Associate Director
Saint Louis University
School of Public Health
Center for the Study of Bioterrorism and Emerging Infections
Safety Officer, Missouri 1 Disaster Medical Response Team
Saint Louis, Missouri

Alvin C. Bronstein, MD, FACEP
Medical Director, Rocky Mountain Poison and Drug Center;
Assistant Professor of Surgery
Colorado Health Sciences Center
Denver, Colorado

THIRD EDITION

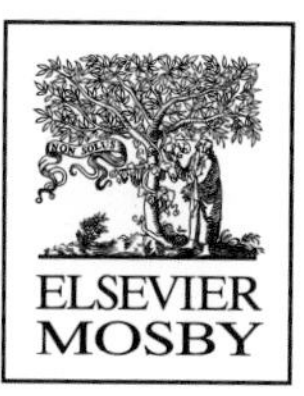

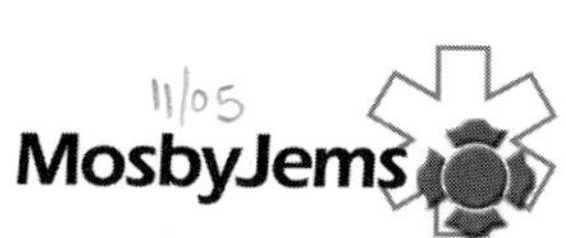

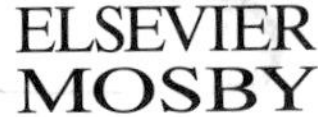

11830 Westline Industrial Drive
St. Louis, Missouri 63146

EMERGENCY CARE FOR HAZARDOUS MATERIALS EXPOSURE, THIRD EDITION

ISBN 0-323-02342-8

NOTICE

EMS is an ever-changing field. Standard safety precautions must be followed, but as new research and clinical experience broaden our knowledge, changes in treatment and drug therapy may become necessary or appropriate. Readers are advised to check the most current product information provided by the manufacturer of each drug to be administered to verify the recommended dose, the method and duration of administration, and contraindications. It is the responsibility of the licensed prescriber, relying on experience and knowledge of the patient, to determine dosages and the best treatment for each individual patient. Neither the publisher nor the author assumes any liability for any injury and/or damage to persons or property arising from this publication. The Publisher.

International Standard Book Number 0-323-02342-8

Acquisitions Editor: Linda Honeycutt
Developmental Editor: Katherine Tomber
Publishing Services Manager: Patricia Tannian
Project Manager: John Casey
Senior Book Designer: Teresa McBryan

Printed in United States of America

Last digit is the print number: 9 8 7 6 5 4 3 2 1

Dedication

A debt of honor and thanks is owed to the people who protect our safety and way of life. Those who unselfishly volunteer to serve in our nation's armed forces, emergency responders from the fire, police, and EMS fields, medical providers from hospitals, clinics, and private practices, public health workers, and emergency management personnel. People from every one of these groups make many personal sacrifices to ensure our health, safety, and freedom. Many place themselves in harm's way each and every day. This text is dedicated to those who serve, especially to those who have made the ultimate sacrifice and to their families and loved ones left behind.

Reviewers

Christian E. Callsen, Jr., LP
Senior Division Commande—Operations
Austin-Travis County Emergency Medical Services
Austin, Texas

Attila J. Hertelendy, BHsc, CCEMT-P, NREMT-P
Instructor
University of Mississippi Medical Center
Jackson, Mississippi

Paul E. Phrampus, MD, FACEP
Assistant Professor
Department of Emergency Medicine
University of Pittsburgh
Pittsburgh, Pennsylvania

Gordon M. Sachs, EFO, MPA
Chief (Ret.)
Fairfield Fire and EMS
Fairfield, Pennsylvania

Preface

While hazardous material medical emergencies continue to be challenge for medical personnel, the threat of weapons of mass destruction (WMD) has captured the focus of media and medical provider attention. The third edition of *Emergency Care for Hazardous Material Exposure* provides amplified and strengthened treatment guidelines for not only hazardous materials exposure but also exposure to agents that may be used in an intentional release or terrorist attack.

The purpose of this edition is to provide a foundation in this vital area for the EMS field provider and the first receivers in the hospital setting. This edition includes an expanded index, updated treatment guidelines, and a new WMD guideline section that adds 31 new treatment guidelines. This new section expands the treatment guidelines to 140 (13 generic hazard class guidelines, 5 acid guidelines, 5 base guidelines, 21 organic solvent/petroleum distillate guidelines, 2 other organic guidelines, 2 nitrogen compound guidelines, 10 insecticide guidelines, 13 herbicide and rodenticide guidelines, 17 metal/metalloid guidelines, 4 asphyxiant guidelines, 2 irritant guidelines, 7 halogen / halogen compound guidelines, 8 miscellaneous chemical guidelines, 3 radiological agent guidelines, 19 biological agent guidelines, and 9 chemical agent guidelines). The treatment protocol section, drug protocol section, and EMS/hazardous materials operating procedures have also been updated and expanded.

The first and second editions provided an organized approach for the care of patients exposed to hazardous materials. We hope that the third edition not only will continue to supply this information but also will provide the same organized approach to the new challenge of WMD response.

Just as individuals react to specific chemical insults with a great degree of variation, each chemical, alone or in combination, is capable of producing a variety of environmental and end-organ effects. This basic principle must be kept in mind when responding to a hazardous material incident. Therefore it is not possible to predict with complete accuracy the total scope of the myriad of toxic effects that may be encountered. We will continue in our research and data collections for future editions and welcome your comments and incident experiences.

We owe major thanks to the people at Elsevier: Andrew Allen, Linda Honeycutt, Katherine Tomber, and John Casey. They are truly dedicated to improving the level of health care through education. We thank them for supporting us in the past and allowing us to produce this text.

Phillip L. Currance
Bruce Clements
Alvin C. Bronstein

User's Guide

This manual has been established as a field reference source on the health effects of hazardous materials exposure. The book has been organized into six sections to facilitate field use.

INDEXES: By hazard class, numerical and alphabetical numerical listing, and chemical grouping
GUIDELINES: Management keyed to specific chemical groups
TREATMENT PROTOCOLS: Treatment for specific hazardous materials–induced medical problems
DRUG PROTOCOLS: Outlines for advanced life support drugs, specific physiological antagonists (antidotes), and antibiotics
EMS/HAZARDOUS MATERIALS OPERATING PROCEDURES: Pre-incident planning, incident response, and post-incident analysis procedures
REFERENCES: Sources used to compile information and suggested additional texts

Section One ■ CHEMICAL INDEXES

The index section has been divided into three parts:
U.S. Department of Transportation (DOT) Hazard Class Section: If only the hazardous material placard is visible
Numerical Index: If the UN/NA (United Nations/North American number) or Product Identification Number (PIN) is known
Alphabetical Index: If the chemical name is known; whenever possible, the alphabetical index should be used for exact chemical name and appropriate guideline identification.

NOTE: If the chemicals in question cannot be located in the index, refer to the general hazard class guidelines that are keyed to the Department of Transportation (DOT) Hazard Classes.

WARNING! Multiple chemical agents may have the same United Nations Number (UN/NA/PIN). Therefore be sure to look up the guideline for the specific material in question by chemical name and not UN/NA/PIN alone.

When only the UN/NA/PIN is known, familiarize yourself with all of the GUIDELINES referenced to that particular UN/NA/PIN until the exact chemical(s) is/are identified. Generally substances with the same UN/NA/PIN have similar kinds of on-site protective equipment cautions. They will usually differ in their toxicology and respective medical management. When multiple guidelines are referenced, incident and patient management should be based on the most conservative information until the specific substance is identified.

The index includes chemicals listed in the North American Emergency Response Guidebook, the Comprehensive Environmental Response, Compensation and Liability Act (CERCLA—Superfund" List), the Superfund Amendment and Reauthorization Act of 1986 (SARA—Extremely Hazardous Substances List), the federal Water Pollution Control Act (Clean Water Act), the Clean Air Act, the Centers for Disease Control and Prevention, Critical Biological Agents for Public Health Preparedness, and the Federal Bureau of Investigation's top ten list of agents most likely to be used in a chemical attack.

Section Two ■ GUIDELINES

The first 13 Guidelines are indexed to the DOT Hazard Classes. If the exact chemical identity is not known, these guidelines supply generic information by Hazard Class. Guidelines 14 to 109 were established for chemicals with similar toxic effects and treatment modalities. Guidelines 110 to 140 were established for agents that could be used as weapons of mass destruction. The guidelines have been divided into representative groups to facilitate use. Each substance/agent listed in the index is either referenced to a specific or a general Hazard Class management guideline. Some substances/agent are referenced to more than one guideline.
The guidelines are organized as follows:

Substance Identification: General description of the chemical(s) covered by this guideline. Product description, uses, and background information are included.

Routes of Exposure: Possible routes of exposure are included.

Target Organs: Affected primary and secondary target organ systems are listed. Primary target organs are those directly affected by the product. Secondary target organs are those affected by compromise of another body system.

Life Threat: The primary life threat usually associated with this group of products is described.

Signs and Symptoms by System: Usual signs and symptoms associated with exposure to this product group are listed.

Symptom Onset for Acute Exposure: To assist with triage and patient treatment decisions, the symptom onset secondary to acute product exposure is listed.

Co-Exposure Concerns: Concomitant exposure to these products may have an additive health effect.

Thermal Decomposition Products: Known thermal decomposition products are described to assist in classification of increased chemical threat in fire situations.

Medical Problems Possibly Aggravated by Exposure: Medical conditions that may be aggravated by exposure to this group of product/s are included

Decontamination: Specific decontamination procedures are described.

Immediate First Aid: Procedures for immediate first aid by trained first responders and first aid squads are described.

Basic Treatment: Basic care procedures for emergency medical technicians are listed; basic level personnel and basic procedures for advanced personnel are described.

Advanced Treatment: Procedures for personnel with advanced levels of training (paramedics, nurses, nurse practitioners, physician assistants, and physicians) are described.

Initial Emergency Department Considerations: Initial hospital emergency department procedures are described. This section includes suggested therapeutic interventions, treatment, and laboratory studies.

Special Considerations: Additional information specific to this group of products is presented.

NOTE: Each of the above sections is included in each guideline as appropriate (not every section is included in each guideline).
Therapeutic interventions are presented as suggestions. All treatment and medication (drug) decisions and protocols must be approved by the local medical control physician.

It is beyond the scope of this text to specify the exact type of protective equipment required for the specific chemical(s) encountered. Experienced hazmat response personnel must use appropriate information resources and protective clothing compatibility charts to identify the exact chemical protective clothing needed. Do not enter hazardous environments or carry out decontamination practices without appropriate training and equipment.

Section Three ■ TREATMENT PROTOCOLS

These were written for treatment of specific medical problems resulting from hazardous materials exposure and problems encountered during response operations such as heat stress. The protocols give detailed information on therapeutic interventions listed in the guidelines. This section also includes general information on inhalation and dermal and ingestion exposures. These protocols should be used in conjunction with, and adapted to, your local field protocols. All treatment protocols must be approved by the local medical control physician.

Section Four ■ DRUG PROTOCOLS

Concise discussions for all drugs referred to in the guidelines section are provided. These include appropriate advanced life support (ALS) medications and specific physiological antagonists (antidotes). Some of these medications are not appropriate for field use. Protocols in this section should be modified to conform to your local standards. All drug protocols must be approved by the local medical control physician.

NOTE: The treatment and drug protocols have been provided only as suggested usage outlines. Your operating procedures and the standing and/or verbal orders established by your local medical control physician take precedence.

Section Five ■ EMS/HAZARDOUS MATERIALS OPERATING PROCEDURES

Procedures for safe response practices, scene operations, and hazmat team support are described. Preplanning, postincident procedures, medical surveillance, and emergency equipment suggestions are given.

Section Six ■ REFERENCES

Sources used in compiling this manual are listed.

Disclaimer

The views and opinions expressed in this text and related materials are solely those of the authors and do not reflect the positions or official policy of any local jurisdiction, state agency, any department of the U.S. Government or any affiliated agencies.

While the authors, editors, publisher, and their agents have made every effort to ensure the accuracy of information contained in this work, they cannot be held responsible for any errors found in this text. The authors, editors, publisher, and their agents do not bear any responsibility or liability for the information contained in this text or for any uses to which it may be put.

The contents of this text and related materials are not intended to be a substitute for professional medical advice, diagnosis or treatment. Always seek the medical advice of a physician or other qualified health provider. Information contained in this text in no way authorizes anyone to perform any of the procedures or protocols that are listed. Operating protocols, standing, and/or verbal orders must be established by local Emergency Medical Service Physician control.

This text is based on current research and to the best of the author's ability, the information, drug indications, dosages, and precautions are current as of publication. The reader is urged to consult the package information provided by the manufacturer for the latest changes.

Do not enter hazardous environments or carry out decontamination procedures without proper protective equipment. It is beyond the scope of this text to advise the exact type of protective equipment needed. Other resources and chemical compatibility charts must be checked. Training in the proper use of protective equipment is essential to your safety.

The use of any product or equipment names in this text is for illustrative purposes only. It in no way endorses or promotes the use of any specific product or company.

Contents

Section One

INDEXES

If the chemicals in question cannot be located in the index, refer to the general hazard class guidelines that are keyed to the Department of Transportation (DOT) Hazard Classes.

WARNING! Multiple chemical agents may have the same United Nations Number (UN/NA/PIN). Therefore be sure to look up the guideline for the specific material in question by chemical name and not UN/NA/PIN alone.

When only the UN/NA/PIN is known, familiarize yourself with all of the GUIDELINES referenced to that particular UN/NA/PIN until the exact chemical(s) is/are identified. Generally, substances with the same UN/NA/PIN have similar kinds of on-site protective equipment cautions. They will usually differ in their toxicology and respective medical management.

Numerical Index

UN/ NA/PIN	Chemical Name	Guideline Number
0004	Ammonium Picrate, dry or wetted with less than 10% water	14
0072	Cyclonite	1
0076	2,4-Dinitrophenol	62
0154	Picric Acid	62
0208	Tetryl	43
0209	Trinitrotoluene	24, 47
0214	Trinitrobenzene	24, 47
0222	Ammonium Nitrate, with more than 0.2% combustible material	47
0223	Ammonium Nitrate Fertilizer, which is more liable to explode than ammonium nitrate with 0.2% combustible material	47
0357	Substances, explosive, n.o.s.	1
0358	Substances, explosive, n.o.s.	1
0359	Substances, explosive, n.o.s.	1
0402	Ammonium Perchlorate	21, 97
1001	Acetylene	33, 92
1001	Acetylene, dissolved	33, 92
1002	Air, compressed	3
1003	Air, refrigerated liquid (cryogenic liquid)	3
1005	Ammonia	21, 133, 138
1005	Ammonia, anhydrous, liquefied	21, 133, 138
1005	Ammonia Solution, with more than 50% ammonia	21
1005	Anhydrous Ammonia	21, 133, 138
1006	Argon, compressed	92
1008	Boron Trifluoride	103, 133, 138
1009	Bromotrifluoromethane	26
1009	Monobromotrifluoromethane	27
1009	Trifluorobromomethane	27
1010	Butadiene, inhibited	33
1010	1,3-Butadiene	33
1011	Butane or Butane Mixture	33
1011	*n*-Butane	33
1012	Butene	33
1012	Butylene	33
1013	Carbon Dioxide	92
1014	Carbon Dioxide–Oxygen Mixture	92
1015	Carbon Dioxide–Nitrous Oxide Mixture	92
1016	Carbon Monoxide	89
1017	Chlorine	98, 133, 138
1018	Chlorodifluoromethane	27
1020	Chloropentafluoroethane	27
1020	Monochloropentafluoroethane	27
1021	Chlorotetrafluoroethane	27
1021	Monochlorotetrafluoroethane	27
1022	Chlorotrifluoromethane	27
1022	Monochlorotrifluoromethane	27
1022	Trifluorochloromethane	27
1023	Coal Gas	2
1026	Cyanogen	90, 132
1026	Cyanogen, liquefied	90, 132
1026	Cyanogen Gas	90, 132

WARNING: More than one chemical agent may have the same UN Number. Look up the guideline for the specific material in question by chemical name and not UN/NA/Pin Number alone.

UN/ NA/PIN	Chemical Name	Guideline Number
1027	Cyclopropane	92
1027	Cyclopropane, liquefied	92
1028	Dichlorodifluoromethane	27
1029	Dichlorofluoromethane	27
1029	Dichloromonofluoromethane	27
1030	Difluoroethane	27
1032	Dimethylamine, anhydrous	20
1033	Dimethyl Ether	38
1035	Ethane, compressed	33
1036	Ethylamine	20
1036	Monoethylamine	20
1037	Ethyl Chloride	26
1038	Ethylene, refrigerated liquid (cryogenic liquid)	33, 92
1039	Ethyl Methyl Ether	38
1039	Methyl Ethyl Ether	38
1040	Ethylene Oxide	45, 133, 138
1040	ETO	45, 133, 138
1041	Carbon Dioxide–Ethylene Oxide Mixture, with more than 6% ethylene oxide	45, 92
1041	Ethylene Oxide–Carbon Dioxide Mixture, with more than 6% ethylene oxide	45, 92
1043	Fertilizer Ammoniating Solution, with more than 35% free ammonia	21, 47
1044	Fire Extinguisher, with compressed or liquefied gas	92
1045	Fluorine	99, 133, 138
1045	Fluorine, compressed	99, 133, 138
1046	Helium	92
1046	Helium, compressed	92

UN/ NA/PIN	Chemical Name	Guideline Number
1048	Hydrogen Bromide	95, 133, 138
1048	Hydrogen Bromide, anhydrous	95, 133, 138
1049	Hydrogen, compressed	2, 92
1050	Hydrochloric Acid	14
1050	Hydrochloric Acid, anhydrous	14
1050	Hydrogen Chloride	14, 133, 138
1050	Hydrogen Chloride, anhydrous	14, 133, 138
1051	Hydrocyanic Acid	90, 132, 138
1051	Hydrocynac Acid	90, 132, 138
1051	Hydrogen Cyanide	90, 132, 138
1051	Hydrogen Cyanide, anhydrous, stabilized	90, 132, 138
1052	Hydrofluoric Acid	16
1052	Hydrofluoric Acid, anhydrous	16, 133, 138
1052	Hydrogen Fluoride	16, 133, 138
1052	Hydrogen Fluoride, anhydrous	16, 133, 138
1053	Hydrogen Sulfide	91, 138
1053	Hydrogen Sulfide, liquefied	91, 138
1055	Isobutylene	33
1056	Krypton	92
1056	Krypton, compressed	92
1057	Cigarette Lighter, with flammable gas	33
1057	Flammable Gas, in lighter for cigars, cigarettes, etc.	33
1057	Lighter, for cigars, etc., with flammable gas	33

WARNING: More than one chemical agent may have the same UN Number. Look up the guideline for the specific material in question by chemical name and not UN/NA/Pin number alone.

UN/ NA/PIN	Chemical Name	Guideline Number
1057	Lighter Refills, for cigarettes, containing flammable gas	33
1058	Liquefied Gas, nonflammable, charged with nitrogen, carbon dioxide, or air	3
1058	Liquefied Nonflammable Gas, charged with nitrogen, carbon dioxide, or air	3
1060	Methyl Acetylene and Propadiene Mixture, stabilized	35
1061	Methylamine	20
1061	Monomethylamine, anhydrous	20
1062	Methyl Bromide	95
1062	Fumigants	10
1063	Methyl Chloride	26
1064	Methyl Mercaptan	105
1065	Neon, compressed	92
1066	Nitrogen, compressed	92
1067	Dinitrogen Tetroxide	48
1067	Nitrogen Dioxide	48
1067	Nitrogen Oxides	48
1067	Nitrogen Peroxide	48
1067	Nitrogen Tetroxide	48
1069	Nitrosyl Chloride	14
1070	Nitrous Oxide, compressed	48
1071	Oil Gas	35
1072	Oxygen, compressed	7
1073	Oxygen, refrigerated liquid (cryogenic liquid)	7
1075	Liquefied Petroleum Gas, LPG	2, 35
1075	Petroleum Gas, liquefied	2, 35
1076	Carbonyl Chloride	101
1076	Phosgene	101, 133, 138
1077	Propylene	33

UN/ NA/PIN	Chemical Name	Guideline Number
1078	Chlorodifluoromethane and Chloropentafluoroethane Mixture	27
1078	Chlorotrifluoromethane and Trifluoromethane Mixture	27
1078	Dichlorodifluoromethane and Chlorodifluoromethane Mixture	27
1078	Dichlorodifluoromethane and Dichlorotetrafluoroethane Mixture	27
1078	Dichlorodifluoromethane and Difluoroethane Mixture	27
1078	Dichlorodifluoromethane, Trichlorofluoromethane, and Chlorodifluoromethane Mixture	27
1078	Dichlorodifluoromethane and Trichlorofluoromethane Mixture	27
1078	Dichlorodifluoromethane and Trichlorotrifluoroethane Mixture	27
1078	Dispersant Gas, n.o.s.	3
1078	Freons/Halons (various)	27
1078	Refrigerant Gases, n.o.s.	27
1078	Trifluoromethane and Chlorotrifluoromethane Mixture	27
1079	Sulfur Dioxide	105, 133, 138
1079	Sulfur Dioxide, liquefied	105, 133, 138
1080	Sulfur Hexafluoride	92
1081	Tetrafluoroethylene, inhibited	26
1082	Trifluorochloroethylene	27
1082	Trifluorochloroethylene, inhibited	27
1083	Trimethylamine	20

WARNING: More than one chemical agent may have the same UN Number. Look up the guideline for the specific material in question by chemical name and not UN/NA/Pin number alone.

UN/ NA/PIN	Chemical Name	Guideline Number
1083	Trimethylamine, anhydrous	20
1085	Vinyl Bromide	95
1085	Vinyl Bromide, inhibited	95
1086	Monochloroethylene	26
1086	Vinyl Chloride	28
1086	Vinyl Chloride, inhibited	28
1087	Vinyl Methyl Ether	38
1087	Vinyl Methyl Ether, inhibited	38
1088	Acetal	41
1089	Acetaldehyde	41
1090	Acetone	42
1091	Acetone Oil	42
1092	Acrolein	59
1092	Acrolein, inhibited	59
1093	Acrylonitrile	90
1093	Acrylonitrile, inhibited	90
1098	Allyl Alcohol	29
1099	Allyl Bromide	61
1100	Allyl Chloride	61, 98
1103	Trimethyl Aluminum	10
1104	Amyl Acetates	37
1105	Amyl Alcohols	30
1105	Isoamyl Alcohols	30
1106	Amylamine	20
1107	Amyl Chloride	26
1108	Amylene	5, 92
1108	1-Pentene	33
1109	Amyl Formate	37
1110	Amyl Methyl Ketone	42
1110	Methyl Amyl Ketone	42
1111	Amyl Mercaptan	105
1112	Amyl Nitrate	47
1113	Amyl Nitrite	47
1114	Benzene	25
1114	Benzol	25
1115	Benzine	25, 35
1118	Brake Fluid, hydraulic	35
1120	Butanol	30
1120	Butyl Alcohol	30
1123	Butyl Acetate	37
1125	Butylamine	20
1125	*n*-Butylamine	20
1126	Butyl Bromide	26
1127	Butyl Chloride	26
1127	Chlorobutane	26
1128	Butyl Formate	37
1129	Butyraldehyde	41
1130	Camphor Oil	36
1131	Carbon Bisulfide	93
1131	Carbon Disulfide	93, 133, 138
1132	Carbon Remover, liquid	35
1133	Adhesive	9
1133	Adhesive, containing flammable liquid	5
1133	Cement	19
1133	Cement, liquid, n.o.s.	19
1133	Cement, containing flammable liquid	19
1134	Chlorobenzene	25
1135	Ethylene Chlorohydrin	28, 61
1136	Coal Tar Distillate	24, 25
1136	Coal Tar Oil	24, 25
1137	Coal Tar Distillate	24, 25
1137	Coal Tar Oil	24, 25
1139	Coating Solution	10
1142	Antifreeze	40
1142	Cleaning Compound	19
1142	Compound, Polishing, liquid, etc. (combustible or flammable)	10

WARNING: More than one chemical agent may have the same UN Number. Look up the guideline for the specific material in question by chemical name and not UN/NA/Pin number alone.

UN/NA/PIN	Chemical Name	Guideline Number
1142	Flammable Liquid Preparations, n.o.s.	5
1142	Reducing Liquid	10
1142	Removing Liquid	10
1143	Crotonaldehyde	59
1143	Crotonaldehyde, inhibited	59
1144	Crotonylene	33
1145	Cyclohexane	33
1146	Cyclopentane	33
1147	Decahydronaphthalene	43
1148	Diacetone Alcohol	42
1149	Butyl Ether	38
1149	Dibutyl Ether	38
1150	Dichloroethylene	27
1150	1,2-Dichloroethylene	27
1152	Dichloropentane	27
1153	Diethoxyethane	38
1153	Diethyl Cellosolve	40
1153	Ethylene Glycol Diethyl Ether	40
1154	Diethylamine	20
1155	Diethyl Ether	38
1155	Ether	38
1155	Ethyl Ether	38
1156	Diethyl Ketone	42
1157	Diisobutyl Ketone	42
1158	Diisopropylamine	20
1159	Diisopropyl Ether	38
1159	Isopropyl Ether	38
1160	Dimethylamine Solution	20
1161	Dimethyl Carbonate	37
1162	Dimethyldichlorosilane	107
1163	Dimethylhydrazine, unsymmetrical	23
1164	Dimethyl Sulfide	105
1164	Methyl Sulfide	105
1165	Dioxane	39

UN/NA/PIN	Chemical Name	Guideline Number
1166	Dioxolane	40
1167	Divinyl Ether, inhibited	38
1168	Drier, paint or varnish, liquid, n.o.s.	10
1169	Extract, aromatic, liquid	24
1170	Alcohol (beverage)	29
1170	Alcohol (ethyl)	29
1170	Alcoholic Beverage	29
1170	Ethanol	29
1170	Ethyl Alcohol	29
1171	2-Ethoxyethanol	40
1171	Ethylene Glycol Monobutyl and Monoethyl Ether	40
1172	2-Ethoxyethanol Acetate	40
1172	Ethylene Glycol Monomethyl Ether Acetate	40
1173	Ethyl Acetate	37
1175	Ethylbenzene	24
1176	Ethyl Borate	103
1177	Ethylbutyl Acetate	37
1178	Ethyl Butyraldehyde	41
1179	Ethylbutyl Ether	38
1180	Ethyl Butyrate	37
1181	Ethyl Chloroacetate	37
1182	Ethyl Chloroformate	37
1183	Ethyldichlorosilane	107
1184	Ethylene Dichloride	26
1185	Ethylene Imine, inhibited	20
1188	Ethylene Glycol Monomethyl Ether and Acetate	40
1189	Ethylene Glycol Monomethyl Ether Acetate	40
1190	Ethyl Formate	37
1191	2-Ethyl Hexaldehyde	41
1191	Octyl Aldehyde	41
1192	Ethyl Lactate	37

WARNING: More than one chemical agent may have the same UN Number. Look up the guideline for the specific material in question by chemical name and not UN/NA/Pin number alone.

UN/ NA/PIN	Chemical Name	Guideline Number
1193	Methyl Ethyl Ketone	42
1194	Ethyl Nitrite, and Solutions	47
1195	Ethyl Propionate	37
1196	Ethyltrichlorosilane	107
1197	Extract, Flavoring, Liquid	5
1198	Formaldehyde (Formalin)	41, 133, 138
1199	Furfural	41
1201	Fusel Oil	30
1202	Gas Oil	35
1203	Diesel Fuel	35
1203	Gasohol	35
1203	Gasoline	35
1203	Motor Fuel, n.o.s.	35
1203	Motor Spirit	35
1203	Petrol	35
1204	Glyceryl Trinitrate Solution	1, 47
1205	Gutta Percha Solution	34
1206	*n*-Heptane	33
1207	Hexaldehyde	41
1208	*n*-Hexane	33
1208	Neohexane	33
1210	Ink	5
1212	Isobutanol	30
1212	Isobutyl Alcohol	30
1213	Isobutyl Acetate	37
1214	Isobutylamine	20
1216	Isooctene	33
1218	Isoprene, inhibited	33
1219	Isopropanol	29
1219	Isopropyl Alcohol	29
1220	Isopropyl Acetate	37
1221	Isopropyl Amine	20
1222	Isopropyl Nitrate	47
1223	Kerosene	35
1224	Ketone, liquid, n.o.s.	42
1226	Cigarette Lighter, with flammable liquid	33
1226	Lighter for Cigars, etc., with flammable liquid	33
1226	Lighter Fluid	33
1228	Mercaptan Mixture, aliphatic	105
1228	Mercaptans and Mixtures, liquid, n.o.s.	105
1229	Mesityl Oxide	42
1230	Methanol	31
1230	Methyl Alcohol	31
1230	Wood Alcohol	31
1231	Methyl Acetate	31
1232	Methyl Acetone	42
1233	Methyl Amyl Acetate	37
1234	Methylal	38
1235	Methylamine	20
1235	Monomethylamine, aqueous solution	20
1237	Methyl Butyrate	37
1238	Methyl Chlorocarbonate	26
1238	Methyl Chloroformate	26
1239	Methyl Chloromethyl Ether	26, 38
1242	Methyl Dichlorosilane	107
1243	Methyl Formate	31
1244	Monomethylhydrazine	23
1245	Methyl Isobutyl Ketone	42
1246	Methyl Isopropenyl Ketone, inhibited	42
1247	Methyl Methacrylate Monomer	37
1248	Methyl Propionate	37
1249	Methyl Propyl Ketone	42
1249	2-Pentanone	42
1250	Methyl Trichlorosilane	107

WARNING: More than one chemical agent may have the same UN Number. Look up the guideline for the specific material in question by chemical name and not UN/NA/Pin number alone.

UN/ NA/PIN	Chemical Name	Guideline Number
1250	Silanes	107
1251	Methyl Vinyl Ketone	42
1255	Naphthas, Petroleum	35
1255	Petroleum Naphtha	35
1256	Naphtha, Solvent	35
1257	Casinghead Gasoline	35
1257	Natural Gasoline	35
1259	Nickel Carbonyl	85
1261	Nitromethane	47
1262	Isooctane	33
1262	Octane	33
1263	Enamel	10, 35
1263	Lacquer	35
1263	Lacquer Base, liquid	35
1263	Paint, etc., flammable liquid	5
1263	Paint-Related Material, flammable liquid	5
1263	Polish, liquid	10
1263	Shellac	35
1263	Stain	35
1263	Thinner	35
1263	Varnish	35
1263	Wood Filler, liquid	35
1264	Paraldehyde	41
1265	Isopentane	33
1265	Pentane	33
1266	Perfumery Products, with flammable solvent	35
1267	Petroleum Crude Oil	35
1268	Petroleum Distillate	35
1268	Road Oil	35
1270	Oil, petroleum, n.o.s.	35
1270	Petroleum Oil	35
1271	Petroleum Ether	38
1271	Petroleum Spirits	35
1272	Pine Oil	34
1274	Normal Propyl Alcohol	29
1274	Propanol	29
1274	*n*-Propyl Alcohol	29
1275	Propionaldehyde	41
1276	*n*-Propyl Acetate	37
1277	Monopropylamine	20
1277	Propylamine	20
1278	Propyl Chloride	26
1279	1,2-Dichloropropane	61
1279	Propylene Dichloride	61
1280	Propylene Oxide	38
1281	Propyl Formate	37
1282	Pyridine	24
1286	Rosin Oil	10
1287	Rubber Solvent	35
1287	Rubber Solution	10
1288	Shale Oil	33
1289	Sodium Methylate, solutions in alcohol	19, 31
1292	Ethyl Silicate	107
1292	Tetraethyl Silicate	107
1293	Tincture, Medicinal	10
1294	Toluene/Toluol	24
1295	Trichlorosilane	107
1296	Triethylamine	20
1297	Trimethylamine, aqueous solution	20
1298	Triethylchlorosilane	107
1298	Trimethylchlorosilane	107
1299	Turpentine	34
1300	Turpentine Substitute	34
1301	Vinyl Acetate	37
1301	Vinyl Acetate, inhibited	37
1302	Vinyl Ethyl Ether	38
1302	Vinyl Ethyl Ether, inhibited	38
1303	Vinylidene Chloride	26

WARNING: More than one chemical agent may have the same UN Number. Look up the guideline for the specific material in question by chemical name and not UN/NA/Pin number alone.

UN/ NA/PIN	Chemical Name	Guideline Number
1303	Vinylidene Chloride, inhibited	26
1304	Vinyl Butyl Ether	38
1304	Vinyl Isobutyl Ether	38
1304	Vinyl Isobutyl Ether, inhibited	38 38
1305	Vinyl Trichlorosilane	107
1306	Wood Preservative, liquid	35
1307	Xylene (xylol)	24
1308	Zirconium Metal, liquid suspension	10
1308	Zirconium Suspended in a Liquid	10
1309	Aluminum Powder, coated	10
1310	Ammonium Picrate, wetted with more than 10% water	14
1312	Borneol	36
1313	Calcium Resinate	6
1314	Calcium Resinate, fused	6
1318	Cobalt Resinate, precipitated	77
1320	Dinitrophenol, wetted with not less than 15% water	62
1321	Dinitrophenolate, wet, with not less than 15% water	62
1322	Dinitroresorcinol, wet, with not less than 15% water	62
1323	Ferrocerium	79
1324	Film, motion picture, nitrocellulose base	6
1324	Film, nitrocellulose base	6
1325	Cosmetics, flammable solid, n.o.s.	6
1325	Flammable Solid, n.o.s.	6
1325	Pyroxylin Plastic, rod, sheet, roll, tube, or scrap	38
1325	Smokeless Powder, small arms	1

UN/ NA/PIN	Chemical Name	Guideline Number
1325	Tetraethylammonium Perchlorate, dry	97
1326	Hafnium Metal, powder, wet	6
1327	Bhusa	10
1327	Hay	6
1327	Straw	6
1328	Hexamine	20
1330	Manganese and Compounds	83
1330	Manganese Resinate	83
1331	Matches, strike anywhere	97
1332	Metaldehyde	41
1333	Cerium, crude	10
1333	Cerium, slabs, ingots, or rods	10
1333	Mischmetal, powder	6, 10
1334	Creosote Salts	44
1334	Naphthalene, crude or refined	43
1336	Nitroguanidine, wet, with not less than 20% water	62
1336	Picrite, wet, with not less than 20% water	62
1337	Nitrostarch, wet, with not less than 30% solvent	47
1337	Nitrostarch, wet, with not less than 20% water	47
1338	Phosphorus, amorphous, red	109
1338	Red Phosphorus	109
1339	Phosphorus Heptasulfide, free from yellow or white phosphorus	105, 109
1340	Phosphorus Pentasulfide, free from yellow or white phosphorus	105, 109
1341	Phosphorus Sesquisulfide, free from yellow or white phosphorus	105, 109
1343	Phosphorus Trisulfide, free from yellow or white phosphorus	105, 109

WARNING: More than one chemical agent may have the same UN Number. Look up the guideline for the specific material in question by chemical name and not UN/NA/Pin number alone.

UN/ NA/PIN	Chemical Name	Guideline Number
1344	Picric Acid, wet, with not less than 10% water	62
1344	Trinitrophenol, wet	62
1345	Rubber Scrap, powdered or granulated	10
1345	Rubber Shoddy, powdered or granulated	10
1346	Silicon, powder, amorphous	9
1347	Silver Picrate, wet, with not less than 30% water	10
1348	Sodium Dinitro-ortho-cresolate, wet, with not less than 15% water	44
1349	Sodium Picramate, wet, with not less than 20% water	6
1350	Sulfur	105
1352	Titanium, metal, powder, wet, with not less than 20% water	10
1353	Toe Puffs, nitrocellulose base	6
1354	Trinitrobenzene, wet	24, 47
1355	Trinitrobenzoic Acid, wet	15, 47
1356	Trinitroluene, wet	24, 47
1357	Urea Nitrate, wet	47
1358	Zirconium Metal, powder, wet	10
1358	Zirconium Powder, wet	10
1360	Calcium Phosphide	108
1361	Carbon, animal or vegetable origin	6, 9
1361	Charcoal	9
1361	Coal, ground bituminous, sea coal, etc.	6
1361	Coal Facings	6
1361	Sea Coal	6
1362	Activated Carbon	9
1362	Carbon, activated	9
1363	Copra	5
1364	Cotton Waste, oily	9

UN/ NA/PIN	Chemical Name	Guideline Number
1365	Cotton, wet	9
1366	Diethylzinc	88
1367	Diethylmagnesium	82
1368	Dimethylmagnesium	82
1369	Dimethyl-*p*-nitrosoaniline	32
1369	Nitrosodimethylaniline	32
1370	Dimethylzinc	88
1371	Drier, paint or varnish, solid, n.o.s.	10
1371	Drier, paint, solid, n.o.s.	10
1372	Fiber, animal or vegetable, burnt, wet or damp, n.o.s.	9
1373	Fabric, animal or vegetable, with oil, n.o.s.	5
1373	Fiber, animal or vegetable, with oil, n.o.s.	5
1374	Fish Meal and Scrap, unstabilized	9
1375	Fuel, pyrophoric, n.o.s.	5
1375	Pyrophoric Fuel, n.o.s.	5
1376	Iron Oxide, spent	79
1376	Iron Sponge, spent	79
1378	Metal Catalyst, finely divided, activated or spent, wet, with not less than 40% water or other suitable liquid	10
1378	Nickel Catalyst, finely divided, activated or spent, wet, with not less than 40% water or other suitable liquid	85
1378	Nickel and Compounds	85
1379	Paper, treated with unsaturated oil	6
1380	Pentaborane	103
1381	Phosphorus, white or yellow, dry or under water or in solution	109
1381	White Phosphorus, dry	109

WARNING: More than one chemical agent may have the same UN Number. Look up the guideline for the specific material in question by chemical name and not UN/NA/Pin number alone.

UN/ NA/PIN	Chemical Name	Guideline Number
1381	White Phosphorus, wet	109
1381	Yellow Phosphorus, dry	109
1381	Yellow Phosphorus, wet	109
1382	Potassium Sulfide, anhydrous or with less than 30% water of hydration	19
1383	Aluminum, powder, pyrophoric	10
1383	Iron and Compounds	79
1383	Pyrophoric Metal or Alloy, n.o.s.	6
1383	Zinc Powder or Dust, pyrophoric	88
1384	Sodium Dithionite	105
1384	Sodium Hydrosulfite	105
1385	Sodium Sulfide, anhydrous, with less than 30% of water of crystallization	91
1387	Wool Waste, wet	9
1389	Alkali Metal Amalgam, n.o.s.	19
1390	Alkali Metal Amide, n.o.s.	19
1391	Alkali Metal Dispersion, n.o.s.	19
1391	Alkaline Earth Metal Dispersion, n.o.s.	19
1392	Alkaline Earth Metal Amalgam, n.o.s.	19
1393	Alkaline Earth Metal Alloy, n.o.s.	19
1394	Aluminum Carbide	10
1395	Aluminum Ferrosilicon, powder	79
1396	Aluminum Powder, uncoated	10
1397	Aluminum Phosphide	108
1398	Aluminum Silicon Powder, uncoated	10
1399	Barium Alloy	74
1400	Barium	74
1400	Barium Metal	74

UN/ NA/PIN	Chemical Name	Guideline Number
1401	Calcium, metal and alloys	10
1402	Calcium Carbide	13
1403	Calcium Cyanamide, with more than 0.1% calcium carbide	10
1404	Calcium Hydride	13
1405	Calcium Silicide	6
1406	Calcium Silicon	6
1407	Caesium, metal	6
1407	Cesium Metal	6
1408	Ferrosilicon	79
1409	Hydride, metal, n.o.s.	10
1410	Lithium Aluminum Hydride	81
1411	Lithium Aluminum Hydride, ether solution	81
1412	Lithium Amide	81
1413	Lithium Borohydride	81, 103
1414	Lithium Hydride	81
1415	Lithium Metal	81
1417	Lithium Silicon	81
1418	Magnesium, powder	82
1418	Magnesium Alloy, with more than 50% magnesium powder	82
1419	Magnesium Aluminum Phosphide	82, 108
1420	Potassium, metal, liquid alloy	10
1420	Potassium Metal, liquid alloy	10
1421	Alkali Metal, liquid alloy	19
1421	Alkali Metal Alloy, liquid, n.o.s.	19
1421	Sodium, metal, liquid, alloy	6
1422	Potassium Sodium Alloy	6
1422	Sodium Potassium Alloy	6
1423	Rubidium Metal	10
1424	Sodium Amalgam	84

WARNING: More than one chemical agent may have the same UN Number. Look up the guideline for the specific material in question by chemical name and not UN/NA/Pin number alone.

UN/ NA/PIN	Chemical Name	Guideline Number
1425	Sodium Amide	19
1426	Sodium Borohydride	103
1427	Sodium Hydride	19
1428	Sodium	6
1428	Sodium Metal	6
1429	Sodium, metal dispersion in organic liquids	6
1431	Sodium Methylate, dry	19, 31
1432	Sodium Phosphide	108
1433	Stannic Phosphide	108
1434	Strontium Alloy	10
1435	Zinc Ashes	88
1436	Zinc Metal, powder or dust	88
1436	Zinc Powder or Dust, nonpyrophoric	88
1437	Zirconium Hydride	88
1438	Aluminum Nitrate	47
1439	Ammonium Dichromate	21
1442	Ammonium Perchlorate	21, 97
1444	Ammonium Persulfate	14
1445	Barium Chlorate	74, 97
1446	Barium Nitrate	47, 74
1447	Barium Perchlorate	74, 97
1448	Barium Permanganate	14, 74
1449	Barium Peroxide	74
1450	Bromate, inorganic, n.o.s.	96
1451	Caesium Nitrate	14, 47
1451	Cesium Nitrate	14, 47
1452	Calcium Chlorate	97
1453	Calcium Chlorite	98
1454	Calcium Nitrate	47
1455	Calcium Perchlorate	97
1456	Calcium Permanganate	14
1457	Calcium Peroxide	8
1458	Boron, Boric Acid, and Borates	103
1458	Borate and Chlorate Mixture	97, 103
1458	Chlorate and Borate Mixture	97, 103
1458	Chlorate Salts	97
1459	Chlorate and Magnesium Chloride Mixture	82, 97
1461	Chlorate, inorganic, n.o.s.	97
1462	Chlorite, inorganic, n.o.s.	98
1463	Chromic Acid, solid	14
1463	Chromic Anhydride	14
1463	Chromium Trioxide, anhydrous	14
1465	Didymium Nitrate	47
1466	Ferric Nitrate	47, 79
1467	Guanidine Nitrate	20
1469	Lead Nitrate	47, 80
1470	Lead Perchlorate	80
1471	Lithium Hypochlorite, dry, including mixtures with more than 39% available chlorine	22, 81
1472	Lithium Peroxide	81
1473	Magnesium Bromate	82, 96
1474	Magnesium Nitrate	47, 82
1475	Magnesium Perchlorate	82, 97
1476	Magnesium Peroxide	82
1477	Nitrate, inorganic, n.o.s.	47
1478	Nitrate of Sodium and Potash mixture	47
1478	Sodium Nitrate and Potash Mixture	47
1479	Cosmetics, oxidizer, n.o.s.	7
1479	Cupric Nitrate	78
1479	Oxidizer, n.o.s.	7
1479	Oxidizing Material, n.o.s.	7
1479	Oxidizing Substance, solid, n.o.s.	7

WARNING: More than one chemical agent may have the same UN Number. Look up the guideline for the specific material in question by chemical name and not UN/NA/Pin number alone.

UN/ NA/PIN	Chemical Name	Guideline Number
1479	Potassium Dichromate	14
1479	Sodium Dichromate	10
1481	Perchlorate, inorganic, n.o.s.	97
1482	Permanganate, inorganic, n.o.s.	14
1483	Peroxide, inorganic, n.o.s.	7
1484	Potassium Bromate	96
1485	Chlorate of Potash	97
1485	Potassium Chlorate	97
1486	Potassium Nitrate	47
1486	Saltpeter	47
1487	Potassium Nitrate and Sodium Nitrite Mixture	47
1487	Sodium Nitrite and Potassium Nitrate Mixture	47
1488	Potassium Nitrite	47
1489	Potassium Perchlorate	97
1490	Potassium Permanganate	14
1491	Potassium Peroxide	7
1492	Potassium Persulfate	9
1493	Silver Nitrate	47
1494	Sodium Bromate	96
1495	Chlorate of Soda	97
1495	Sodium Chlorate	97
1496	Sodium Chlorite	22
1498	Sodium Nitrate	47
1499	Sodium Nitrate and Potassium Nitrate Mixture	47
1500	Sodium Nitrite	47
1502	Sodium Perchlorate	97
1503	Sodium Permanganate	14
1504	Sodium Peroxide	7
1505	Sodium Persulfate	105
1506	Strontium Chlorate	97
1507	Strontium Nitrate	47
1508	Strontium Perchlorate	97

UN/ NA/PIN	Chemical Name	Guideline Number
1509	Strontium Peroxide	7
1510	Tetranitromethane	47
1511	Urea Hydrogen Peroxide	8
1511	Urea Peroxide	8
1512	Zinc Ammonium Nitrite	47, 88
1513	Zinc Chlorate	88, 97
1514	Zinc Nitrate	47, 88
1515	Zinc Permanganate	82, 88
1516	Zinc Peroxide	88
1517	Zirconium Picramate, wet	6, 10
1541	Acetone Cyanohydrin	90
1544	Alkaloid, solid, n.o.s., or Alkaloid Salt, solid, n.o.s. (poisonous)	20
1545	Allyl Isothiocyanate, inhibited	94
1545	Allyl Isothiocyanate, stabilized	94
1546	Ammonium Arsenate	72
1547	Aniline	32
1547	Aromatic Nitrogen Compounds	32
1547	Aryl Amines	32
1548	Aniline Hydrochloride	32
1549	Antimony Compound, inorganic, n.o.s.	10
1549	Antimony Tribromide	95
1549	Antimony Tribromide Solution	95
1549	Antimony Trifluoride	99
1549	Antimony Trifluoride Solution	99
1550	Antimony Lactate	10
1551	Antimony Potassium Tartrate	10
1553	Arsenic Acid, liquid	72
1554	Arsenic Acid, solid	72
1555	Arsenic Bromide	72, 95
1556	Arsenic Compound, liquid, n.o.s.	72

WARNING: More than one chemical agent may have the same UN Number. Look up the guideline for the specific material in question by chemical name and not UN/NA/Pin number alone.

UN/ NA/PIN	Chemical Name	Guideline Number
1556	Methyldichloroarsine	73
1556	Phenyldichloroarsine	72, 73
1557	Arsenic Compound, solid, n.o.s.	72
1557	Arsenic Disulfide	72
1557	Arsenic Iodide, solid	72
1557	Arsenic Trisulfide	72
1558	Arsenic	72
1558	Arsenic Metal	72
1559	Arsenic Pentoxide	72
1560	Arsenic Chloride	72, 98
1560	Arsenic Trichloride	72, 98
1561	Arsenic, white, solid	72
1561	Arsenic Trioxide	72
1562	Arsenical Dust	72
1562	Arsenical Flue Dust	72
1564	Barium Compound, n.o.s.	74
1564	Barium and Compounds	74
1565	Barium Cyanide	74, 90, 132
1566	Beryllium Chloride	75
1566	Beryllium Compound, n.o.s.	75
1566	Beryllium Fluoride	75
1567	Beryllium and Compounds	75
1567	Beryllium, powder	75
1569	Bromoacetone	42, 95
1570	Brucine	69
1571	Barium Azide, wet, with not less than 50% water	74
1572	Cacodylic Acid	72
1573	Calcium Arsenate	72
1574	Calcium Arsenate and Calcium Arsenite Mixture, solid	72
1574	Calcium Arsenite	72
1575	Calcium Cyanide	90, 132
1577	1,2-Chloro Dinitrobenzene	24, 47
1577	Chlorodinitrobenzene	24, 47
1577	Dinitrochlorobenzene	24, 47
1578	Chloronitrobenzene	24, 47
1578	Nitrochlorobenzene, liquid	24, 47
1578	Nitrochlorobenzene, solid	24, 47
1579	4-Chloro-*o*-toluidine Hydrochloride	20
1580	Chloropicrin	9, 26, 136
1581	Chloropicrin and Methyl Bromide Mixture	26, 95, 136
1581	Methyl Bromide and Chloropicrin Mixture	26, 95, 136
1582	Chloropicrin and Methyl Chloride Mixture	9, 26, 136
1582	Methyl Chloride and Chloropicrin Mixture	9, 26, 136
1583	Chloropicrin Mixture, n.o.s.	9, 26, 136
1584	Cocculus, solid	10
1585	Copper Acetoarsenite	78
1586	Copper Arsenite	72, 78
1587	Copper Cyanide	78, 90, 132
1588	Cyanide, inorganic, n.o.s.	90, 132
1588	Cyanide or Cyanide Mixture, dry	90, 132
1589	Cyanogen Chloride, inhibited	90, 132
1590	Dichloroaniline	32
1591	Dichlorobenzene	57
1591	*o*-Dichlorobenzene	57
1592	*p*-Dichlorobenzene	57
1592	Paradichlorobenzene	57
1593	Dichloromethane	27
1593	Methylene Chloride	26, 89
1593	Dichloromethane	27
1594	2-(2,4-Dichlorophenoxy)ethyl Sulfate Sodium Salts	60

WARNING: More than one chemical agent may have the same UN Number. Look up the guideline for the specific material in question by chemical name and not UN/NA/Pin number alone.

UN/ NA/PIN	Chemical Name	Guideline Number
1594	Diethyl Sulfate	105
1594	Ethyl Sulfate	15, 105
1595	Dimethyl Sulfate	105
1595	Methyl Sulfate	105
1596	Dinitroaniline	32
1597	Dinitrobenzene	32
1597	Dinitrobenzene Solution	32
1598	Dinitro-*o*-cresol	44
1599	Dinitrophenol Solution, in water or flammable liquid	62
1600	Dinitrotoluene, molten	32
1601	Disinfectant, solid, n.o.s., poisonous	10
1602	Dye, n.o.s. (poisonous)	10
1602	Dye, intermediate, n.o.s. (poisonous)	10
1603	Ethyl Bromoacetate	96
1604	Ethylenediamine	20
1605	1,2-Dibromoethane	27
1605	Dibromoethane	27
1605	Ethylene Dibromide	95
1606	Ferric Arsenate	72, 79
1607	Ferric Arsenite	72, 79
1608	Ferrous Arsenate	72, 79
1610	Halogenated Irritating Liquid, n.o.s.	26
1610	Halogenated Solvents/ Degreasers	26
1611	Hexaethyl Tetraphosphate	49
1612	Hexaethyl Tetraphosphate and Compressed Gas Mixture	49
1613	Hydrocyanic Acid, aqueous solution, with less than 5% hydrocyanic acid	90, 132, 138
1613	Hydrocyanic Acid, aqueous solution, with not less than 5% hydrocyanic acid	90, 132, 138
1614	Hydrogen Cyanide, anhydrous, stabilized, (absorbed)	90, 132, 138
1616	Lead Acetate	80
1617	Lead Arsenate	72, 80
1618	Lead Arsenite	72, 80
1620	Lead Cyanide	80, 90, 132
1621	London Purple	32, 72
1622	Magnesium Arsenate	72, 82
1623	Mercuric Arsenate	72, 84
1624	Mercuric Chloride	84
1624	Mercury, inorganic	84
1625	Mercuric Nitrate	47, 84
1626	Mercuric Potassium Cyanide	84, 90, 132
1627	Mercurous Nitrate	47, 84
1628	Mercurous Sulfate	84
1629	Mercurous Acetate	84
1629	Mercuric Acetate	84
1629	Mercury Acetate	84
1630	Mercury Ammonium Chloride	84
1631	Mercury Benzoate	84
1633	Mercury Bisulfate	84
1634	Mercuric Bromide	84, 95
1634	Mercurous Bromide	84, 95
1634	Mercury Bromide	84, 95
1636	Mercuric Cyanide	84, 90, 132
1636	Mercury Cyanide	84, 90, 132
1637	Mercury Gluconate	84
1638	Mercury Iodide	84, 100
1639	Mercurol	84
1639	Mercury Nucleate	84
1640	Mercury Oleate	84
1641	Mercury Oxide	84
1642	Mercuric Oxycyanide	84, 90, 132

WARNING: More than one chemical agent may have the same UN Number. Look up the guideline for the specific material in question by chemical name and not UN/NA/Pin number alone.

UN/ NA/PIN	Chemical Name	Guideline Number
1642	Mercury Oxycyanide, desensitized	84, 90, 132
1643	Mercury Potassium Iodide	84, 100
1644	Mercury Salicylate	84
1645	Mercuric Sulfate	84
1645	Mercury Sulfate	84
1646	Mercury Thiocyanate	84, 94
1647	Methyl Bromide and Ethylene Dibromide Mixture, liquid	95
1648	Acetonitrile	90
1648	Methyl Cyanide	90, 132
1649	Anti-Knock Compound	80
1649	Ethyl Fluid	33
1649	Lead Tetraethyl	80
1649	Lead Tetramethyl	80
1649	Motor Fuel Anti-Knock Compound	35, 80
1649	Motor Fuel Anti-Knock Mixture	35, 80
1649	Tetraethyl Lead	80
1649	Tetramethyl Lead	80
1650	Naphthylamine (beta)	20
1651	Naphthylthiourea	43
1652	Naphthylurea	43
1653	Nickel Cyanide	85, 90, 132
1654	Nicotine	51
1655	Nicotine Compound, solid, n.o.s.	51
1655	Nicotine Preparation, solid, n.o.s.	51
1656	Nicotine Hydrochloride, and solutions	51
1657	Nicotine Salicylate	51
1658	Nicotine Sulfate, liquid	51
1658	Nicotine Sulfate, solid	51
1659	Nicotine Tartrate	51

UN/ NA/PIN	Chemical Name	Guideline Number
1660	Nitric Oxide	48
1661	Nitroaniline	32
1662	Nitrobenzene	24, 47
1663	Nitrophenol	62
1664	Nitrotoluene	24, 47
1665	Nitroxylene	24, 47
1665	Nitroxylol	44, 47
1669	Pentachloroethane	26
1670	Perchloromethyl Mercaptan	105
1671	Carbolic Acid	44
1671	Phenol, solid	44
1672	Phenylcarbylamine Chloride	32
1673	Paradiaminobenzene	32
1673	Phenylenediamine	20
1674	Phenylmercuric Acetate, liquid	84
1677	Potassium Arsenate	72
1678	Potassium Arsenite	72
1679	Potassium Cuprocyanide	90, 132
1680	Cyanide	90, 132
1680	Potassium Cyanide, solid	90, 132
1680	Potassium Cyanide Solution	90, 132
1681	Rodenticides, n.o.s.	10
1683	Silver Arsenite	72
1684	Silver Cyanide	90, 132
1685	Sodium Arsenate	72
1686	Sodium Arsenite Solution	72
1687	Sodium Azide	18
1688	Sodium Cacodylate	72
1689	Cyanide	90, 132
1689	Sodium Cyanide	90, 132
1690	Sodium Fluoride, solid	16
1690	Sodium Fluoride Solution	16
1691	Strontium Arsenite	72
1692	Strychnine, and salts	69

WARNING: More than one chemical agent may have the same UN Number. Look up the guideline for the specific material in question by chemical name and not UN/NA/Pin number alone.

UN/ NA/PIN	Chemical Name	Guideline Number
1693	Irritating Agent, n.o.s.	9
1693	ORM-A, n.o.s.	10
1693	Tear Gas Devices	9, 136
1693	Tear Gas Substance, liquid, n.o.s.	9, 136
1693	Tear Gas Substances, solid, n.o.s.	9, 136
1694	Bromobenzyl Cyanide	90, 132
1695	Chloroacetone, stabilized	42
1695	Monochloroacetone, inhibited	42
1695	Monochloroacetone, stabilized	42
1697	Chloroacetophenone	42
1698	Diphenylaminechloroarsine	72
1699	Diphenylchloroarsine	73
1700	Tear Gas Candles	9, 136
1700	Tear Gas Grenades	9, 136
1701	Xylyl Bromide	24, 95
1702	Tetrachloroethane	26
1703	Tetraethyl Dithiopyrophosphate and Compressed Gas Mixture	49
1703	Tetraethyl Dithiopyrophosphate and Gases, mixtures or in solution	49
1704	Sulfotep	49
1704	Tetraethyl Dithiopyrophosphate, dry, liquid, or mixture	49
1705	Tetraethyl Pyrophosphate, and compressed gas mixture	49
1707	Thallium Compound, n.o.s.	87
1707	Thallium Salt, n.o.s.	87
1707	Thallium Sulfate, solid	87
1708	Toluidines (*o*-, *m*-, and *p*-)	32
1709	Toluenediamine	32
1709	Toluylenediamine	32
1710	Trichloroethylene	28
1711	Xylidine	24
1712	Zinc Arsenate	72, 88
1712	Zinc Arsenate and Zinc Arsenite Mixture	72, 88
1712	Zinc Arsenite	72, 88
1713	Zinc Cyanide	88, 90, 132
1714	Zinc Phosphide	88, 108
1715	Acetic Anhydride	15
1716	Acetyl Bromide	15
1717	Acetyl Chloride	15
1718	Acid Butyl Phosphate	15
1718	Butyl Acid Phosphate	15
1718	Butyl Phosphoric Acid	15
1719	Alkaline Corrosive Liquid, n.o.s.	19
1719	Caustic Alkali Liquid, n.o.s.	19
1722	Allyl Chlorocarbonate	15
1722	Allyl Chloroformate	37
1723	Allyl Iodide	61, 100
1724	Allyl Trichlorosilane, stabilized	107
1725	Aluminum Bromide, anhydrous	95
1726	Aluminum Chloride, anhydrous	10, 98
1727	Ammonium Bifluoride, solid	99
1727	Ammonium Hydrogen Fluoride, solid	99
1728	Amyltrichlorosilane	107
1729	Anisoyl Chloride	15
1730	Antimony Pentachloride, liquid	10
1731	Antimony Pentachloride Solution	10
1732	Antimony Pentafluoride	99

WARNING: More than one chemical agent may have the same UN Number. Look up the guideline for the specific material in question by chemical name and not UN/NA/Pin number alone.

UN/ NA/PIN	Chemical Name	Guideline Number
1733	Antimony Chloride	10
1733	Antimony Trichloride	10
1733	Antimony Trichloride Solution	10
1736	Benzoyl Chloride	9, 24
1737	Benzyl Bromide	24
1738	Benzyl Chloride	24
1739	Benzyl Chloroformate	37
1740	Bifluoride, n.o.s.	99
1741	Boron Trichloride	103, 133, 138
1742	Boron Trifluoride Acetic Acid Complex	103
1743	Boron Trifluoride Propionic Acid Complex	103
1744	Bromine	95
1744	Bromine Solution	95
1745	Bromine Pentafluoride	95
1746	Bromine Trifluoride	95
1747	Butyl Trichlorosilane	107
1748	Calcium Hypochlorite, dry, including mixtures with more than 39% available chlorine (8.8% available oxygen)	22
1749	Chlorine Trifluoride	16, 98
1750	Chloroacetic Acid, liquid	15
1751	Chloroacetic Acid, solid	15
1752	Chloroacetyl Chloride	98
1753	Chlorophenol Trichlorosilane	107
1754	Chlorosulfonic Acid	14
1754	Chlorosulfonic Acid and Sulfur Trioxide Mixture	14, 105
1755	Chromic Acid	14
1755	Chromic Acid Solution	14
1756	Chromic Fluoride, solid	99
1757	Chromic Fluoride Solution	99
1758	Chromium Oxychloride	14
1759	Aluminum Sulfate	14

UN/ NA/PIN	Chemical Name	Guideline Number
1759	Corrosive Solid, n.o.s.	13
1759	Cosmetics, corrosive solid, n.o.s.	13
1759	Ferrous Chloride, solid	79
1759	Fungicide, corrosive, n.o.s.	10, 13
1759	Stannous Chloride, solid	14
1760	Acid, liquid, n.o.s.	14, 15
1760	Aluminum Phosphate Solution	14
1760	Aluminum Sulfate Solution	14
1760	Aminoethoxyethanol	20, 29
1760	Aminopropyldiethanolamine	20
1760	Aminopropylmorpholine	20
1760	Aminopropylpiperazine	20
1760	Bis(aminopropyl) Amine	20
1760	Caproic Acid (hexanoic acid)	15
1760	Chemical Kit	10
1760	Cleaning Compound, liquid, corrosive	19
1760	Compound, tree- or weed-killing liquid (corrosive)	10, 13
1760	Corrosive Acids (various)	14, 15
1760	Corrosive Liquid, n.o.s.	13
1760	Cosmetics, corrosive liquid, n.o.s.	13
1760	Dichloropropionic Acid	15
1760	2,2-Dichloropropionic Acid	15
1760	Ethylphosphonothioic-dichloride, anhydrous	13
1760	Ethyl Phosphorodichloridate	13
1760	Ferrous Chloride Solution	79
1760	Hexanoic Acid	15
1760	Isopentanoic Acid	15
1760	Methyl Phosphonothioic Dichloride	109
1760	Morpholine, aqueous, mixture	20
1760	Nitric Acid, other than fuming, with not more than 40% acid	14

NUMERICAL INDEX

WARNING: More than one chemical agent may have the same UN Number. Look up the guideline for the specific material in question by chemical name and not UN/NA/Pin number alone.

UN/ NA/PIN	Chemical Name	Guideline Number
1760	ORM-B, n.o.s.	10
1760	Paint, etc., corrosive liquid	13
1760	Paint-Related Material, corrosive liquid	13
1760	Pentanoic Acid	15
1760	Sulfuric Acid	14
1760	Textile Treating Compound	10
1760	Titanium Sulfate Solution	10
1760	Valeric Acid (*n*-Pentanoic Acid)	15
1761	Cupriethylenediamine Solution	20, 78
1762	Cyclohexenyl Trichlorosilane	107
1763	Cyclohexyl Trichlorosilane	107
1764	Dichloroacetic Acid	15
1765	Dichloroacetyl Chloride	15
1766	Dichlorophenyl Trichlorosilane	107
1767	Diethyl Dichlorosilane	107
1768	Difluorophosphoric Acid, anhydrous	14
1769	Diphenyl Dichlorosilane	107
1770	Diphenylmethyl Bromide	95
1771	Dodecyl Trichlorosilane	107
1773	Ferric Chloride, anhydrous	79
1773	Iron Chloride, solid	79
1774	Fire Extinguisher Charge, corrosive liquid	13
1775	Fluoboric Acid	16, 103
1776	Fluorophosphoric Acid, anhydrous	14
1776	Monofluorophosphoric Acid	14
1777	Fluorosulphonic Acid	14
1778	Fluosilicic Acid	16
1778	Hydrofluosilicic Acid	16
1778	Hydrosilicofluoric Acid	16
1778	Silicofluoric Acid	99

UN/ NA/PIN	Chemical Name	Guideline Number
1779	Formic Acid	15
1780	Fumaryl Chloride	15
1781	Hexadecyl Trichlorosilane	107
1782	Hexafluorophosphoric Acid	14
1783	Hexamethylendiamine Solution	20
1784	Hexyl Trichlorosilane	107
1786	Acid Mixture, Hydrofluoric and Sulfuric Acids	14, 16
1786	Hydrofluoric and Sulfuric Acid Mixture	14, 16
1786	Sulfuric and Hydrofluoric Acid Mixture	14, 16
1787	Hydriodic Acid	14, 100
1787	Hydriodic Acid, and Solutions	14, 100
1787	Hydrogen Iodide	100
1787	Hydrogen Iodide Solution	100
1788	Hydrobromic Acid	95
1788	Hydrobromic Acid, and Solutions	95
1788	Hydrogen Bromide Solution	95
1789	Hydrogen Chloride Solution	14
1789	Hydrochloric Acid Solution	14
1789	Muriatic Acid	14
1790	Etching Acid, liquid	14, 16
1790	Fluoric Acid	16
1790	Hydrofluoric Acid	16, 133, 138
1790	Hydrogen Fluoride Solution	16
1791	Hypochlorite Solution, with more than 5% available chlorine	22
1791	Potassium Hypochlorite Solution	22
1791	Sodium Hypochlorite Solution	22
1792	Iodine Monochloride	100

WARNING: More than one chemical agent may have the same UN Number. Look up the guideline for the specific material in question by chemical name and not UN/NA/Pin number alone.

UN/ NA/PIN	Chemical Name	Guideline Number
1793	Isopropyl Acid Phosphate	37
1794	Lead Sulfate, with more than 3% free acid	80
1796	Acid Mixture, nitrating	14
1796	Mixed Acid	14
1796	Nitrating Acid	47
1796	Nitrating Acid, mixture	47
1798	Nitrohydrochloric Acid	14
1798	Nitromuriatic Acid	14
1799	Nonyl Trichlorosilane	107
1800	Octadecyl Trichlorosilane	107
1801	Octyl Trichlorosilane	107
1802	Perchloric Acid, not more than 50% acid, by weight	7, 14
1803	Phenolsulfonic Acid, liquid	15, 44
1804	Phenyl Trichlorosilane	107
1805	Phosphoric Acid	14
1806	Phosphorus Pentachloride	98, 109
1807	Phosphoric Anhydride	14
1807	Phosphorus Pentoxide	109
1808	Phosphorus Tribromide	95, 109
1809	Chloride of Phosphorus	98, 109
1809	Phosphorus Trichloride	98, 109, 133, 138
1810	Phosphoryl Chloride	98, 109
1810	Phosphorus Oxychloride	98, 109
1811	Potassium Bifluoride	16
1811	Potassium Hydrogen Fluoride	16
1812	Potassium Fluoride	16
1813	Battery, electric, storage, dry, containing potassium hydroxide	19
1813	Caustic Potash, dry, solid	19
1813	Potassium Hydroxide, dry, solid	19
1814	Caustic Potash, liquid or solution	19
1814	Potash Liquor	19
1814	Potassium Hydroxide	19
1814	Potassium Hydroxide Solution	19
1815	Propionyl Chloride	26
1816	Propyl Trichlorosilane	107
1817	Pyrosulfuryl Chloride	14
1818	Silicon Chloride	98
1818	Silicon Tetrachloride	98
1819	Sodium Aluminate Solution	10
1821	Sodium Bisulfate, solid	105
1821	Sodium Hydrogen Sulfate, solid	105
1823	Caustic Soda, dry, solid	19
1823	Lye, dry, solid	19
1823	Sodium Hydroxide, dry, solid	19
1824	Caustic Soda Liquor	19
1824	Caustic Soda, solution	19
1824	Caustic Soda Solution	19
1824	Lye Solution	19
1824	Sodium Hydrate	19
1824	Sodium Hydroxide Solution	19
1825	Sodium Monoxide	19
1826	Acid Mixture, spent, nitrating	14
1826	Mixed Acid, spent	14
1826	Nitrating Acid Mixture, spent	47
1826	Spent Mixed Acid	14
1827	Stannic Chloride, anhydrous	14
1827	Tin and Inorganic Tin Compounds	10
1827	Tin Chloride, fuming	10
1827	Tin Tetrachloride	10
1828	Chloride of Sulfur	14
1828	Sulfur Chloride	14
1829	Sulfuric Anhydride	14
1829	Sulfuric Trioxide	14
1829	Sulfur Trioxide, inhibited	14

WARNING: More than one chemical agent may have the same UN Number. Look up the guideline for the specific material in question by chemical name and not UN/NA/Pin number alone.

UN/ NA/PIN	Chemical Name	Guideline Number
1829	Sulfur Trioxide, stabilized	14
1830	Sulfuric Acid, with more than 51% but not more than 95% acid	14
1830	Sulfuric Acid, with not more than 51% acid	14
1831	Oleum	14, 133, 138
1831	Pyrosulfuric Acid	14, 133, 138
1831	Sulfuric Acid, fuming	14, 133, 138
1832	Sulfuric Acid, spent	14
1833	Sulfurous Acid	14
1834	Sulfuryl Chloride	14
1835	Tetramethyl Ammonium Hydroxide	20
1836	Thionyl Chloride	105
1837	Thiophosphoryl Chloride	109
1838	Titanium and Compounds	10
1838	Titanium Tetrachloride	10
1839	Trichloroacetic Acid	15
1840	Zinc Chloride Solution	88
1841	Acetal Ammonia	21, 41
1841	Acetaldehyde Ammonia	21, 41
1843	Ammonium Dinitro-*o*-cresolate	21
1845	Carbon Dioxide, solid	92
1845	Dry Ice	92
1846	Carbon Tetrachloride	28
1847	Potassium Sulfide, hydrated, with not less than 30% water of hydration	19
1848	Propanoic Acid	15
1848	Propionic Acid	15
1849	Sodium Sulfide, hydrated, with not less than 30% water	91
1849	Sodium Sulfide Solution	91
1850	Eradicator, paint or grease, flammable liquid	5
1851	Drugs, n.o.s.	10
1851	Medicines, n.o.s.	10
1854	Barium Alloy, pyrophoric	74
1855	Calcium, metal, and alloys, pyrophoric	6, 10
1855	Calcium Alloy, pyrophoric	6, 10
1855	Calcium, pyrophoric	6
1857	Textile Waste, wet, n.o.s.	87, 97
1858	Hexafluoropropylene	26
1859	Silicon Tetrafluoride	99
1860	Vinyl Fluoride	26
1860	Vinyl Fluoride, inhibited	26
1862	Ethyl Crotonate	37
1863	Fuel, Aviation, turbine engine	35
1863	Jet Fuel	35
1864	Gas Drips, hydrocarbon	35
1865	Propyl Nitrate	47
1866	Resin Compound, liquid, flammable	5
1866	Resin Solution	5
1866	Resin Solution, flammable	5
1866	Resin Solution (Resin Compound), liquid	10
1867	Cigarette, self-lighting	51
1868	Decaborane	103
1869	Magnesium, pellets, turnings, or ribbon	82
1869	Magnesium Alloy, with more than 50% magnesium, pellets, turnings, or ribbon	82
1870	Potassium Borohydride	103
1871	Titanium Hydride	10
1872	Lead Dioxide	80

WARNING: More than one chemical agent may have the same UN Number. Look up the guideline for the specific material in question by chemical name and not UN/NA/Pin number alone.

UN/ NA/PIN	Chemical Name	Guideline Number
1872	Lead Peroxide	80
1873	Perchloric Acid, more than 50% but not more than 72% acid, by weight	7, 14
1884	Barium Oxide	74
1885	Benzidine	32
1886	Benzylidene Chloride	24
1887	Bromochloromethane	27
1888	Chloroform	26
1889	Cyanogen Bromide	90, 132
1891	Ethyl Bromide	95
1892	Ethyl Dichloroarsine	73
1893	Organophosphates, poisonous, n.o.s.	49, 135
1894	Phenylmercuric Hydroxide	84
1895	Phenylmercuric Nitrate	47, 84
1896	Resin Solution, poisonous	10
1897	Perchloroethylene	26
1897	Tetrachloroethylene	28
1898	Acetyl Iodide	100
1899	Alkane Sulfonic Acid	15
1902	Di(2-ethylhexyl)-Phosphoric Acid	15
1902	Diisooctyl Acid Phosphate	15
1903	Disinfectant, corrosive, liquid, n.o.s.	13
1905	Selenic Acid	14, 86
1906	Sludge Acid	14
1907	Soda Lime	19
1908	Sodium Chlorite Solution, with more than 5% available chlorine	22
1910	Calcium Oxide	19
1911	Diborane or Diborane Mixture	103, 133, 138
1912	Methyl Chloride and Methylene Chloride Mixture	26, 89

UN/ NA/PIN	Chemical Name	Guideline Number
1913	Neon, refrigerated liquid (cryogenic liquid)	92
1914	Butyl Propionate	37
1915	Cyclohexanone	42
1916	Dichlorodiethyl Ether	38
1916	Dichloroethyl Ether	38
1916	sym-Dichloroethyl Ether	38
1917	Ethyl Acrylate, inhibited	37
1918	Cumene	24
1918	Isopropylbenzene	24
1919	Methylacrylate, inhibited	37
1920	Nonane	33
1921	Propyleneimine, inhibited	20
1922	Pyrrolidine	20
1923	Calcium Dithionite	105
1923	Calcium Hydrosulfite	105
1924	Ethyl Aluminum Dichloride	10
1925	Ethyl Aluminum Sesquichloride	10
1926	Methyl Aluminum Sesquibromide	95
1927	Methyl Aluminum Sesquichloride	98
1928	Methyl Magnesium Bromide in Ethyl Ether	38, 95
1929	Potassium Dithionite	105
1929	Potassium Hydrosulfite	105
1930	Tributyl Aluminum	10
1930	Triisobutyl Aluminum	10
1931	Zinc Dithionite	88
1931	Zinc Hydrosulfite	88, 105
1932	Zirconium Scrap	10
1935	Cyanide	90, 132
1935	Cyanide Solution, n.o.s.	90, 132
1938	Bromoacetic Acid, solid	95
1938	Bromoacetic Acid Solution	95

WARNING: More than one chemical agent may have the same UN Number. Look up the guideline for the specific material in question by chemical name and not UN/NA/Pin number alone.

UN/ NA/PIN	Chemical Name	Guideline Number
1939	Phosphorus Oxybromide, solid	95, 109
1940	Thioglycolic Acid	15
1941	Dibromodifluoromethane	27
1942	Ammonium Nitrate, with not more than 0.2% combustible material	47
1942	Ammonium Nitrate, with organic coating	47
1944	Matches, safety	97
1945	Matches, wax (Vesta)	97
1950	Aerosols	9, 10
1951	Argon, refrigerated liquid (cryogenic liquid)	92
1952	Carbon Dioxide–Ethylene Oxide Mixture, with not more than 6% ethylene oxide	45, 92
1952	Ethylene Oxide–Carbon Dioxide Mixture, with not more than 6% ethylene oxide	45, 92
1953	Compressed Gas, flammable, poisonous, n.o.s.	2, 10
1953	Liquefied Gas, flammable, poisonous, n.o.s.	2, 10
1953	Poisonous Gas, flammable, n.o.s.	2, 10
1953	Poisonous Liquid, flammable, n.o.s.	5, 10
1954	Compressed Gas, flammable, n.o.s.	2
1954	Dispersant Gas, flammable, n.o.s	2
1954	Flammable Gas, n.o.s.	2
1954	Liquefied Gas, flammable, n.o.s.	2
1954	Refrigerant Gas, flammable, n.o.s.	2
1954	Refrigerating Machine, containing flammable, nonpoisonous, liquefied gas	2, 92
1955	Chloropicrin and Nonflammable Gas Mixture	9, 26, 136
1955	Compressed Gas, poisonous, n.o.s.	10
1955	Liquefied Gas, poisonous, n.o.s	2, 10
1955	Methyl Bromide and Nonflammable Compressed Gas Mixture	95
1955	Organic Phosphorus Compound, mixed with Compressed Gas	49, 135
1955	Poisonous Gas, n.o.s.	10
1955	Poisonous Liquid, n.o.s.	10
1955	Tetrafluorohydrazine	23
1956	Accumulators, pressurized	2
1956	Compressed Gas, n.o.s.	3
1956	Hexafluoropropylene Oxide	26, 38
1956	Liquefied Gas, n.o.s.	2
1956	Nonflammable Gas, n.o.s.	3
1957	Deuterium	2, 92
1958	Dichlorotetrafluoroethane	27
1959	Difluoroethylene	27
1959	1,1-Difluoroethylene	27
1959	Vinylidene Fluoride	26
1960	Engine-Starting Fluid	35
1961	Ethane, refrigerated liquid (cryogenic liquid)	33
1961	Ethane-Propane Mixture, refrigerated liquid (cryogenic liquid)	33
1962	Ethylene, compressed	33, 92
1963	Helium, refrigerated liquid (cryogenic liquid)	92

WARNING: More than one chemical agent may have the same UN Number. Look up the guideline for the specific material in question by chemical name and not UN/NA/Pin number alone.

UN/ NA/PIN	Chemical Name	Guideline Number
1964	Hydrocarbon Gas, compressed, n.o.s.	2, 33
1965	Hydrocarbon Gas, liquefied, n.o.s.	2, 33
1966	Hydrogen, refrigerated liquid (cryogenic liquid)	2, 92
1967	Insecticide Gas, poisonous, n.o.s.	10, 49
1967	Methyl Parathion and Compressed Gas Mixture	49, 135
1967	Parathion and Compressed Gas Mixture	49, 135
1968	Insectide Gas, n.o.s.	10
1969	Isobutane or Isobutane Mixture	92
1970	Krypton, refrigerated liquid (cryogenic liquid)	92
1971	Methane, compressed	33, 92
1971	Natural Gas, compressed, with a high methane content	33, 92
1972	Liquefied Natural Gas	33, 92
1972	LNG, liquefied natural gas	33, 92
1972	Methane, refrigerated liquid (cryogenic liquid)	33, 92
1972	Natural Gas, refrigerated liquid, (cryogenic liquid) with a high methane content	33, 92
1973	Chlorodifluoromethane and Chloropentafluoroethane Mixture	27
1974	Bromochlorodifluoromethane	27
1974	Chlorodifluorobromomethane	27
1975	Nitric Oxide and Dinitrogen Tetroxide Mixture	48
1975	Nitric Oxide and Nitrogen Dioxide Mixture	48
1975	Nitric Oxide and Nitrogen Tetroxide Mixture	48
1976	Octafluorocyclobutane	26

UN/ NA/PIN	Chemical Name	Guideline Number
1977	Nitrogen, refrigerated liquid (cryogenic liquid)	92
1978	Propane	33
1979	Rare Gas Mixture	10, 92
1980	Helium	92
1980	Helium-Oxygen Mixture	92
1980	Rare Gas–Oxygen Mixture	10, 92
1981	Rare Gas–Nitrogen Mixture	10, 92
1982	Tetrafluoromethane	27
1983	Chlorotrifluoroethane	27
1984	Trifluoromethane	27
1986	Alcohol, denatured (toxic)	31
1986	Alcohol, toxic, n.o.s.	31
1986	Propargyl Alcohol	30
1987	Alcohol, denatured	31
1987	Alcohol, nontoxic, n.o.s.	29, 30
1987	Alcohol, n.o.s.	29, 30
1988	Aldehyde, toxic, n.o.s.	41
1989	Aldehyde, n.o.s.	41
1989	Benzaldehyde	41
1991	Chloroprene, inhibited	9, 33
1992	Flammable Liquid, poisonous, n.o.s.	5, 10
1993	Combustible Liquid, n.o.s.	4
1993	Compound, Tree- or Weed-Killing, liquid (combustible or flammable)	4, 10
1993	Cosmetics, flammable, n.o.s.	5
1993	Creosote, coal tar	44
1993	Ethyl Nitrate	47
1993	Flammable Liquid, n.o.s.	5
1993	Fuel Oil	35
1993	Insecticide, liquid, n.o.s.	10
1993	Organic Peroxide, liquid or solution, n.o.s.	8
1993	Wax, liquid	33

WARNING: More than one chemical agent may have the same UN Number. Look up the guideline for the specific material in question by chemical name and not UN/NA/Pin number alone.

UN/ NA/PIN	Chemical Name	Guideline Number
1994	Iron and Compounds	79
1994	Iron Carbonyl	79
1994	Iron Pentacarbonyl	79
1999	Asphalt	35
1999	Road Asphalt, liquid	35
1999	Tar, liquid	24, 25
2000	Celluloid, in blocks, rods, rolls, sheets, tubes, etc., except celluloid scrap	6
2001	Cobalt Naphthenate, powder	77
2002	Celluloid Scrap	6
2003	Aluminum Alkyl	10
2003	Metal Alkyl, n.o.s.	10
2004	Magnesium Diamide	82
2005	Magnesium Diphenyl	82
2006	Plastics, nitrocellulose-based, spontaneously combustible, n.o.s.	6
2008	Zirconium	10
2008	Zirconium Metal, powder, dry	10
2008	Zirconium Powder, dry	10
2009	Zirconium Metal, wire, sheet, or strips (thinner than 18 microns)	10
2010	Magnesium Hydride	82
2011	Magnesium Phosphide	82, 108
2012	Potassium Phosphide	108
2013	Strontium Phosphide	108
2014	Hydrogen Peroxide Solution, with not less than 20% but not more than 52% peroxide	7
2015	Hydrogen Peroxide, stabilized, with more than 52% peroxide	7
2016	Ammunition, toxic, nonexplosive	10
2016	Chemical Ammunition, nonexplosive with poisonous material	9, 10
2016	Grenade, without bursting charge, with poisonous gas	10
2017	Ammunition, tear-producing, nonexplosive	9, 136
2017	Chemical Ammunition, nonexplosive, with irritant	9, 136
2017	Grenade, tear gas	9, 136
2018	Chloroaniline, solid	32
2019	Chloroaniline, liquid	32
2020	2-Chlorophenol	44
2020	Chlorophenol, solid	44
2020	Pentachlorophenol	67
2020	Trichlorophenol	44
2021	Chlorophenol, liquid	44
2021	2,4-Dichlorophenol	44
2021	2,6-Dichlorophenol	44
2022	Cresylic Acid	44
2022	Mining Reagent, liquid	35
2023	Epichlorohydrin	61
2024	Mercury Compound, liquid, n.o.s.	84
2025	Mercury Compound, solid, n.o.s.	84
2026	Phenylmercuric Compound, solid, n.o.s.	84
2027	Sodium Arsenite, solid	72
2028	Bomb, smoke, nonexplosive, with corrosive liquid, without initiating device	9, 13
2029	Hydrazine, anhydrous	23
2029	Hydrazine Aqueous Solution, with more than 64% hydrazine, by weight	23
2030	Hydrazine Aqueous Solution, with not more than 64% hydrazine by weight	23
2030	Hydrazine Hydrate	23

WARNING: More than one chemical agent may have the same UN Number. Look up the guideline for the specific material in question by chemical name and not UN/NA/Pin number alone.

UN/ NA/PIN	Chemical Name	Guideline Number
2030	Hydrazine Solution, with not more than 64% hydrazine by weight	23
2031	Nitric Acid, other than fuming, with more than 40% acid	14
2032	Nitric Acid, fuming	14, 133, 138
2032	Nitric Acid, red fuming	14, 133, 138
2033	Potassium Monoxide	19
2033	Potassium Oxide	19
2034	Hydrogen and Methane Mixture, compressed	92
2035	Trifluoroethane, compressed	27
2036	Xenon	92
2037	Receptacles, small, with flammable compressed gas	2
2038	Dinitrotoluene, solid	32
2044	Dimethylpropane	33
2044	Neopentane	33
2045	Butyl Aldehyde	41
2045	Isobutyl Aldehyde	41
2045	Isobutyraldehyde	41
2046	Cymene	24
2046	Methyl Propyl Benzene	24
2047	Dichloropropene	61
2047	Dichloropropene and Propylene Dichloride Mixture	61
2047	1,3-Dichloropropene	61
2048	Dicyclopentadiene	33
2049	Diethylbenzene	24
2050	Diisobutylene	33
2051	Dimethylaminoethanol	20
2051	Dimethylethanolamine	20
2052	Dipentene	34
2053	Methyl Amyl Alcohol	30
2053	Methyl Isobutyl Carbinol	30
2053	MIBC	30
2054	Morpholine	20
2055	Styrene	24
2055	Styrene Monomer, inhibited	24
2056	Tetrahydrofuran	38
2057	Tripropylene	33
2058	Valeraldehyde	41
2058	Amyl Aldehyde	41
2059	Collodion	29, 38
2059	Nitrocellulose, wet, with more than 40% flammable liquid by weight	5
2059	Nitrocellulose, solution in a flammable liquid	5
2059	Pyroxylin Solution	38
2060	Nitrocellulose, solution in a flammable liquid	5
2067	Ammonium Nitrate Fertilizer	47
2068	Ammonium Nitrate Fertilizer, with calcium carbonate	47
2069	Ammonium Nitrate Fertilizer, with ammonium sulfate	47
2069	Ammonium Nitrate–Sulfate Mixture	47
2070	Ammonium Nitrate Fertilizer, with phosphate or potash	47
2071	Ammonium Nitrate Fertilizer, with not more than 45% ammonium nitrate	47
2071	Ammonium Nitrate Fertilizer, with not more than 0.4% of combustible material	47
2072	Ammonium Nitrate Fertilizer, n.o.s.	47
2073	Ammonia Solution, with more than 44% ammonia	21
2074	Acrylamide	106

WARNING: More than one chemical agent may have the same UN Number. Look up the guideline for the specific material in question by chemical name and not UN/NA/Pin number alone.

UN/ NA/PIN	Chemical Name	Guideline Number
2075	Chloral, anhydrous, inhibited	26
2076	Cresols	44
2076	Cresol (*o*-, *m*-, and *p*-)	44
2077	Naphthylamine (alpha)	20
2078	Toluene Diisocyanate (TDI)	94
2079	Diethylene Triamine	20
2080	Acetyl Acetone Peroxide	8, 42
2080	3,5-Dimethyl-3,5-Dihydroxydioxolane-1,2	40
2081	Acetyl Benzoyl Peroxide	8
2082	Acetyl Cyclohexane Sulfonyl Peroxide	8
2083	Acetyl Cyclohexane Sulfonyl Peroxide	8
2084	Acetyl Peroxide	8
2084	Diacetyl Peroxide	8, 42
2085	Benzoyl Peroxide	8
2085	Dibenzoyl Peroxide	8
2086	Benzoyl Peroxide	8
2087	Benzoyl Peroxide	8
2087	Dibenzoyl Peroxide	8
2088	Benzoyl Peroxide	8
2088	Dibenzoyl Peroxide	8
2089	Benzoyl Peroxide	8
2089	Dibenzoyl Peroxide	8
2090	Benzoyl Peroxide	8
2090	Dibenzoyl Peroxide	8
2091	*tert*-Butyl Cumene Peroxide	8
2091	*tert*-Butyl Cumyl Peroxide	8
2091	*tert*-Butyl Isopropyl Benzene Hydroperoxide	8
2092	*tert*-Butyl Hydroperoxide, not more than 80% in di-tert-butyl peroxide and/ or solvent	8
2093	*tert*-Butyl Hydroperoxide	8
2094	*tert*-Butyl Hydroperoxide	8

UN/ NA/PIN	Chemical Name	Guideline Number
2095	*tert*-Butyl Peroxyacetate	8, 15
2096	*tert*-Butyl Peroxyacetate	8, 15
2097	*tert*-Butyl Peroxybenzoate	8, 15
2098	*tert*-Butyl Peroxybenzoate	8, 15
2099	*tert*-Butyl Monoperoxymaleate, technical pure	8, 15
2099	*tert*-Butyl Peroxymaleate, technical pure	8, 15
2100	*tert*-Butyl Monoperoxymaleate, solution or paste	8, 15
2100	*tert*-Butyl Peroxymaleate, solution or paste	8, 15
2101	*tert*-Butyl Monoperoxymaleate	8, 15
2101	*tert*-Butyl Peroxymaleate	8, 15
2102	*tert*-Butyl Peroxide	8
2102	Di-*tert*-butyl Peroxide, technical pure	8
2103	*tert*-Butyl Peroxyisopropyl Carbonate, technical pure	8, 15
2104	*tert*-Butyl Peroxyisononanoate	8, 15
2104	*tert*-Butyl Peroxy-3,5,5-trimethylhexanoate	8, 15
2105	*tert*-Butyl Monoperoxyphthalate	8, 15
2105	*tert*-Butyl Peroxyphthalate	8, 15
2106	Di-*tert*-butylperoxyphthalate	37
2107	Di-*tert*-butylperoxyphthalate	37
2108	Di-*tert*-butylperoxyphthalate	37
2110	*tert*-Butyl Peroxypivalate	8, 15
2111	2,2-Di(*tert*-butylperoxy)-butane	8, 33
2112	Di-(2-*tert*-butylperoxyisopropyl) Benzene	8, 24

WARNING: More than one chemical agent may have the same UN Number. Look up the guideline for the specific material in question by chemical name and not UN/NA/Pin number alone.

UN/ NA/PIN	Chemical Name	Guideline Number
2112	1,4-Di(2-*tert*-butylperoxyisopropyl) Benzene and 1,3-Di (2-*tert*-butylperoxy-isopropyl) Benzene	8, 24
2113	*p*-Chlorobenzoyl Peroxide	8
2113	Di-(4-chlorobenzoyl) Peroxide	8
2114	*p*-Chlorobenzoyl Peroxide	8
2114	Di-(4-chlorobenzoyl) Peroxide	8
2115	*p*-Chlorobenzoyl Peroxide	8
2114	Di-4-(chlorobenzoyl) Peroxide	8
2116	Cumyl Hydroperoxide	8, 24
2116	Cumene Hydroperoxide, technical pure	8, 24
2117	Cyclohexanone Peroxide, more than 90% with less than 10% water	8
2117	1-Hydroxy-1′-hydroperoxy-dicyclohexyl Peroxide, more than 90% with less than 10% water	8
2118	Cyclohexanone Peroxide, not more than 72% in solution	8
2118	1-Hydroxy-1′-hydroperoxy–dicyclohexyl Peroxide	8
2119	Cyclohexanone Peroxide, not more than 90%, with not less than 10% water	8
2119	1-Hydroxy-1′-hydroperoxy Dicyclohexyl Peroxide	8
2120	Decanoyl Peroxide, technical pure	8
2120	Didecanoyl Peroxide, technical pure	8
2121	Dicumyl Peroxide	8
2122	Di-(2-ethylhexyl)peroxy-dicarbonate	8
2123	Di-(2-ethylhexyl)peroxy-dicarbonate	8
2124	Dilauroyl Peroxide, technical pure	8
2124	Lauroyl Peroxide, technical pure	8
2125	Menthane Hydroperoxide, para, technical pure	8
2125	Menthyl Hydroperoxide, para, technical pure	8
2125	Paramenthane Hydroperoxide	8
2126	Isobutyl Methyl Ketone Peroxide	8, 42
2126	Methyl Isobutyl Ketone Peroxide	8, 42
2127	Ethyl Methyl Ketone Peroxide	8, 42
2127	Methyl Ethyl Ketone Peroxide, with not more than 60%, in solution	8, 42
2127	Methyl Ethyl Ketone Peroxide, with not more than 60% peroxide	8, 42
2128	Di(3,5,5-trimethylhexanoyl) Peroxide	8
2128	Isononanoyl Peroxide, technical pure or in solution	8
2129	Caprylyl Peroxide	8
2129	Di–octanoyl Peroxide	8
2129	Octanoyl Peroxide	8
2130	Di–nonanoyl Peroxide	8
2130	Pelargonyl Peroxide	8
2131	Peracetic Acid, solution	8, 15
2131	Peroxyacetic Acid, solution	8, 15
2132	Dipropionyl Peroxide	8
2132	Propionyl Peroxide	8
2133	Diisopropyl Peroxydicarbonate, technical pure	8

WARNING: More than one chemical agent may have the same UN Number. Look up the guideline for the specific material in question by chemical name and not UN/NA/Pin number alone.

UN/ NA/PIN	Chemical Name	Guideline Number
2133	Isopropyl Peroxydicarbonate	8
2133	Propyl Peroxydicarbonate	8
2134	Diisopropyl Peroxydicarbonate	8
2134	Isopropyl Peroxydicarbonate	8
2135	Disuccinic Acid Peroxide, technical pure	8
2135	Succinic Acid Peroxide, technical pure	15
2136	Tetrahydronaphthyl Hydroperoxide, technical pure	8, 43
2136	Tetralin Hydroperoxide, technical pure	8, 43
2137	2,4-Dichlorobenzoyl Peroxide	8
2137	Di-2,4-dichlorobenzoyl Peroxide, not more than 75% in water	8
2138	2,4-Dichlorobenzoyl Peroxide	8
2138	Di-2,4-dichlorobenzoyl Peroxide, not more than 52% as paste	8
2139	2,4-Dichlorobenzoyl Peroxide	8
2139	Di-2,4-dichlorobenzoyl Peroxide, not more than 52% in solution	8
2140	*n*-Butyl-4,4-di(*tert*-butyl-peroxy) Valerate	15
2141	*n*-Butyl-4,4-di(*tert*-butyl-peroxy) Valerate	15
2142	*tert*-Butyl Peroxyisobutyrate	8, 15
2143	*tert*-Butyl Peroxy-2-ethyl-hexanoate, technical pure	8, 15
2144	*tert*-Butyl Peroxydiethylacetate	8, 15
2145	1,1-Di(*tert*-butylperoxy)-3,3,5-trimethylcyclohexane	8, 33
2146	1,1-Di(*tert*-butylperoxy)-3,3,5-trimethylcyclohexane	8, 33
2147	1,1-Di(*tert*-butylperoxy)-3,3,5-trimethylcyclohexane	8, 33
2148	Di(1-hydroxycyclohexyl) Peroxide	8
2149	Dibenzyl Peroxydicarbonate	8
2150	Di-*sec*-butyl Peroxydicarbonate	8
2151	Di-*sec*-butyl Peroxydicarbonate	8
2152	Dicyclohexyl Peroxydicarbonate	8
2153	Dicyclohexyl Peroxydicarbonate	8
2154	Di(4-*tert*-butylcyclohexyl) Peroxydicarbonate	8
2155	2,5-Dimethyl-2,5-di(*tert*-butylperoxy)hexane, technical pure	8
2156	2,5-Dimethyl-2,5-di(t*ert*-butylperoxy)hexane	8
2157	2,5-Dimethyl-2,5-di(2-ethyl-hexanoyl-peroxy)hexane, technical pure	8
2158	2,5-Dimethyl-2,5-di(*tert*-butylperoxy)hexyne-3, technical pure	*8*
2159	2,5-Dimethyl-2,5-di(*tert*-butylperoxy)hexyne-3, with not more than 52% peroxide in inert solid	8
2160	*tert*-Octyl Hydroperoxide	8
2160	1,1,3,3-Tetramethylbutyl Hydroperoxide, technical pure	8
2161	*tert*-Octyl Peroxy-2-ethylhexanoate	8, 15
2161	1,1,3,3-Tetramethylbutyl-peroxy-2-ethyl Hexanoate, technical pure	8

WARNING: More than one chemical agent may have the same UN Number. Look up the guideline for the specific material in question by chemical name and not UN/NA/Pin number alone.

UN/ NA/PIN	Chemical Name	Guideline Number
2162	Pinane Hydroperoxide, technical pure	8
2162	Pinanyl Hydroperoxide, technical pure	8
2162	Trimethyl Norpinanyl Hydroperoxide, technical pure	24
2163	Diacetone Alcohol Peroxide	8, 42
2164	Dicetyl Peroxydicarbonate, technical pure	8
2165	3,3,6,6,9,9-Hexamethyl-1,2,4,5-tetraoxocyclononane, technical pure	8
2166	3,3,6,6,9,9-Hexamethyl-1,2,4,5-tetraoxocyclononane	8
2167	3,3,6,6,9,9-Hexamethyl-1,2,4,5-tetraoxocylcononane	8
2168	2,2-Di(4,4-di-(*tert*-butylperoxy)cyclohexyl) propane	8
2169	Butyl Peroxydicarbonate	8, 15
2169	Di–butyl Peroxydicarbonate	8, 15
2170	Butyl Peroxydicarbonate <27% in solution	8, 15
2170	Di–butyl Peroxydicarbonate <27% in solution	8, 15
2171	Diisopropylbenzene Hydroperoxide	8
2171	Isopropylcumyl Hydroperoxide	8, 24
2172	2,5-Dimethyl-2,5-di-(benzoylperoxy)hexane, technical pure	8
2173	2,5-Dimethyl-2,5-di-(benzoylperoxy)hexane	8
2174	2,5-Dimethyl-2,5-dihydro-peroxy-hexane	8
2175	Diethyl Peroxydicarbonate	8
2176	Di-n-propyl Peroxydicarbonate, technical pure	8

UN/ NA/PIN	Chemical Name	Guideline Number
2177	*tert*-Butyl Peroxy-neodecanoate	8, 15
2178	2,2-Dihydroperoxy Propane	8
2179	1,1-Di(tert-butylperoxy) cyclohexane	8, 33
2180	1,1-Di(tert-butylperoxy) cyclohexane	8, 33
2181	1,2-Di(tert-butylperoxy) cyclohexane	8, 33
2182	Diisobutyryl Peroxide	8
2183	*tert*-Butyl Peroxycrotonate	8, 15
2184	Ethyl 3,3-Di(*tert*-Butylperoxy) Butyrate	8
2185	Ethyl 3,3-Di(tert-Butylperoxy) Butyrate, not more than 77%	8
2186	Hydrogen Chloride, refrigerated liquid (cryogenic liquid)	14, 133, 138
2187	Carbon Dioxide, refrigerated liquid (cryogenic liquid)	92
2188	Arsine	73, 138
2189	Dichlorosilane	107
2190	Oxygen Difluoride	99, 104
2191	Fumigants	10
2191	Sulfuryl Fluoride	99, 105
2192	Germane, germanium hydride	73
2192	Germanium Hydride	73
2193	Hexafluoroethane	26
2194	Selenium Hexafluoride	86, 99
2195	Tellurium Hexafluoride	10
2196	Tungsten Hexafluoride	99, 133, 138
2197	Hydrogen Iodide, anhydrous	100
2198	Phosphorus Pentafluoride	99, 109
2199	Phosphine	108,133
2200	Allene	33
2200	Propadiene	33

WARNING: More than one chemical agent may have the same UN Number. Look up the guideline for the specific material in question by chemical name and not UN/NA/Pin number alone.

UN/NA/PIN	Chemical Name	Guideline Number
2200	Propadiene, inhibited	33
2201	Nitrous Oxide, refrigerated liquid (cryogenic liquid)	48
2202	Hydrogen Selenide, anhydrous	86
2202	Hydroselenic Acid	14, 86
2203	Silane	107
2204	Carbonyl Sulfide	91
2205	Adiponitrile	90
2206	Isocyanates and solutions, n.o.s., b.p. less than 300° C	94
2207	Isocyanates and solutions, n.o.s., b.p. not less than 300° C	94
2208	Bleaching Powder	22
2208	Calcium Hypochlorite Mixture, dry, with more than 10% but not more than 39% available chlorine	22
2208	Chlorinated Lime	22
2209	Formaldehyde	41, 133, 138
2209	Formaldehyde Solution (Formalin)	41
2210	Maneb	63
2210	Maneb or Maneb Preparation(s), with 50% or more Maneb	63
2210	Pesticide, water-reactive, containing manganese ethylene-bisdithiocarbamate (Maneb)	63
2211	Plastic Moulding Material, evolving flammable vapor	6
2211	Polystyrene Beads, expandable, evolving a flammable vapor	5
2212	Asbestos, blue or brown	102
2212	Blue Asbestos	102

UN/NA/PIN	Chemical Name	Guideline Number
2212	Brown Asbestos	102
2213	Parformaldehyde	41
2214	Phthalic Anhydride	15
2215	Maleic Acid	15
2215	Maleic Anhydride	15
2216	Fish Meal and Scrap, stabilized	9
2218	Acrylic Acid	15
2219	Allyl Glycidyl Ether	38
2220	Aluminum Alkyl Halide Solution	10
2221	Aluminum Alkyl Chloride	10, 98
2221	Aluminum Alkyl Halide	10
2222	Anisole	24
2224	Benzonitrile	90
2225	Benzene Sulfonyl Chloride	15
2226	Benzotrichloride	9, 24
2227	Butyl Methacrylate	37
2228	Butyl Phenol, liquid	44
2228	*o-sec*-Butylphenol	44
2229	Butyl Phenol, solid	44
2232	Chloroacetaldehyde	41
2233	Chloroanisidine	24, 47
2234	Chlorobenzotrifluoride	24
2235	Chlorobenzyl Chloride	24
2236	Chloromethylphenyl-isocyanate	94
2237	Chloronitroaniline	32
2238	Chlorotoluene	24
2238	*o*-Chlorotoluene	24
2239	Chlorotoluidine, liquid or solid	20
2240	Chromosulfuric Acid	14
2241	Cycloheptane	33
2242	Cycloheptene	33

WARNING: More than one chemical agent may have the same UN Number. Look up the guideline for the specific material in question by chemical name and not UN/NA/Pin number alone.

UN/ NA/PIN	Chemical Name	Guideline Number
2243	Cyclohexyl Acetate	37
2244	Cyclopentanol	30
2245	Cyclopentanone	42
2246	Cyclopentene	33
2247	Decane	33
2248	Dibutylamine	20
2249	Bis(2-chloromethyl) Ether	38
2249	Dichlorodimethyl Ether, symmetrical	38
2250	Dichlorophenylisocyanate	94
2251	Dicycloheptadiene	33
2251	Norborandiene	33
2252	Dimethoxyethane	40
2252	1,2-Dimethoxyethane	40
2253	Dimethylaniline	32
2253	*N,N*-Dimethylaniline	32
2254	Matches, fusee	97
2255	Organic Peroxide, sample, n.o.s.	8
2255	Polyester Resin Kits	10
2256	Cyclohexene	33
2257	Potassium	10
2257	Potassium Metal	10
2258	Propylenediamine	20
2259	Triethylene Tetramine	10
2260	Tripropylamine	20
2261	Xylenol	24, 44
2262	Dimethylcarbamoyl Chloride	10
2263	Dimethylcyclohexane	33
2264	2,3-Dimethylcyclohexyl Amine	10, 20
2265	Dimethylformamide	10
2265	*N,N*-Dimethylformamide	10
2266	Dimethyl–Propylamine	20
2267	Dimethyl Chlorothiophosphate	49
2267	Dimethyl Phosphorochloridothioate	49
2267	Dimethyl Thiophosphoryl Chloride	49
2269	Dipropylene Triamine	20
2269	Iminobispropylamine	20
2269	Iminodipropylamine	20
2270	Ethylamine	20
2270	Ethylamine Solution	20
2271	Ethyl Amyl Ketone	42
2271	5-Methyl-3-Heptanone	42
2272	Ethylaniline	32
2273	2-Ethylaniline	32
2274	Ethylbenzylaniline	32
2275	Ethylbutanol	30
2276	Ethyl Hexylamine	20
2277	Ethyl Methacrylate	37
2278	Heptene	33
2279	Hexachlorobutadiene	26
2280	Hexamethylendiamine, solid	20
2281	Hexamethylene Diisocyanate	94
2282	Hexanol	30
2283	Isobutyl Methacrylate	37
2284	Isobutyronitrile	90
2285	Isocyanatobenzo-trifluoride	94, 99
2286	Isododecane	33
2286	Pentamethyl Heptane	33
2287	Isoheptene	33
2288	Isohexene	33
2289	Isophoronediamine	20
2290	IPDI	94
2290	Isophorone Diisocyanate	94
2291	Lead Chloride	80
2291	Lead Compound, soluble, n.o.s.	80
2291	Lead Fluoborate	80, 103

WARNING: More than one chemical agent may have the same UN Number. Look up the guideline for the specific material in question by chemical name and not UN/NA/Pin number alone.

UN/NA/PIN	Chemical Name	Guideline Number
2293	Methoxymethylpentanone	33, 92
2294	Methylaniline	32
2294	*N*-Methylaniline	32
2295	Methyl Chloroacetate	37
2296	Methylcyclohexane	33
2297	Methyl Cyclohexanone	42
2297	2-Methylcyclohexanone	42
2298	Methyl Cyclopentane	33
2299	Methyl Dichloroacetate	37
2300	Methyl Ethyl Pyridine	24
2300	2-Methyl-5-ethyl Pyridine	24
2301	Methylfuran	33
2302	Methylhexanone	42
2302	Methyl Isoamyl Ketone	42
2303	Isopropenyl Benzene	24
2304	Naphthalene, molten	43
2305	Nitrobenzenesulfonic Acid	15
2306	Nitrobenzotrifluoride	24, 47
2307	Nitrochlorobenzo-trifluoride	24, 47
2308	Nitrosylsulfuric Acid	14
2309	Octadiene	33
2310	Pentane-2,4-Dione	42
2311	Phenetidine	32
2312	Phenol, molten	44
2313	Picoline	24
2313	2-Picoline	24
2315	PCBs	46
2315	Polychlorinated Biphenyls (PCBs)	46
2316	Sodium Cuprocyanide, solid	90, 132
2317	Sodium Cuprocyanide Solution	90, 132
2318	Sodium Hydrosulfide, solid, with less than 25% water of crystallization	91
2319	Terpene Hydrocarbons, n.o.s.	34
2320	Tetraethylenepentamine	20
2321	Trichlorobenzene, liquid	24
2322	Trichlorobutene	26
2323	Triethyl Phosphite	109
2324	Triisobutylene	33
2325	Mesitylene	24
2325	Trimethyl Benzene	24
2326	Trimethylcyclohexylamine	20
2327	Trimethylhexamethylene-diamine	20
2328	Trimethylhexamethylene-diisocyanate	94
2329	Trimethyl Phosphite	109
2330	Hendecane	35
2330	Undecane	33
2331	Zinc Chloride, anhydrous	88
2332	Acetaldehyde Oxime	5
2333	Allyl Acetate	37
2334	Allyl Amine	20
2335	Allyl Ethyl Ether	38
2336	Allyl Formate	37
2337	Phenyl Mercaptan	105
2338	Benzotrifluoride	9, 24
2339	2-Bromobutane	26
2340	Bromoethyl Ethyl Ether	38
2341	Bromoethylbutane	26
2341	Bromomethylbutane	26
2342	Bromoethylpropane	26
2342	Bromomethylpropane	26
2343	Bromopentane	26
2344	Bromopropane	26
2345	Bromopropyne	26
2346	Butanedione	45
2346	Diacetyl	42

WARNING: More than one chemical agent may have the same UN Number. Look up the guideline for the specific material in question by chemical name and not UN/NA/Pin number alone.

UN/ NA/PIN	Chemical Name	Guideline Number
2347	Butanethiol	33
2347	Butyl Mercaptan	105
2347	Butane-Thiol	33, 105
2348	Butyl Acrylate	37
2348	*n*-Butyl Acrylate	37
2350	Butyl Methyl Ether	38
2351	Butyl Nitrite	47
2352	Butyl Vinyl Ether	38
2353	Butyryl Chloride	15
2354	Chloromethyl Ethyl Ether	38
2356	Chloropropane	33
2357	Cyclohexylamine	20
2358	Cyclooctatetraene	33
2359	Diallylamine	20
2360	Diallylether	38
2361	Di-Isobutylamine	20
2362	1,1-Dichloroethane	27
2363	Ethyl Mercaptan	105
2364	Propyl Benzene	24
2366	Diethyl Carbonate	37
2367	Methyl Valeraldehyde	41
2368	Pinene	34
2369	Ethylene Glycol Monobutyl Ether	40
2370	Hexene	33
2371	Isopentene	33
2372	*bis*(Dimethylamino) Ethane	33
2372	1,2-Di-(dimethylamino) Ethane	32, 33
2373	Diethoxymethane	38
2374	Diethoxypropene	59
2375	Diethyl Sulfide	105
2376	Dihydropyran	24
2377	1,1-Dimethoxyethane	40
2377	Dimethoxyethane	40
2378	Dimethylamino-acetonitrile	90
2379	Dimethylbutylamine	20
2379	1,3-Dimethylbutylamine	20
2380	Dimethyldiethoxysilane	107
2381	Dimethyldisulfide	105
2382	Dimethylhydrazine, symmetrical	23
2383	Dipropylamine	20
2384	Dipropyl Ether	38
2385	Ethyl Isobutyrate	37
2386	Ethyl Piperidine	20
2387	Fluorobenzene	25
2388	Fluorotoluene	24
2389	Furan	33
2390	Iodo Butane	26
2391	Iodo Methylpropane	26
2392	Iodo Propane	26
2393	Isobutyl Formate	37
2394	Isobutyl Propionate	37
2395	Isobutyryl Chloride	26
2396	Methacrylaldehyde	41
2397	Methyl Butanone	42
2397	Methyl Isopropyl Ketone	42
2398	Methyl Butyl Ether	38
2398	Methyl-*tert*-Butyl Ether	38
2399	Methylpiperidine	20
2400	Methyl Isovalerate	37
2401	Piperidine	20
2402	Isopropyl Mercaptan	105
2402	Propanethiol	105
2402	Propyl Mercaptan	105
2403	Isopropenyl Acetate	37
2404	Proprionitrile	90
2405	Isopropyl Butyrate	37
2406	Isopropyl Isobutyrate	37
2407	Isopropyl Chloroformate	37

WARNING: More than one chemical agent may have the same UN Number. Look up the guideline for the specific material in question by chemical name and not UN/NA/Pin number alone.

UN/ NA/PIN	Chemical Name	Guideline Number
2408	Isopropyl Formate	37
2409	Isopropyl Propionate	37
2410	Tetrahydropyridine	24
2411	Butyronitrile	90
2412	Tetrahydrothiophene	105
2413	Tetrapropyl-ortho-titanate	10
2414	Thiophene	105
2416	Trimethylborate	103
2417	Carbonyl Fluoride	16
2418	Sulfur Tetrafluoride	16, 105
2419	Bromotrifluoroethylene	26
2420	Hexafluoroacetone	42
2421	Nitrogen Trioxide	48
2422	Octafluorobutene	26
2424	Octafluoropropane	26
2424	Perfluoropropane	26
2426	Ammonium Nitrate, liquid (hot concentrated solution)	47
2426	Ammonium Nitrate Solution, with not less than 15% water	47
2427	Potassium Chlorate Solution	97
2428	Sodium Chlorate Solution	97
2429	Calcium Chlorate Solution	97
2430	Alkyl Phenol, n.o.s.	44
2431	Anisidine	25
2432	Diethyl Aniline	32
2433	Chloronitrotoluene	24
2434	Dibenzyldichlorosilane	107
2435	Ethyl Phenyl Dichlorosilane	107
2436	Thioacetic Acid	15, 105
2437	Methylphenyldichloro-silane	107
2438	Pivaloyl Chloride	26

UN/ NA/PIN	Chemical Name	Guideline Number
2438	Trimethylacetyl Chloride	15
2439	Sodium Bifluoride, solid	99
2439	Sodium Bifluoride Solution	99
2439	Sodium Hydrogen Fluoride	16
2440	Stannic Chloride, hydrated	14
2441	Titanium Trichloride, pyrophoric	10
2441	Titanium Trichloride Mixture, pyrophoric	10
2442	Trichloroacetyl Chloride	26
2443	Vanadium Oxytrichloride	10
2443	Vanadium Oxytrichloride and Titanium Tetrachloride Mixture	10
2444	Vanadium Tetrachloride	10
2445	Butyl Lithium	81
2445	Lithium Alkyl	81
2446	Nitrocresol	44, 47
2447	Phosphorus, white, molten	109
2448	Sulfur, molten	105
2449	Ammonium Oxalate	17, 21
2449	Cupric Oxalate	78
2449	Oxalates, water soluble	17
2451	Nitrogen Trifluoride	99
2452	Ethyl Acetylene, inhibited	33, 92
2453	Ethyl Fluoride	27
2454	Methyl Fluoride	27
2455	Methyl Nitrite	47
2456	Chloropropene	33
2457	Dimethylbutane	33
2458	Hexadiene	33
2459	2-Methyl-1-butene	33
2460	Methylbutene	33
2460	2-Methyl-2-butene	33
2461	Methylpentadiene	33
2462	Methylpentane	33

WARNING: More than one chemical agent may have the same UN Number. Look up the guideline for the specific material in question by chemical name and not UN/NA/Pin number alone.

UN/ NA/PIN	Chemical Name	Guideline Number
2463	Aluminum Hydride	10
2464	Beryllium Nitrate	75
2465	Dichloroisocyanuric Acid, and its salts, dry	15
2465	Dichloro-*s*-triazinetrione, and its salts, dry	9
2465	Potassium Dichloroisocyanurate	22
2465	Potassium Dichloro-*s*-triazinetrione	22
2465	Sodium Dichloroisocyanate	22
2465	Sodium Dichloroisocyanurate	22
2465	Sodium Dichloro-*s*-triazinetrione	22
2466	Potassium Superoxide	10
2467	Sodium Percarbonate	7
2468	Mono-(trichloro)-tetra-(monopotassium dichloro)-penta-*s*-triazinetrione, dry	9
2468	Trichloroisocyanuric Acid, dry	22
2468	Trichlorotriazinetrione and its salts, dry	22
2468	Trichloro-*s*-Triazinetrione, dry	22
2469	Zinc Bromate	88, 96
2470	Phenylacetonitrile, liquid	90
2471	Osmium Compounds	10
2471	Osmium Tetroxide	10
2472	Pindone	71
2473	Sodium Arsanilate	72
2474	Thiophosgene	101
2475	Vanadium Trichloride	10
2477	Methyl Isothiocyanate	94
2478	Isocyanates and solutions, n.o.s. (flammable)	94
2480	Methyl Isocyanate	94, 133, 138
2481	Ethyl Isocyanate	94
2482	Propyl Isocyanate	94
2483	Isopropyl Isocyanate	94
2484	*tert*-Butyl Isocyanate	94
2485	*n*-Butyl Isocyanate	94
2486	Isobutyl Isocyanate	94
2487	Phenyl Isocyanate	94
2488	Cyclohexyl Isocyanate	94
2489	Diphenylmethane-4, 4′-diisocyanate (MDI)	94
2489	Methylene Bis(4-phenyl Isocyanate) (MDI)	94
2490	Bis (2-chloroisopropyl) Ether	38
2490	Dichloroisopropyl Ether	38
2491	Ethanolamines, and solutions	20
2491	Monoethanolamine	20
2493	Hexamethyleneimine	20
2495	Iodine Pentafluoride	16, 100
2496	Propionic Anhydride	15
2497	Sodium Phenolate, solid	44
2498	Tetrahydrobenzaldehyde	41
2501	1-Aziridinyl Phosphine Oxide (TRIS)	10
2501	Phosphoric Acid Triethyleneimine	10
2501	Tri(1-aziridinyl) Phosphine Oxide	10
2501	Tris(1-aziridinyl) Phosphine Oxide	10
2502	Valeryl Chloride	15
2503	Zirconium	10
2503	Zirconium Tetrachloride	10
2504	Acetylene Tetrabromide	33, 92

WARNING: More than one chemical agent may have the same UN Number. Look up the guideline for the specific material in question by chemical name and not UN/NA/Pin number alone.

UN/ NA/PIN	Chemical Name	Guideline Number
2504	Tetrabromoethane	26
2505	Ammonium Fluoride	99
2506	Ammonium Hydrogen Sulfate	14
2507	Chloroplatinic Acid, solid	14
2508	Molybdenum Pentachloride	10
2509	Potassium Bisulfate	14
2509	Potassium Hydrogen Sulfate	14
2511	Chloropropionic Acid	15
2512	Aminophenol	32
2513	Bromoacetyl Bromide	95
2514	Bromobenzene	26
2515	Bromoform	26
2516	Carbon Tetrabromide	28
2517	Chlorodifluoroethane	27
2517	Difluoromonochloroethane	27
2518	Cyclododecatriene	33
2520	Cyclooctadiene	33
2521	Diketene	42
2522	Dimethylaminoethyl Methacrylate	37
2524	Ethyl Orthoformate	37
2525	Ethyl Oxalate	17
2526	Furfurylamine	20
2527	Isobutyl Acrylate	37
2528	Isobutyl Isobutyrate	37
2529	Isobutyric Acid	15
2530	Isobutyric Anhydride	15
2531	Methacrylic Acid, inhibited	15
2533	Methyl Trichloroacetate	37
2534	Methylchlorosilane	107
2535	Methylmorpholine	20
2536	Methyl Tetrahydrofuran	38
2538	Nitronaphthalene	43
2541	Terpinolene	34
2542	Tributylamine	20
2545	Hafnium Compounds	6
2545	Hafnium Metal, powder, dry	6
2546	Titanium	10
2546	Titanium, metal, powder, dry	10
2547	Sodium Superoxide	7
2548	Chlorine Pentafluoride	98, 99
2550	Ethyl Methyl Ketone Peroxide	8, 42
2550	Methyl Ethyl Ketone Peroxide	8, 42
2551	*tert*-Butyl Peroxy-diethylacetate with *tert*-Butyl Peroxybenzoate	8, 15
2552	Hexafluoroacetone Hydrate	42
2553	Coal Tar Naphtha	43
2553	Naphtha	35
2553	Painter's Naphtha	35
2554	Methyl Allyl Chloride	61
2555	Nitrocellulose, wet, with not less than 20% water	6
2556	Nitrocellulose, wet, with not less than 25% Alcohol	5
2557	Lacquer Base, dry	35
2557	Nitrocellulose, with plasticizing substance	6, 10
2558	Epibromohydrin	61
2560	Methylpentanol	30
2561	3-Methyl-1-butene	33
2562	*tert*-Butyl Peroxyisobutyrate	8, 15
2563	Methyl Ethyl Ketone Peroxide, with not more than 52% peroxide	8, 42
2564	Trichloroacetic Acid Solution	15

WARNING: More than one chemical agent may have the same UN Number. Look up the guideline for the specific material in question by chemical name and not UN/NA/Pin number alone.

UN/ NA/PIN	Chemical Name	Guideline Number
2565	Dicyclohexylamine	62
2567	Sodium Pentachlorophenate	67
2570	Cadmium Compound	76
2570	Cadmium Acetate	76
2570	Cadmium Bromide	76
2570	Cadmium Chloride	76
2571	Ethyl Sulfuric Acid	15
2572	Phenylhydrazine	23
2573	Thallium Chlorate	87, 97
2574	Tricresylphosphate	106
2576	Phosphorus Oxybromide, molten	95, 109
2577	Phenylacetyl Chloride	24
2578	Phosphorus Trioxide	109
2579	Piperazine	20
2580	Aluminum Bromide, Solution	95
2581	Aluminum Chloride, Solution	10, 98
2582	Ferric Chloride Solution	79
2582	Iron Chloride Solution	79
2583	Alkyl Sulfonic Acid, solid	15
2583	Aryl Sulfonic Acid, solid	15
2583	Toluene Sulfonic Acid, solid	15
2584	Alkyl Sulfonic Acid, liquid	15
2584	Aryl Sulfonic Acid, liquid	15
2584	Dodecylbenzenesulfonic Acid	15
2584	Toluene Sulfonic Acid, liquid	15
2585	Alkyl Sulfonic Acid, solid	15
2585	Aryl Sulfonic Acid, solid	15
2585	Toluene Sulfonic Acid, solid	15
2586	Alkyl Sulfonic Acid, liquid	15
2586	Aryl Sulfonic Acid, liquid	15
2586	Toluene Sulfonic Acid, liquid	15

UN/ NA/PIN	Chemical Name	Guideline Number
2587	Benzoquinone	24
2588	Insecticide, dry, n.o.s.	10
2588	Pesticide, solid, poisonous, n.o.s.	10
2588	Propoxur	50
2588	Ronnel	49
2588	Rotenone	53
2589	Vinyl Chloroacetate	37
2590	Asbestos, white	102
2590	White Asbestos	102
2591	Xenon, refrigerated liquid (cryogenic liquid)	92
2592	Distearyl Peroxydicarbonate	8
2593	Di(2-methylbenzoyl) Peroxide	8
2594	*tert*-Butyl Peroxyneodecanoate	8, 15
2595	Dimyristyl Peroxydicarbonate	8
2596	*tert*-Butyl Peroxy-3-phenylphthalide	8, 15
2597	Di(3,5,5-trimethyl-1,2-dioxolanyl-3) Peroxide	8
2598	Ethyl 3,3-Di(*tert*--butylperoxy) Butyrate	8
2599	Chlorotrifluoromethane and Trifluoromethane Mixture	27
2599	Trifluoromethane and Chlorotrifluoromethane Mixture	27
2600	Carbon Monoxide–Hydrogen Mixture	89
2601	Cyclobutane	92
2602	Dichlorodifluoro-methane and Difluoroethane Azeotropic Mixture	27
2603	Cycloheptatriene	33

WARNING: More than one chemical agent may have the same UN Number. Look up the guideline for the specific material in question by chemical name and not UN/NA/Pin number alone.

UN/ NA/PIN	Chemical Name	Guideline Number
2604	Boron Trifluoride Diethyl Etherate	103
2605	Methoxymethyl Isocyanate	94
2606	Methyl Orthosilicate	107
2606	Methyl Silicate	107
2606	Tetramethoxysilane	107
2607	Acrolein Dimer, stabilized	59
2608	Nitropropane	47
2609	Triallyl Borate	103
2610	Triallylamine	20
2611	Chloropropanol	30
2611	2-Chloro-1-propanol	30
2611	Propylene Chlorohydrin	61
2612	Methyl Propyl Ether	38
2614	Methallyl Alcohol	30
2615	Ethoxypropane	38
2615	Ethyl Propyl Ether	38
2616	Triisopropyl Borate	103
2617	Hexahydrocresol	44
2617	Methyl Cyclohexanol	30
2618	Vinyl Toluene	24
2618	Vinyl Toluene, inhibited	24
2619	Benzyl Dimethylamine	32
2620	Amyl Butyrate	15
2621	Acetyl Methyl Carbinol	42
2622	Glycidaldehyde	41
2623	Fire Lighter, solid with flammable liquid	33
2624	Magnesium Silicide	82
2626	Chloric Acid Solution	14
2627	Nitrite, inorganic, n.o.s.	47
2628	Potassium Fluoroacetate	64
2629	Sodium Fluoroacetate	64
2630	Barium Selenate	74, 86
2630	Barium Selenite	74, 86
2630	Calcium Selenate	86
2630	Copper Selenate	78, 86
2630	Copper Selenite	78, 86
2630	Potassium Selenate	86
2630	Potassium Selenite	86
2630	Selenates and Selenites	86
2630	Sodium Selenate	86
2630	Sodium Selenite	86
2630	Zinc Selenate	86, 88
2630	Zinc Selenite	86, 88
2642	Fluoracetic Acid	64
2643	Methyl Bromoacetate	95
2644	Methyl Iodide	52
2645	Phenacyl Bromide	95
2646	Hexachlorocyclopentadiene	26
2647	Malonic Dinitrile	90
2647	Malononitrile	90
2648	Dibromobutanone	42
2649	1,3-Dichloroacetone	42
2649	Dichloropropanone	42
2650	Dichloronitroethane	27
2651	Diaminodiphenyl Methane	47
2653	Benzyl Iodide	24
2655	Potassium Fluorosilicate, solid	99
2655	Potassium Silicofluoride, solid	99
2656	Quinoline	24
2657	Selenium Disulfide	86, 105
2658	Selenium Metal, powder	86
2659	Sodium Chloroacetate	37
2660	Nitrotoluidine (mono)	24, 47
2661	Hexachloroacetone	42
2662	Hydroquinone	32, 44
2664	Dibromomethane	27
2664	Methylene Bromide	95
2666	Ethyl Cyanoacetate	37

WARNING: More than one chemical agent may have the same UN Number. Look up the guideline for the specific material in question by chemical name and not UN/NA/Pin number alone.

UN/ NA/PIN	Chemical Name	Guideline Number
2666	Malonic Ethyl Ester Nitrile	90
2667	Butyl Toluene	24
2668	Chloroacetonitrile	90
2669	Chlorocresol	44
2670	Cyanuric Chloride	15
2671	Aminopyridine	24
2672	Ammonium Hydroxide	19
2672	Ammonia Solution, with not less than 12% and not more than 44% ammonia	21
2673	Aminochlorophenol	44
2674	Sodium Fluorosilicate	99
2674	Sodium Silicofluoride, solid	99
2676	Stibine	10
2677	Rubidium Hydroxide Solution	10
2678	Rubidium Hydroxide, solid	10
2679	Lithium Hydroxide Solution	19, 81
2680	Lithium Hydroxide Monohydrate	19, 81
2681	Caesium Hydroxide Solution	19
2681	Cesium Hydroxide Solution	19
2682	Caesium Hydroxide	19
2682	Cesium Hydroxide	19
2683	Ammonium Hydrosulfide Solution	21
2683	Ammonium Sulfide Solution	21, 105
2684	Diethylaminopropylamine	20
2685	Diethylene Diamine	20
2686	Diethylaminoethanol	20
2687	Dicyclohexylammonium Nitrite	47, 62
2688	Chlorobromopropane	27

UN/ NA/PIN	Chemical Name	Guideline Number
2689	Glycerol-alpha-mono-chlorohydrin	61
2690	Butyl Imidazole	33
2691	Phosphorus Pentabromide	95, 109
2692	Boron Tribromide	103
2693	Ammonium Bisulfite, solid	21, 105
2693	Ammonium Bisulfite Solution	21, 105
2693	Bisulfite, inorganic, aqueous solution, n.o.s.	105
2693	Calcium Bisulfite Solution	105
2693	Calcium Hydrogen Sulfite Solution	105
2693	Magnesium Bisulfite Solution	82, 105
2693	Potassium Bisulfite Solution	105
2693	Sodium Bisulfite Solution	105
2693	Zinc Bisulfite Solution	88, 105
2698	Tetrahydrophthalic Anhydride	15
2699	Trifluoroacetic Acid	15
2703	Isopropyl Mercaptan	105
2704	Propyl Mercaptan	105
2705	Pentol	30
2707	Dimethyldioxane	39
2708	Butoxyl	37
2709	Butyl Benzene	24
2710	Butyrone	42
2710	Dipropyl Ketone	42
2711	Dibromobenzene	24
2713	Acridine	24
2714	Zinc Resinate	88
2715	Aluminum Resinate	10
2716	Butynediol	30

WARNING: More than one chemical agent may have the same UN Number. Look up the guideline for the specific material in question by chemical name and not UN/NA/Pin number alone.

UN/ NA/PIN	Chemical Name	Guideline Number
2717	Camphor	36
2717	Camphor, synthetic	36
2718	Tripropylaluminum	10
2719	Barium Bromate	74, 96
2720	Chromium Nitrate	47
2721	Copper Chlorate	78, 97
2722	Lithium Nitrate	47, 81
2723	Magnesium Chlorate	82, 97
2724	Manganese Nitrate	47, 83
2725	Nickel Nitrate	47, 85
2726	Nickel Nitrite	47, 85
2727	Thallium Nitrate	47, 87
2728	Zirconium Nitrate	47
2729	Hexachlorobenzene	57
2730	Nitroanisole	24, 47
2732	Nitrobromobenzene	47, 95
2733	Alkylamine, n.o.s.	20
2733	Alkylamines or Polyalkylamines, n.o.s.	20
2733	Polyalkylamine, flammable, corrosive, n.o.s.	5, 20
2734	Alkylamine, n.o.s.	20
2734	Alkylamines or Polyalkylamines, n.o.s	20
2734	Polyalkylamine, corrosive, flammable, n.o.s.	20
2735	Alkylamine, n.o.s. (corrosive)	20
2735	Alkylamines or Polyalkylamines, n.o.s. (corrosive)	20
2735	Polyalkylamine, corrosive, n.o.s.	20
2738	Butylaniline	32
2739	Butyric Anhydride	15
2740	*n*-Propyl Chloroformate	26
2741	Barium Hypochlorite	22, 74
2742	*sec*-Butyl Chloroformate	37
2742	Chloroformate, n.o.s.	37
2742	Isobutyl Chloroformate	15
2743	Butyl Chloroformate	37
2744	Cyclobutylchloroformate	37
2745	Chloromethylchloroformate	37
2746	Phenylchloroformate	37
2747	*tert*-Butylcyclohexyl Chloroformate	37
2748	Ethyl Hexylchloroformate	37
2749	Tetramethyl Silane	107
2750	Dichloropropanol	30
2751	Diethylthiophosphoryl Chloride	49
2752	Epoxyethoxypropane	38
2752	1,2-Epoxy-3-ethoxypropane	38
2752	1,2-Epoxy-3-ethyloxypropane	38
2753	Ethylbenzyl Toluidine	32
2754	Ethyl Toluidine	32
2755	3-Chloroperoxybenzoic Acid	15
2756	Organic Peroxide Mixture	8
2757	Benomyl	63
2757	Carbamate Pesticide, solid, poisonous, n.o.s.	50
2757	Carbaryl	50
2757	Carbofuran	50
2757	Lannate	50
2757	Methomyl	50
2757	Mexacarbate	50
2757	Mercaptodimethur	50
2758	Carbamate Pesticide, liquid, flammable, poisonous, n.o.s.	50
2759	Arsenical Pesticide, solid, poisonous, n.o.s.	72

WARNING: More than one chemical agent may have the same UN Number. Look up the guideline for the specific material in question by chemical name and not UN/NA/Pin number alone.

UN/ NA/PIN	Chemical Name	Guideline Number
2759	Bordeaux Arsenite, liquid or solid	72, 78
2760	Arsenical Pesticide, liquid, flammable, poisonous, n.o.s.	72
2761	Aldrin and its Mixtures	56
2761	DDT	55
2761	Dichlorodiphenyl-trichloroethane, DDT	55
2761	Dieldrin	56
2761	Endosulfan	56
2761	Endrin Mixture, dry or liquid	56
2761	Heptachlor	54
2761	Hexachlorocyclohexane	57
2761	Kepone	57
2761	Lindane	57
2761	Methoxychlor	56
2761	Organochlorine Pesticide, solid, poisonous, n.o.s.	56
2761	TDE (1,1-dichloro-2,2-bis-(p-chlorophenyl)ethane)	55
2761	Toxaphene	58
2762	Chlordane, flammable liquid	54
2762	Organochlorine Pesticide, liquid, flammable, poisonous, n.o.s.	54
2763	Triazine Pesticide, solid, poisonous, n.o.s.	9
2764	Triazine Pesticide, liquid, flammable, poisonous, n.o.s.	9
2765	2,4-D	60
2765	2,4-D Esters	60
2765	2,4-Dichlorophenoxyacetic Acid	60
2765	Phenoxy Pesticide, solid, poisonous, n.o.s.	60
2765	2,4,5-T	60
2765	2,4,5-TP	60
2765	Trichlorophenoxyacetic Acid	60
2765	2,4,5-Trichlorophenoxy-acetic Acid	60
2765	2,4,5-Trichlorophenoxy-propionic Acid	60
2766	Phenoxy Pesticide, liquid, flammable, poisonous, n.o.s.	60
2767	Phenyl Urea Pesticide, solid, poisonous, n.o.s.	43
2768	Phenyl Urea Pesticide, liquid, flammable, poisonous, n.o.s.	43
2769	Benzoic Derivative Pesticide, solid, poisonous, n.o.s.	15
2770	Benzoic Derivative Pesticide, liquid, flammable, poisonous, n.o.s.	15
2771	Dithiocarbamate Pesticide, solid, n.o.s.	63
2771	Thiram	63
2772	Dithiocarbamate Pesticide, flammable liquid, n.o.s.	63
2773	Phthalimide Derivative Pesticide, solid, poisonous, n.o.s.	9
2774	Phthalimide Derivative Pesticide, liquid, flammable, poisonous, n.o.s.	9
2775	Copper-Based Pesticide, solid, poisonous, n.o.s.	78

WARNING: More than one chemical agent may have the same UN Number. Look up the guideline for the specific material in question by chemical name and not UN/NA/Pin number alone.

UN/ NA/PIN	Chemical Name	Guideline Number
2776	Copper-Based Pesticide, liquid, flammable, poisonous, n.o.s.	78
2777	Mercury-Based Pesticide, solid, poisonous, n.o.s.	84
2778	Mercury-Based Pesticide, liquid, flammable, poisonous, n.o.s.	84
2779	Substituted Nitrophenol Pesticide, solid, poisonous, n.o.s.	62
2780	Substituted Nitrophenol Pesticide, liquid, flammable, poisonous, n.o.s.	62
2781	Bipyridilium Pesticide, solid, poisonous, n.o.s.	66
2781	Diquat	66
2781	Paraquat	66
2782	Bipyridilium Pesticide, liquid, flammable, poisonous, n.o.s.	66
2783	Abate	49
2783	Azinphos-Methyl	49
2783	Azinphos Methyl (Guthion)	49
2783	Chlorpyrifos	49
2783	Coumaphos	49
2783	Demeton	49
2783	Demeton-Methyl	49
2783	Diazinon	49
2783	Dichlorvos	49
2783	Dicrotophos	49
2783	Dioxathion	49
2783	Disulfoton	49
2783	EPN	49
2783	Ethion	49
2783	Guthion	49
2783	Hexaethyl Tetraphosphate Mixture	49
2783	Malathion	49
2783	Methyl Parathion, liquid	49
2783	Methyl Parathion Mixture, dry	49
2783	Mevinphos	49
2783	Monocrotophos	49
2783	Naled	49
2783	Organic Phosphate Compound, liquid (Poison B)	49
2783	Organic Phosphate Compound, solid (Poison B)	49
2783	Organophosphorus Pesticide, solid, poisonous, n.o.s.	49
2783	Parathion Mixture, liquid or dry	49, 138
2783	Phorate	49
2783	Temaphos	49
2783	TEPP	49
2783	Tetraethyl Pyrophosphate Mixture, dry, liquid or mixture	49
2783	Trichlorfon	49
2784	Organophosphorus Pesticide, liquid, flammable, poisonous, n.o.s.	49
2784	Parathion, flammable liquid	49, 138
2784	Tetraethyl Pyrophosphate, flammable liquid	49
2785	Thiapentanal	10
2786	Organotin Pesticide, solid, poisonous, n.o.s.	65

WARNING: More than one chemical agent may have the same UN Number. Look up the guideline for the specific material in question by chemical name and not UN/NA/Pin number alone.

UN/ NA/PIN	Chemical Name	Guideline Number
2787	Organotin Pesticide, liquid, flammable, poisonous, n.o.s.	65
2788	Organotin Compounds, n.o.s.	65
2789	Acetic Acid, Glacial	15
2789	Acetic Acid Solution, more than 80% acid	15
2790	Acetic Acid	15
2790	Acetic Acid Solution, more than 10% but not more than 80% acid	15
2792	Igniter for Aircraft Thrust Device	6
2793	Ferrous Metal, borings, cuttings, shavings, or turnings	79
2793	Iron Swarf	79
2793	Steel Swarf	79
2794	Battery, electric, storage, wet, filled with acid	14
2794	Battery, wet, filled with acid (electric storage)	14
2795	Battery, electric, storage, wet, filled with alkali	19
2795	Battery, wet, filled with alkali (electric storage)	19
2796	Battery Fluid, acid	14
2796	Electrolyte, Battery Fluid, acid	10, 13
2797	Battery Fluid, alkali	19
2797	Electrolyte, alkali, with battery	19
2797	Battery Fluid, alkali, with electronic equipment or actuating device	19
2798	Benzene Phosphorus Dichloride	109
2798	Phenyl Phosphorus Dichloride	109
2799	Benzene Phosphorus Thiodichloride	109
2799	Phenyl Phosphorus Thiodichloride	109
2800	Battery, electric, storage wet, nonspillable	14, 19
2800	Battery, wet, nonspillable (electric storage)	14, 19
2801	Dye, n.o.s. (corrosive)	13
2801	Dye Intermediate, n.o.s. (corrosive)	13
2802	Copper Chloride	78
2803	Gallium, metal	10
2805	Lithium Hydride, fused, solid	81
2806	Lithium Nitride	47, 81
2809	Mercury	84
2809	Mercury Metal	84
2810	Poison B Liquid, n.o.s.	10
2810	Poisonous Liquid, n.o.s. (Poison B)	10
2811	Flue Dust, poisonous	10
2811	Lead Fluoride	80, 99
2811	Poisonous Solid, n.o.s.	10
2811	Selenium Oxide	86
2812	Sodium Aluminate, solid	10
2813	Lithium Acetylide–Ethylenediamine Complex	81
2813	Substances that, when in contact with water, emit flammable gases, n.o.s.	2
2813	Water-Reactive Solid, n.o.s.	6
2814	Etiologic Agent, n.o.s.	11
2814	Infectious Substance, affecting humans	11
2815	Aminoethylpiperazine	20

WARNING: More than one chemical agent may have the same UN Number. Look up the guideline for the specific material in question by chemical name and not UN/NA/Pin number alone.

UN/ NA/PIN	Chemical Name	Guideline Number
2817	Ammonium Bifluoride, solution	99
2817	Ammonium Hydrogen Fluoride Solution	99
2818	Ammonium Polysulfide Solution	21, 105
2819	Amyl Acid Phosphate	9
2820	Butyric Acid	15
2821	Phenol Solution	44
2822	Chloropyridine	24
2823	Crotonic Acid	15
2825	Diisopropylethanolamine	20
2826	Ethyl Chlorothioformate	37
2829	Caproic Acid	15
2830	Lithium Ferrosilicon	81
2831	Methyl Chloroform	26
2831	Trichloroethane	26
2831	1,1,1-Trichloroethane	26
2834	Phosphorous Acid (ortho)	14
2835	Sodium Aluminum Hydride	10
2837	Sodium Bisulfate Solution	105
2837	Sodium Hydrogen Sulfate Solution	105
2838	Vinyl Butyrate	37
2838	Vinyl Butyrate, inhibited	37
2839	Aldol	41
2840	Butyraldoxime	41
2841	Diamylamine	20
2842	Nitroethane	33, 47
2844	Calcium Manganese Silicon	83
2845	Aluminum Alkyl	10
2845	Ethyl Phosphonous Dichloride, anhydrous	109
2845	Methyl Phosphonous Dichloride	109

UN/ NA/PIN	Chemical Name	Guideline Number
2845	Pyrophoric Liquid, n.o.s.	5
2846	Pyrophoric Solid, n.o.s.	6
2849	3-Chloropropanol	30
2849	3-Chloropropanol-1	30
2849	Trimethylene Chlorohydrin	61
2850	Propylene Tetramer	33
2851	Boron Trifluoride Dihydrate	103
2852	Dipicryl Sulfide, wet with not less than 10% water	47
2853	Magnesium Fluorosilicate	82, 99
2853	Magnesium Silicofluoride, solid	82, 99
2854	Ammonium Fluosilicate	99
2854	Ammonium Silicofluoride, solid	99
2855	Zinc Fluorosilicate	88, 99
2856	Fluosilicates, n.o.s.	99
2856	Silicofluoride, solid, n.o.s.	99
2857	Refrigerating Machine, containing nonflammable, nonpoisonous, liquefied gas	3
2858	Zirconium Metal, wire, sheet, or strips (thinner than 254 microns but not thinner than 18 microns)	10
2859	Ammonium Metavanadate	10
2860	Vanadium Trioxide	10
2861	Ammonium Polyvanadate	10
2862	Vandium Pentoxide	10
2863	Sodium Ammonium Vanadate	10
2864	Potassium Metavanadate	10
2865	Hydroxylamine Sulfate	20
2869	Titanium Trichloride Mixture	10

WARNING: More than one chemical agent may have the same UN Number. Look up the guideline for the specific material in question by chemical name and not UN/NA/Pin number alone.

UN/NA/PIN	Chemical Name	Guideline Number
2870	Aluminum Borohydride	103
2870	Aluminum Borohydride in Devices	103
2871	Antimony, powder	10
2871	Antimony Powder	10
2872	Dibromochloropropane	61
2873	Dibutylaminoethanol	30
2874	Furfuryl Alcohol	30
2875	Hexachlorophene	26, 44
2876	Resorcinol	44
2876	Resorcinol Monoacetate	44
2877	Thiourea	43
2878	Titanium Sponge, granules or powder	10
2879	Selenium Oxychloride	86
2880	Calcium Hypochlorite, hydrated, including mixtures with not less than 5.5% but not more than 10% water	22
2881	Metal Catalyst, dry	10
2881	Nickel Catalyst, dry	85
2883	2,2-Di(*tert*-butylperoxy)-propane	8, 33
2884	2,2-Di(*tert*-butylperoxy)-propane	8, 33
2885	1,1-Di(*tert*-butylperoxy) cyclohexane	8, 33
2886	*tert*-Butyl Peroxy-2-ethyl-hexanoate with 2, 2-Di(*tert*-butylperoxy) Butane	8, 15
2887	*tert*-Butyl Peroxy-2-ethyl-hexanoate with 2,2-Di(*tert*-butylperoxy) Butane	8, 15
2888	*tert*-Butyl Peroxy-2-ethyl-hexanoate, not more than 50%, with phlegmatizer	8, 15
2889	Diisotridecylperoxy-dicarbonate	8
2890	*tert*-Butyl Peroxybenzoate	8, 15
2891	*tert*-Amyl Peroxy-neodecanoate	8, 15
2892	Dimyristyl Peroxy-dicarbonate, not more than 42% in water	8
2893	Dilauroyl Peroxide, not more than 42% stable dispersion in water	8
2893	Lauroyl Peroxide, not more than 42% stable dispersion in water	8
2894	Di(4-*tert*-butylcyclohexyl) Peroxydicarbonate	8
2895	Dicetyl Peroxydicarbonate, not more than 42% stable dispersion in water	8
2896	Cyclohexanone Peroxide, not more than 72% as paste	8
2897	1,1-Di(*tert*-butylperoxy) Cyclohexane	8, 33
2898	*tert*-Amyl Peroxy-2-ethylhexanoate	8, 15
2899	Organic Peroxide, n.o.s. (including trial quantities)	8
2900	Infectious Substance, affecting animals only	11
2901	Bromine Chloride	95
2902	Allethrin	52
2902	Fungicide, poisonous, n.o.s.	10
2902	Insecticide, liquid, poisonous, n.o.s.	10

WARNING: More than one chemical agent may have the same UN Number. Look up the guideline for the specific material in question by chemical name and not UN/NA/Pin number alone.

UN/ NA/PIN	Chemical Name	Guideline Number
2902	Pesticide, liquid, poisonous, n.o.s.	10
2903	Pesticide, liquid, poisonous, flammable, n.o.s.	5, 10
2904	Chlorophenate, liquid	44
2905	Chlorphenate, solid	44
2906	Triisocyanatoisocyanurate of Isophoronediisocyante, 70% solution	10
2907	Isosorbide Dinitrate Mixture	47
2908	Radioactive Material, empty packages	12
2909	Radioactive Material, articles manufactured from natural or depleted uranium or natural thorium	12
2910	Radioactive Material, excepted package	12
2910	Radioactive Material, limited quantity, n.o.s.	12
2911	Radioactive Material, instruments and articles	12
2912	Radioactive Material, low specific activity (LSA), n.o.s.	12
2918	Radioactive Material, fissile, n.o.s.	12
2920	Corrosive Liquid, flammable, n.o.s.	5, 13
2921	Corrosive Solid, flammable, n.o.s.	6, 13
2922	Corrosive Liquid, poisonous, n.o.s.	10, 13
2922	Sodium Hydrosulfide Solution	91
2923	Corrosive Solid, poisonous, n.o.s.	10, 13
2923	Sodium Hydrosulfide, solid, with not less than 25% water of crystallization	91
2924	Dichlorobutene	27
2924	Flammable Liquid, corrosive, n.o.s.	5, 13
2925	Flammable Solid, corrosive, n.o.s.	6, 13
2926	Flammable Solid, poisonous, n.o.s.	6, 10
2927	Poisonous Liquid, corrosive, n.o.s.	10, 13
2928	Poisonous Solid, corrosive, n.o.s.	10, 13
2929	Chloropicrin Mixture, flammable	9, 26, 136
2929	Poisonous Liquid, flammable, n.o.s.	5, 10
2930	Poisonous Solid, flammable, n.o.s.	6, 10
2931	Vanadyl Sulfate	10
2933	Methyl Chloropropionate	26
2934	Isopropyl Chloropropionate	37
2935	Ethyl Chloropropionate	37
2936	Thiolactic Acid	15
2937	Methylbenzyl Alcohol (alpha)	30
2938	Methyl Benzoate	15
2940	Cyclooctadiene Phosphine	108
2940	Phosphabicyclononane	10
2941	Fluoroaniline	32
2942	2-Trifluoromethylaniline	32
2943	Tetrahydrofurfurylamine	20
2944	Fluoroaniline	32
2945	Methylbutylamine	20

WARNING: More than one chemical agent may have the same UN Number. Look up the guideline for the specific material in question by chemical name and not UN/NA/Pin number alone.

UN/ NA/PIN	Chemical Name	Guideline Number
2946	2-Amino-5-diethylaminopentane	20, 33
2947	Isopropyl Chloroacetate	37
2948	3-Trifluoromehylaniline	32
2949	Sodium Hydrosulfide, with not less than 25% water of crystallization	91
2949	Sodium Hydrosulfide Solution	91
2950	Magnesium Granules, coated	82
2951	Diphenyloxide-4,4′-disulfohydrazide	23
2952	Azodiisobutyronitrile	90
2953	2,2′-Azodi-(2,4-dimethylvaleronitrile)	10
2954	1,1′-Azodi-(hexahydrobenzonitrile)	10
2955	2,2′-Azodi-(2,4-dimethyl-4-methoxyvaleronitrile)	10
2956	*tert*-Butyl-2,4,6-trinitro-*m*-xylene	24
2956	Musk Xylene	24
2957	*tert*-Amylperoxypivalate	8, 15
2958	Diperoxy Azelaic Acid	8
2959	2,5-Dimethyl-2,5-di-(benzoylperoxy) Hexane	8
2960	Di-(2-ethylhexyl) Peroxydicarbonate	8
2961	2,4,4-Trimethylpentyl-2-peroxyphenoxyacetate	37
2962	Disuccinic Acid Peroxide, not more than 72% in water	8
2962	Succinic Acid Peroxide, not more than 72% in water	15

UN/ NA/PIN	Chemical Name	Guideline Number
2963	Cumyl Peroxy-neo-decanoate	8, 24
2964	Cumyl Peroxypivalate	8, 24
2965	Boron Trifluoride Dimethyl Etherate	103
2966	Thioglycol	105
2967	Sulfamic Acid	14
2968	Maneb or Maneb Preparation(s), stabilized against self-heating	63
2969	Castor Beans, Meal, Pomace, or Flake	10
2970	Benzene Sulfohydrazide	15
2971	Benzene-1,3-disulfohydrazide	24
2972	Dinitrosopentamethylene Tetramine	20
2973	Dinitroso-dimethyl Terephthalamide	10
2974	Radioactive Material, special form, n.o.s.	12
2975	Thorium Metal, pyrophoric	6, 10
2976	Thorium Nitrate, solid	47
2977	Uranium Hexafluoride, fissile (containing more than 1% U-235)	12, 99
2978	Uranium Hexafluoride, fissile excepted or nonfissile	12, 99
2978	Uranium Hexafluoride, low specific activity	12, 99
2979	Uranium Metal, pyrophoric	12
2980	Uranium Nitrate Hexahydrate Solution	12, 47
2981	Uranyl Nitrate, solid	12, 47
2982	Radioactive Material, n.o.s.	12

WARNING: More than one chemical agent may have the same UN Number. Look up the guideline for the specific material in question by chemical name and not UN/NA/Pin number alone.

UN/ NA/PIN	Chemical Name	Guideline Number
2983	Ethylene Oxide–Propylene Oxide Mixture	45
2984	Hydrogen Peroxide Solution with not less than 8% but less than 20% peroxide	7
2985	Chlorosilane, n.o.s. (flammable, corrosive)	107
2986	Chlorosilane, n.o.s. (flammable, corrosive)	107
2987	Chlorosilane, n.o.s. (corrosive)	107
2988	Chlorosilane, n.o.s. (emits flammable gas when wet, corrosive)	107
2989	Lead Phosphite, dibasic	80
2991	Carbamate Pesticide, liquid, poisonous, flammable, n.o.s.	50
2992	Carbamate Pesticide, liquid, poisonous, n.o.s.	50
2993	Arsenical Pesticide, liquid, poisonous, flammable, n.o.s.	72
2994	Arsenical Pesticide, liquid, poisonous, n.o.s.	72
2995	Organochlorine Pesticide, liquid, poisonous, flammable, n.o.s.	54
2996	Organochlorine Pesticide, liquid, poisonous, n.o.s.	54
2997	Triazine Pesticide, liquid, poisonous, flammable, n.o.s.	9
2998	Triazine Pesticide, liquid poisonous, n.o.s.	9
2999	Phenoxy Pesticide, liquid, poisonous, flammable, n.o.s.	60
3000	Phenoxy Pesticide, liquid, poisonous, n.o.s.	60
3001	Phenyl Urea Pesticide, liquid, poisonous, flammable, n.o.s.	43
3002	Phenyl Urea Pesticide, liquid, poisonous, n.o.s.	43
3003	Benzoic Derivative Pesticide, liquid, poisonous, flammable, n.o.s.	15
3004	Benzoic Derivative Pesticide, liquid, poisonous, n.o.s.	15
3005	Dithiocarbamate Pesticide, flammable liquid, n.o.s.	63
3006	Dithiocarbamate Pesticide, liquid, n.o.s.	63
3007	Phthalimide Derivative Pesticide, liquid, poisonous, flammable, n.o.s.	9
3008	Phthalimide Derivative Pesticide, liquid, poisonous, n.o.s.	9
3009	Copper-Based Pesticide, liquid, poisonous, flammable, n.o.s.	78
3010	Copper-Based Pesticide, liquid, poisonous, n.o.s.	78
3011	Mercury-Based Pesticide, liquid, poisonous, flammable, n.o.s.	84
3012	Mercury-Based Pesticide, liquid, poisonous, n.o.s.	84
3013	Substituted Nitrophenol Pesticide, liquid, poisonous, flammable, n.o.s.	62

WARNING: More than one chemical agent may have the same UN Number. Look up the guideline for the specific material in question by chemical name and not UN/NA/Pin number alone.

UN/ NA/PIN	Chemical Name	Guideline Number
3014	Substituted Nitrophenol Pesticide, liquid, poisonous, n.o.s.	62
3015	Bipyridilium Pesticide, liquid, poisonous, flammable, n.o.s.	66
3016	Bipyridilium Pesticide, liquid poisonous, n.o.s.	66
3017	Organophosphorus Pesticide, liquid, poisonous, flammable, n.o.s.	49
3018	Organophosphorus Pesticide, liquid, poisonous, n.o.s.	49
3019	Organotin Pesticide, liquid, poisonous, flammable, n.o.s.	65
3020	Organotin Pesticide, liquid, poisonous, n.o.s.	65
3021	Pesticide, liquid, flammable, poisonous, n.o.s.	5, 10
3022	Butylene Oxide, stabilized	45
3022	1,2-Butylene Oxide, stabilized	45
3023	*tert*-Octyl Mercaptan	105
3024	Coumarin Derivative Pesticide, flammable liquid, n.o.s.	42
3025	Coumarin Derivative Pesticide, flammable liquid, n.o.s.	42
3026	Coumarin Derivative Pesticide, liquid, n.o.s.	42
3027	Coumarin Derivative Pesticide, solid, n.o.s.	42
3028	Battery, electric, storage, dry, containing potassium hydroxide	19
3030	2,2′-Azodi-(2-methyl-butyronitrile)	10
3031	Self-Reactive Substances, samples, n.o.s.	10
3032	Self-Reactive Substances, trial quantities, n.o.s.	10
3033	3-Chloro-4-diethylamino-benzenediazonium Zinc Chloride	88
3034	4-Dipropylaminobenzene-diazonium Zinc Chloride	88
3035	3-(2-Hydroxyethoxy)-4-pyrrolidin-1-ylbenzene-diazonium Zinc Chloride	88
3036	2,5-Diethoxy-4-morpho-linobenzenediazonium Zinc Chloride	10
3037	4-(Benzyl(ethyl)amino)-3-ethoxybenzenediazonium Zinc Chloride	10, 88
3038	4-(Benzyl(methyl)amino)-3-ethoxybenzenediazonium Zinc Chloride	10, 88
3039	4-Dimethylamino-6(2-di-methylaminoethoxy) Toluene-2-diazonium Zinc Chloride	88
3040	Sodium 2-Diazo-1-naph-thol-4-sulfonate	44
3041	Sodium 2-Diazo-1-naph-thol-5-sulfonate	44
3042	2-Diazo-1-naphthol-4-sulfochloride	43
3043	2-Diazo-1-naphthol-5-sulfochloride	43
3044	*Tert*-Amylperoxybenzoate	8, 15
3045	Peroxyacetic Acid solution	8, 15
3046	Methyl Cyclohexanone Peroxide	8, 42

NUMERICAL INDEX

WARNING: More than one chemical agent may have the same UN Number. Look up the guideline for the specific material in question by chemical name and not UN/NA/Pin number alone.

UN/ NA/PIN	Chemical Name	Guideline Number
3047	*Tert*-Butyl Peroxypivalate	8, 15
3048	Aluminum Phosphide Pesticide	108
3049	Metal Alkyl Halide, n.o.s.	10
3050	Metal Alkyl Hydride, n.o.s.	10
3051	Aluminum Alkyl	10
3052	Aluminum Alkyl Halide	10
3053	Magnesium Alkyl	82
3054	Cyclohexyl Mercaptan	105
3055	Aminoethoxyethanol	20, 29
3056	*n*-Heptaldehyde	41
3057	Trifluoroacetyl Chloride	15
3058	Di-(2-phenoxyethyl) Peroxydicarbonate, technically pure	8
3059	Di-(2-phenoxyethyl) Peroxydicarbonate, not more than 85% with water	8
3060	2,5-Dimethyl-2,5-di-(isononanoylperoxy) Hexane, not more than 77% in solution	8
3060	2,5-Dimethyl-2,5-di-(3,5,5-trimethylhexanoylperoxy) Hexane, not more than 77% in solution	8
3061	Acetyl Acetone Peroxide, not more than 32% as a paste	8, 42
3061	3,5-Dimethyl-3,5-dihydroxy-dioxolane-1,2, not more than 32% as a paste	40
3062	*tert*-Butyl Peroxystearyl Carbonate, technical pure	8, 15
3063	Diperoxydodecane Diacid, not more than 42% with not less than 56% sodium sulfate	8, 105

UN/ NA/PIN	Chemical Name	Guideline Number
3064	Nitroglycerin, solution in alcohol, with more than 1% but not more than 5% nitroglycerin	29, 47
3065	Alcoholic Beverage	29
3066	Paint, etc., corrosive liquid	13
3066	Paint-Related Material, corrosive liquid	13
3067	*tert*-Amyl Hydroperoxide, not more than 88% in solution	8
3068	Methyl Ethyl Ketone Peroxide, with not more than 40% peroxide	8, 42
3069	1,1-Di-(*tert*-butylperoxy) Cyclohexane	8, 33
3070	Dichlorodifluoromethane and Ethylene Oxide Mixture, with not more than 12% ethylene oxide	27, 45
3070	Ethylene Oxide and Dichlorodifluoromethane Mixture, with not more than 12% ethylene oxide	27, 45
3071	Mercaptan, liquid, n.o.s.	105
3071	Mercaptan Mixture, liquid, n.o.s.	105
3073	Vinyl Pyridines, inhibited	24
3074	Benzoyl Peroxide, not more than 62%, with not less than 28% inert solid and not less than 10% water	8
3074	Dibenzoyl Peroxide, not more than 62%, with not less than 28% inert solid and not less than 10% water	8

WARNING: More than one chemical agent may have the same UN Number. Look up the guideline for the specific material in question by chemical name and not UN/NA/Pin number alone.

UN/ NA/PIN	Chemical Name	Guideline Number
3075	*tert*-Butyl Hydroperoxide, not more than 82%, with not less than 7% water and not less than 9% di-*tert*-butyl peroxide	8
3076	Aluminum Alkyl Hydride	10
3077	Environmentally Hazardous Substance, solid, n.o.s.	10
3078	Cerium, turnings or gritty powder	10
3079	Methacrylonitrile, inhibited	90
3080	Isocyanates and Solutions, n.o.s., flash point not less than 23° C and not more than 60.5° C	94
3081	3-Chloroperoxybenzoic Acid, not more than 57% with water and 3-chlorobenzoic acid	15
3082	Environmentally Hazardous Substance, liquid, n.o.s.	10
3083	Perchloryl Fluoride	7, 99
3084	Corrosive Solid, oxidizing, n.o.s.	7, 13
3085	Oxidizing Substance, solid corrosive, n.o.s.	7, 13
3086	Poisonous Solid, oxidizing, n.o.s.	7, 10
3087	Oxidizing Substance, solid, poisonous, n.o.s.	7, 10
3088	Self-Heating Substances, solid n.o.s.	10
3089	Metal Powder, flammable, n.o.s.	6, 10
3090	Lithium Battery	81
3091	Lithium Batteries, contained in equipment	81
3092	1-Methoxy-2-Propanol	40
3093	Corrosive Liquid, oxidizing, n.o.s.\	7, 13
3094	Corrosive Liquid, which in contact with water emits a flammable gas, n.o.s.	2, 13
3095	Corrosive Solid, self-heating, n.o.s.	13
3096	Corrosive Solid, which in contact with water emits a flammable gas, n.o.s.	2, 13
3097	Flammable Solid, oxidizing, n.o.s.	6, 7
3098	Oxidizing Substance, liquid corrosive, n.o.s.	7, 13
3099	Oxidizing Substance, liquid poisonous, n.o.s.	7, 10
3100	Oxidizing Substance, solid, self-heating, n.o.s.	7
3101	Organic Peroxide Type B, liquid	8
3102	Organic Peroxide Type B, solid	8
3103	Organic Peroxide Type C, liquid	8
3104	Organic Peroxide Type C, solid	8
3105	Organic Peroxide Type D, liquid	8
3106	Organic Peroxide Type D, solid	8
3107	Organic Peroxide Type E, liquid	8
3108	Organic Peroxide Type E, solid	8
3109	Organic Peroxide Type F, liquid	8
3110	Organic Peroxide Type F, solid	8
3111	Organic Peroxide Type B, liquid, temperature-controlled	8

WARNING: More than one chemical agent may have the same UN Number. Look up the guideline for the specific material in question by chemical name and not UN/NA/Pin number alone.

UN/ NA/PIN	Chemical Name	Guideline Number
3112	Organic Peroxide Type B, solid, temperature-controlled	8
3113	Organic Peroxide Type C, liquid, temperature controlled	8
3114	Organic Peroxide Type C, solid, temperature-controlled	8
3115	Organic Peroxide Type D, liquid, temperature-controlled	8
3116	Organic Peroxide Type D, solid, temperature-controlled	8
3117	Organic Peroxide Type E, liquid, temperature-controlled	8
3118	Organic Peroxide Type E, solid, temperature-controlled	8
3119	Organic Peroxide Type F, liquid, temperature-controlled	8
3120	Organic Peroxide Type F, solid, temperature-controlled	8
3121	Oxidizing Substance, solid, which, in contact with water, emits a flammable gas, n.o.s.	7
3122	Poisonous Liquid, oxidizing, n.o.s.	7, 10
3123	Poisonous Liquid, which, in contact with water, emits a flammable gas, n.o.s.	2, 10
3124	Poisonous Solid, self-heating, n.o.s.	10
3125	Poisonous Solid, which,, in contact with water, emits a flammable gas, n.o.s.	2, 10
3126	Self-Heating Substance, solid, corrosive, n.o.s.	13
3127	Self-Heating Substance, solid, oxidizing, n.o.s.	7
3128	Self-Heating Substance, solid, poisonous, n.o.s.	10
3129	Substance that, in contact with water, emits a flammable gas, liquid, corrosive, n.o.s.	2, 13
3130	Substance that, in contact with water, emits a flammable gas, liquid, poisonous, n.o.s.	2, 10
3131	Substance that, in contact with water, emits a flammable gas, solid, corrosive, n.o.s.	2, 13
3132	Substance that, in contact with water, emits a flammable gas; solid, flammable, n.o.s.	2, 6
3133	Substance that, in contact with water, emits a flammable gas, solid, oxidizing, n.o.s.	2, 7
3134	Substance that, in contact with water, emits a flammable gas, solid, poisonous, n.o.s.	2, 10
3135	Substance that, in contact with water, emits a flammable gas, solid, self-heating, n.o.s.	2

WARNING: More than one chemical agent may have the same UN Number. Look up the guideline for the specific material in question by chemical name and not UN/NA/Pin number alone.

UN/ NA/PIN	Chemical Name	Guideline Number
3136	Trifluoromethane, refrigerated liquid (cryogenic liquid)	27
3137	Oxidizing Substance, solid, flammable, n.o.s.	6, 7
3138	Ethylene, Acetylene and Propylene Mixture, refrigerated liquid (cryogenic liquid), containing at least 71.5% ethylene with not more than 22.5% acetylene and not more than 6% propylene	33, 92
3139	Oxidizing Substance, liquid, n.o.s.	7
3140	Alkaloid, liquid, n.o.s., or Alkaloid Salt, liquid, n.o.s. (poisonous)	20
3141	Antimony Compound, inorganic liquid, n.o.s.	10
3142	Disinfectant, Liquid, n.o.s., poisonous	10
3143	Dye, solid, n.o.s., or Dye Intermediate, solid, n.o.s., poisonous	10
3144	Nicotine Compound, liquid, n.o.s.	51
3144	Nicotine Preparation, liquid, n.o.s.	51
3145	Alkyl Phenol, liquid, n.o.s.	44
3146	Organotin Compound, solid, n.o.s.	65
3147	Dye, solid, n.o.s,. or Dye Intermediate, solid, n.o.s., corrosive	13
3148	Substance that, in contact with water, emits a flammable gas, liquid, n.o.s.	2

UN/ NA/PIN	Chemical Name	Guideline Number
3149	Hydrogen Peroxide–Peroxyacetic Acid Mixture, with acid(s), water and not more than 5% peroxyacetic acid, stabilized	7
3150	Device, small, hydrocarbon gas–powered, with release device	92
3151	Polyhalogenated Biphenyl, liquid, or Polyhalogenated Terphenyl, liquid	46
3152	Polyhalogenated Biphenyl, solid, or Polyhalogenated Terphenyl, solid	46
3153	Perfluoromethylvinyl Ether	38
3154	Perfluoroethylvinyl Ether	38
9011	Camphene	36
9018	Dichlorodifluoroethylene	27
9026	Dinitrocyclohexyl Phenol	62
9026	4,6-Dinitro-*o*-cyclohexylphenol	62
9037	Hexachloroethane	26
9069	Tetramethylmethylene-Diamine	20
9077	Adipic Acid	15
9083	Ammonium Carbamate	21
9084	Ammonium Carbonate	21
9085	Ammonium Chloride	21
9086	Ammonium Chromate	21
9088	Ammonium Fluoroborate	103
9163	Zirconium Sulfate	10
9170	Thorium Metal, pyrophoric	6, 10
9171	Thorium Nitrate, solid	47
9180	Uranyl Acetate	12, 37
9180	Uranium acetate	12, 37

WARNING: More than one chemical agent may have the same UN Number. Look up the guideline for the specific material in question by chemical name and not UN/NA/Pin number alone.

UN/ NA/PIN	Chemical Name	Guideline Number
9183	Organic Peroxide, liquid or solution, n.o.s.	8
9187	Organic Peroxide, solid, n.o.s.	8
9188	Hazardous Substance, liquid or solid, n.o.s.	10
9188	ORM-E, liquid or solid, n.o.s.	10
9189	Hazardous Waste, liquid or solid, n.o.s.	10
9190	Ammonium Permanganate	14
9191	Chlorine Dioxide Hydrate, frozen	98
9192	Fluorine, refrigerated liquid (cryogenic liquid)	99, 133, 138
9193	Oxidizer, corrosive liquid, n.o.s.	7, 13
9194	Oxidizer, corrosive solid, n.o.s.	7, 13
9195	Metal Alkyl Solution, n.o.s.	10
9199	Oxidizer, poisonous liquid, n.o.s.	7, 10
9200	Oxidizer, poisonous solid, n.o.s.	7, 10
9202	Carbon Monoxide, cryogenic liquid	89
9205	Lithium Battery	81

UN/ NA/PIN	Chemical Name	Guideline Number
9206	Methyl Phosphonic Dichloride	109
9261	Aldicarb and Dichloromethane Mixture	26, 50
9262	Aminodimethylbutyronitrile	90
9263	Chloropivaloyl Chloride	10
9264	3,5-Dichloro-2,4-6-trifluoropyridine	24
9265	Methanesulfonyl Chloride	49
9266	Methylphosphonic Difluoride	109
9267	Sulfur Chloride and Carbon Tetrachloride Mixture	28, 105
9268	3-Trifluoromethyl-Phenylisocyanate	94
9269	Trimethoxysilane	107
9270	Chlorotrifluoropyridine	24
9271	Nitrogen Fluoride Oxide	48, 99
9271	Trifluoroamine Oxide	99
9272	Sulfur Chloride Pentafluoride	99, 105
9273	Phosphorus Trifluoride	99, 109
9274	1,1-Dichloro-1-fluoroethane	27

WARNING: More than one chemical agent may have the same UN Number. Look up the guideline for the specific material in question by chemical name and not UN/NA/Pin number alone.

Alphabetical Index

Chemical Name	UN/ NA/PIN	Guideline Number
Abate	2783	49
Abattoir Fever		123
AC	1051	90, 132
Accumulators, pressurized	1956	2
Acenaphthene		43
Acenaphthylene		43
Acenocoumarol		71
Acephate		49
Acetal	1088	41
Acetal Ammonia	1841	21, 41
Acetaldehyde	1089	41
Acetaldehyde Ammonia	1841	21, 41
Acetaldehyde Oxime	2332	5
Acetamide		15
Acetic Acid, glacial	2789	15
Acetic Acid Solution, more than 80% acid	2789	15
Acetic Acid Solution, more than 10% but not more than 80% acid	2790	15
Acetic Anhydride	1715	15
Acetone	1090	42
Acetone Cyanohydrin	1541	90
Acetone Oil	1091	42
Acetone Thiosemicarbazide		23
Acetonitrile	1648	90
Acetonyl bromide	1569	136
Acetophenone		42
Acetyl Acetone Peroxide	2080	8, 42
Acetyl Acetone Peroxide, not more than 32% as a paste	3061	8, 42
2-Acetylaminofluorene		10
Acetyl Benzoyl Peroxide	2081	8
Acetyl Bromide	1716	15
Acetyl Chloride	1717	15
Acetyl Cyclohexane Sulfonyl Peroxide	2082	8
Acetyl Cyclohexane Sulfonyl Peroxide	2083	8
1-Acetyl-2-thiourea		48
Acetylene	1001	33, 92
Acetylene, dissolved	1001	33, 92
Acetylene Dichloride		33, 92
Acetylene Tetrabromide	2504	33, 92
Acetyl Iodide	1898	100
Acetyl Methyl Carbinol	2621	42
Acetylmethyl bromide	1569	136
Acetyl Peroxide	2084	8
Acid, liquid, n.o.s.	1760	14, 15
Acid Butyl Phosphate	1718	15
Acid Mixture, hydrofluoric and sulfuric acids	1786	14, 16
Acid Mixture, nitrating	1796	14
Acid Mixture, spent, nitrating	1826	14
Acid Liquid, n.o.s.	1760	14, 15
Acid Sludge	1906	14
Acridine	2713	24
Acrolein, inhibited	1092	59
Acrolein Dimer, stabilized	2607	59
Acquinite	1580	136
Acrylamide	2074	106
Acrylic Acid	2218	15
Acrylonitrile, inhibited	1093	90
Acrylyl Chloride		9
Activated Carbon	1362	9
Adamsite	1698	72,140
Adhesive	1133	9

Chemical Name	UN/ NA/PIN	Guideline Number
Adhesive, containing flammable liquid	1133	5
Adipic Acid	9077	15
Adiponitrile	2205	90
Aerosols	1950	9, 10
African Hemorrhagic Fever		130
Agent W		124
Air, compressed	1002	3
Air, refrigerated liquid (cryogenic liquid)	1003	3
Aircraft Hydraulic Power Unit Fuel Tank (containing M86 fuel)		35
Alcohols (beverage)	1170	29
Alcohols, denatured	1987	31
Alcohols, denatured (toxic)	1986	31
Alcohols, ethyl	1170	29
Alcohol, nontoxic, n.o.s.	1987	29, 30
Alcohol, n.o.s.	1987	29, 30
Alcohol, toxic, n.o.s.	1986	29, 30
Alcoholic Beverage	1170	29
Alcoholic Beverage	3065	29
Aldehyde, n.o.s.	1989	41
Aldehyde, toxic, n.o.s.	1988	41
Aldicarb	2757	50
Aldicarb and Dichloromethane Mixture	9261	26, 50
Aldol	2839	41
Aldrin	2761	56
Aldrin and Its Mixtures	2761	56
Aliphatic Hydrocarbons		33
Aliphatic Thiocyanates		94
Alkali Metal, liquid alloy	1421	19
Alkali Metal Alloy, liquid n.o.s	1421	19
Alkali Metal Amalgam, n.o.s.	1389	19
Alkali Metal Amide, n.o.s.	1390	19

Chemical Name	UN/ NA/PIN	Guideline Number
Alkali Metal Dispersion, n.o.s.	1391	19
Alkaline Corrosive Liquid n.o.s.	1719	19
Alkaline Earth Metal Alloy n.o.s.	1393	19
Alkaline Earth Metal Amalgam n.o.s.	1392	19
Alkaline Earth Metal Dispersion, n.o.s.	1391	19
Alkaloid, liquid, n.o.s., or Alkaloid Salt, liquid, n.o.s. (poisonous)	3140	20
Alkaloid, solid, n.o.s. or Alkaloid Salt, solid, n.o.s. (poisonous)	1544	20
Alkanes (C5-C8)		33
Alkane Sulfonic Acid		15
Alkyl Mercuric Chloride		84
Alkyl aluminums		10
Alkylamine, n.o.s.	2733	20
Alkylamine, n.o.s.	2734	20
Alkylamine, n.o.s. (corrosive)	2735	20
Alkylamines or Polyalkylamines, n.o.s.	2733	20
Alkylamines or Polyalkyamines, n.o.s.	2734	20
Alkylamines or Polyalkylamines, n.o.s. (corrosive)	2735	20
Alkyl Phenol, liquid, n.o.s.	3145	44
Alkyl Phenol, n.o.s.	2430	44
Alkyl Sulfonic Acid, liquid	2584	15
Alkyl Sulfonic Acid, liquid	2586	15
Alkyl Sulfonic Acid, solid	2583	15
Alkyl Sulfonic Acid, solid	2585	15
Allene	2200	33
Allethrin	2902	52
Allyl Acetate	2333	37

Chemical Name	UN/ NA/PIN	Guideline Number
Allyl Alcohol	1098	29
Allyl Amine	2334	20
Allyl Bromide	1099	61
Allyl Chloride	1100	61, 98
Allyl Chlorocarbonate	1722	15
Allyl Chloroformate	1722	37
Allyl Ethyl Ether	2335	38
Allyl Formate	2336	37
Allyl Glycidyl Ether	2219	38
Allyl Iodide	1723	61, 100
Allyl Isothiocyanate, inhibited	1545	94
Allyl Isothiocyanate, stabilized	1545	94
Allyl Trichlorosilane, stabilized	1724	107
alpha-Hydroxy-alpha-phenylbenzeneacetic acid	2810	134
Alum		14
Aluminum, powder, pyrophoric	1383	6
Aluminum Alkyl	2003	10
Aluminum Alkyl	2845	10
Aluminum Alkyl	3051	10
Aluminum Alkyl Chloride	2221	10, 98
Aluminum Alkyl Halide	2221	10
Aluminum Alkyl Halide	3052	10
Aluminum Alkyl Halide, solution	2220	10
Aluminum Alkyl Hydride	3076	10
Aluminum Borohydride	2870	103
Aluminum Borohydride in devices	2870	103
Aluminum Bromide, anhydrous	1725	95
Aluminum Bromide, solution	2580	95
Aluminum Carbide	1394	10
Aluminum Chloride, anhydrous	1726	10, 98
Aluminum Chloride, solution	2581	10, 98
Aluminum Ferrosilicon, powder	1395	79
Aluminum Hydride	2463	10
Aluminum Nitrate	1438	47
Aluminum Oxide (fibrous forms)		10
Aluminum Phosphate Solution	1760	14
Aluminum Phosphide	1397	108
Aluminum Phosphide Pesticide	3048	108
Aluminum Powder, coated	1309	10
Aluminum Powder, uncoated	1396	10
Aluminum Resinate	2715	10
Aluminum Silicon Powder, uncoated	1398	10
Aluminum Sulfate	1760	14
Aluminum Sulfate, solid	1759	14
Aluminum Sulfate Solution	1760	14
2-Aminoanthraquinone		10
4-Aminoazobenzene		32
4-Aminobiphenyl		47
Aminocarb		50
Aminochlorophenol	2673	44
2-Amino-5-diethylamino-pentane	2946	20, 33
Aminodimethyl-butyronitrile	9262	90
2-Amino Ethyl Ethanol Amine		20, 29
Aminoethoxyethanol	1760	20, 29
Aminoethoxyethanol	3055	20, 29
Aminoethylpiperazine	2815	20
1-Amino-2-methylanthraquinone		20

Chemical Name	UN/ NA/PIN	Guideline Number
5-(Aminomethyl)-3-isoxazolol		10
4-Amino-2-Nitrophenol		32
Aminophenol	2512	32
Aminopropyldiethanol-amine	1760	20
Aminopropylmorpholine	1760	20
Aminopropylpiperazine	1760	20
Aminopterin		10
Aminopyridine	2671	24
p-Aminosalicyclic Acid		15
Amiton		49, 135
Amiton Oxalate		49, 135
Amitrole		10
Ammonia	1005	21, 133, 138
Ammonia, anhydrous, liquefied	1005	21, 133, 138
Ammonia Solution with not less than 12% and not more than 44% ammonia	2672	21
Ammonia Solution, with more than 44% ammonia	2073	21
Ammonia Solution, with more than 50% ammonia	1005	21
Ammoniated Mercury		84
Ammonium Acetate		21
Ammonium Arsenate	1546	72
Ammonium Benzoate		21
Ammonium Bicarbonate		21
Ammonium Bichromate		20
Ammonium Bifluoride, solid	1727	99
Ammonium Bifluoride, solution	2817	99
Ammonium Bisulfite, solid	2693	21, 105
Ammonium Bisulfite Solution	2693	21, 105
Ammonium Bromide		95

Chemical Name	UN/ NA/PIN	Guideline Number
Ammonium Carbamate	9083	21
Ammonium Carbonate	9084	21
Ammonium Chloride	9085	21
Ammonium Chromate	9086	21
Ammonium Citrate, dibasic		21
Ammonium Dichromate	1439	21
Ammonium Dinitro-*o*-cresolate	1843	21
Ammonium Fluororate		103
Ammonium Fluoride	2505	99
Ammonium Fluoroborate	9088	103
Ammonium Fluorosilicate	2854	99
Ammonium Hydrogen Fluoride, solution	2817	99
Ammonium Hydrogen Fluoride, solid	1727	99
Ammonium Hydrogen Sulfate	2506	14
Ammonium Hydrosulfide Solution	2683	21
Ammonium Hydroxide	2672	19
Ammonium Metavanadate	2859	10
Ammonium Nitrate, liquid (hot concentrated solution)	2426	47
Ammonium Nitrate, with more than 0.2% combustible material	0222	47
Ammonium Nitrate, with not more than 0.2% combustible material	1942	47
Ammonium Nitrate, with organic coating	1942	47
Ammonium Nitrate Fertilizer	2067	47
Ammonium Nitrate Fertilizer, containing not more than 45% ammonium nitrate	2071	47
Ammonium Nitrate Fertilizer, n.o.s.	2072	47

Chemical Name	UN/ NA/PIN	Guideline Number
Ammonium Nitrate Fertilizer, which is more liable to explode than ammonium nitrate with 0.2% combustible material	0223	47
Ammonium Nitrate Fertilizer, with ammonium sulfate	2069	47
Ammonium Nitrate Fertilizer, with calcium carbonate	2068	47
Ammonium Nitrate Fertilizer, with not more than 0.4% of combustible material	2071	47
Ammonium Nitrate Fertilizer,with phosphate or potash	2070	47
Ammonium Nitrate–Fuel Oil Mixtures		1, 47
Ammonium Nitrate Solution, with not less than 15% water	2426	47
Ammonium Nitrate–Sulfate Mixture	2069	47
Ammonium Oxalate	2449	17, 21
Ammonium Perchlorate	1442	21, 97
Ammonium Perchlorate	0402	21, 97
Ammonium Permanganate	9190	14
Ammonium Persulfate	1444	14
Ammonium Picrate, wet, with more than 10% water	1310	14
Ammonium Picrate, dry or wet, with less than 10% water	0004	14
Ammonium Polysulfide Solution	2818	21, 105
Ammonium Polyvanadate	2861	10
Ammonium Salts		21
Ammonium Silicofluoride, solid	2854	99
Ammonium Sulfamate	9089	21, 105

Chemical Name	UN/ NA/PIN	Guideline Number
Ammonium Sulfate (solution)		21, 105
Ammonium Sulfide Solution	2683	21, 105
Ammonium Sulfite	9090	21, 105
Ammonium Tartrate	9091	15
Ammonium Thiocyanate	9092	94
Ammonium Vanadate		10
Ammosite, brown asbestos	2212	102
Ammunition, tear-producing nonexplosive	2017	9
Ammunition, toxic, nonexplosive	2016	10
Amphetamine		10
Amygdalin		90
Amyl Acetates	1104	37
iso-Amyl Acetate		37
sec-Amyl Acetate		37
tert-Amyl Acetate		37
Amyl Acid Phosphate	2819	9
Amyl Alcohols	1105	30
Amyl Aldehyde	2058	41
Amylamine	1106	20
Amyl Butyrate	2620	15
Amyl Chloride	1107	26
Amylene	1108	92
Amyl Formate	1109	37
tert-Amyl Hydroperoxide, not more than 88% in solution	3067	8
Amyl Mercaptan	1111	105
Amyl Methyl Ketone	1110	42
Amyl Nitrate	1112	47
Amyl Nitrite	1113	47
tert-Amylperoxybenzoate	3044	8, 15
tert-Amyl Peroxy-2-ethyl-hexanoate	2898	8, 15

Chemical Name	UN/ NA/PIN	Guideline Number
tert-Amyl Peroxy Neodecanoate	2891	8, 15
tert-Amylperoxypivalate	2957	8, 15
Amyl Phenol		44
Amyltrichlorocyclane		26
Amyltrichlorosilane	1728	107
Anethole		24
Angel Dust		134
Anhydrous Ammonia	1005	21, 133, 138
Aniline	1547	32
Aniline Hydrochloride	1548	32
Anisidines	2431	25
o-Anisidine Hydrochloride		25
Anisindione		71
Anisole	2222	24
Anisoyl Chloride	1729	15
Anthophyllite	2212	102
Anthracene		24
Anthrax		113
Anti-Freeze	1142	40
Anti-Knock Compound	1649	80
Antimony, powder	2871	10
Antimony Chloride	1733	10
Antimony Compound, inorganic, liquid, n.o.s.	3141	10
Antimony Compounds, inorganic, n.o.s.	1549	10
Antimony Hydride	2676	10
Antimony Lactate	1550	10
Antimony Pentachloride, liquid	1730	10
Antimony Pentachloride Solution	1731	10
Antimony Pentafluoride	1732	99
Antimony Pentasulfide		10
Antimony Potassium	1551	10
Antimony Potassium Tartrate	1551	10

Chemical Name	UN/ NA/PIN	Guideline Number
Antimony Powder	2871	10
Antimony Salts		10
Antimony Tribromide	1549	95
Antimony Trichloride	1733	10
Antimony Trifluoride	1549	99
Antimony Trioxide		10
Antu (alpha naphthylthiourea)		43
Apl-Luster		70
Arbotect		70
Argon, compressed	1006	92
Argon, refrigerated liquid (cryogenic liquid)	1951	92
Aroclor 1016		46
Aroclor 1221		46
Aroclor 1232		46
Aroclor 1242		46
Aroclor 1248		46
Aroclor 1254		46
Aroclor 1260		46
Aroclors		46
Aromatic Hydrocarbon Solvent		24
Aromatic Nitrogen Compounds	1547	32
Aromatic Solvent Naphtha		43
Arsanilic Acid		72
Arsenates		72
Arsenic	1558	72
Arsenic Acid, liquid	1553	72
Arsenic Acid, solid	1554	72
Arsenical Dust	1562	72
Arsenical Flue Dust	1562	72
Arsenical Pesticide, liquid, flammable, poisonous	2760	72
Arsenical Pesticide, liquid, poisonous, flammable, n.o.s.	2993	72
Arsenical Pesticide, liquid, poisonous, n.o.s.	2994	72

Chemical Name	UN/ NA/PIN	Guideline Number
Arsenical Pesticide, solid, poisonous, n.o.s.	2759	72
Arsenic Bromide	1555	72, 95
Arsenic Chloride	1560	72, 98
Arsenic Compound, liquid, n.o.s.	1556	72
Arsenic Compound, solid, n.o.s.	1557	72
Arsenic Disulfide	1557	72
Arsenic hydride	2188	73, 138
Arsenic Iodide, solid	1557	72
Arsenic Metal	1558	72
Arsenic Pentoxide	1559	72
Arsenic Trichloride	1560	72, 98
Arsenic Trihydride	2188	73, 138
Arsenic Trioxide	1561	72
Arsenic Trisulfide	1557	72
Arsenic, white, solid	1561	72
Arsenites		72
Arseniuretted Hydrogen	2188	73, 138
Arsenous Hydride	2188	73, 138
Arsenous Oxide		72
Arsenous Trichloride		72. 98
Arsine	2188	73, 138
Arsine, (2-chlorovinyl)-dichloro-	2810	72, 139
Arsine, dichloro (2-chlorovinyl)-	2810	72, 139
Arsenous Dichloride, (2-chloroethenyl)-	2810	72, 139
Aryl Amines	1547	32
Aryl Sulfonic Acid, liquid	2584	15
Aryl Sulfonic Acid, liquid	2586	15
Aryl Sulfonic Acid, solid	2583	15
Aryl Sulfonic Acid, solid	2585	15
Asbestos, blue or brown	2212	102
Asbestos, white	2590	102
Asphalt	1999	35
Auramine		32

Chemical Name	UN/ NA/PIN	Guideline Number
Azaserine		10
Azinphos-Ethyl		49
Azinphos Methyl (Guthion)	2783	49
Aziridine		20
Aziridine, 2-Methyl		20
1-Aziridinyl Phosphine Oxide (tris)	2501	10
Azobenzene		32
2,2′-Azodi-(2,4-dimethyl-4-methoxyvaleronitrile)	2955	10
2,2′-Azodi-(2,4-dimethyl-valeronitrile)	2953	10
1,1′-Azodi-(hexahydro-benzonitrile)	2954	10
Azodiisobutyronitrile	2952	90
2,2′-Azodi-(2-methyl-butyronitrile)	3030	10
Bacillary Dysentery		117
Bacillus Anthracis		113
Balkan Grippe		123
Balkan Influenza		123
Bandane		54
Barium	1400	74
Barium Alloy	1399	74
Barium Alloy, pyrophoric	1854	74
Barium Azide, wet, with not less than 50% water	1571	74
Barium Bromate	2719	74, 96
Barium Chlorate	1445	74, 97
Barium Compounds, n.o.s.	1564	74
Barium Cyanide	1565	74, 90
Barium Fluosilicate		53, 74
Barium Hypochlorite	2741	22, 74
Barium Metaborate		74, 103
Barium Metal	1400	74
Barium Nitrate	1446	47, 74
Barium Oxide	1884	74
Barium Perchlorate	1447	74, 97
Barium Permanganate	1448	14, 74

Chemical Name	UN/ NA/PIN	Guideline Number
Barium Peroxide	1449	74
Barium Salts		74
Barium Selenate	2630	74, 86
Barium Selenite	2630	74, 86
Barthrin		52
Battery, electric, storage, dry, containing potassium hydroxide	1813	19
Battery, electric, storage, potassium hydroxide	3028	19
Battery, electric, storage, wet, filled with acid	2794	14
Battery, electric, storage, wet, filled with alkali	2795	19
Battery, electric, storage, wet, nonspillable	2800	14, 19
Battery, wet, filled with acid (electric storage)	2794	14
Battery, wet, filled with alkali (electric storage)	2795	19
Battery, wet, nonspillable (electric storage)	2800	14, 19
Battery Fluid, acid	2796	14
Battery Fluid, alkali	2797	19
Battery Fluid, alkali, with battery	2797	19
Battery Fluid, alkali, with electronic equipment or actuating device	2797	19
Baygon		50
Bendiocarb		50
Benomyl	2757	63
Bensulfide		49
Benz(c)acridine		10
Benzal Chloride		24
Benzaldehyde	1989	41
Benzamide		15
Benzamide, 3,5-dichloro-*N*-(1,1-dimethyl-2-propynyl)		57
Benz(a)anthracene		43

Chemical Name	UN/ NA/PIN	Guideline Number
Benzeneamine, 3-(trifluoromethyl)		32
Benzenearsonic Acid		72
Benzene	1114	25
Benzene-1,3-disulfohydrazide	2971	24
Benzeneethanamine, alpha, alpha-dimethyl		32
Benzene Hexachloride		57
Benzene Phosphorus Dichloride	2798	109
Benzene Phosphorus Thiodichloride	2799	109
Benzene Sulfohydrazide	2970	15
Benzene Sulfonyl Chloride	2225	15
Benzenethiol		33
Benzidine	1885	32
Benzine	1115	25, 35
Benzimidazole, 4,5-dichloro-2-(trifluorome)		24
Benzo(b)fluoranthene		24
Benzo(k)fluoranthene		24
Benzoic Acid	9094	15
Benzoic Derivative Pesticide, liquid, flammable, poisonous, n.o.s.	2770	15
Benzoic Derivative Pesticide, liquid, poisonous, flammable, n.o.s.	3003	15
Benzoic Derivative Pesticide, liquid, poisonous, n.o.s.	3004	15
Benzoic Derivative Pesticide, solid, poisonous, n.o.s.	2769	15
Benzoic Trichloride		15
Benzol	1114	25
Benzonitrile	2224	90
Benzo(ghi)perylene		24

Chemical Name	UN/ NA/PIN	Guideline Number
Benzo(a)pyrene		24
Benzoquinone	2587	24
Benzotrichloride	2226	9, 24
Benzotrifluoride	2338	9, 24
Benzoyl Chloride	1736	9, 24
Benzoyl Peroxide	2085	8
Benzoyl Peroxide	2086	8
Benzoyl Peroxide	2087	8
Benzoyl Peroxide	2088	8
Benzoyl Peroxide	2089	8
Benzoyl Peroxide	2090	8
Benzoyl Peroxide, not more than 62%, with not less than 28% inert solid and not less than 10% water	3074	8
Benzyl Bromide	1737	24
Benzyl Chloride	1738	24
Benzyl Chloroformate	1739	37
o-Benzyl-*p*-Chlorophenol		24
Benzyl Cyanide, liquid	2470	90
Benzyl Dimethylamine	2619	32
4-(Benzyl(ethyl)amino)3-ethoxybenzenediazonium Zinc Chloride	3037	10, 88
Benzylidene Chloride	1886	24
Benzyl Iodide	2653	24
4-(Benzyl(methyl)amino)-3-ethoxybenzenediazonium Zinc Chloride	3038	10, 88
Bertholite	1017	98, 133
Beryllium, powder	1567	75
Beryllium Chloride	1566	75
Beryllium Compound	1566	75
Beryllium and Compounds	1567	75
Beryllium Fluoride	1566	75
Beryllium Nitrate	2464	75
Beta-Chlorovinyldichloroarsine	2810	72, 139

Chemical Name	UN/ NA/PIN	Guideline Number
alpha-BHC		57
beta-BHC		57
delta-BHC		57
Bhusa	1327	10
Bicyclo(2.2.1)heptane-2-carbonitrile, 5-chloro-6-((((methylamino)carbonyl) oxy)imino)-, (1S(1 alpha, 2 beta, 4 alpha, 5 alpha, 6E))-		50
Bidrin		49
Bifluoride, n.o.s.	1740	99
2,2′-Bioxirane		38
Biphenyl		24
Bipyridilium Pesticide, liquid, flammable, poisonous, n.o.s.	2782	66
Bipyridilium Pesticide, liquid, flammable, poisonous, n.o.s.	3015	66
Bipyridilium Pesticide, liquid, poisonous, n.o.s.	3016	66
Bipyridilium Pesticide, solid, poisonous, n.o.s.	2781	66
Bis(aminopropyl)Amine	1760	20
Bis(beta-chloroethyl)sulfide		139
Bis(2(-chlorethyl-thio)ester		139
Bis(2-chloroethoxy) Methane		38
Bis(2-chloroethyl) Ether		38
Bis-(2-chloroethyl) Methyl Amine		139
Bis-(2-chloroethyl) Ethyl Amine		139
Bis-(2-chloroethyl)sulfide		139
Bis(2-chloroethylthio) methane		139
Bis(2-chloroethylthioethyl) ether		139
Bis(2-chloroethylthiomethyl) ether		139
Bis(2-chloro-1-methyl(ethyl) Ether		38

Chemical Name	UN/ NA/PIN	Guideline Number
tert-Butyl Hydroperoxide, not more than 82%, with not less than 7% water and not less than 9% di-*tert*-butyl peroxide	3075	8
Butyl Hydroxytoluene		24
Butyl Imidazole	2690	33
n-Butyl Isocyanate	2485	94
tert-Butyl Isocyanate	2484	94
tert-Butyl Isopropyl Benzene Hydroperoxide	2091	8
Butyl Lithium	2445	81
Butyl Mercaptan	2347	105
Butyl Methacrylate	2227	37
Butyl Methyl Ether	2350	38
tert-Butyl Monoperoxy-maleate	2101	8, 15
tert-Butyl Monoperoxy-maleate, solution or paste	2100	8, 15
tert-Butyl Monoperoxy-maleate, technical pure	2099	8, 15
tert-Butyl Monoperoxy-phthalate	2105	8, 15
Butyl Nitrite	2351	47
tert-Butyl Peroxide	2102	8
Butyl Perbenzoate		8, 15
tert-Butyl Peroxyacetate	2095	8, 15
tert-Butyl Peroxyacetate	2096	8, 15
tert-Butyl Peroxybenzoate	2097	8, 15
tert-Butyl Peroxybenzoate	2098	8, 15
tert-Butyl Peroxybenzoate	2890	8, 15
tert-Butyl Peroxycrotonate	2183	8, 15
Butyl Peroxydicarbonate	2169	8, 15
Butyl Peroxydicarbonate	2170	8, 15
tert-Butyl Peroxydiethyl-acetate	2144	8, 15
tert-Butyl Peroxydiethyl-acetate with *tert*-butyl Peroxybenzoate	2551	8, 15
tert-Butyl Peroxy-2-Ethyl Hexanoate, not more than 50%, with phlegmatizer	2888	8, 15
tert-Butyl Peroxy-2-Ethyl Hexanoate, technical pure	2143	8, 15
tert-Butyl Peroxy-2-Ethyl Hexanoate, with 2,2-di-(*tert*-butylperoxy) butane	2886	8, 15
tert-Butyl Peroxy-isobutyrate	2562	8, 15
tert-Butyl Peroxy-isobutyrate	2142	8, 15
tert-Butyl Peroxyisononanoate	2104	8, 15
tert-Butyl Peroxyisopropyl Carbonate, technical pure	2103	8, 15
tert-Butyl Peroxymaleate	2101	8, 15
tert-Butyl Peroxymaleate, solution or paste	2100	8, 15
tert-Butyl Peroxymaleate, technical pure	2099	8, 15
tert-Butyl Peroxyneodecanoate	2177	8, 15
tert-Butyl Peroxy-neodecanoate	2594	8, 15
tert-Butyl Peroxy-3-phenylphthalide	2596	8, 15
tert-Butyl Peroxyphthalate	2105	8, 15
tert-Butyl Peroxypivalate	2110	8, 15
tert-Butyl Peroxypivalate	3047	8, 15
tert-Butyl Peroxystearyl Carbonate, technical pure	3062	8, 15
tert-Butyl Peroxy-3,5,5-trimethylhexanoate	2104	8, 15
Butyl Phenol, liquid	2228	44
Butyl Phenol, solid	2229	44
o-sec-Butylphenol	2228	44
Butyl Phosphoric Acid	1718	15
n-Butyl Phthalate		37
Butyl Propionate	1914	37

Chemical Name	UN/ NA/PIN	Guideline Number
Butyl Toluene	2667	24
Butyl Trichlorosilane	1747	107
tert-Butyl-2,4,6-trinitro-xylene	2956	24
Butyl Vinyl Ether	2352	38
Butynediol	2716	30
Butyraldehyde	1129	41
Butyraldoxime	2840	41
Butyric Acid	2820	15
iso-Butyric Acid		15
Butyric Anhydride	2739	15
Butyrone	2710	42
n-Butyronitrile	2411	90
Butyryl Chloride	2353	15
Buzz	2810	134
BZ	2810	134
CA	1694	136
Cacodylic Acid	1572	72
Cadmium and Compounds	2570	76
Cadmium Acetate	2570	76
Cadmium Bromide	2570	76
Cadmium Chloride	2570	76
Cadmium Oxide		76
Cadmium Stearate		76
Caesium, Metal	1407	6
Caesium Hydroxide	2682	19
Caesium Hydroxide, solution	2681	19
Caesium Nitrate	1451	14, 47
Calcium, metal and alloys	1401	10
Calcium, metal and alloys, pyrophoric	1855	6, 10
Calcium Alloy, pyrophoric	1855	6, 10
Calcium Arsenate	1573	72
Calcium Arsenate and Calcium Arsenite Mixture, solid	1574	72
Calcium Arsenite	1574	72
Calcium Bisulfite Solution	2693	105
Calcium Carbide	1402	13
Calcium Chlorate	1452	97
Calcium Chlorate Solution	2429	97
Calcium Chlorite	1453	98
Calcium Chromate		10
Calcium Cyanamide, with more than 0.1% calcium carbide	1403	10
Calcium Cyanide	1575	90
Calcium Dithionite	1923	105
Calcium Dodeculbenzenesulfonate		15
Calcium Hydride	1404	13
Calcium Hydrogen Sulfite Solution	2693	105
Calcium Hydrosulfite	1923	105
Calcium Hydroxide		19
Calcium Hypochlorite, dry, including mixtures with more than 39% available chlorine (8.8% available oxygen)	1748	22
Calcium Hypochlorite, hydrated, including mixtures with not less than 5.5% but not more than 10% water	2880	22
Calcium Hypochlorite Mixture, dry, with more than 10% but not more than 39% available chlorine	2208	22
Calcium Manganese Silicon	2844	83
Calcium Nitrate	1454	47
Calcium Oxide	1910	19
Calcium Perchlorate	1455	97
Calcium Permanganate	1456	14
Calcium Peroxide	1457	8
Calcium Phosphide	1360	108

Chemical Name	UN/ NA/PIN	Guideline Number
Calcium Polysulfide		105
Calcium, pyrophoric	1855	6
Calcium Resinate	1313	6
Calcium Resinate, fused	1314	6
Calcium Selenate	2630	86
Calcium Silicide	1405	6
Calcium Silicon	1406	6
Camphene	9011	36
Camphechlor		58
Camphor	2717	36
Camphor, synthetic	2717	36
Camphor Oil	1130	36
Cantharidin		9
Caproic Acid	2829	15
Caproic Acid (hexanoic acid)	1760	15
Caprolactam		9, 10
Caprylic Alcohol		30
Caprylyl Peroxide	2129	8
Captan	9099	63
Carbachol Chloride		50
Carbamate Pesticide, liquid, flammable, poisonous, n.o.s.	2758	50
Carbamate Pesticide liquid, poisonous, flammable, n.o.s.	2991	50
Carbamate Pesticide liquid, poisonous, n.o.s.	2992	50
Carbamate Pesticide solid, poisonous, n.o.s.	2757	50
Carbamic Acid, Ethyl Ester		37
Carbamic Acid, Methyl-Propoxur		50
Carbanolate		50
Carbaryl	2757	50
Carbitol		40
Carbitol Esters		37
Carbofuran	2757	50

Chemical Name	UN/ NA/PIN	Guideline Number
Carbolic Acid	1671	44
Carbon, Activated	1362	9
Carbon, animal or vegetable origin	1361	6, 9
Carbon Bisulfide	1131	93
Carbon Dioxide	1013	92
Carbon Dioxide, refrigerated liquid (cryogenic liquid)	2187	92
Carbon Dioxide, solid	1845	92
Carbon Dioxide–Ethylene Oxide Mixture, with more than 6% ethylene oxide	1041	45, 92
Carbon Dioxide–Ethylene Oxide Mixture, with not more than 6% ethylene oxide	1952	45, 92
Carbon Dioxide–Nitrous Oxide Mixture	1015	92
Carbon Dioxide–Oxygen Mixture	1014	92
Carbon Disulfide	1131	93, 133, 138
Carbonic Acid, Trichloromethyl Ester		101, 133
Carbonic Dichloride		101, 133
Carbonic Difluoride		99
Carbon Monoxide	1016	89
Carbon Monoxide, cryogenic liquid	9202	89
Carbon Monoxide–Hydrogen Mixture	2600	89
Carbon Monoxide, from methylene chloride		26, 89
Carbonochloridic Acid, trimethyl ester	1076	101, 133
Carbon Oxychloride	1076	101, 133
Carbon Oxysulfide	2204	91
Carbon Remover, liquid	1132	35
Carbon Tetrabromide	2516	28
Carbon Tetrachloride	1846	28
Carbonyl Chloride	1076	101, 133

Chemical Name	UN/ NA/PIN	Guideline Number
Chlorinated Hydrocarbons		26
Chlorinated Lime	2208	22
Chlorinated Naphthalene		43
Chlorinated Phenols		44
Chlorinated Solvents	1610	26
Chlorinated Trisodium Phosphate		22
Chlorine	1017	98, 133, 138
Chlorine Dioxide	9091	98, 133
Chlorine Dioxide Hydrate, frozen	9191	98, 133
Chlorine Pentafluoride	2548	98, 99, 133
Chlorine Trifluoride	1749	16, 98, 133
Chlorite, inorganic, n.o.s.	1462	98, 133
Chlormephos		49
Chlormequat Chloride		10
Chlornaphazine		10
Chloroacetaldehyde	2232	41
Chloroacetic Acid, liquid	1750	15
Chloroacetic Acid, solid	1751	15
alpha-Chloroacetophenone	1697	42, 136
2-Chloroacetophenone	1697	42, 136
Chloroacetone, stabilized	1695	42
Chloroacetonitrile	2668	90
Chloroacetophenone	1697	42
Chloroacetyl Chloride	1752	98
Chloroaniline, liquid	2019	32
Chloroaniline, solid	2018	32
Chloroanisidine	2233	24, 47
2-Chlorobenzalmalonitrile	2810	136
Chlorobenzene	1134	25
Chlorobenzilate		57
Chlorobenzotrifluoride	2234	24
p-Chlorobenzoyl Peroxide	2113	8
p-Chlorobenzoyl Peroxide	2114	8
p-Chlorobenzoyl Peroxide	2115	8

Chemical Name	UN/ NA/PIN	Guideline Number
Chlorobenzyl Chloride	2235	24
o-Chlorobenzylidene Malonitrile	2810	136
1-chloro-2(beta-chloroethylthio)ethane	2810	139
2-Chlorobmn	2810	136
Chlorobromomethane	1887	26
Chlorobromopropane	2688	27
Chlorobutane	1127	27
p-Chloro-m-cresol	2669	44
4-Chloro-2-cyclopentylphenol		44
Chlorodibromomethane		26
1-Chloro-2-di-chloroarsinoethane		72, 139
Chlorodiethylaluminum		6, 10
3-Chloro-4-diethylamino-benediazonium Zinc Chloride	3033	88
Chlorodifluorobromo-methane	1974	27
Chlorodifluoroethane	2517	27
Chlorodifluoromethane	1018	27
Chlorodifluoromethane and Chloropentafluoroethane Mixture	1973	27
Chlorodifluoromethane and Chloropentafluoroethane Mixture	1078	27
Chlorodinitrobenzene	1577	24, 47
1-Chloro-2,4-dinitrobenzene	1577	24, 47
Chlorodiphenyl		46
Chloroethane		26
Chloroethanol		38
Tris(2-chloroethyl) Amine	2810	139
Chloroethyl Chloroformate		37
N,N-Bis(2-chloroethyl) Methylamine	2810	139
2-Chloroethylchloro-methylsulfide		139

ALPHABETICAL INDEX

Chemical Name	UN/ NA/PIN	Guideline Number
Di-2-chloroethyl Sulfide, beta,beta′-dichloroethyl	2810	139
1,2-Bis(2-chloroethylthio) ethane		139
1,3-Bis(2-chloroethylthio)-*n*-propane		139
1,4-Bis(2-chloroethylthio)-*n*-butane		139
1,5-Bis(2-chloroethylthio)-*n*-pentane		139
2-Chloroethyl Vinyl Ether		38
Chlorofluorocarbons (CFCs)	1018	27
	1020	27
	1021	27
	1022	27
	1028	27
	1029	27
	1030	27
	1078	27
Chloroform	1888	26
Chloroformate, n.o.s.	2742	37
Chloroformyl Chloride	1076	101, 133
Chloromethane		26
3-Chloro-4-methylaniline		32
Chloromethyl-chloroformate	2745	37
Chloromethyl Ethyl Ether	2354	38
Chloromethyl Methyl Ether	1239	38
Chloromethyl-plenylisocyanate	2236	94
Chloromethyl Phenyl Ketone	1697	136
3-Chloro-2-methyl-1-propene		61
Chloromethyoxypropyl-mercuric Acetate		37
2-Chloronaphthalene		43

Chemical Name	UN/ NA/PIN	Guideline Number
2-Chloro-*N*-(2-chloroethyl)-*N*-ethylethanamine	2810	139
Chloronitroaniline	2237	32
Chloronitrobenzenes	1578	24, 47
1-Chloro-1-nitropropane		26, 47
Chloronitrotoluene	2433	24
2-Chloro-*N,N*-Bis(2-chloroethyl) ethanamine	2810	139
Chloropentafluoroethane	1020	27
3-Chloroperoxybenzoic Acid	2755	15
3-Chloroperoxybenzoic Acid, not more than 57% with water and 3-chlorobenzoic acid	3081	15
Chlorophacinone		71
Chlorophenate, liquid	2904	44
Chlorophenate, solid	2905	44
2-Chlorophenol	2020	44
2-Chloro-4(hydroxymercuri)-phenol		84
Chlorophenols, solids	2020	44
Chlorophenols, liquids	2021	44
2-chloro-1-phenylethanone	1697	136
Chloro-2-phenylphenol		44
4-Chlorophenyl phenylether		38, 44
Chlorophenyl Trichlorosilane	1753	107
p-Chlorophenoxyacetic Acid		60
Chloropicrin	1580	26, 136
Chloropicrin and Methyl Bromide Mixture	1581	26, 95, 136
Chloropicrin and Methyl Chloride Mixture	1582	26, 136
Chloropicrin Mixture, flammable	2929	26, 136
Chloropicrin and Nonflammable Gas Mixture	1955	26, 136

Chemical Name	UN/ NA/PIN	Guideline Number
Chloropicrin Mixture, n.o.s.	1583	26, 136
Chloropivaloyl Chloride	9263	10
Chloroplatinic Acid, solid	2507	14
Chloroprene	1991	9, 33
Chloropropane	2356	33
Chloropropanol	2611	30
2-Chloro-1-propanol	2611	30
3-Chloropropanol	2849	30
3-Chloropropanol-1	2849	30
Chloropropene	2456	33
Chloropropionic Acid	2511	15
3-Chloropropionitrile		90
Chloropyridine	2822	24
Chlorosilane, n.o.s. (corrosive)	2987	107
Chlorosilane, n.o.s. (emits flammable gas when wet, corrosive)	2988	107
Chlorosilane, n.o.s. (flammable, corrosive)	2985, 2986	107
N-Chlorosuccinimide		44
Chlorosulfonic Acid	1754	14, 137
Chlorosulfonic Acid and Sulfur Trioxide Mixture	1754	14, 105, 137
Chlorosulphonic Acid		14, 137
Chlorotetrafluoroethane	1021	27
Chlorothalonil		10
Chlorothion		49
Chlorothymol		44
Chlorotoluene	2238	24
o-Chlorotoluene	2238	24
Chlorotoluidine, liquid or solid	2239	20
4-Chloro-o-toluidine Hydrochloride	1579	20
Chlorotrifluoroethane	1983	27
Chlorotrifluoromethane	1022	27
Chlorotrifluoromethane and Trifluoromethane Mixture	1078, 2599	27
Chlorotrifluoropyridine	9270	24
Tris(2-chlorovinyl)arsine		72, 139
Chlorovinylarsine Dichloride	2810	72, 139
beta-Chlorovinylbichloroarsine	2810	72, 139
beta-Chlorovinyldichloroarsine	2810	72, 139
beta-Chlorovinyldichloroarsine	2810	72, 139
2-Chlorovinyl-dichloroarsine	2810	72, 139
Chloroxuron		10
4-Chloro-3,5-xylenol		44
Chlorpyrifos	2783	49
Chlorthiophos		49
Cholera		131
Chromate Salts		14
Chromic Acetate		14
Chromic Acid, solid	1463	14
Chromic Acid, solution	1755	14
Chromic Anhydride	1463	14
Chromic Chloride		14
Chromic Fluoride, solution	1757	99
Chromic Fluoride, solid	1756	99
Chromic Sulfate	9100	14
Chromium		14
Chromium Nitrate	2720	47
Chromium Oxychloride	1758	14
Chromium Trioxide, anhydrous	1463	14
Chromosulfuric Acid	2240	14
Chromous Chloride		14
Chrysene		43
Chrysotile, blue or brown	2212	102
Chrysotile, white	2590	102

Chemical Name	UN/ NA/PIN	Guideline Number
Cigarette, self-lighting	1867	51
Cigarette Lighter, with flammable gas	1057	33
Cigarette Lighter, with flammable liquid	1226	33
CK	1589	90, 132
CL	1017	98, 133
Clark I	1699	140
Clark II	2810	140
Cleaning Compound	1142	19
Cleaning Compound, liquid, corrosive	1760	19
Clostridium Botulinum		114
CN	1697	136
Coal, Ground Bituminous, Sea Coal, etc.	1361	6
Coal Facings	1361	6
Coal Gas	1023	2
Coal Tar Creosote		24
Coal Tar Distillates	1136	24, 25
Coal Tar Distillates	1137	24, 25
Coal Tar Naphtha	2553	43
Coal Tar Oil	1136	24, 25
Coal Tar Oil	1137	24, 25
Coating Solution	1139	10
Cobalt Carbonyl		77
Cobalt Hydrocarbonyl		77
Cobalt Naphthenate, powder	2001	77
Cobalt Resinate, precipitated	1318	77
Cobalt Salts		77
Cobaltous Bromide		77, 95
Cobaltous Formate		77
Cobaltous Sulfamate		77
Cocculus, solid	1584	10
Colchicine		10
Collodion	2059	29, 38
Combustible Liquid, n.o.s.	1993	4

Chemical Name	UN/ NA/PIN	Guideline Number
Compound, polishing, liquid, etc. (combustible or flammable)	1142	10
Compound, tree- or weed-killing, liquid (combustible or flammable)	1993	4, 10
Compound, tree- or weed-killing, liquid (corrosive)	1760	10, 13
Compound X		114
Compressed Gas, flammable, n.o.s.	1954	2
Compressed Gas, flammable, poisonous, n.o.s.	1953	2, 10
Compressed Gas, n.o.s.	1956	3
Compressed Gas, poisonous, n.o.s.	1955	10
Copper and Compounds		78
Copper Acetoarsenite	1585	78
Copper Arsenate		72, 78
Copper Arsenite	1586	72, 78
Copper-Based Pesticide liquid, flammable, poisonous, n.o.s.	2776	78
Copper-Based Pesticide liquid, poisonous, flammable, n.o.s.	3009	78
Copper-Based Pesticide liquid, poisonous, n.o.s.	3010	78
Copper-Based Pesticide, solid, poisonous, n.o.s.	2775	78
Copper Chlorate	2721	78, 97
Copper Chloride	2802	78
Copper Cyanide	1587	78, 90
Copper Naphthenates		78, 43
Copper Oxychloride Sulfate		78
Copper 3-phenylsalicylate		78
Copper Quinolinolate		78
Copper Selenate	2630	78, 86
Copper Selenite	2630	78, 86

Chemical Name	UN/ NA/PIN	Guideline Number
Copra	1363	5
Corrosives, acids	1760	14, 15
Corrosives, ammonia	1005	21
Corrosives, ammonium hydroxide	2672	21
Corrosive Liquid, flammable, n.o.s.	2920	5, 13
Corrosive Liquid, n.o.s.	1760	13
Corrosive Liquid, oxidizing, n.o.s.	3093	7, 13
Corrosive Liquid, poisonous, n.o.s.	2922	10, 13
Corrosive Liquid That, When in Contact with Water, Emits a Flammable Gas, n.o.s.	3094	2, 13
Corrosive Solid, flammable, n.o.s.	2921	6, 13
Corrosive Solid, n.o.s.	1759	13
Corrosive, poisonous, n.o.s.	2923	10, 13
Corrosive Solid, oxidizing	3084	7, 13
Corrosive Solid, self-heating, n.o.s.	3095	13
Corrosive Solid, that, when in contact with water, emits a flammable gas, n.o.s.	3096	2, 13
Cosmetics, corrosive liquid, n.o.s.	1760	13
Cosmetics, corrosive solid, n.o.s.	1759	13
Cosmetics, flammable liquid, n.o.s.	1993	5
Cosmetics, flammable solid, n.o.s.	1325	6
Cosmetics, oxidizer, n.o.s.	1479	7
Cotton, wet	1365	9
Cotton Waste, oily	1364	9
Coumachlor		71
Coumafuryl		71
Coumaphos	2783	49
Coumarin Derivative Pesticide, flammable liquid, n.o.s.	3024	42
Coumarin Derivative Pesticide, flammable liquid, n.o.s.	3025	42
Coumarin Derivative Pesticide, liquid, n.o.s.	3026	42
Coumarin Derivative Pesticide, solid, n.o.s.	3027	42
Coumatetralyl		71
Coxiella Burnetii		123
p-Cresidine		24
Creolin		59
Creosol		44
Creosote, coal tar	1993	44
Creosote Salts	1334	44
Cresol (*o*-, *m*-, and *p*-)	2076	44
m-Cresyl Acetate		37
Cresylic Acid	2022	44
Crimean Congo Hemorrhagic Fever		116
Crimidine		10
Crotonaldehyde, inhibited	1143	59
Crotonic Acid	2823	15
Crotonylene	1144	33
Crufomate	2765	49
Cryolite		99
Cryptosporidium parvum		131
CS	2810	136
CSA		137
CS Gas	2810	136
CS2	2810	136
Cube		53
Cumene	1918	24
Cumene Hydroperoxide, technical pure	2116	8, 24

ALPHABETICAL INDEX

Chemical Name	UN/ NA/PIN	Guideline Number
Cumyl Hydroperoxide	2116	8, 24
Cumyl Peroxy-neo-decanoate	2963	8, 24
Cumyl Peroxypivalate	2964	8, 24
Cupferron		20
Cupric Acetate	9106	78
Cupric Acetoarsenite		78
Cupric Arsenite		72, 78
Cupric Chloride		78
Cupric Nitrate	1479	78
Cupric Oxalate	2449	78
Cupric Sulfate	9109	78
Cupric Sulfate, ammoniated	9110	78
Cupric Tartrate		78
Cupriethylenediamine Solution	1761	20, 78
Cuprous Chloride		78
Cuprous Oxide		78
CX	2811	139
Cyanic Acid		94
Cyanide, inorganic, n.o.s.	1588	90
Cyanide or Cyanide mixture, dry	1588	90
Cyanide, potassium, solution	1680	90
Cyanide, sodium	1689	90
Cyanide, solution, n.o.s.	1935	90
Cyanogen	1026	90
Cyanogen, liquefied	1026	90
Cyanogen Bromide	1889	90
Cyanogen Chloride, inhibited	1589	90
Cyanogen Gas	1026	90
Cyanogen Iodide		90
Cyano Organic Compounds		90
Cyanophos		49
Cyanuric Chloride	2670	15

Chemical Name	UN/ NA/PIN	Guideline Number
Cyanuric Fluoride		16
Cyclethrin		52
Cyclobutane	2601	92
Cyclobutylchloroformate	2744	37
Cyclocoumarol		71
Cyclododecatriene	2518	33
Cycloheptane	2241	33
Cycloheptatriene	2603	33
Cycloheptene	2242	33
Cyclohexane	1145	33
Cyclohexanol		30
Cyclohexanone	1915	42
Cyclohexanone Peroxide, more than 90%, with less than 10% water	2117	8
Cyclohexanone Peroxide, not more than 72% as a paste	2896	8
Cyclohexanone Peroxide, not more than 72% in solution	2118	8
Cyclohexanone Peroxide, not more than 90%, with not less than 10% water	2119	8
Cyclohexene	2256	33
Cyclohexenyl Trichlorosilane	1762	107
Cycloheximide		9, 10
Cyclohexyl Acetate	2243	37
Cyclohexylamine	2357	20
2-Cyclohexyl-4,6-dinitrophenol		62
Cyclohexyl Isocyanate	2488	94
Cyclohexyl Mercaptan	3054	105
Cyclohexyl Methyl-phosphonpofluoridate	2810	135
Cyclohexyl Trichlorosilane	1763	107
Cyclonite (RDX, T4, or C4)	0072	1
Cyclooctadiene	2520	33

ALPHABETICAL INDEX

Chemical Name	UN/ NA/PIN	Guideline Number
Dibenz(b,f)(1,4)oxazepine		136
Dibenzofuran		46
Dibenz(a,i)pyrene		24
Dibenzoyl Peroxide	2085	8
Dibenzoyl Peroxide	2087	8
Dibenzoyl Peroxide	2088	8
Dibenzoyl Peroxide	2089	8
Dibenzoyl Peroxide	2090	8
Dibenzoyl Peroxide, not more than 62%, with not less than 28% inert solid and not less than 10% water	3074	8
Dibenzyldichlorosilane	2434	107
Dibenzyl Peroxydicarbonate	2149	8
Diborane or Diborane Mixture	1911	103, 133, 138
Dibromobenzene	2711	24
Dibromobutanone	2648	42
Dibromochloropropane	2872	61
1,2-Dibromo-3-chloropropane		61
Dibromodifluoromethane	1941	27
Dibromoethane	1605	27
1,2-Dibromoethane	1605	27
Dibromotetrafluoroethane (Halon 2402)		27
Dibromomethane	2664	27
Diborane	1911	103, 133, 138
Dibutylamine	2248	20
Dibutylaminoethanol	2873	30
Di(4-*tert*-butylcyclohexyl) Peroxydicarbonate	2154	8
Di(4-*tert*-butylcyclohexyl) Peroxydicarbonate	2894	8
Dibutyl Ether	1149	38
Dibutyl Peroxide		8
Dibutyl Phthalate		37

Chemical Name	UN/ NA/PIN	Guideline Number
Di-*tert*-butyl Peroxide, technical pure	2102	8
2,2-Di-(*tert*-butylperoxy)-butane	2111	8, 33
1,1-Di-(*tert*-butylperoxy)-cyclohexane	2179	8, 33
1,1-Di-(*tert*-butylperoxy)-cyclohexane	2180	8, 33
1,1-Di-(*tert*-butylperoxy)-cyclohexane	2885	8, 33
1,1-Di-(*tert*-butylperoxy)-cyclohexane	2897	8, 33
1,1-Di-(*tert*-butylperoxy)-cyclohexane	3069	8, 33
1,2-Di-(*tert*-butylperoxy)-cyclohexane	2181	8, 33
Di-*n*-Butyl Peroxy-dicarbonate	2169	8
Di-*n*-Butyl Peroxy-dicarbonate	2170	8
Di-*sec*-Butyl Peroxy-Dicarbonate	2150	8
Di-*sec*-Butyl Peroxy-Dicarbonate	2151	8
Di-(2-*tert*-butylperoxy-isopropyl)benzene	2112	8, 24
1,4-Di-(2-*tert*-butylperoxy-isopropyl)benzene and 1,3-Di-(2-*tert*-butylperoxy-isopropyl)benzene	2112	8, 24
Di-*tert*-butylperoxyphthalate	2106	37
Di-*tert*-butylperoxyphthalate	2107	37
Di-*tert*-butylperoxyphthalate	2108	37
2,2-Di-(*tert*-butylperoxy)-propane	2884	8, 33
2,2-Di-(*tert*-butylperoxy)-propane	2883	8, 33

Chemical Name	UN/ NA/PIN	Guideline Number
1,1-Di-(*tert*-butylperoxy)-3,3,5-trimethylcyclohexane	2146	8, 33
1,1-Di-(*tert*-butylperoxy)-3,3,5-trimethylcyclohexane	2147	8, 33
1,1-Di-(*tert*-butylperoxy)-3,3,5-trimethylcyclohexane	2145	8, 33
Dicamba		60
Dicetyl Peroxydicarbonate, not more than 42%	2895	8
Dicetyl Peroxydicarbonate, technical pure	2164	8
Dichlobenil		10
Dichlofenthion		49
Dichlone		10
Dichloran		25
Dichloren	2810	139
Dichloroacetic Acid	1764	15
1,3-Dichloroacetone	2649	42
Dichloroacetyl Chloride	1765	15
Dichloro Acetylene		33, 92
Dichloroaniline	1590	32
o-Dichlorobenzene	1591	57
p-Dichlorobenzene	1592	57
3,3′-Dichlorobenzidine Dichlorobenzidine		32
2,4-Dichlorobenzoyl Peroxide	2137	8
2,4-Dichlorobenzoyl Peroxide	2138	8
2,4-Dichlorobenzoyl Peroxide	2139	8
Di-(4-chlorobenzoyl) Peroxide	2113	8
Di-(4-chlorobenzoyl) Peroxide	2114	8
Di-(4-chlorobenzoyl) Peroxide	2115	8

Chemical Name	UN/ NA/PIN	Guideline Number
1,1-Dichloro-2,2-bis(*p*-chlorophenyl)ethane		57
Dichlorobromomethane		27
Dichlorobutene	2924	27
Trans-1,4-dichlorobutene		27
Dichloro(2-chlorovinyl) arsine	2810	72, 139
Dichlorodiethyl Ether	1916	38
2,2′-Dichlorodiethyl Sulfide	2810	139
beta,beta′-Dichlorodiethyl Sulfide	2810	139
Dichlorodifluoroethylene	9018	27
Dichlorodifluoromethane (Freon 12)	1028	27
Dichlorodifluoromethane and Chlorodifluoromethane Mixture	1078	27
Dichlorodifluoromethane and Dichlorotetrafluoroethane Mixture	1078	27
Dichlorodifluoromethane and Difluoroethane Azeotropic Mixture	2602	27
Dichlorodifluoromethane and Difluoroethane Mixture	1078	27
Dichlorodifluoromethane and Ethylene Oxide Mixture, with not more than 12% ethylene oxide	3070	27, 45
Dichlorodifluoromethane, Trichlorofluoromethane, and Chlorodifluoromethane Mixture	1078	27
Dichlorodifluoromethane and Trichlorofluoromethane Mixture	1078	27
Dichlorodifluoromethane and Trichlorotrifluoroethane Mixture	1078	27

Chemical Name	UN/ NA/PIN	Guideline Number
Dichlorodimethyl Ether, symmetrical	2249	38
1,3-Dichloro-5, 5-dimethyl Hydantoin		10
Dichlorodiphenyl-trichlorethane (DDT)	2761	55, 57
1,1-Dichloroethane	2362	27
1,2-Dichloroethane		27
Dichloroethylene	1150	27
1,2-Dichloroethylene	1150	27
1,1-Dichlorethylene		27
Dichloroethyl Ether	1916	38
1,1-Dichloro-1-fluoroethane	9274	27
Dichlorofluoromethane	1029	27
Dichloroisocyanuric Acid, and its salts, dry	2465	15
Dichloroisopropyl Ether	2490	38
Dichloromethane	1593	27
Dichloromethyl Ether		38
Dichloromethylphenylsilane		107
Dichloromono-fluoromethane	1029	27
Dichloronitroethane	2650	27
1,1-Dichloro-1-nitroethane	2650	27
2,2'-Dichloro-*N*-methyldiethylamine	2810	139
Dichloropentane	1152	27
Dichlorophen(e)		44
2,4-Dichlorophenol	2021	44
2,6-Dichlorophenol	2021	44
2,4-Dichlorophen-oxyacetic Acid	2765	60
4-(2,4-Dichlorophenoxy) Butyric Acid		60
2-(2,4-Dichlorophenoxy) Ethyl Sulfate Sodium Salts	1594	60
2-(2,4-Dichlorophenoxy) Propionic Acid		60
Dichlorophenylarsine		73
Dichlorophenylisocyanate	2250	94
Di-(*p*-chlorophenyl) methylcarbinol (DMC)		55
Dichlorophenyl Trichlorosilane	1766	107
Dichloropropane	1279	61
1,1-Dichloropropane		61
1,2-Dichloropropane	1279	61
1,3-Dichloropropane		61
Dichloropropanol	2750	30
1,3-Dichloro-2-propanol	2750	30
Dichloropropanone	2649	42
Dichloropropene	2047	61
Dichloropropene and Propylene Dichloride Mixture	2047	61
1,3-Dichloropropene	2047	61
2,3-Dichloropropene		61
Dichloropropionic Acid	1760	15
2,2-Dichloropropionic Acid	1760	15
1,3-Dichloropropylene		61
Dichlorosilane	2189	107
Dichlorotetrafluorethane	1958	27
Dichloro-*s*-triazinetrione, and its salts, dry	2465	9
2,2′-Dichlorotriethylamine	2810	139
3,5-Dichloro-2,4, 6-trifluoropyridine	9264	24
Dichlorvos	2783	49
Dichromate Salts		10
Dicofol		54
Dicrotophos	2783	49
Dicumyl Peroxide	2121	8
Dicycloheptadiene	2251	33
Dicylohexylamine	2565	62

Chemical Name	UN/NA/PIN	Guideline Number
Dicyclohexylamine 4,6-dinitro-*o*-cyclohexylphenolate		62
Dicyclohexylamine Nitrite	2687	47, 62
Dicyclohexylammonium Nitrite	2687	47
Dicyclohexyl Peroxy-dicarbonate	2152	8
Dicyclohexyl Peroxydicarbonate	2153	8
Dicyclopentadiene	2048	33
Didecanoyl Peroxide, technical pure	2120	8
9,10-Didehydro-*N,N*-diethyl-6-methyl-8-beta-ergoline-8-carboxamide	2811	134
2,2-Di-(4,4-di-*tert*-butylperoxycyclohexyl) Propane	2168	8
Di-2,4-Dichlorobenzoyl Peroxide, not more than 52% as paste	2138	8
Di-2,4-Dichlorobenzoyl Peroxide, not more than 52% in solution	2139	8
Di-2,4-Dichlorobenzoyl Peroxide, not more than 75% in water	2137	8
1,2-Di-(dimethylamino) ethane	2372	32, 33
Didymium Nitrate	1465	47
Dieldrin	2761	56
Dienochlor		54
Diepoxybutane		45
Diesel Fuel	1203	35
Diesel Oil		35
Diethanolamine		20
Diethoxyethane	1153	38
Diethoxymethane	2373	38

Chemical Name	UN/NA/PIN	Guideline Number
2,5-Diethoxy-4-morpholinobenzene-diazonium Zinc Chloride	3036	10
Diethoxypropene	2374	59
Diethylamine	1154	20
Diethylaminoethanol	2686	20
Diethylaminopropylamine	2684	20
Diethyl Aniline	2432	32
Diethylarsine		73
Diethylbenzene	2049	24
Diethylcarbamazine Citrate		10
Diethyl Carbonate	2366	37
Diethyl Cellosolve	1153	40
Diethyl Chlorophosphate		49
Diethyl 2-chlorovinyl Phosphate		49
Diethyl Dichlorosilane	1767	107
Di(2-ethylhexyl)phthalate		37
Diethylene Glycol		40
Diethylene Glycol Abietate		40
Diethylene Glycol Mono and Di Esters		40
Diethylene Triamine	2079	20
Diethyl Ether	1155	38
Diethylethylene Diamine	2685	20
Di-(2-ethylhexyl) Peroxydicarbonate	2122	8
Di-(2-ethylhexyl) Peroxydicarbonate	2123	8
Di-(2-ethylhexyl) Peroxydicarbonate	2960	8
Di-(2-ethylhexyl) Phosphoric Acid	1902	15
Diethyl Isopropylthiomethyl Dithiophosphate		49
Diethyl Ketone	1156	42
N,N-Diethyl Lysergamide	2811	134
Diethylmagnesium	1367	82

Chemical Name	UN/ NA/PIN	Guideline Number
Diethyl-*p*-nitrophenyl Phosphate (Paraoxon)		49
Diethyl Peroxydicarbonate	2175	8
Diethyl Phthalate		37
Diethyl Propylmethyl-pyrimidyl Thiophosphate		49
O,O-Diethyl O-Pyrazinyl Phosphorothioate		49
Diethylstilbestrol		10
O,O-Diethyl S-[2-(Diethylamino)ethyl] Phosphorothiolate		49, 135
Diethyl Sulfate	1594	105
Diethyl Sulfide	2375	105
Diethylthiophosphoryl Chloride	2751	49
Diethylzinc	1366	88
Difluorochloroethane	2517	27
Difluoroethane	1030	27
Difluoroethylene	1959	27
1,1-Difluoroethylene	1959	27
Difluoromonochloroethane	2517	27
Difluorophosphoric Acid, anhydrous	1768	14
Digitoxin		10
Diglycidyl Ether		38
Digoxin		10
2,2-Dihydroperoxy Propane	2178	8
Dihydropyran	2376	24
Dihydrorotenone		53
Dihydrosafrole		44
Di(1-hydroxycyclohexyl) Peroxide	2148	8
2,6-Diiodo-4-nitrophenol		62
Diisobutylamine	2361	20
Diisobutyl Carbinol		30
Diisobutylene	2050	33
Diisobutyl Ketone	1157	42

Chemical Name	UN/ NA/PIN	Guideline Number
Diisobutyryl Peroxide	2182	8
Diisooctyl Acid Phosphate	1902	15
Diisopropylamine	1158	20
S-(2-Diisopropyl-aminoethyl) Methylphosphonothiolate	2810	135
S-(2-Diisopropyl-aminoethyl) O-Ethyl Methyl Phosphonothiolate	2810	135
S-2((2-Diisopropyl-amino)ethyl) O-Ethyl Methylphosphonothiolate	2810	135
S-2-Diisopropyl-aminoethyl O-Ethyl Methylphosphonothioate	2810	135
Diisopropylbenzene Hydroperoxide	2171	8
Diisopropylethanolamine	2825	20
Diisopropyl Ether	1159	38
Diisopropyl Fluorophosphate		49
Diisopropyl Peroxydicarbonate	2134	8
Diisopropyl Peroxy-dicarbonate, technical pure	2133	8
Diisotridecylperoxy-dicarbonate	2889	8
Diketene	2521	42
Dilan		55
Dilauroyl Peroxide, not more than 42%, in water	2893	8
Dilauroyl Peroxide, technical pure	2124	8
Dimefox	2783	49
Di-1-*p*-menthene		34
Dimetan		50
Dimethlaminoethanol	2051	20
Dimethoate		49
3,3′-Dimethoxybenzidine		32

Chemical Name	UN/ NA/PIN	Guideline Number
Dimethoxyethane	2252	40
Dimethoxyethane	2377	40
1,1-Dimethoxyethane	2377	40
1,2-Dimethoxyethane	2252	40
Dimethrin		52
Dimethylamidoethoxy-phosphoryl Cyanide	2810	135
Dimethylamine, anhydrous	1032	20
Dimethylamine Solution	1160	20
Dimethylaminoacetonitrile	2378	90
4-Dimethylaminoazobenzene		32
Dimethylaminoazobenzene		32
4-Dimethylamino-6 (2-dimethylaminoethoxy) toluene-2-diazonium Zinc Chloride	3039	88
Dimethylaminoethanol	2051	20
Dimethylaminoethoxy-cyanophosphine Oxide	2810	135
Dimethylaminoethyl Methacrylate	2522	37
Dimethylaniline	2253	32
N,N-Dimethylaniline	2253	32
7,12-Dimethylbenz(a)-anthracene		24
3,3'-Dimethylbenzidine		32
Di(2-methylbenzoyl) Peroxide	2593	8
Dimethylbutane	2457	33
1,3-Dimethylbutylamine	2379	20
Dimethylbutylamine	2379	20
Dimethylcarbamoyl Chloride	2262	10
Dimethyl Carbonate	1161	37
Dimethyl Chlorothiophosphate	2267	49
Dimethylcyclohexane	2263	33
2,3-Dimethylcyclohexyl Amine	2264	10, 20
2,5-Dimethyl-2,5-di-(benzoylperoxy) Hexane	2173	8
2,5-Dimethyl-2,5-di-(benzoylperoxy) Hexane	2959	8
2,5-Dimethyl-2,5-di-(benzoylperoxy) Hexane, technical pure	2172	8
2,5-Dimethyl-2,5-di-(*tert*-butylperoxy) Hexane	2156	8
2,5-Dimethyl-2,5-di-(*tert*-butylperoxy) Hexane, technical pure	2155	8
2,5-Dimethyl-2,5-di-(*tert*-butylperoxy) Hexyne-3, technical pure	2158	8
2,5-Dimethyl-2,5-di-(*tert*-butylperoxy) Hexyne-3, with not more than 52% peroxide in inert solid	2159	8
Dimethyldichlorosilane	1162	107
Dimethyldiethoxysilane	2380	107
2,5-Dimethyl-2,5-di-(2-ethyl-hexanoylperoxy) Hexane, technical pure	2157	8
2,5-Dimethyl-2,5-dihydro-peroxy Hexane	2174	8
3,5-Dimethyl-3,5-dihydroxy-dioxolane-1,2	2080	40
3,5-Dimethyl-3,5-dihydroxy-dioxolane-1,2, not more than 32% as a paste	3061	40
2,5-Dimethyl-2,5-di-(iso-nonanoylperoxy) Hexane, not more than 77% in solution	3060	8
Dimethyldioxane	2707	39
Dimethyldisulfide	2381	105

Chemical Name	UN/ NA/PIN	Guideline Number
2,5-Dimethyl-2,5-di-(3,5,5-trimethyl-hexanoylperoxy) Hexane, not more than 77% in solution	3060	8
Dimethylethanolamine	2051	20
Dimethyl Ether	1033	38
Dimethylformamide	2265	10
N,N-Dimethylformamide	2265	10
Dimethylamine, anhydrous		20
Dimethylhydrazine, symmetrical	2382	23
Dimethylhydrazine, unsymmetrical	1163	23
1,1-Dimethylhydrazine	1163	23
Dimethylmagnesium	1368	82
3,3-Dimethyl-*n*-but-2-yl Methylphosphonofluridate	2810	135
Dimethyl-*p*-nitrosoaniline	1369	32
2,4-Dimethylphenol		44
Dimethyl-*p*-phenylenediamine		20
Dimethyl Phosphoro-chloridothioate	2267	49
Dimethyl Phthalate		37
Dimethylpropane	2044	33
Dimethyl–Propylamine	2266	20
Dimethyl Sulfate	1595	105
Dimethyl Sulfide	1164	105
Dimethyl Thiophosphoryl Chloride	2267	49
Dimethylzinc	1370	88
Dimetilan		50
Dimyristyl Peroxydicarbonate	2595	8
Dimyristyl Peroxy-dicarbonate, not more than 42%, in water	2892	8
4,6-Dinitro-o-amylphenol		62
Dinitroaniline	1596	32
Dinitrobenzenes	1597	32
Dinitrobenzene Solution	1597	32
Dinitrochlorobenzene	1577	32
Dinitro-*o*-cresol	1598	44
4,6-Dinitro-*o*-cresol		44
4,6-Dinitro-*o*-cresol and salts		44
Dinitrocyclohexyl Phenol	9026	62
4,6-Dinitro-*o*-cyclohexylphenol		62
Dinitrogen Tetroxide	1067	48
Dinitrophenol	1320	62
Dinitrophenol, wet, with not less than 15% water	1320	62
Dinitrophenol, solution, in water or flammable liquids	1599	62
2,4-Dinitrophenol	0076	62
2,4-Dinitrophenol, wet, with not less than 15% water	1320	62
2,4-Dinitrophenol, solution, in water or flammable liquids	1599	62
2,5-Dinitrophenol		62
2,6-Dinitrophenol		62
Dinitrophenolate, wet, with not less than 15% water	1321	62
Dinitroresorcinol, wet, with not less than 15% water	1322	62
Dinitroso-dimethyl Terephthalamide	2973	10
Dinitrosopentamethylene Tetramine	2972	20
Dinitrotoluene, molten	1600	32
Dinitrotoluene, solid	2038	32
2,4-Dinitrotoluene		32
2,6-Dinitrotoluene		32
3,4-Dinitrotoluene		32
Dinocap		62

Chemical Name	UN/ NA/PIN	Guideline Number
Di–Nonanoyl Peroxide	2130	8
Di–Octanoyl Peroxide	2129	8
Dinoseb		62
Dinoterb		62
n-Dioctylphthalate		37
Di–Octyl Phthalate		37
Dioxacarb		50
1,4-Dioxane		39
Dioxane	1165	39
Dioxathion	2783	49
Dioxolane	1166	40
Dipentene	2052	34
Diperoxy Azelaic Acid	2958	8
Diperoxydodecane Diacid, not more than 42%, with not less than 56% sodium sulfate	3063	8, 105
Diphacinone		71
Diphenadione		71
Di-(2-phenoxyethyl) Peroxydicarbonate, not more than 85% with water	3059	8
Di-(2-phenoxyethyl) Peroxydicarbonate, technical pure	3058	8
Diphenylamine		32
Diphenylamine-chloroarsine	1698	72
Diphenylarsinous Chloride	1699	72, 140
Diphenylarsinous Cyanide	2810	72, 140
Diphenylchloroarsine	1699	72, 140
Diphenylcyanoarsine	2810	72, 140
Diphenyl Dichlorosilane	1769	107
1,2-Diphenylhydrazine		23
Diphenylmethyl Bromide	1770	95
Diphenylmethane-4,4′-diisocyanate (MDI)	2489	94
Diphenyloxide-4,4′-disulfohydrazide	2951	23

Chemical Name	UN/ NA/PIN	Guideline Number
Diphosgen	1076	101, 133
Diphosgene	1076	101, 133
Diphosphoramide, octamethyl		49
Dipicryl Sulfide, wet, with not less than 10% water	2852	47
Diproprionyl Peroxide	2132	8
Dipropylamine	2383	20
4-Dipropylaminobenzene-diazonium Zinc Chloride	3034	88
Dipropylene Glycol		40
Dipropylene Triamine	2269	20
Dipropyl Ether	2384	38
Dipropyl Ketone	2710	42
Di–propyl Peroxy-dicarbonate, technical pure	2176	8
Diquat	2781	66
Diquat Dibromide		66, 95
Disinfectant, liquid, corrosive, n.o.s.	1903	13
Disinfectant, liquid, poisonous, n.o.s.	3142	10
Disinfectant, solid, poisonous, n.o.s.	1601	10
Disodium Methanearsonate		72
Dispersant Gas, flammable, n.o.s.	1954	2
Dispersant Gas, n.o.s.	1078	3
Distearyl Peroxydicarbonate	2592	8
Distilled Mustard	2810	139
Disuccinic Acid Peroxide, not more than 72%, in water	2962	8
Disuccinic Acid Peroxide, technical pure	2135	8
Disulfoton	2783	49
Dithiazanine Iodide		10
Dithiobiuret		105

Chemical Name	UN/ NA/PIN	Guideline Number
Dithiocarbamate Pesticide, n.o.s	2711	63
Dithiocarbamate Pesticide, flammable liquid, n.o.s.	2772	63
Dithiocarbamate Pesticide, flammable liquid, n.o.s.	3005	63
Dithiocarbamate Pesticide, liquid, n.o.s.	3006	63
Dithiocarbamate Pesticide, solid, n.o.s.	2771	63
Di-(3,5,5-trimethyl-1,2-dioxolanyl-3) Peroxide	2597	8
Di-(3,5,5-trimethyl-hexanoyl) Peroxide	2128	8
Diuron		10
Divinyl Ether, inhibited	1167	38
D-Lysergic Acid Diethylamide	2811	134
DM	1698	140
DMC (Di-(*p*-chlorophenyl) methylcarbinol)		55
Dodecylbenzene-Sulfonic Acid	2584	15
Dodecyl Trichlorosilane	1771	107
Donovan's Solution		72, 84
Dowicides		44
DP	1076	101, 133
Drier, paint or varnish, liquid, n.o.s	1168	10
Drier, paint or varnish, solid, n.o.s.	1371	10
Drier, paint, solid, n.o.s.	1371	10
2,4-D Salts		60
Drugs, n.o.s.	1851	10
Dry Ice	1845	92
Dye, corrosive, n.o.s.	2801	13
Dye, poisonous, n.o.s.	1602	10
Dye, solid, n.o.s., or Dye Intermediate, solid, corrosive, n.o.s.	3147	13
Dye, solid, n.o.s., or Dye Intermediate, solid, poisonous, n.o.s.	3143	10
Dye Intermediate, corrosive, n.o.s.	2801	13
Dye Intermediate, poisonous, n.o.s.	1602	10
EA 1033	2810	139
EA 1034	2810	72, 139
EA 1205	2810	135
EA 1210	2810	135
EA 1701	2810	135
Eastern Equine Encephalitis (EEE)		129
Ebola Virus		130
E coli		117
ED	1892	72, 139
EDE		28
EEE		129
Electrolyte, acid	1735	14
Electrolyte, alkaline	2797	19
Electrolyte, battery fluid acid	2796	10, 13
Emetine, dihydrochloride		10
EMMI		84
Enamel	1263	10, 35
Endemic Typhus Fever		128
Endosulfan	2761	56
alpha-Endosulfan		56
beta-Endosulfan		56
Endosulfan Sulfate		56
Endothal		63
Endothall		63
Endothion		49
Endrin mixture, dry or liquid	2761	56

Chemical Name	UN/ NA/PIN	Guideline Number
Endrin Aldehyde		56
Engine Starting Fluid	1960	35
Environmentally Hazardous Substance, liquid, n.o.s.	3082	10
Environmentally Hazardous Substance, solid, n.o.s.	3077	10
Epibromohydrin	2558	61
Epichlorohydrin	2023	61
Epidemic Typhus Fever		128
Epinephrine		10
EPN	2783	49
Epoxyethane	1040	45
Epoxyethoxypropane	2752	38
1,2-Epoxy-3-ethoxypropane	2752	38
1,2-Epoxy-3-ethyloxy-propane	2752	38
EPTC		63
Eradicator, paint or grease, flammable liquid	1850	5
Erbon		60
Ergocalciferol		10
Ergotamine Tartrate		10
Escherichia coli O157:H7		117
ET-15		49
Etching Acid, liquid	1790	14, 16
Ethane, compressed	1035	33
Ethane, refrigerated liquid (cryogenic liquid)	1961	33
Ethane-Propane Mixture, refrigerated liquid (cryogenic liquid)	1961	33
Ethanesulfonyl Chloride		26
Ethanol, and solutions	1170	29
Ethanolamine, and solutions	2491	20
Ether	1155	38
Ethiofencarb		50
Ethion (ETO)	2783	49
Ethoxyethanol	1171	40
2-Ethoxyethanol	1171	40
Ethoxyethyl Acetate	1172	40
2-Ethoxyethyl Acetate	1172	40
Ethoxypropane	2615	38
Ethyl Acetate	1173	37
Ethyl Acetylene, inhibited	2452	33, 92
Ethyl Acrylate, inhibited	1917	37
Ethyl Alcohol	1170	29
Ethyl Aluminum Dichloride	1924	10
Ethyl Aluminum Sesquichloride	1925	10
Ethylamine	1036	20
Ethylamine solution	2270	20
Ethyl Amyl Ketone	2271	42
Ethylaniline	2272	32
2-Ethylaniline	2273	32
Ethylbenzene	1175	24
Ethylbenzylaniline	2274	32
Ethylbenzyl Toluidine	2753	32
Ethylbis(2-chloroethyl) amine	2810	139
Ethyl Biscoumacetate		71
Ethyl Borate	1176	103
Ethyl Bromide	1891	95
Ethyl Bromoacetate	1603	96
Ethylbutanol	2275	30
Ethylbutyl Acetate	1177	37
Ethyl Butyl Ether	1179	38
Ethyl Butyraldehyde	1178	41
Ethyl Butyrate	1180	37
Ethyl Chloride	1037	26
Ethyl Chloroacetate	1181	37
Ethyl Chloroformate	1182	37
Ethyl Chloropropionate	2935	37
Ethyl Chlorothioformate	2826	37
Ethyl Crotonate	1862	37

Chemical Name	UN/ NA/PIN	Guideline Number
Ethyl Cyanoacetate	2666	37
Ethyl 3,3-di(*tert*-butylperoxy)butyrate	2184	8
Ethyl 3,3-di(*tert*-butylperoxy)butyrate	2598	8
Ethyl 3,3-di(*tert*-butylperoxy)butyrate, not more than 77%	2185	8
Ethyl Dichloroarsine	1892	72, 136
Ethyldichlorosilane	1183	107
Ethyldimethylamino-cyanophosphonate	2810	135
Ethyl Dimethyl-phosphoramidocyanidate	2810	135
Ethylene, compressed	1962	33, 92
Ethylene, refrigerated liquid (cryogenic liquid)	1038	33, 92
Ethylene, Acetylene, and Propylene Mixture, refrigerated liquid (cryogenic liquid), containing at least 71.5% ethylene, with not more than 22.5% acetylene and not more than 6% propylene	3138	33, 92
Ethylene Chlorohydrin	1135	28, 61
Ethylene, compressed	1962	33
Ethylenediamine	1604	20
Ethylenediamine Tetra-acetic Acid	9117	20
Ethylene Dibromide	1605	95
Ethylene Dichloride	1184	26
Ethylene Fluorohydrin		64
Ethylene Glycol		40
Ethylene Glycol Alkyl and (Aryl) Esters		40
Ethylene Glycol Diethyl Ether	1153	40
Ethylene Glycol Dinitrate		47
Ethylene Glycol Monobutyl Ether	2369	40
Ethylene Glycol Monoethyl Ether	1171	40
Ethylene Glycol Monoethyl Ether Acetate	1172	40
Ethylene Glycol Monomethyl Ether	1188	40
Ethylene Glycol Monomethyl Ether and Acetate	1189	40
Ethyleneimine, inhibited	1185	20
Ethylene Oxide	1040	45, 133, 138
Ethylene Oxide–Carbon Dioxide Mixture, with more than 6% ethylene oxide	1041	45, 92
Ethylene Oxide–Carbon Dioxide Mixture, with not more than 6% ethylene oxide	1952	45, 92
Ethylene Oxide and Dichlorodifluoro Methane Mixture, with not more than 12% ethylene oxide	3070	27, 45
Ethylene, refrigerated liquid (cryogenic liquid)	1038	33, 92
Ethylene Oxide–Propylene Oxide Mixture	2983	45
Ethyl Ester of Dimethyl-phosphoroamidocyanidic Acid	2810	135
Ethyl Ether	1155	38
Ethyl Fluid	1649	33
Ethyl Fluoride	2453	27
Ethyl Formate	1190	37
Ethyl Hexaldehyde	1191	41
2-Ethyl Hexaldehyde	1191	41
2-Ethylhexyl Alcohol		30
Ethyl Hexylamine	2276	20

Chemical Name	UN/ NA/PIN	Guideline Number
Ethyl Hexylchloroformate	2748	37
Ethyl Isobutyrate	2385	37
Ethyl Isocyanate	2481	94
Ethyl Lactate	1192	37
Ethyl Mercaptan	2363	105
Ethyl Mercuric Chloride		84
Ethyl Mercuri-2-3-dihydroxypropylmercaptide		84
N-Ethylmercuri-*p*-toluene Sulfonanilide		84
Ethyl Mercury Phosphate		84
Ethyl Methacrylate	2277	37
Ethyl Methyl Ether	1039	38
Ethyl Methyl Ketone	1193	42
Ethyl Methyl Ketone Peroxide	2550	8, 42
Ethyl Methyl Ketone Peroxide, with not more than 60%, in solution	2127	8, 42
Ethyl *N,N*-dimethyl-phosphoramidocyanidate	2810	135
Ethyl Nitrate	1993	47
Ethyl Nitrite, and solutions	1194	47
Ethyl Orthoformate	2524	37
Ethyl Oxalate	2525	17
Ethyl Phenyl Dichlorosilane	2435	107
Ethylphosphonothioic-Dichloride, Anhydrous	1760	13
Ethyl Phosphonous Dichloride Anhydrous	2845	109
Ethyl Phosphorodi-chloridate	1760	13
Ethyl Phosphorodimethyl-amidocyanidate	2810	135
Ethyl Piperidine	2386	20
Ethyl Propionate	1195	37
2-Ethyl-3-propyl Acrolein		59
Ethyl Propyl Ether	2615	38

Chemical Name	UN/ NA/PIN	Guideline Number
O-Ethyl S-(Diisopropylaminoethyl) methylphosphonothioate	2810	135
Ethyl S-Dimethylaminoethyl-methylphosphonothiolate	2810	135
O-Ethyl S-(2-Diisopropylaminoethyl) methylthiophosphonoate	2810	135
O-Ethyl S-(2-Diisopropylaminoethyl) methylphosphonothiolate	2810	135
Ethyl Silicate	1292	107
O-Ethyl S,S-Dipropyl Phosphorodithioate		49
Ethyl Sulfate	1594	15
Ethyl Sulfuric Acid	2571	15
Ethyl Toluidine	2754	32
Ethyltrichlorosilane	1196	107
Etiologic Agent, n.o.s.	2814	11
ETO	1040	45, 133, 138
Eucalyptol		36
Eugenol		44
Explosive A		1
Explosive B		1
Explosive C		1
Extract, aromatic, liquid	1169	24
Extract, flavoring, liquid	1197	5
Fabric, animal or vegetable with oil, n.o.s.	1373	5
Fenac		60
Fenamiphos		49
Fenitrothion		49
Fensulfothion	2765	49
Fenthion	2765	49
Fenvalerate		52
Ferbam		63
Ferric Ammonium Citrate	9118	79
Ferric Arsenate	1606	72, 79

ALPHABETICAL INDEX

Chemical Name	UN/ NA/PIN	Guideline Number
Ferric Arsenite	1607	72, 79
Ferric Chloride, anhydrous	1773	79
Ferric Chloride Solution	2582	79
Ferric Cyanide		90
Ferric Fluoride	9120	79, 99
Ferric Nitrate	1466	47, 79
Ferric Salts		79
Ferric Subsulfate		79
Ferric Sulfate	9121	79
Ferrocerium	1323	79
Ferrocholinate		79
Ferrosilicon	1408	79
Ferrous Arsenate	1608	72, 79
Ferrous Chloride, solid	1759	79
Ferrous Chloride Solution	1760	79
Ferrous Metal, borings, cuttings, shavings, or turnings	2793	79
Ferrous Salts		79
Ferrous Sulfate	9125	79
Fertilizer Ammoniating Solution, with more than 35% free ammonia	1043	21, 47
Fiber, animal or vegetable, burnt, wet, or damp, n.o.s.	1372	9
Fiber, animal or vegetable, with oil, n.o.s.	1373	5
Film, motion picture, nitrocellulose base	1324	6
Film, nitrocellulose base	1324	6
Fire Extinguisher, with compressed or liquefied gas	1044	92
Fire Extinguisher Charge, corrosive liquid	1774	13
Fire Lighter, solid, with flammable liquid	2623	33
Fish Meal and Scrap, stabilized	2216	9

Chemical Name	UN/ NA/PIN	Guideline Number
Fish Meal and Scrap, unstabilized	1374	9
Flammable Gas, in lighter, for cigars, cigarettes, etc.	1057	33
Flammable Gas, n.o.s.	1954	2
Flammable Liquid, corrosive, n.o.s.	2924	5, 13
Flammable Liquid, n.o.s.	1993	5
Flammable Liquid, poisonous, n.o.s.	1992	5, 10
Flammable Liquid Preparations n.o.s.	1142	5
Flammable Solid, corrosive, n.o.s.	2925	6, 13
Flammable Solid, n.o.s	1325	6
Flammable Solid, oxidizing, n.o.s.	3097	6, 7
Flammable Solid, poisonous, n.o.s.	2926	6, 10
Flea-borne Typhus Fever		128
Flue Dust, poisonous	2811	10
Fluoboric Acid	1775	16, 103
Fluoracetic Acid	2642	64
Fluoric Acid	1790	16
Fluorides		99
Fluorine, compressed	1045	99, 133, 138
Fluorine, refrigerated liquid (cryogenic liquid)	9192	99, 133, 138
Fluoroacetamide		64
Fluoroacetate (1080)	2642	64
Fluoroacetic Acid	2642	64
Fluoroaniline	2941	32
Fluoroaniline	2944	32
Fluorobenzene	2387	25
Fluoromethyl-pinacolyloxphosphine Oxide	2810	135

Chemical Name	UN/ NA/PIN	Guideline Number
Fluorophosphoric Acid, anhydrous	1776	14
Fluorosilicates, n.o.s.	2856	99
Fluorosulfonic Acid	1777	14
Fluorosulphonic Acid	1777	14
Fluorotoluene	2388	24
Fluosilicate Salts	2856	99
Fluosilicic Acid	1778	16
FM		137
Fog Oil		137
Formaldehyde solution (formalin)	2209	41
Formaldehyde solution (formalin)	1198	41
Formalin	1078	41
Formetanate		50
Formic Acid	1779	15
Four Corners Virus		119
Fowler's Solution		72
Francis Disease		127
Francisella Tularensis		127
Freon		27
Fuel, aviation, turbine engine	1863	35
Fuel, pyrophoric, n.o.s.	1375	5
Fuel Oil	1993	35
Fumaric Acid	9126	15
Fumaryl Chloride	1780	15
Fumigants	1062	10
Fumigants	2191	10
Fungicide, corrosive, n.o.s.	1759	10, 13
Fungicide, poisonous, n.o.s.	2902	10
Furan	2389	33
Furfural	1199	41
Furfuryl Alcohol	2874	30
Furfurylamine	2526	20
Fusel Oil	1201	30

Chemical Name	UN/ NA/PIN	Guideline Number
GA	2810	135
Gallic Acid		15
Gallium, metal	2803	10
Gas Drips, hydrocarbon	1864	35
Gasohol	1203	35
Gas Oil	1202	35
Gasoline	1203	35
GB	2810	135
GD	2810	135
Germane, Germanium Hydride	2192	73
Germanium Hydride	2192	73
GF	2810	135
Glanders		118
Glifonox		68
Glutaraldehyde		41
Glycerol-alpha-mono-chlorohydrin	2689	61
Glyceryl Trinitrate Solution	1204	1, 47
Glycidaldehyde	2622	41
Glycofurol		40
Glycolic Acid		15
Glyphosate		68
Glyphosate Isopropylamine Salt		68
Glyphosate Mono (Isopropylamine) Salt		68
Gold Bronze Powder		78
Green Monkey Disease		130
Grenade, tear gas	2017	9, 136
Grenade, without bursting charge, with poisonous gas	2016	10
Guaiacol		44
Guanidine Nitrate	1467	20
Guthion	2783	49
Gutta-Percha Solution	1205	34
H	2810	139
Hafnium and Compounds	2545	6

Chemical Name	UN/ NA/PIN	Guideline Number
Hafnium Metal, powder, dry	2545	6
Hafnium Metal, powder, wet	1326	6
Halogenated Irritating Liquid, n.o.s.	1610	26
Halogenated Solvents	1610	26
Halons	1078	27
Hantavirus		119
Hay	1327	6
Hazardous Substance, liquid or solid, n.o.s.	9188	10
Hazardous Waste, liquid or solid, n.o.s.	9189	10
HC		137
HD	2810	139
Helium, compressed	1046	92
Helium-Oxygen Mixture	1980	92
Helium, refrigerated liquid (cryogenic liquid)	1963	92
Hendecane	2330	35
Heptachlor	2761	54
Heptachlor Epoxide		54
n-Heptaldehyde	3056	41
Heptane	1206	33
n-Heptane	1206	33
Heptene	2278	33
Hexachloroacetone	2661	42
Hexachlorobenzene	2729	57
Hexachloro-1,3-butadiene		26
Hexachlorobutadiene	2279	26
Hexachlorocyclohexane	2761	57
Hexachlorocyclopentadiene	2646	26
Hexachloro-epoxy-octahydro-dimethanonaphthalene		56
Hexachloroethane	9037	137
Hexachloronaphthalene		43
Hexachlorophene	2875	26, 44
Hexachloropropene		26

Chemical Name	UN/ NA/PIN	Guideline Number
Hexadecyl Alcohol		30
Hexadecyl Trichlorosilane	1781	107
Hexadiene	2458	33
Hexaethyl Tetraphosphate	1611	49
Hexaethyl Tetraphosphate and Compressed Gas Mixture	1612	49
Hexaethyl Tetraphosphate Mixture	2783	49
Hexafluoroacetone	2420	42
Hexafluoroacetone Hydrate	2552	42
Hexafluoroethane	2193	26
Hexafluorophosphoric Acid	1782	14
Hexafluoropropylene	1858	26
Hexafluoropropylene Oxide	1956	26, 38
Hexahydrocresol	2617	44
Hexaldehyde	1207	41
Hexanoic Acid	1760	15
Hexamethylene Diamine, solid	2280	20
Hexamethylene Diamine, solution	1783	20
3,3,6,6,9,9-Hexamethyl-1,2,4,5-tetraoxocylcononane	2166	8
3,3,6,6,9,9-Hexamethyl-1,2,4,5-tetraoxocylcononane	2167	8
3,3,6,6,9,9-Hexamethyl-1,2,4,5-tetraoxocylcononane, technical pure	2165	8
Hexamethylene Diamine, solid	2280	20
Hexamethylene Diamine, solution	1783	20
Hexamethylene Diisocyanate	2281	94
Hexamethyleneimine	2493	20
Hexamethylenetetramine		20

Chemical Name	UN/ NA/PIN	Guideline Number
Hydrogen Chloride Solution	1789	14
Hydrogen, compressed	1049	2, 92
Hydrogen, refrigerated liquid (cryogenic liquid)	1966	2, 92
Hydrogen Cyanide, anhydrous, stabilized	1051	90, 132, 138
Hydrogen Cyanide, anhydrous, stabilized (absorbed)	1614	90, 132 138
Hydrogen Fluoride, anhydrous	1052	16, 133, 138
Hydrogen Fluoride Solution	1790	16, 133, 138
Hydrogen Iodide, anhydrous	2197	100
Hydrogen Iodide Solution	1787	100
Hydrogen and Methane Mixture, compressed	2034	92
Hydrogen Peroxide–Peroxyacetic Acid Mixture, with acid(s), water, and not more than 5% peroxyacetic acid, stabilized	3149	7
Hydrogen Peroxide, stabilized, with more than 52% peroxide	2015	7
Hydrogen Peroxide Solution, with not less than 8% but less than 20% peroxide	2984	7
Hydrogen Peroxide Solution, with not less than 20% but more than 52% peroxide	2014	7
Hydrogen Phosphide	2199	108
Hydrogen Selenide, anhydrous	2202	86
Hydrogen Sulfide	1053	91, 138
Hydrogen Sulfide, liquefied	1053	91,138

Chemical Name	UN/ NA/PIN	Guideline Number
Hydroperoxide		7
Hydroquinone	2662	32, 44
Hydroselenic Acid	2202	14, 86
Hydrosilicofluoric Acid	1778	16
3-(2-Hydroxyethoxy)-4-pyrrolidin-1-ylbenzene-diazonium Zinc Chloride	3035	88
1-Hydroxy-1′-Hydroperoxy Dicyclohexyl Peroxide	2118	8
1-Hydroxy-1′-Hydroperoxy Dicyclohexyl Peroxide	2119	8
1-Hydroxy-1′-Hydroperoxy Dicyclohexyl Peroxide, more than 90%, with less than 10% water	2117	8
Hydroxylamine		20
Hydroxylamine Sulfate	2865	20
Hydroxymercuricresol		84
Hydroxymercurinitrophenol		47, 84
Hydroxyphenyl-mercurichloride		84
4-Hydroxy-3-nitrophenylarsonic Acid		72
Hypochlorite Solution, with more than 5% available chlorine	1791	22
Igniter for Aircraft Thrust Device	2792	6
Imidan		49
Iminobispropylamine	2269	20
Iminodipropylamine	2269	20
Indeno(1,2,3-cd)pyrene		24
Infectious Substance, affecting animals only	2900	11
Infectious Substance, affecting humans	2814	11
Ink	1210	5
Insecticide, dry, n.o.s.	2588	10
Insecticide, liquid, n.o.s.	1993	10

Chemical Name	UN/ NA/PIN	Guideline Number
Insecticide, liquid, poisonous, n.o.s.	2902	10
Insecticide Gas, n.o.s.	1968	10
Insecticide Gas, poisonous, n.o.s.	1967	10, 49
Iodine Monochloride	1792	100
Iodine Pentafluoride	2495	16, 100
Iodo Butane	2390	26
Iodo Methylpropane	2391	26
Iodo Propane	2392	26
IPDI	2290	94
Iprit S-Lost	2810	139
Iron Carbonyl	1994	79
Iron Chloride, solid	1773	79
Iron Chloride Solution	2582	79
Iron Oxide, spent	1376	79
Iron Pentacarbonyl	1994	79
Iron Sponge, spent	1376	79
Iron Swarf	2793	79
Irritating Agent, n.o.s.	1693	9
Isoamyl Acetate		37
Isoamyl Alcohol	1105	30
Isobenzan		57
Isobutane or Isobutane Mixture	1969	92
Isobutanol	1212	30
Isobutyl Acetate	1213	37
Isobutyl Acrylate	2527	37
Isobutyl Alcohol	1212	30
Isobutyl Aldehyde	2045	41
Isobutylamine	1214	20
Isobutyl Chloroformate	2742	15
Isobutylene	1055	33
Isobutyl Formate	2393	37
Isobutyl Isobutyrate	2528	37
Isobutyl Isocyanate	2486	94
Isobutyl Methacrylate	2283	37

Chemical Name	UN/ NA/PIN	Guideline Number
Isobutyl Methyl Ketone Peroxide	2126	8, 42
Isobutyl Propionate	2394	37
Isobutyraldehyde	2045	41
Isobutyric Acid	2529	15
Isobutyric Anhydride	2530	15
Isobutyronitrile	2284	90
Isobutyryl Chloride	2395	26
Isocyantes and solutions, flammable, n.o.s.	2478	94
Isocyantes and Solutions, n.o.s., b.p. less than 300° C	2206	94
Isocyantes and Solutions, n.o.s., b.p. not less than 300° C	2207	94
Isocyantes and Solutions, n.o.s., FP not less than 23° C and not more than 60.5° C	3080	94
Isocyanato-benzotrifluoride	2285	94, 99
Isocyanic Acid		94
Isocyanuric Acid, chlorinated	2468	15
Isododecane	2286	33
Isodrin		56
Isofluorphate		49
Isoheptene	2287	33
Isohexene	2288	33
Isolan		50
Isononanoyl Peroxide, technical pure or in solution	2128	8
Isononyl Alcohol		30
Isooctane	1262	33
Isooctene	1216	33
Isooctyl Alcohol		30
Isopentane	1265	33
Isopentanoic Acid	1760	15

Chemical Name	UN/ NA/PIN	Guideline Number
Isopentene	2371	33
Isophoronediamine	2289	20
Isophorone		42
Isophorone Diisocyanate	2290	94
Isoprene, inhibited	1218	33
Isoprocarb		50
Isopropanolamine Dodecylbenzene Sulfonate		10
Isopropanol	1219	29
Isopropenyl Acetate	2403	37
Isopropenyl Benzene	2303	24
Isopropoxymethyl-phosphonyl Fluoride	2810	135
Isopropoxymethyl-phosphoryl Fluoride	2810	135
Isopropyl Acetate	1220	37
Isopropyl Acid Phosphate	1793	37
Isopropyl Alcohol	1219	29
Isopropyl Amine	1221	20
Isopropylbenzene	1918	24
Isopropyl Butyrate	2405	37
Isopropyl Chloroacetate	2947	37
Isopropyl Chloroformate	2407	37
Isopropyl Chloropropionate	2934	37
Isopropylcumyl Hydroperoxide	2171	8, 24
Isopropyl Ester of Methylphosphono-fluoridic Acid	2810	135
Isopropyl Ether	1159	38
Isopropyl Formate	2408	37
4,4′-Isopropylidenedi-phenol		44
Isopropyl Isobutyrate	2406	37
Isopropyl Isocyanate	2483	94
Isopropyl Mercaptan	2402	105
Isopropyl Mercaptan	2703	105

Chemical Name	UN/ NA/PIN	Guideline Number
Isopropyl Methylfluorophosphate	2810	135
Isopropyl Methyl-fluorophosphonate	2810	135
O-Isopropyl Methyl-isopropoxfluorophosphine Oxide	2810	135
O-Isopropyl Methyl-isopropoxfluorophosphine Oxide	2810	135
O-Isopropyl Methyl-phosphonochloride		135
Isopropyl Methyl-phosphonofluoridate	2810	135
Isopropylmethylpyrazolyl Dimethylcarbamate		50
Isopropyl Nitrate	1222	47
Isopropyl Peroxy-dicarbonate	2133	8
Isopropyl Peroxy-dicarbonate	2134	8
Isopropyl Propionate	2409	37
Isosafrole		44
Isosorbide Dinitrate Mixture	2907	47
Jet Fuel	1863	35
Kanechlor S		46
Kelthane		57
Kepone	2761	57
Kerosene	1223	35
Ketene		41
Ketone, liquid, n.o.s.	1224	42
Krypton, compressed	1056	92
Krypton, refrigerated liquid (cryogenic liquid)	1970	92
L	2810	72, 139
Lacquer	1263	35
Lacquer Base, dry	2557	35
Lacquer Base, liquid	1263	35
Lactic Acid		15

Chemical Name	UN/ NA/PIN	Guideline Number
Lactonitrile		90
Lannate	2757	50
Landrin		50
Lasiocarpine		10
Lassa Virus		130
Lauroyl Peroxide, not more than 42%	2893	8
Lauroyl Peroxide, technical pure	2124	8
Lauryl Alcohol		30
Lauryl Thiocyanate		94
Lead		80
Lead Acetate	1616	80
Lead Arsenate	1617	72, 80
Lead Arsenite	1618	72, 80
Lead Chloride	2291	80
Lead Chromate		80
Lead Compound, soluble, n.o.s.	2291	80
Lead Cyanide	1620	80, 90
Lead Dioxide	1872	80
Lead Fluoborate	2291	80, 103
Lead Fluoride	2811	80, 99
Lead, inorganic		80
Lead Iodide		80, 100
Lead Nitrate	1469	47, 80
Lead, organic		80
Lead Perchlorate	1470	80
Lead Peroxide	1872	80
Lead Phosphate		80
Lead Phosphite, dibasic	2989	80
Lead Stearate		80
Lead Subacetate		80
Lead Sulfate, with more than 3% free acid	1794	80
Lead Sulfide		80
Lead Tetraethyl	1649	80
Lead Tetramethyl	1649	80

Chemical Name	UN/ NA/PIN	Guideline Number
Lead Thiocyanate		80, 94
Leptophos		49
Lethane 60		94
Lewisite	2810	72, 139
Lewisite (liquid arsenic compound)	2810	72, 139
Lewisite 2	2810	72, 139
Lewisite 3	2810	72, 139
Lighter, for cigarettes, with flammable gas	1057	33
Lighter, for cigarettes, with flammable liquid	1226	33
Lighter Fluid	1226	33
Lighter Refills, with flammable gas	1057	33
Lime		19
Limonene		34
Linamarin		90
Lindane	2761	57
Liquefied Gas, flammable, n.o.s.	1954	2
Liquefied Gas, flammable, poisonous, n.o.s.	1953	2, 10
Liquefied Gas, nonflammable, charged with nitrogen, carbon dioxide, or air	1058	3
Liquefied Gas, n.o.s.	1956	2
Liquefied Gas, poisonous, n.o.s.	1955	2, 10
Liquefied Natural Gas	1972	33, 92
Liquefied Nonflammable Gas, charged with nitrogen, carbon dioxide, or air	1058	3
Liquefied Petroleum Gas	1075	2, 35
Lithium Acetylide–Ethylenediamine Complex	2813	81
Lithium Alkyl	2445	81

ALPHABETICAL INDEX

Chemical Name	UN/ NA/PIN	Guideline Number
Lithium Aluminum Hydride	1410	81
Lithium Aluminum Hydride, ether solution	1411	81
Lithium Amide	1412	81
Lithium Batteries, contained in equipment	3091	81
Lithium Battery	9205	81
Lithium Battery	3090	81
Lithium Borohydride	1413	81, 103
Lithium Chromate		81
Lithium Ferrosilicon	2830	81
Lithium Hydride	1414	81
Lithium Hydride, fused, solid	2805	81
Lithium Hydroxide Monohydrate	2680	19, 81
Lithium Hydroxide Solution	2679	19, 81
Lithium Hypochlorite, dry, including mixtures with more than 39% available chlorine	1471	22, 81
Lithium Metal	1415	81
Lithium Nitrate	2722	47, 81
Lithium Nitride	2806	47, 81
Lithium Peroxide	1472	81
Lithium Silicon	1417	81
Lithopone		74, 88
LNG, Liquefied Natural Gas	1972	33
London Purple	1621	32, 72
LPG, Liquefied Petroleum Gas	1075	2, 35
LSD	2811	134
Lye, dry, solid	1823	19
Lysergic Acid Diethylamide	2811	134
Lye Solution	1824	19
Mace	1697	136

Chemical Name	UN/ NA/PIN	Guideline Number
Machupo Virus		130
Magnesium, pellets, turnings, or ribbon	1869	82
Magnesium Powder	1418	82
Magnesium Alkyl	3053	82
Magnesium Alloy, with more than 50% magnesium pellets, turnings, or ribbon	1869	82
Magnesium Alloy, with more than 50% magnesium, powder	1418	82
Magnesium Aluminum Phosphide	1419	82, 108
Magnesium Arsenate	1622	72, 82
Magnesium Bisulfite Solution	2693	82, 105
Magnesium Bromate	1473	82, 96
Magnesium Chlorate	2723	82, 97
Magnesium Diamide	2004	82
Magnesium Diphenyl	2005	82
Magnesium Fluorosilicate	2853	82, 99
Magnesium Granules, coated	2950	82
Magnesium Hydride	2010	82
Magnesium Nitrate	1474	47, 82
Magnesium Perchlorate	1475	82, 97
Magnesium Peroxide	1476	82
Magnesium Phosphide	2011	82, 108
Magnesium Silicide	2624	82
Magnesium Silicofluoride, solid	2853	82, 99
Malathion	2783	49
Maleic Acid	2215	15
Maleic Anhydride	2215	15
Maleic Hydrazide		15
Malonic Dinitrile	2647	90
Malonic Ethyl Ester Nitrile	2666	90
Malononitrile	2647	90

Chemical Name	UN/ NA/PIN	Guideline Number
Malta Fever		115
Mancozeb		50
Maneb	2210	63
Maneb, or Maneb Preparation(s), stabilized against self-heating	2968	63
Maneb, or Maneb Preparation(s), with 50% or more Maneb	2210	63
Manganese Nitrate	2724	47, 83
Manganese Resinate	1330	83
Manganese, Tricarbonyl-methylcyclopentadienyl		83
Marburg Virus		130
Matches, fusee	2254	97
Matches, safety	1944	97
Matches, strike anywhere	1331	97
Matches, wax (Vesta)	1945	97
Mba	2810	139
MBOCA		32
MCPA		60
MDI		94
Mechloroethamine	2810	139
Mecoprop		60
Medicines, n.o.s.	1851	10
Mediterranean Fever		115
Melioidosis		120
Melphalan		10
Menthane Hydroperoxide, para, technical pure	2125	8
Menthol		24
Menthyl Hydroperoxide, para, technical pure	2125	8
Mercaptan, liquid, n.o.s.	3071	105
Mercaptan Mixture, aliphatic	1228	105
Mercaptan Mixture, liquid, n.o.s.	3071	105
Mercaptans and Mixtures, liquid, n.o.s.	1228	105
Mercaptan and Mixtures, liquid, n.o.s.	1228	105
Mercaptan, liquid, n.o.s.	3071	105
Mercaptodimethur	2757	50
Mercuric Acetate	1629	84
Mercuric Arsenate	1623	72, 84
Mercuric Bromide	1634	84, 95
Mercuric Chloride	1624	84
Mercuric Cyanide	1636	84, 90
Mercuric Nitrate	1625	47, 84
Mercuric Oxide		84
Mercuric Oxycyanide	1642	84, 90
Mercuric Potassium Cyanide	1626	84, 90
Mercuric Sulfate	1645	84
Mercuric Thiocyanate		84, 94
Mercurol	1639	84
Mercurous Acetate	1629	84
Mercurous Bromide	1634	84, 95
Mercurous Chloride		84
Mercurous Nitrate	1627	47, 84
Mercurous Sulfate	1628	84
Mercury	2809	84
Mercury Acetate	1629	84
Mercury Ammonium Chloride	1630	84
Mercury-Based Pesticide, liquid, flammable, poisonous, n.o.s.	2778	84
Mercury-Based Pesticide, liquid, poisonous, flammable, n.o.s.	3011	84
Mercury-Based Pesticide, liquid poisonous, n.o.s.	3012	84
Mercury-Based Pesticide, solid, poisonous, n.o.s.	2777	84

Chemical Name	UN/ NA/PIN	Guideline Number
Mercury Benzoate	1631	84
Mercury Bisulfate	1633	84
Mercury Bromide	1634	84, 95
Mercury Compound, liquid, n.o.s.	2024	84
Mercury Compound, solid, n.o.s.	2025	84
Mercury Cyanide	1636	84, 90
Mercury, elemental	2809	84
Mercury Fulminate		84
Mercury Gluconate	1637	84
Mercury Iodide	1638	84, 100
Mercury, inorganic	1624	84
Mercury Metal	2809	84
Mercury Nucleate	1639	84
Mercury Oleate	1640	84
Mercury Oxide	1641	84
Mercury Oxycyanide	1642	84, 90
Mercury Oxycyanide, desensitized	1642	84, 90
Mercury Potassium Iodide	1643	84, 100
Mercury Salicylate	1644	84
Mercury Sulfate	1645	84
Mercury Thiocyanate	1646	84, 94
Merodicein		84
Mertect		70
Mertect 160		70
Mesitylene	2325	24
Mesityl Oxide	1229	42
Metal Alkyl, n.o.s.	2003	10
Metal Alkyl Halide, n.o.s.	3049	10
Metal Alkyl Hydride, n.o.s.	3050	10
Metal Alkyl Solution, n.o.s.	9195	10
Metal Catalyst, dry	2881	10
Metal Catalyst, finely divided, activated, or spent, wet, with not less than 40% water or other suitable liquid	1378	10
Metaldehyde	1332	41
Metal Powder, flammable, n.o.s.	3089	6, 10
Meta-Systox	2783	49
Methacrolein Diacetate		10
Methacrylaldehyde	2396	41
Methacrylic Acid, inhibited	2531	15
Methacrylic Anhydride		15
Methacrylonitrile, inhibited	3079	90
Methacryloyl Chloride		10
Methacryloyloxyethyl Isocyanate		94
Methallyl Alcohol	2614	30
Methamidophos		49
Methanamine		20
Methane, compressed	1971	33, 92
Methane, refrigerated liquid, (cryogenic liquid)	1972	33, 92
Methanesulfonyl Chloride	9265	49
Methanesulfonyl Fluoride		49
Methanol	1230	31
Methapyrilene		10
Methenamine		41
Methidathion		49
Methiocarb		50
Methomyl	2757	50
Methoxychlor	2761	56
2-Methoxyethanol		40
Methoxyethylmercuric Acetate		84
Methoxyethylmercuric Chloride		84

Chemical Name	UN/ NA/PIN	Guideline Number
Methoxymethyl Isocyanate	2605	94
Methoxymethylpentanone	2293	33, 92
4-Methoxyphenol		44
1-Methoxy-2-propanol	3092	40
Methyl Acetate	1231	31
Methyl Acetone	1232	42
Methyl Acetylene/ Propadiene Mixture, stabilized	1060	35
Methylacrylate, inhibited	1919	37
Methyl Acrylonitrile		90
Methylal	1234	38
Methyl Alcohol	1230	31
Methyl Allyl Chloride	2554	61
Methyl Aluminum Sesquibromide	1926	95
Methyl Aluminum Sesquichloride	1927	98
Methylamine, anhydrous	1061	20
Methylamine, aqueous solution	1235	20
p-Methylaminophenol Sulfate		32, 44
Methyl Amyl Acetate	1233	37
Methyl Amyl Alcohol	2053	30
Methyl Amyl Ketone	1110	42
Methylaniline	2294	32
Methyl Benzoate	2938	15
Methylbenzyl Alcohol (alpha)	2937	30
Methyl Bromide	1062	95
Methyl Bromide and Chloropicrin Mixture	1581	26, 95, 136
Methyl Bromide and Ethylene Dibromide Mixture, liquid	1647	95
Methyl Bromide and Nonflammable Compressed Gas Mixture	1955	95

Chemical Name	UN/ NA/PIN	Guideline Number
Methyl Bromoacetate	2643	95
Methyl Butanone	2397	42
Methylbutene	2460	33
2-Methyl-1-butene	2459	33
2-Methyl-2-butene	2460	33
3-Methyl-1-butene	2561	33
Methylbutylamine	2945	20
Methyl-*tert*-butyl Ether	2398	38
Methyl *n*-butyl Ketone		42
Methyl Butyrate	1237	37
Methyl Cellosolve Acetate		40
Methyl Chloride	1063	26
Methyl Chloride and Chloropicrin Mixture	1582	9, 26
Methyl Chloride and Methylene Chloride Mixture	1912	26, 89
Methyl Chloroacetate	2295	37
Methyl 2-chloroacrylate		37
Methyl Chlorocarbonate	1238	26
Methyl Chloroform	2831	26
Methyl Chloroformate	1238	26
Methyl Chloromethyl Ether	1239	26, 38
4-(2, Methyl-4-chlorophenoxy) Butyric Acid		60
Methyl Chloropropionate	2933	26
Methylchlorosilane	2534	107
3-Methylcholanthrene		24
Methyl Cyanide	1648	90
Methylcyclohexane	2296	33
Methylcyclohexanol	2617	30
2-Methylcyclohexanone	2297	42
Methyl Cyclohexanone Peroxide	3046	8, 42
Methyl Cyclopentane	2298	33
Methyl Demeton		49
Methyl Dichloroacetate	2299	37

ALPHABETICAL INDEX

Chemical Name	UN/ NA/PIN	Guideline Number
Methyl Dichloroarsine	1556	73
Methyl Dichlorosilane	1242	107
4,4′-Methylene-bis (2-chloroaniline)		32
Methylene bis(4-phenyl isocyanate)	2489	94
4,4′-Methylene-bis (*N,N*-dimethyl)benzenamine		10
Methylene Bromide	2664	95
Methylene Chloride	1593	26, 89
Methylene Iodide		100
4,4′-Methylenedianiline		32
S-[2 bis (1-methylethylamino) ethyl] O-Ethyl Ester O-Ethyl	2810	135
Methyl Ethyl Ether	1039	38
Methyl Ethyl Ketone	1193	42
Methyl Ethyl Ketone Peroxide	2550	8, 42
Methyl Ethyl Ketone Peroxide, with not more than 40% peroxide	3068	8, 42
Methyl Ethyl Ketone Peroxide, with not more than 52% peroxide	2563	8, 42
Methyl Ethyl Ketone Peroxide, with not more than 60% peroxide	2127	8, 42
Methyl Ethyl Pyridine	2300	24
2-Methyl-5-Ethyl Pyridine	2300	24
Methyl Fluoride	2454	27
Methyl Fluoroacetate		64
Methylfluorophosphoric acid, isopropyl ester	2810	135
Methylfluoropinacoly-phosphonate	2810	135
Methyl Fluorosulfate		26
Methyl Formate	1243	31
Methylfuran	2301	33

Chemical Name	UN/ NA/PIN	Guideline Number
5-Methyl-3-heptanone	2271	42
Methylhexanone	2302	42
Methylhydrazine	1244	23
Methyl Iodide	2644	52
Methyl Isoamyl Ketone	2302	42
Methyl Isobutyl Carbinol	2053	30
Methyl Isobutyl Ketone	1245	42
Methyl Isobutyl Ketone Peroxide	2126	8, 42
Methyl Isocyanate	2480	94
Methylisopropoxy-fluorophosphine Oxide	2810	135
Methyl Isopropenyl Ketone, inhibited	1246	42
Methyl Isopropyl Ketone	2397	42
Methyl Isothiocyanate	2477	94
Methyl Isovalerate	2400	37
Methyl Magnesium Bromide in Ethyl Ether	1928	38, 95
Methyl Mercaptan	1064	105
Methylmercuric Dicyanamide		84
Methyl Methacrylate, monomer inhibited	1247	37
Methylmorpholine	2535	20
Methyl Naphthalene		43
Methyl Nitrite	2455	47
Methyl Orthosilicate	2606	107
Methyl Parathion, liquid	2783	49
Methyl Parathion Mixture, dry	2783	49
Methyl Parathion and Compressed Gas Mixture	1967	49
Methylpentadiene	2461	33
Methylpentane	2462	33
Methylpentanol	2560	30
Methyl Phenkapton		49
Methylphenyl-dichlorosilane	2437	107

Chemical Name	UN/ NA/PIN	Guideline Number
Monochloroethylene	1086	26
Monochloropenta-fluoroethane	1020	27
Monochlorotetra-fluoroethane	1021	27
Monochlorotri-fluoromethane	1022	27
Monocrotophos	2783	49
Monoethanolamine	2491	20
Monoethylamine	1036	20
Monofluorophosphoric Acid	1776	14
Monomethylamine, anhydrous	1061	20
Monomethylamine, aqueous solution	1235	20
Monomethylhydrazine	1244	23
Monopropylamine	1277	20
Mono-(trichloro)-tetra--(monopotassium dichloro)-penta-*s*-triazinetrione, dry	2468	9
Morpholine	2054	20
Morpholine, aqueous, mixture	1760	20
Motor Fuel, n.o.s.	1203	35
Motor Fuel Anti-Knock Compound	1649	35, 80
Motor Fuel Anti-Knock Mixture	1649	35, 80
Motor Spirit	1203	35
MPMC		50
Muerto Canyon Virus		119
Muriatic Acid	1789	14
Murine Typhus	128	128
Muscimol		10
Musk Xylene	2956	24
O-Mustard		139
Mustard Gas	2810	139
Mustard Lewsite	2810	139
Mustine Note	2810	139

Chemical Name	UN/ NA/PIN	Guideline Number
Nabam		63
Nairovirus		116
Naled	2783	49
Naphtha	2553	35
Naphtha, petroleum	1255	35
Naphtha, solvent	1256	35
Naphthalene, crude or refined	1334	43
Naphthalene, molten	2304	43
Naphthenic Acid		15
b-Naphthol		44
1,4-Naphthoquinone		44
Naphthylamine (alpha)	2077	20
Naphthylamine (beta)	1650	20
Naphthylthiourea	1651	43
Naphthylurea	1652	43
Natural Gas, compressed, with a high methane content	1971	33, 92
Natural Gas, refrigerated liquid (cryogenic liquid), with a high methane content	1972	33, 92
Natural Gas, compressed, with a high methane content	1971	33, 92
Natural Gasoline	1257	35
Navadel		49
N-Butyl Isocyanate	2485	94
Neohexane	1208	33
Neon, compressed	1065	92
Neon, refrigerated liquid (cryogenic liquid)	1913	92
Neopentane	2044	33
Neotran		60
N-Ethylaniline	2272	32
Nickel and Soluble Compounds	1378	85
Nickel Ammonium Sulfate		85

Chemical Name	UN/ NA/PIN	Guideline Number
Nickel Carbonyl	1259	85
Nickel Catalyst, dry	2881	85
Nickel Catalyst, finely divided, activated, or spent, wet, with not less than 40% water or other suitable liquid	1378	85
Nickel Chloride		85
Nickel Cyanide	1653	85, 90
Nickel Hydroxide		85
Nickel Nitrate	2725	47, 85
Nickel Nitrite	2726	47, 85
Nickel Sulfate		85
Nicotine	1654	51
Nicotine Compound, liquid, n.o.s.	3144	51
Nicotine Compound, solid n.o.s.	1655	51
Nicotine Hydrochloride, and solutions	1656	51
Nicotine Preparation, liquid, n.o.s.	3144	51
Nicotine Preparation, solid, n.o.s.	1655	51
Nicotine Salicylate	1657	51
Nicotine Sulfate, liquid	1658	51
Nicotine Sulfate, solid	1658	51
Nicotine Tartrate	1659	51
Nitrate, inorganic, n.o.s.	1477	47
Nitrate Salts		47
Nitrate of Sodium and Potash, mixture	1478	47
Nitrate, n.o.s.	1477	47
Nitrating Acid	1796	47
Nitrating Acid, mixture	1796	47
Nitrating Acid Mixture, spent	1826	47
Nitric Acid	1760	14
Nitric Acid, fuming	2032	14, 133, 138

Chemical Name	UN/ NA/PIN	Guideline Number
Nitric Acid, other than fuming, with more than 40% acid	2031	14
Nitric Acid, other than fuming, with not more than 40% acid	1760	14
Nitric Acid, red fuming	2032	14, 133, 138
Nitric Oxide	1660	48
Nitric Oxide and Dinitrogen Tetroxide Mixture	1975	48
Nitric Oxide and Nitrogen Dioxide Mixture	1975	48
Nitric Oxide and Nitrogen Tetroxide Mixture	1975	48
Nitrilotriacetic Acid		15
Nitrite, inorganic, n.o.s.	2627	47
p-Nitroaniline	1661	32
Nitroanisole	2730	24, 47
Nitrobenzene	1662	24, 47
Nitrobenzenesulfonic Acid	2305	15
Nitrobenzotrifluoride	2306	24, 47
4-Nitrobiphenyl		44, 47
Nitrobromobenzene	2732	47, 95
Nitrocellulose, solution in a flammable liquid	2059	5
Nitrocellulose, solution in a flammable liquid	2060	5
Nitrocellulose, wet, with more than 40% flammable liquid by weight	2559	5
Nitrocellulose, wet, with not less than 25% alcohol	2556	5
Nitrocellulose, wet, with not less than 20% water	2555	6
Nitrocellulose, with plasticizing substance	2557	6, 10
Nitrochlorobenzene, liquid	1578	24, 47
Nitrochlorobenzene, solid	1578	24, 47

Chemical Name	UN/ NA/PIN	Guideline Number
o-Nitrochlorobenzene	1578	24, 47
p-Nitrochlorobenzene	1578	24, 47
Nitrochlorobenzotri-fluoride	2307	24, 47
Nitrochloroform	1580	136
Nitro Compounds	1477	47
Nitro Compounds	1796	47
Nitrocresol	2446	44, 47
Nitrocyclohexane		33, 37
Nitroethane	2842	33, 47
Nitrofen		24, 47
Nitrogen, compressed	1066	92
Nitrogen, refrigerated liquid (cryogenic liquid)	1977	92
Nitrogen Dioxide	1067	48
Nitrogen Fluoride Oxide	9271	48, 99
Nitrogen Lost	2810	139
Nitrogen Mustard	2810	139
Nitrogen Mustard 3	2810	139
Nitrogen Oxide	1067	48
Nitrogen Peroxide	1067	48
Nitrogen Tetroxide	1067	48
Nitrogen Trifluoride	2451	99
Nitrogen Trioxide	2421	48
Nitroglycerin		47
Nitroglycerin Solution in Alcohol, with not more than 1% nitroglycerin	1204	29, 47
Nitroglycerin Solution in Alcohol, with more than 1% but not more than 5% nitroglycerin	3064	29, 47
Nitroguanidine, wet, with not less than 20% water	1336	62
Nitrohydrochloric Acid	1798	14
Nitromethane	1261	47
Nitromuriatic Acid	1798	14
Nitronaphthalene	2538	43

Chemical Name	UN/ NA/PIN	Guideline Number
Nitrophenol	1663	62
p-Nitrophenol		62
Nitropropane	2608	47
2-Nitropropane		47
Nitroprusside Salts		90
Nitrotrichloromethane	1580	136
N-Nitrosodi-*n*-butylamine		20, 47
N-Nitrosodiethanolamine		20, 47
N-Nitrosodiethylamine		20, 47
N-Nitrosodimethylamine		20, 47
Nitrosodimethylamine		20, 47
Nitrosodimethylaniline	1369	32
N-Nitrosodiphenylamine		20, 47
p-Nitrosodiphenylamine		20, 47
N-Nitrosodi–propylamine		20, 47
N-Nitroso-*N*-ethylurea		47, 48
N-Nitroso-*N*-methylurea		47, 48
N-Nitrosomethylvinylamine		20, 27
N-Nitrosomorpholine		20, 47
N-Nitroso-*N*-methylurethane		47, 94
N-Nitrosonornicotine		51
N-Nitrosopiperidine		47
N-Nitrosopyrrolidine		47
Nitrostarch, wet, with not less than 30% solvent	1337	47
Nitrostarch, wet, with not less than 20% water	1337	47
Nitrosyl Chloride	1069	14
Nitrosylsulfuric Acid	2308	14
Nitrotoluene	1664	24, 47
Nitrotoluidine (mono)	2660	24, 47
Nitrous Oxide, compressed	1070	48
Nitrous Oxide, refrigerated liquid (cryogenic liquid)	2201	48
Nitroxylene	1665	24, 47
Nitroxylol	1665	44, 47

Chemical Name	UN/ NA/PIN	Guideline Number
N,N-Dimethylaniline	2253	32
N,N-Dimethylformamide	2265	15
Nonane	1920	33
Nonflammable Gas, n.o.s.	1956	3
Nonyl Trichlorosilane	1799	107
Norbormide		10
Norbornadiene	2251	33
Normal Propyl Alcohol	1274	29
Nux Vomica		69
O_3 (ozone)		104
OCBM	2810	136
Octachloronaphthalene		43
Octadecyl Trichlorosilane	1800	107
Octadiene	2309	33
Octafluorobutene	2422	26
Octafluorocyclobutane	1976	26
Octafluoropropane	2424	26
Octamethyl Pyro-phosphoramide		49
Octane	1262	33
1-Octanol		30
Octanoyl Peroxide	2129	8
Octyl Aldehyde	1191	41
Octyl Ammonium Metharsonate		72
Octyl Cresols		44
tert-Octyl Hydroperoxide	2160	8
tert-Octyl Mercaptan	3023	105
tert-Octyl Peroxy-2-ethylhexanoate	2161	8, 15
Octyl Trichlorosilane	1801	107
Ohara Disease		127
Oil Gas	1071	35
Oil, Petroleum, n.o.s.	1270	35
Oleum	1831	14, 133, 138
Organic Peroxide, liquid or solution, n.o.s.	1993	8
Organic Peroxide, liquid or solution, n.o.s.	9183	8
Organic Peroxide Mixture	2756	8
Organic Peroxide, n.o.s. (including trial quantities)	2899	8
Organic Peroxide, sample, n.o.s.	2255	8
Organic Peroxide, solid, n.o.s.	9187	8
Organic Peroxide Type B, liquid	3101	8
Organic Peroxide Type B, liquid, temperature-controlled	3111	8
Organic Peroxide Type B, solid	3102	8
Organic Peroxide Type B, solid, temperature-controlled	3112	8
Organic Peroxide Type C, liquid	3103	8
Organic Peroxide Type C, liquid, temperature-controlled	3113	8
Organic Peroxide Type C, solid	3104	8
Organic Peroxide Type C, solid, temperature-controlled	3114	8
Organic Peroxide Type D, liquid	3105	8
Organic Peroxide Type D, liquid, temperature controlled	3115	8
Organic Peroxide Type D, solid	3106	8
Organic Peroxide Type D, solid, temperature-controlled	3116	8
Organic Peroxide Type E, liquid	3107	8

Chemical Name	UN/ NA/PIN	Guideline Number
Organic Peroxide Type E, liquid, temperature-controlled	3117	8
Organic Peroxide Type E, solid	3108	8
Organic Peroxide Type E, solid, temperature-controlled	3118	8
Organic Peroxide Type F, liquid	3109	8
Organic Peroxide Type F, liquid, temperature-controlled	3119	8
Organic Peroxide Type F, solid	3110	8
Organic Peroxide Type F, solid, temperature-controlled	3120	8
Organic Phosphate Compound liquid (Poison B)	2783	49
Organic Phosphate Compound solid (Poison B)	2783	49
Organic Phosphorus Insecticides		49
Organic Phosphorus Compound Mixed with Compressed Gas	1955	49
Organochlorine Pesticide, liquid, flammable, poisonous, n.o.s.	2762	54
Organochlorine Pesticide, liquid, poisonous, flammable, n.o.s.	2995	54
Organochlorine Pesticide, liquid, poisonous, flammable, n.o.s.	2996	54
Organochlorine Pesticide, solid, poisonous, n.o.s.	2761	56
Organomercury Compounds		84
Organophosphates, poisonous, n.o.s.	1893	49

Chemical Name	UN/ NA/PIN	Guideline Number
Organophosphorus Pesticide, liquid, flammable, poisonous, n.o.s.	2784	49
Organophosphorus Pesticide liquid, poisonous, flammable, n.o.s.	3017	49
Organophosphorus Pesticide liquid, poisonous, n.o.s.	3018	49
Organophosphorus Pesticide solid, poisonous, n.o.s.	2783	49
Organotin Compounds, n.o.s.	2788	65
Organotin Compound, solid, n.o.s.	3146	65
Organotin Pesticide, n.o.s.	2786	65
Organotin Pesticide, liquid,flammable, poisonous, n.o.s.	2787	65
Organotin Pesticide, liquid, poisonous, flammable, n.o.s.	3019	65
Organotin Pesticide, liquid, poisonous, n.o.s.	3020	65
Organotin Pesticide, solid, poisonous, n.o.s.	2786	65
ORM-A, n.o.s.	1693	10
ORM-B, n.o.s.	1760	10
ORM-E, liquid or solid, n.o.s.	9188	10
ortho-Chlorobenzylidine Malononitrile	2810	136
Osmic Acid		14
Osmium and Compounds	2471	10
Osmium Oxide (OsO_4)		10
Osmium Tetroxide	2471	10

Chemical Name	UN/ NA/PIN	Guideline Number
Ouabain		10
Oxalates, water-soluble	2449	17
Oxalic Acid		17
Oxamyl		50
Oxetane		38
Oxidizer, corrosive liquid, n.o.s.	9193	7, 13
Oxidizer, corrosive solid n.o.s.	9194	7, 13
Oxidizer, n.o.s.	1479	7
Oxidizer, poisonous liquid, n.o.s.	9199	7, 10
Oxidizer, poisonous solid, n.o.s.	9200	7, 10
Oxidizing Material, n.o.s.	1479	7
Oxidizing Substance, corrosive liquid	3098	7, 13
Oxidizing Substance, liquid, n.o.s.	3139	7
Oxidizing Substance, poisonous liquid, n.o.s.	3099	7, 10
Oxidizing Substance, corrosive solid, n.o.s.	3085	7, 13
Oxidizing Substance, solid, flammable, n.o.s.	3137	6, 7
Oxidizing Substance, solid, n.o.s	1479	7
Oxidizing Substance, solid, poisonous, n.o.s.	3087	7, 10
Oxidizing Substance, solid, self-heating, n.o.s.	3100	7
Oxidizing Substance, solid that, when in contact with water, emits a flammable gas, n.o.s.	3121	7
Oxirane		45
Oxydisulfoton		49
Oxygen, compressed	1072	7
Oxygen, refrigerated liquid (cryogenic liquid)	1073	7
Oxygen Difluoride	2190	99, 104
Ozone		104
Ozone and Cyclohexene		33, 104
Ozone Mixed with Nitrogen Oxides (53%:47%)		48, 104
Ozone Mixed with Sulfur Dioxide (1:1)		104, 105
Paint, etc., corrosive liquid	1760	13
Paint, etc., corrosive liquid	3066	13
Paint, etc., flammable liquid	1263	5
Paint-Related Material, corrosive liquid	1760	13
Paint-Related Material, corrosive liquid	3066	13
Paint-Related Material, flammable liquid	1263	5
Paint Stripper	1610	35
Painters' Naphtha	2553	35
Paper, treated with unsaturated oil	1379	6
Paradiaminobenzene	1673	32
Paradichlorobenzene	1592	57
Paraffin		33
Paraformaldehyde	2213	41
Paraldehyde	1264	41
Paramenthane Hydroperoxide	2125	8
Paraoxon		49
Paraquat	2781	66
Paraquat Methosulfate		66
Parathion, flammable liquid	2784	49
Parathion and Compressed Gas Mixture	1967	49

Chemical Name	UN/ NA/PIN	Guideline Number
Parathion Mixture, liquid or dry	2783	49
Parathion-methyl		49
Paris Green		72, 78
PBB		46
PCBs	2315	46
PCNB		67
PCP		134
PD	1556	101, 133
Pelargonyl Peroxide	2130	8
Pentaborane	1380	103
Pentachlorobenzene		24
Pentachloroethane	1669	26
Pentachloronitrobenzene		67
Pentachlorophenol (PCP)	2020	67
Pentadecylamine		20
1,3-Pentadiene		33
Pentaerythritol		40
Pentamethyl Heptane	2286	33
Pentane	1265	33
Pentane-2,4-dione	2310	42
Pentanoic Acid	1760	15
2-Pentanone	1249	42
1-Pentene	1108	33
Pentol	2705	30
PERC	1897	26
Peracetic Acid, solution	2131	8, 15
Perchlorate, inorganic, n.o.s.	1481	97
Perchloric Acid, more than 50% but not more than 72% acid, by weight	1873	7, 14
Perchloric acid, not more than 50% acid by weight	1802	7, 14
Perchloroethylene	1897	26
Perchloromethyl Mercaptan	1670	105

Chemical Name	UN/ NA/PIN	Guideline Number
Perchloryl Fluoride	3083	7, 99
Perfluoroethylvinyl Ether	3154	38
Perfluoroisobutene		10
Perfluoromethyvinyl Ether	3153	38
Perfluoropropane	2424	26
Perfumery Products, with flammable solvent	1266	35
Permanganate, inorganic, n.o.s.	1482	14
Permethrin		52
Peroxide, inorganic, n.o.s.	1483	7
Peroxyacetic Acid, solution	2131	8, 15
Peroxyacetic Acid Solution	3045	8, 15
Persulfate Salts		22
Perthane		55
Pesticide, carbamates, liquid, flammable, poisonous, n.o.s.	2758	50
Pesticide, carbamates, liquid, flammable, poisonous, n.o.s.	2991	50
Pesticide, carbamates, liquid, poisonous, n.o.s.	2992	50
Pesticide, liquid, flammable, poisonous, n.o.s.	3021	5, 10
Pesticide, liquid, poisonous, flammable, n.o.s.	2903	5, 10
Pesticide, liquid, poisonous, n.o.s.	2902	10
Pesticide, organophosphates	2783	49
Pesticide, solid, poisonous, n.o.s.	2588	10
Pesticide, water-reactive, containing Maneb	2210	63

Chemical Name	UN/ NA/PIN	Guideline Number
Petrol	1203	35
Petroleum Crude Oil	1267	35
Petroleum Distillate, n.o.s.	1268	35
Petroleum Ether	1271	38
Petroleum Gas, liquefied	1075	2, 35
Petroleum Naphtha	1255	35
Petroleum Oil	1270	35
Petroleum Spirits	1271	35
PFIB		10
PFMP	2810	135
Phenacetin		32
Phenacyl Bromide	2645	95
Phenacyl Chloride	1697	136
Phenamiphos		49
Phenanthrene		24
Phenarsazine Chloride	1698	136
Phenazopyridine Hydrochloride		32, 43
Phencyclidine		134
Phenetidine	2311	32
Phenindione		71
Phenol, molten	2312	44
Phenol, solid	1671	44
Phenol Solution	2821	44
Phenolsulfonic Acid, liquid	1803	15, 44
Phenoxarsine		73
Phenoxy Pesticide, liquid, flammable, poisonous, n.o.s.	2766	60
Phenoxy Pesticide, liquid, poisonous, flammable, n.o.s.	2999	60
Phenoxy Pesticide, liquid, poisonous, n.o.s.	3000	60
Phenoxy Pesticide, solid, poisonous, n.o.s.	2765	60
Phenprocoumon		71
Phenylacetonitrile, liquid	2470	90
Phenylacetyl Chloride	2577	24
Phenylarsenic Dichloride	1556	139

Chemical Name	UN/ NA/PIN	Guideline Number
Phenyl-arsonous Dichloride	1556	139
Phenylcarbylamine Chloride	1672	32
Phenyl Cellosolve		40
Phenyl Chloroformate	2746	26
Phenyl Chloromethyl Ketone	1697	136
1-(1-Phenylcyclohexyl) piperidine		134
Phenyldichloroarsine	1556	139
Phenyldichloroarsine and Phosgene	1556	101, 133, 139
Phenylenediamine	1673	20
Phenylhydrazine	2572	23
Phenylhydrazine Hydrochloride		23
Phenyl Isocyanate	2487	94
Phenyl Mercaptan	2337	105
Phenylmercuric Acetate, liquid	1674	84
Phenylmercuric Compound, solid, n.o.s.	2026	84
Phenylmercuric Hydroxide	1894	84
Phenylmercuric Nitrate	1895	47, 84
Phenylmercuric Salts of Organic Acids		84
Phenylmercuric Salts of Inorganic Acids		84
Phenylmercuric Triethanol Ammonium Lactate		84
Phenylmercury Acetate		84
Phenylphenol		44
Phenylphosphine		108
Phenyl Phosphorus Dichloride	2798	109
Phenyl Phosphorus Thiodichloride	2799	109
Phenylsilatrane		10
Phenylthiourea		43

Chemical Name	UN/ NA/PIN	Guideline Number
Phenyltrichlorosilane	1804	107
Phenyl Urea Pesticide, n.o.s.	2767	43
Phenyl Urea Pesticide, liquid, flammable, poisonous, n.o.s.	2768	43
Phenyl Urea Pesticide, liquid, poisonous, flammable, n.o.s.	3001	43
Phenyl Urea Pesticide, liquid poisonous, n.o.s.	3002	43
Phenyl Urea Pesticide, solid, poisonous, n.o.s.	2767	43
Phorate	2783	49
Phosacetim		49
Phosdrin		49
Phosfolan		49
Phosgene	1076	101, 133 138
Phosgene Oxime	2811	101, 138, 139
Phosmet		49
Phosphabicyclononane	2940	10
Phosphamidon		49
Phosphine	2199	108
Phosphonochloridic Acid		135
Phosphonofluoridic Acid, methyl-, 1-methylethyl ester	2810	135
Phosphonofluoridic Acid, methyl-, isopropyl ester	2810	135
Phosphonofluoridic Acid, methyl-,1,2,2-trimethylpropyl ester	2810	135
Phosphonothioic Acid		49
Phosphonothioic Acid, methyl-	2810	135
Phosphonothioic Acid, methyl-, S[2-[bis (1-methylethyl)amino] ethyl] O-ethyl ester	2810	135

Chemical Name	UN/ NA/PIN	Guideline Number
Phosphoric Acid	1805	14
Phosphoric Acid Triethyleneimine	2501	10
Phosphoric Anhydride	1807	14
Phosphorous Acid (ortho)	2834	14
Phosphorus	1381	109
Phosphorus, amorphous, red	1338	109
Phosphorus Heptasulfide, free from yellow or white phosphorus	1339	105, 109
Phosphorus Oxybromide, molten	2576	95, 109
Phosphorus Oxybromide, solid	1939	95, 109
Phosphorus Oxychloride	1810	98, 109
Phosphorus Pentabromide	2691	95, 109
Phosphorus Pentachloride	1806	98, 109
Phosphorus Pentafluoride	2198	99, 109
Phosphorus Pentasulfide, free from yellow or white phosphorus	1340	105, 109
Phosphorus Pentoxide	1807	109
Phosphorus Sesquisulfide, free from yellow or white phosphorus	1341	105, 109
Phosphorus Tribromide	1808	95, 109
Phosphorus Trichloride	1809	98, 109, 133, 138
Phosphorus Trifluoride	9273	99, 109
Phosphorus Trioxide	2578	109
Phosphorus Trisulfide, free from yellow or white phosphorus	1343	105, 109
Phosphorus, white, molten	2447	109
Phosphorus, white or yellow, dry or under water, or in solution	1381	109
Phosphoryl Chloride	1810	98, 109
Phostex		49

Chemical Name	UN/ NA/PIN	Guideline Number
PHP		134
Phthalic Anhydride	2214	15
Phthalimide Derivative Pesticide, liquid, flammable, poisonous, n.o.s.	2774	9
Phthalimide Derivative 3007 Pesticide, liquid, poisonous, flammable, n.o.s.	9	
Phthalimide Derivative Pesticide, liquid, poisonous, n.o.s.	3008	9
Phthalimide Derivative Pesticide, solid, poisonous, n.o.s	2773	9
Phthalonitrile		90
Physostigmine		10
Picoline	2313	24
Picric Acid, wet, with not less than 10% water	1344	62
Picrite, wet, with not less than 20% water	1336	62
Picrotoxin		10
Pinacolyl Methanefluoro-phosphonate	2810	135
Pinacolyl Methylfluoro-phosphonate	2810	135
O-Pinacolyl Methyl-phosphonochloride, Phosphonochloridic Acid		135
Pinalcolyl Methyl-phosphonofluoridate	2810	135
Pinalcolyl Methyl Phosphonofluoridate	2810	135
O-Pinalcolyl Methylphosphonofluoridate	2810	135
Pinacolyloxymethyl-phosphonyl Fluoride	2810	135
Pinane Hydroperoxide, technical pure	2162	8
Pinanyl Hydroperoxide, technical pure	2162	8
Pindone	2472	71
alpha-Pinene	2368	34
Pine Oil	1272	34
Piperazine	2579	20
Piperidine	2401	20
Piperonyl Butoxide		10
Piperonyl Cyclonene		10
Pirimicarb		50
Pirimifos-ethyl		49
Pivaloyl Chloride	2438	26
2-Pivaly-1,3-indandione		71
Plague		121
Plastic Moulding Material, evolving flammable vapor	2211	6
Plastics, nitrocellulose based, spontaneously combustible, n.o.s.	2006	6
Pneumorickettsiosis		123
Poison B Liquid, n.o.s.	2810	10
Poisonous Gas, flammable, n.o.s.	1953	2, 10
Poisonous Gas, n.o.s.	1955	10
Poisonous Liquid, corrosive n.o.s.	2927	10, 13
Poisonous Liquid, flammable, n.o.s.	1953	5, 10
Poisonous Liquid, flammable, n.o.s.	2929	5, 10
Poisonous Liquid, n.o.s.	1955	10
Poisonous Liquid, n.o.s. (Poison B)	2810	10
Poisonous Liquid, oxidizing, n.o.s.	3122	7, 10
Poisonous Liquid that, when in contact with emits a flammable water, gas, n.o.s.	3123	2, 10

Chemical Name	UN/ NA/PIN	Guideline Number
Poisonous Solid, corrosive, n.o.s.	2928	10, 13
Poisonous Solid, flammable, n.o.s.	2930	6, 10
Poisonous Solid, n.o.s.	2811	10
Poisonous Solid, oxidizing, n.o.s.	3086	7, 10
Poisonous Solid, self-heating, n.o.s.	3124	10
Poisonous Solid that, when in contact with water, emits a flammable gas, n.o.s.	3125	2, 10
Polish, liquid	1263	10
Polyalkylamine, corrosive, flammable, n.o.s.	2734	5, 20
Polyalkylamine, corrosive, n.o.s.	2735	20
Polyalkylamine, flammable, corrosive, n.o.s.	2733	5, 20
Polybrominated Biphenyl		46
Polychlorinated Biphenyl	2315	46
Polyester Resin Kits	2255	10
Polyethylene Glycols		40
Polyhalogenated Biphenyl, liquid, or Polyhalogenated Terphenyl, liquid	3151	46
Polyhalogenated Biphenyl, solid, or Polyhalogenated Terphenyl, solid	3152	46
Polynuclear Aromatic Hydrocarbons		10
Polyol		40
Polystyrene Beads, expandable, evolving a flammable vapor	2211	5
Polytetrafluoroethylene		26
Portland Cement		19
Potash Liquor	1814	19
Potassium	2257	10

Chemical Name	UN/ NA/PIN	Guideline Number
Potassium, metal, liquid alloy	1420	10
Potassium Arsenate	1677	72
Potassium Arsenite	1678	72
Potassium Bichromate		14
Potassium Bifluoride	1811	16
Potassium Bisulfate	2509	14
Potassium Biosulfite Solution	2693	105
Potassium Borohydride	1870	103
Potassium Bromate	1484	96
Potassium Chlorate	1485	97
Potassium Chlorate Solution	2427	97
Potassium Chromate	9142	14
Potassium Cuprocyanide	1679	90
Potassium Cyanide, solid	1680	90
Potassium Cyanide Solution	1680	90
Potassium Dichloro-isocyanurate	2465	22
Potassium Dichloro-s-triazinetrione	2465	22
Potassium Dichromate	1479	14
Potassium Dithionite	1929	105
Potassium Fluoborate		99, 103
Potassium Fluoride	1812	16
Potassium Fluoroacetate	2628	64
Potassium Fluorosilicate, solid	2655	99
Potassium Hydrogen Fluoride	1811	16
Potassium Hydrogen Sulfate	2509	14
Potassium Hydrosulfite	1929	105
Potassium Hydroxide, dry, solid	1813	19
Potassium Hydroxide Solution	1814	19

Chemical Name	UN/ NA/PIN	Guideline Number
Potassium Hypochlorite Solution	1791	22
Potassium Metal	2257	10
Potassium Metal, liquid alloy	1420	10
Potassium Metavanadate	2864	10
Potassium Monopersulfate		9
Potassium Monoxide	2033	19
Potassium Nitrate	1486	47
Potassium Nitrate and Sodium Nitrite Mixture	1487	47
Potassium Nitrite	1488	47
Potassium Oxide	2033	19
Potassium Perchlorate	1489	97
Potassium Permanganate	1490	14
Potassium Peroxide	1491	7
Potassium Persulfate	1492	9
Potassium Phosphate		19
Potassium Phosphide	2012	108
Potassium Selenate	2630	86
Potassium Selenite	2630	86
Potassium Silicofluoride, solid	2655	99
Potassium Silver Cyanide		90
Potassium Sodium Alloy	1422	6
Potassium Sulfide, anhydrous or with less than 30% water of hydration	1382	19
Potassium Sulfide, hydrated, with not less than 30% water of hydration	1847	19
Potassium Superoxide	2466	10
Preplant Soil Fumigant	1581	136
Pri-Brom	1581	136
Prolan		57
Promecarb		50
Propadiene	2200	33

Chemical Name	UN/ NA/PIN	Guideline Number
Propadiene, inhibited	2200	33
Propane	1978	33
Propane Sultone		15
Propanethiol	2402	105
Propanil		32
Propanoic Acid	1848	15
Propanol	1274	29
Propargite		10
Propargyl Alcohol	1986	30
Propargyl Bromide		95
beta-Propiolactone		42
Propionaldehyde	1275	41
Propionic Acid	1848	15
Propionic Anhydride	2496	15
Propionitrile	2404	90
Propionyl Chloride	1815	26
Propionyl Peroxide	2132	8
Propiophenone		44
Propoxur	2588	50
Propyl Acetate	1276	37
Propyl Alcohol	1274	29
Propylamine	1277	20
Propyl Benzene	2364	24
Propyl Chloride	1278	26
Propyl Chloroformate		26
n-Propyl Chloroformate	2740	26
Propylene	1077	33
Propylene Chlorohydrin	2611	61
Propylenediamine	2258	20
Propylene Dichloride	1279	61
Propylene Glycol		40
Propylene Gylcol Monomethyl Ether		40
Propylene Glycol Monostearate		40
Propyleneimine, inhibited	1921	20
Propylene Oxide	1280	38

Chemical Name	UN/ NA/PIN	Guideline Number
Propylene Tetramer	2850	33
Propyl Formate	1281	37
n-Propyl Gallate		44
Propyl Isocyanate	2482	94
n-Propyl Isome		43
Propyl Mercaptan	2402	105
Propyl Mercaptan	2704	105
Di–propylnitrosamine		47
Propyl Nitrate	1865	47
Propyl Peroxydicarbonate	2133	8
Propyl Trichlorosilane	1816	107
Prothoate		49
PS	1580	136
Psittacosis		122
Pyramat		50
Pyrazothion		49
Pyrazoxon		49
Pyrene		24
Pyrenone		52
Pyrethrins or Pyrethrum	9184	52
Pyrethroids		52
Pyridine	1282	24
Pyriminil		10
Pyrocatechol		44
Pyrogallol		44
Pyrolan		50
Pyrolysis Products		10
Pyrophoric Fuel, n.o.s.	1375	5
Pyrophoric Liquid, n.o.s.	2845	5
Pyrophoric Metal or Alloy, n.o.s.	1383	6
Pyrophoric Solid, n.o.s.	2846	6
Pyrosulfuric Acid	1831	14, 133, 138
Pyrosulfuryl Chloride	1817	14
Pyroxylin Plastic, rod, sheet, roll, tube, or scrap	1325	38
Pyroxylin Solution	2059	38

Chemical Name	UN/ NA/PIN	Guideline Number
Pyrrolidine	1922	20
Q (chemical weapon)		139
Q Fever		123
Query Fever		123
Quinoline	2656	24
Quinone		42
Quintozene		67
3-Quinuclidinyl Benzilate	2810	134
Rabbit Fever		127
Radioactive Material, articles manufactured from natural or depleted uranium or natural thorium	2909	12
Radioactive Material, empty packages	2908	12
Radioactive Material, excepted package	2910	12
Radioactive Material, fissile, n.o.s.	2918	12
Radioactive Material, instruments and articles	2911	12
Radioactive Material, limited quantity, n.o.s.	2910	12
Radioactive Material, low specific activity (LSA), n.o.s.	2912	12
Radioactive Material, n.o.s.	2982	12
Radioactive Material, special form, n.o.s.	2974	12
Rare Gas Mixture	1979	10, 92
Rare Gas–Nitrogen Mixture	1981	10, 92
Rare Gas–Oxygen Mixture	1980	10, 92
Receptacles, small, with flammable compressed gas	2037	2
Red Phosphorus	1338	109
Reducing Liquid	1142	10

Chemical Name	UN/ NA/PIN	Guideline Number
Refrigerant Gas, flammable, n.o.s.	1954	2
Refrigerant Gases, n.o.s.	1078	27
Refrigerating Machine, containing flammable, nonpoisonous, liquefied gas	1954	2, 92
Refrigerating Machine, containing nonflammable, nonpoisonous, liquefied gas	2857	3
Removing Liquid	1142	10
Reserpine		10
Residual Oils		35
Resin Compound liquid, flammable	1866	5
Resin Solution, flammable	1866	5
Resin Solution, poisonous	1896	10
Resin Solution, (resin compound), liquid	1866	10
Resmethrin		52
Resorcinol	2876	44
Rhodia-6200		49, 135
Ricin		124
Rickettsia prowazekii		128
Rickettsia rickettsii		128
Rickettsia typhi		128
Road Asphalt, liquid	1999	35
Road Oil	1268	35
Rocky Mountain Spotted Fever		128
Rodenticides, n.o.s.	1681	10
Rolicyclidine		134
Ronnel	2588	49
Rosin Oil	1286	10
Rotenone	2588	53
Rotenoids		53
Roundup		68

Chemical Name	UN/ NA/PIN	Guideline Number
Rubber Scrap, powdered or granulated	1345	10
Rubber Shoddy, powdered or granulated	1345	10
Rubber Solution	1287	10
Rubber Solvent (naphtha)	1287	35
Ruelene		49
Rubidium Hydroxide, solid	2678	10
Rubidium Hydroxide Solution	2677	10
Rubidium Metal	1423	10
SA	2188	73, 138
Saccharin		10
Saccharin, and its salts		10
Safrole		44
Salcomine		10
Saltpeter	1486	47
Salmonella typhi		117
Saprol		44
Sarin	2810	135
Schewefel-lost	2810	139
Sea Coal	1361	6
Selenates and Selenites	2630	86
Selenic Acid	1905	14, 86
Selenious Acid		14, 86
Selenious Acid, dithallium (1+) salt		86, 87
Selenium Dioxide		86
Selenium Disulfide	2657	86, 105
Selenium Hexafluoride	2194	86, 99
Selenium Metal, powder	2658	86
Selenium Oxide	2811	86
Selenium Oxychloride	2879	86
Selenium Sulfide		86, 105
Selenourea		86
Self-Heating Substance, solid, corrosive, n.o.s.	3126	13

Chemical Name	UN/ NA/PIN	Guideline Number
Self-Heating Substance, solid, oxidizing, n.o.s.	3127	7
Self-Heating Substance, solid, poisonous, n.o.s.	3128	10
Self-Heating Substance, solid, n.o.s.	3088	10
Self-Reactive Substances, samples, n.o.s.	3031	10
Self-Reactive Substances, trial quantities, n.o.s.	3032	10
Semicarbazide Hydrochloride		23
Senfgas	2810	139
Serrylan		134
Sesquimustard		139
Shale Oil	1288	33
Shellac	1263	35
Shigella dysenteriae		117
Shigellosis		117
Silanes	2203	107
Silicofluoric Acid	1778	99
Silicofluoride, solid, n.o.s.	2856	99
Silicon	1346	9
Silicon Chloride	1818	98
Silicon Powder, amorphous	1346	9
Silicon Tetrachloride	1818	98
Silicon Tetrafluoride	1859	99
Silver		10
Silver Arsenite	1683	72
Silver Cyanide	1684	90
Silver Nitrate	1493	47
Silver Pictrate, wet, with not less than 30% water	1347	10
Silvex		60
Sin Nombre Virus		119
Sludge Acid	1906	10

Chemical Name	UN/ NA/PIN	Guideline Number
Smallpox		125
Smokeless Powder, small arms	1325	1
Smokes, military		137
Soda Lime	1907	19
Sodium	1428	6
Sodium Acid Sulfate		14
Sodium Aluminate, solid	2812	10
Sodium Aluminate Solution	1819	10
Sodium Aluminum Hydride	2835	10
Sodium Amalgam	1424	84
Sodium Amide	1425	19
Sodium Ammonium Vanadate	2863	10
Sodium Arsanilate	2473	72
Sodium Arsenate	1685	72
Sodium Arsenite, solid	2027	72
Sodium Arsenite solution	1686	72
Sodium Azide	1687	18
Sodium Bichromate		14
Sodium Bifluoride, solid	2439	99
Sodium Bifluoride Solution	2439	99
Sodium Binoxalate		17
Sodium Bisulfate		10
Sodium Bisulfate, solid	1821	105
Sodium Bisulfate Solution	2837	105
Sodium Bisulfite	2693	105
Sodium Borohydride	1426	103
Sodium Bromate	1494	96
Sodium Cacodylate	1688	72
Sodium Carbonate		19
Sodium Chlorate	1495	97
Sodium Chlorate Solution	2428	97
Sodium Chlorite	1496	22

Chemical Name	UN/ NA/PIN	Guideline Number
Sodium Chlorite Solution, with more than 5% available chlorine	1908	22
Sodium Chloroacetate	2659	37
Sodium Chromate		10
Sodium Cuprocyanide, solid	2316	90
Sodium Cuprocyanide Solution	2317	90
Sodium Cyanide	1689	90
Sodium 2-diazo-1-naph-thol-4-sulfonate	3040	44
Sodium 2-diazo-1-naph-thol-5-sulfonate	3041	44
Sodium Dichloroisocyanurate	2465	22
Sodium Dichloroisocyanate	2465	22
Sodium Dichloro-*s*-triazinetrione	2465	22
Sodium Dichromate	1479	10
Sodium Dinitro-ortho Cresolate, wet, with not less than 15% water	1348	44
Sodium Dithionite	1384	105
Sodium Dodecylbenzenesulfonate		10
Sodium Fluoride, solid	1690	16
Sodium Fluoride Solution	1690	16
Sodium Fluoroacetate	2629	64
Sodium Fluorosilicate	2674	99
Sodium Hydrate	1824	19
Sodium Hydride	1427	19
Sodium Hydrogen Fluoride	2439	16
Sodium Hydrogen Sulfate, solid	1821	105
Sodium Hydrogen Sulfate Solution	2837	105

Chemical Name	UN/ NA/PIN	Guideline Number
Sodium Hydrosulfide, solid, with less than 25% water of crystallization	2318	91
Sodium Hydrosulfide, solid, with not less than 25% water of crystallization	2923	91
Sodium Hydrosulfide, with not less than 25% water of crystallization	2949	91
Sodium Hydrosulfide Solution	2922	91
Sodium Hydrosulfide Solution	2949	91
Sodium Hydrosulfite	1384	105
Sodium Hydroxide, dry, solid	1823	19
Sodium Hydroxide Solution	1824	19
Sodium Hypochlorite Solution	1791	22
Sodium Metal	1428	6
Sodium Metal, dispersion in organic liquids	1429	6
Sodium Metal, liquid alloy	1421	6
Sodium Metasilicate		19
Sodium Methylate, dry	1431	19, 31
Sodium Methylate, solutions in alcohol	1289	19, 31
Sodium Monoxide	1825	19
Sodium Nitrate	1498	47
Sodium Nitrate and Potash Mixture	1478	47
Sodium Nitrate and Potassium Nitrate, mixture	1499	47
Sodium Nitrite	1500	47
Sodium Nitrite and Potassium Nitrate, mixture	1487	47

Chemical Name	UN/ NA/PIN	Guideline Number
Sodium Pentachlorophenate	2567	67
Sodium Percarbonate	2467	7
Sodium Perchlorate	1502	97
Sodium Permanganate	1503	14
Sodium Peroxide	1504	7
Sodium Persulfate	1505	105
Sodium Phenolate, solid	2497	44
Sodium Phosphate		14
Sodium Phosphide	1432	108
Sodium Picramate, wet, with not less than 20% water	1349	6
Sodium Potassium Alloy	1422	6
Sodium Selenate	2630	86
Sodium Selenite	2630	86
Sodium Sesquicarbonate		20
Sodium Silicate		19
Sodium Silicofluoride, solid	2674	99
Sodium Sulfide, anhydrous, with less than 30% water of crystallization	1385	91
Sodium Sulfide, hydrated, with not less than 30% water	1849	91
Sodium Sulfide Solution	1849	91
Sodium Superoxide	2547	7
Sodium Tellurite		10
Sodium Thioglycolate		19
Solox		30, 35
Solvents, Chlorinated	1610	26
Soman		135
Spent Mixed Acid	1826	14
Spirits of Nitroglycerine	1204	47
Stain	1263	35

Chemical Name	UN/ NA/PIN	Guideline Number
Stannane		65
Stannic Chloride, anhydrous	1827	14
Stannic Chloride, hydrated	2440	14
Stannic Phosphide	1433	108
Stannous Chloride, solid	1759	14
Staphylococcal Enterotoxin B		126
Staphylococcal Gastroenteritis		117
Staphylococcus aureus		117
Stearyl Alcohol		30
Steel Swarf	2793	79
Stibine	2676	10
Stoddard Solvent		35
Straw	1327	6
Strobane		26
Strontium Alloy	1434	10
Strontium Arsenite	1691	72
Strontium Chlorate	1506	97
Strontium Chromate		10
Strontium Nitrate	1507	47
Strontium Perchlorate	1508	97
Strontium Peroxide	1509	7
Strontium Phosphide	2013	108
Strontium Sulfide		91
Strychnine, and its salts	1692	69
Styrene	2055	24
Styrene Monomer, inhibited	2055	24
Styrene Oxide		24
Substance, liquid, that, in contact with water, emits flammable gas, corrosive, n.o.s.	3129	2, 13
Substance, liquid, that, in contact with water, emits flammable gas, n.o.s.	3148	2

Chemical Name	UN/ NA/PIN	Guideline Number
Substance, liquid, that, in contact with water, emits flammable gas, poisonous, n.o.s.	3130	2, 10
Substance, solid, that, in contact with water, emits flammable gas, corrosive, n.o.s.	3131	2, 13
Substance, solid, that, in contact with water, emits flammable gas, flammable, n.o.s.	3132	2, 6
Substance solid, that, in contact with water, emits flammable gas, oxidizing, n.o.s.	3133	2, 7
Substance, solid, that, in contact with water, emits flammable gas, poisonous, n.o.s.	3134	2, 10
Substance, solid, that, in contact with water, emits flammable gas, self-heating, n.o.s.	3135	2
Substances, liquid and solid, that, in contact with water, emit flammable gases, n.o.s.	2813	2
Substances, explosive, n.o.s.	0357	1
Substances, explosive, n.o.s.	0358	1
Substances, explosive, n.o.s.	0359	1
Substituted Nitrophenol Pesticide, liquid, flammable, poisonous, n.o.s.	2780	62
Substituted Nitrophenol Pesticide, liquid, poisonous, flammable, n.o.s.	3013	62

Chemical Name	UN/ NA/PIN	Guideline Number
Substituted Nitrophenol Pesticide, liquid, poisonous, n.o.s.	3014	62
Substituted Nitrophenol Pesticide, solid, poisonous, n.o.s.	2779	62
Succinic Acid Peroxide, not more than 72%, in water	2962	15
Succinic Acid Peroxide, technical pure	2135	15
Succinonitrile		90
Sulfallate		50
Sulfamic Acid	2967	14
Sulfide, bis(2-chloroethyl)	2810	139
Sulfides		91
Sulfide Salts		91
Sulfotep	1704	49
Sulfoxide		105
Sulfur	1350	105
Sulfur, molten	2448	105
Sulfur Chloride	1828	105
Sulfur Chloride and Carbon Tetrachloride Mixture	9267	28, 105
Sulfur Chloride Pentafluoride	9272	99, 105
Sulfur Dioxide	1079	105
Sulfur Dioxide, liquefied	1079	105, 133, 138
Sulfur Hexafluoride	1080	92, 133, 138
Sulfur Monochloride		105
Sulfur Mustard	2810	139
Sulfur Pentafluoride		99, 105
Sulfur Phosphide		108
Sulfur Tetrafluoride	2418	16, 105
Sulfur Trioxide, inhibited	1829	14
Sulfur Trioxide, stabilized	1829	14

Chemical Name	UN/ NA/PIN	Guideline Number
Sulfuric Acid, fuming	1831	14, 133, 138
Sulfuric Acid, spent	1832	14
Sulfuric Acid, with more than 51% but not more than 95% acid	1830	14
Sulfuric Acid, with not more than 51% acid	1830	14
Sulfuric Anhydride	1829	14
Sulfuric and Hydrofluoric Acid Mixture	1786	14, 16
Sulfuric Trioxide	1829	14
Sulfurous Acid	1833	14
Sulfurous Acid, 2-(*p-tert*-butylphenoxy)-1 methylethyl-2-chloroethyl ester		10
Sulfuryl Chloride	1834	14
Sulfuryl Fluoride	2191	99, 105
Sulphur Mustard Gas	2810	139
Superphosphates		14
2,4,5-T	2765	60
2,4,5-T Acid		60
2,4,5-T Amines		60
2,4,5-T Esters		60
2,4,5-T Salts		60
Tabun		135
Tannic Acid		15
Tar, liquid	1999	24, 25
TBZ		70
TDE (1,1-dichloro-2,2-bis-(*p*-chlorophenyl) ethane)	2761	55
Tear Gas	1693	136
Tear Gas Candle	1700	136
Tear Gas CR		136
Tear Gas CS		136
Tear Gas Devices	1693	136
Tear Gas Grenades	1700	136

Chemical Name	UN/ NA/PIN	Guideline Number
Tear Gas Substances, n.o.s.	1693	136
Tecto		70
Tecto 60		70
Tellurium		10
Tellurium Hexafluoride	2195	10
Temephos	2783	49
TEPP	2783	49
Terbufos		49
Terebene		34
Terpenes		34
Terpene Hydrocarbons, n.o.s.	2319	34
Terphenyl		34
Terpineol		34
Terpin Hydrate		34
Terpinolene	2541	34
Terr-O-Gas	1581	136
tert-Butyl Isocyante	2484	94
Tetrabromo-*o*-cresol		44
Tetrabromoethane	2504	26
1,1,2,2-Tetrabromoethane		26
1,2,4,5-Tetrachlorobenzene		24
2,3,7,8-Tetrachlorodibenzo-*p*-dioxin (TCDD)		60
Tetrachloroethane	1702	26
1,1,1,2-Tetrachloroethane	1702	26
1,1,2,2-Tetrachloroethane	1702	26
Tetrachloroethylene	1897	28
Tetrachlorodifluoroethane	1078	27
2,3,4,6-Tetrachlorophenol		44
Tetrachlorvinfos		49
Tetrachlorvinphos		49
Tetraethylammonium Perchlorate, dry	1325	97
Tetraethyl Dithiopyro-phosphate and Compressed Gas Mixture	1703	49

Chemical Name	UN/ NA/PIN	Guideline Number
Tetraethyl Dithiopyrophosphate, and gases, mixtures, or in solution	1703	49
Tetraethyl Dithiopyrophosphate, dry, liquid, or mixture	1704	49
Tetraethylenepentamine	2320	20
Tetraethyl Lead	1649	80
Tetraethyl Pyrophosphate, flammable liquid	2784	49
Tetraethyl Pyrophosphate and Compressed Gas Mixture	1705	49
Tetraethyl Pyrophosphate Mixture, dry, liquid, or mixture	2783	49
Tetraethyl Silicate	1292	107
1,1,1,2 Tetrafluoroethane (R134A)		27
Tetrafluoroethylene, inhibited	1081	26
Tetraethyltin		65
Tetrafluorohydrazine	1955	23
Tetrafluoromethane	1982	27
Tetrahydrobenzaldehyde	2498	41
Tetrahydrofuran	2056	38
Tetrahydrofurfurylamine	2943	20
Tetrahydronaphthyl Hydroperoxide, technical pure	2136	8, 43
Tetrahydronaphthalene		43
Tetrahydrophthalic Anhydride	2698	15
Tetrahydropyridine	2410	24
Tetrahydrothiophene	2412	105
Tetralin Hydroperoxide, technical pure	2136	8, 43
Tetram		49, 135
Tetram 75		49, 135
Tetram Monooxalate		49, 135

Chemical Name	UN/ NA/PIN	Guideline Number
Tetramethoxysilane	2606	107
Tetramethrin		52
Tetramethyl Ammonium Hydroxide	1835	20
1,1,3,3-Tetramethylbutyl Hydroperoxide, technical pure	2160	8
1,1,3,3-Tetramethylbutylperoxy-2-ethyl Hexanoate, technical pure	2161	8
Tetramethyl Lead	1649	80
Tetramethylmethylenediamine	9069	20
Tetramethyl Silane	2749	107
Tetramine		69
Tetranitromethane	1510	47
Tetra–propyl Dithionopyrophosphate		49
Tetrapropyl-orthotitanate	2413	10
Tetryl	0208	43
Textile Treating Compound	1760	10
Textile Waste, wet, n.o.s.	1857	87, 97
Thallic Oxide		87
Thallium Acetate		87
Thallium Carbonate		87
Thallium Chlorate	2573	87, 97
Thallium Chloride		87
Thallium Compound, n.o.s.	1707	87
Thallium Nitrate	2727	47, 87
Thallium Salt, n.o.s.	1707	87
Thallium Sulfate, solid	1707	87
Thallous Carbonate		87
Thallous Chloride		87
Thallous Malonate		87
Thallous Sulfate		87
Thanite		94
Thiabendazole		70
Thiapentanal	2785	10

Chemical Name	UN/ NA/PIN	Guideline Number
Trichlorotrifluoroethane (Freon 13)	1078	27
Tri-Con	1581	136
Tricresyl Phosphates	2574	106
Triethanolamine Dodecylbenzene Sulfonate		10
Triethoxysilane		107
Triethylamine	1296	20
Triethylene Glycol		40
Triethylene Tetramine	2259	10
Triethyl Phosphite	2323	109
O,O,O-Triethyl Phosphorothioate		49
Trifluoroacetic Acid	2699	15
Trifluoroacetyl Chloride	3057	15
Trifluoroamine Oxide	9271	99
Trifluorobromomethane	1009	27
Trifluorochloroethylene	1082	27
Trifluorochloroethylene, inhibited	1082	27
Trifluorochloromethane	1022	27
Trifluoroethane, compressed	2035	27
Trifluoromethane	1984	27
Trifluoromethane, refrigerated liquid (cryogenic liquid)	3136	27
Trifluoromethane and Chlorotrifluoromethane Mixture	1078	27
Trifluoromethane and Chlorotrifluoromethane Mixture	2599	27
2-Trifluoromethylaniline	2942	32
3-Trifluoromethylaniline	2948	32
3-Trifluoromethyl-phenylisocyanate	9268	94
Trifluralin		9
Triisobutyl Aluminum	1930	10
Triisobutylene	2324	33
Triisocyanatoisocyanurate of Isophoronediisocyanate, 70% solution	2906	10
Triisopropyl Borate	2616	103
Trimethoxysilane	9269	107
Trimethylacetyl Chloride	2438	15
Trimethyl Aluminum	1103	10
Trimethylamine, anhydrous	1083	20
Trimethylamine, aqueous solution	1297	20
Trimethylbenzene	2325	24
Trimethylborate	2416	103
Trimethylchlorosilane	1298	107
Trimethylcyclohexylamine	2326	20
Trimethylene Chlorohydrin	2849	61
Trimethylhexamethyl-enediamine	2327	20
Trimethylhexamethylene di-isocyanate	2328	94
Trimethyl Norpinanyl Hydroperoxide, technical pure	2162	24
Trimethylolpropane Phosphite		10
Trimethyoxysilane		107
2,2,4-Trimethylpentane		33
2,4,4-Trimethylpentyl-2-peroxyphenoxyacetate	2961	37
1,2,2-Trimethylpropoxy-fluoromethylphosphine Oxide	2810	135
1,2,2-Trimethylpropyl Methylphosphono-fluoridate	2810	135
Trimethyl Phosphite	2329	109
Trimethyltin Chloride		65
Trinitrobenzene, wet	1354	24, 47
Trinitrobenzoic Acid, wet	1355	15, 47
Trinitrophenol, wet	1344	62
Trinitrotoluene, wet	1356	24, 47

Chemical Name	UN/ NA/PIN	Guideline Number
2,4,6-Trinitrotoluene	0209	24, 47
Tri-o-cresyl Phosphate		106
Triphenyl Phosphate		106
Triphenyltin Chloride		65
Triphosgene		101, 133
Tripropylaluminum	2718	10
Tripropylamine	2260	20
Tripropylene	2057	33
Trisodium Phosphate		19
Tris(1-aziridinyl)phosphine Oxide	2501	10
Tris(2-chloroethyl)amine		20
Tris(2,3-dibromopropyl) Phosphate		109
Trypan Blue		43
Tularemia		127
Tungsten Hexafluoride	2196	99, 133, 138
Turpentine	1299	34
Turpentine Substitute	1300	34
TX60	2810	135
Typhoid Fever		117
Typhus fever		128
Undecane	2330	33
Undulant Fever		115
Uracil Mustard		10
Uranium Acetate	9180	12, 37
Uranium Hexafluoride	9174	12, 99
Uranium Hexafluoride, fissile	9173	12, 99
Uranium Hexafluoride, fissile (containing more than 1% U-235)	2977	12, 99
Uranium Hexafluoride, fissile excepted or nonfissile	2978	12, 99
Uranium Hexafluoride, low specific activity	2978	12, 99
Uranium Metal, pyrophoric	2979	12
Uranium Metal, pyrophoric	9175	12
Uranium Nitrate Hexahydrate Solution	2980	12, 47
Uranyl Acetate	9180	12, 37
Uranyl Nitrate, solid	2981	12, 47
Uranyl Nitrate, solid	9177	12, 47
Urban Typhus		128
Urea Hydrogen Peroxide	1511	8
Urea Nitrate, wet	1357	47
Urea Peroxide	1511	8
Urethane		94
Valeraldehyde	2058	41
Valeric Acid, (*n*-pentanoic acid)	1760	15
Valeryl Chloride	2502	15
Valinomycin		10
Valone		71
Vanadium Oxytrichloride	2443	10
Vanadium Oxytrichloride and Titanium Tetrachloride Mixture	2443	10
Vanadium Pentoxide	2862	10
Vanadium Tetrachloride	2444	10
Vanadium Trichloride	2475	10
Vanadium Trioxide	2860	10
Vanadyl Sulfate	2931	10
Vanillin		44
Variola Virus		125
Varnish	1263	35
VEE		129
Venezuelan Equine Encephalitis		129
Vervet Monkey Disease		130
V-gas		135
Vibrio Cholerae		131
Vinyl Acetate	1301	37

Chemical Name	UN/ NA/PIN	Guideline Number
Vinyl Acetate, inhibited	1301	37
Vinyl Bromide	1085	95
Vinyl Bromide, inhibited	1085	95
Vinyl Butyl Ether	1304	38
Vinyl Butyrate	2838	37
Vinyl Butyrate, inhibited	2838	37
Vinyl Chloride	1086	28
Vinyl Chloride, inhibited	1086	28
Vinyl Chloroacetate	2589	37
Vinyl Ether		38
Vinyl Ethyl Ether	1302	38
Vinyl Ethyl Ether, inhibited	1302	38
Vinyl Fluoride	1860	26
Vinyl Fluoride, inhibited	1860	26
Vinylidene Chloride	1303	26
Vinylidene Chloride, inhibited	1303	26
Vinylidene Fluoride	1959	26
Vinyl Isobutyl Ether	1304	38
Vinyl Isobutyl Ether, inhibited	1304	38
Vinyl Methyl Ether	1087	38
Vinyl Methyl Ether, inhibited	1087	38
Vinyl Pyridines, inhibited	3073	24
Vinyl Toluene	2618	24
Vinyl Toluene, inhibited	2618	24
Vinyl Trichlorosilane	1305	107
VM &P Naphtha		35
VX	2810	135
Warfarin	2476	71
Warfarin, and its salts		71
Warfarin Sodium		71
Water-Reactive Solid, n.o.s.	2813	6
Wax, liquid	1993	33
WEE		129

Chemical Name	UN/ NA/PIN	Guideline Number
Western Equine Encephalitis		129
White Asbestos	2590	102
White Phosphorus, dry	1381	109
White Phosphorus, wet	1381	109
Wood Alcohol	1230	31
Wood Filler, liquid	1263	35
Wood Preservative, liquid	1306	35
Wool Waste, wet	1387	9
Xenon	2036	92
Xenon, refrigerated liquid (cryogenic liquid)	2591	92
Xylene (xylol)	1307	24
Xylenol	2261	24, 44
Xylidine	1711	24
Xylol	1307	24
Xylyl Bromide	1701	24, 95
Xylylene Dichloride		24
Y	2810	139
Yellow Cross Liquid	2810	139
Yellow Phosphorus, dry	1381	109
Yellow Phosphorus, wet	1381	109
Yersinia pestis	121	121
Yperite	2810	139
S-yperite	2810	139
Zarin	2810	135
Zinc		88
Zinc Acetate		88
Zinc Ammonium Chloride		88
Zinc Ammonium Nitrite	1512	47, 88
Zinc Arsenate	1712	72, 88
Zinc Arsenate and Zinc Arsenite Mixture	1712	72, 88
Zinc Arsenite	1712	72, 88
Zinc Ashes	1435	88
Zinc Bisulfite Solution	2693	88, 105
Zinc Borate		88, 103
Zinc Bromate	2469	88, 96

Chemical Name	UN/ NA/PIN	Guideline Number
Zinc Bromide		88, 95
Zinc Carbonate		88
Zinc Chlorate	1513	88, 97
Zinc Chloride, anhydrous	2331	88
Zinc Chloride Solution	1840	88
Zinc Chromate		88
Zinc Cyanide	1713	88, 90
Zinc Dithionite	1931	88
Zinc Fluoride		88, 99
Zinc Fluorosilicate	2855	88, 99
Zinc Formate		88
Zinc Hydrosulfite	1931	88, 105
Zinc Metal, powder or dust	1436	88
Zinc Nitrate	1514	47, 88
Zinc Permanganate	1515	14, 88
Zinc Peroxide	1516	88
Zinc Phenolsulfonate	9160	88, 105
Zinc Phosphide	1714	88, 108
Zinc Powder or Dust, nonpyrophoric	1436	88
Zinc Powder or Dust, pyrophoric	1383	88
Zinc Resinate	2714	88
Zinc Salts		88
Zinc Selenate	2630	86, 88
Zinc Selenite	2630	86, 88
Zinc Silicofluoride		88, 99
Zinc Sulfate		88
Zineb		63

Chemical Name	UN/ NA/PIN	Guideline Number
Ziram		63
Zirconium Hydride	1437	10
Zirconium Metal, liquid suspension	1308	10
Zirconium Metal, powder, dry	2008	10
Zirconium Metal, powder, wet	1358	10
Zirconium Metal, wire, sheet, or strips (thinner than 18 microns)	2009	10
Zirconium Metal, wire, sheet, or strips (thinner than 254 microns but not thinner than 18 microns)	2858	10
Zirconium Nitrate	2728	47
Zirconium Picramate, wet	1517	6, 10
Zirconium Potassium Fluoride		99
Zirconium Powder, dry	2008	10
Zirconium Powder, wet	1358	10
Zirconium Scrap	1932	10
Zirconium Sulfate	9163	10
Zirconium Suspended in a liquid	1308	10
Zirconium Tetrachloride	2503	10
Zoman	2810	135
Zytron	9	49

Section Two

GUIDELINES

*Metalloids

Do not enter hazardous environments or carry out decontamination procedures without proper protective equipment. It is beyond the scope of this text to recommend the exact type of protective equipment required for such hazardous material indexed. Other resources (i.e., CHRIS manual, material safety data sheets) and chemical compatibility charts must be checked. Equipment must be appropriate and compatible with the chemical(s) involved. Selection should be made by an experienced, knowledgeable person using appropriate reference materials. Training in the proper use of protective equipment is essential to your safety.

Individual patients exposed to particular toxicants may not exhibit all of the signs and symptoms described. In addition, because of patient variability, an exposed patient may exhibit signs and symptoms other than those listed.

The decision not to use emetics has been based on recent studies regarding their use and the often uncontrolled environment of field operations. Do not orally administer any fats, oils, or alcohols for ingested toxins; dilute with water only when indicated.

To the best of our knowledge, drug indications, dosages, and precautions are current as of publication. The reader is urged to consult the package information provided by the manufacturer for the latest changes. Medication use in pregnant patients should be guided by physician control.

These guidelines contain suggested treatments. Operating protocols, standing, and/or verbal orders must be established by local emergency medical service (EMS) physician control.

Explosives

UN Class 1

SUBSTANCE IDENTIFICATION

Any chemical compound, mixture, or device that is designed to function by explosion or detonation (with instantaneous release of gas and heat) or that, by chemical reaction within itself, is able to function in a similar manner, even if not designed to function by explosion. Found in liquid or solid forms. Includes dynamite, TNT, black powder, fireworks, and ammunition.

ROUTES OF EXPOSURE

Skin and eye contact
Inhalation
Ingestion
Skin absorption

LIFE THREAT

Explosion, causing multisystem trauma. Resulting chemical exposure may be highly toxic.

SIGNS AND SYMPTOMS BY SYSTEM

Cardiovascular: Circulatory collapse and arrhythmias.
Respiratory: Tachypnea and dyspnea.
CNS: Headache, dizziness, progressive stupor, and coma.
Gastrointestinal: Nausea, vomiting, diarrhea, and gastroenteritis.
Eye: Chemical conjunctivitis and ocular damage.
Skin: Dermatitis and skin eruptions.
Other: Nitrogen compounds may cause methemoglobinemia.

Medical responders must have an understanding of the types of physical injuries that explosives can cause. Effective triage principles can be based on these specific effects. Four different injury classes are commonly seen from blast scenarios.

Primary Blast Injury

Explosive devices when detonated turn from a solid into a superheated gas in 1/10,000 of a second. These gases expand at a rate of 13,000 mph (Mach 17.6). After the device explodes, waves of pressure are sent out from the seat of the blast, called *blast waves.* These are the first to cause injury to patients by smashing and shattering anything in the way. Four main target organs are affected by this wave:

- Ears
- Lungs
- Gastrointestinal
- Central nervous system

Secondary Injury

Secondary injuries are injuries caused by shrapnel from the fragments of the device and from things that have been attached to the explosive device. This trauma is like any other penetrating trauma. The patient may also have bruising, bleeding, broken bones, and shock.

Tertiary Injuries

Tertiary injuries are those caused by the patient being thrown like a projectile. The injuries are similar to those resulting from falls or motor vehicle accidents. The treatment is also the same for these injuries. These patients may also have primary and secondary blast injuries.

Type IV Injuries (Miscellaneous)

These are all the other injuries caused by the incident, including burns, chemical exposure, and psychological injuries. Burns and psychological injures are the most common types of type IV injuries. The symptoms from the psychological trauma may not be evident for months or even years.

DECONTAMINATION

- Wear positive-pressure SCBA and protective equipment specified by references such as the *North American Emergency Response Guidebook.* If special chemical protective clothing is required, consult the chemical manufacturer or specific protective clothing compatibility charts. A qualified, experienced person should make decisions regarding the type of personal protective equipment necessary.
- Delay entry until trained personnel and proper protective equipment are available.
- Remove patient from contaminated area.
- Quickly remove and isolate patient's clothing, jewelry, and shoes.
- Gently brush away dry particles and blot excess liquids with absorbent material.
- Rinse patient with warm water, 32° C to 35° C (90° F to 95° F), if possible.
- Wash patient with a mild liquid soap and large quantities of water.
- Refer to decontamination protocol in Section Three.

IMMEDIATE FIRST AID

- Ensure that adequate decontamination has been carried out.
- If patient is not breathing, start artificial respiration, preferably with a demand-valve resuscitator, bag-valve-mask device, or pocket mask, as trained. Perform CPR as necessary.
- Immediately flush contaminated eyes with gently flowing water.
- Do not induce vomiting. If vomiting occurs, lean patient forward or place on left side (head-down position, if possible) to maintain an open airway and prevent aspiration.
- Keep patient quiet and maintain normal body temperature.
- Obtain medical attention.

BASIC TREATMENT

- Establish a patent airway (oropharyngeal or nasopharyngeal airway, if needed). Suction if necessary.
- Watch for signs of respiratory insufficiency and assist ventilations if necessary.
- Administer oxygen by nonrebreather mask at 10 to 15 L/min.
- Monitor for pulmonary edema and treat if necessary (refer to pulmonary edema protocol in Section Three).
- Monitor for shock and treat if necessary (refer to shock protocol in Section Three).
- Anticipate seizures and treat if necessary (refer to seizure protocol in Section Three).

- For eye contamination, flush eyes immediately with water. Irrigate each eye continuously with 0.9% saline (NS) during transport (refer to eye irrigation protocol in Section Three.)
- Do not use emetics. For ingestion, rinse mouth and administer 5 ml/kg up to 200 ml of water for dilution if the patient can swallow, has a strong gag reflex, and does not drool (refer to ingestion protocol in Section Three).

ADVANCED TREATMENT

- Consider orotracheal or nasotracheal intubation for airway control in the patient who is unconscious, has severe pulmonary edema, or is in severe respiratory distress.
- Positive-pressure ventilation techniques with a bag-valve-mask device may be beneficial.
- Consider drug therapy for pulmonary edema (refer to pulmonary edema protocol in Section Three).
- Monitor cardiac rhythm and treat arrhythmias as necessary (refer to cardiac protocol in Section Three).
- Start IV administration of D_5W TKO. Use 0.9% saline (NS) or lactated Ringer's if signs of hypovolemia are present. For hypotension with signs of hypovolemia, administer fluid cautiously. Watch for signs of fluid overload (refer to shock protocol in Section Three).
- Treat seizures with diazepam (Valium) or lorazepam (Ativan) (refer to diazepam and lorazepam protocols in Section Four and seizure protocol in Section Three).
- Use proparacaine hydrochloride to assist eye irrigation (refer to proparacaine hydrochloride protocol in Section Four).

SPECIAL CONSIDERATIONS

- Be aware of explosion hazard. Minimum safe distance is 1 mile. Be prepared to treat multisystem trauma injuries.

Flammable Gases

UN Class 2.1

SUBSTANCE IDENTIFICATION

Any compressed or liquefied gas that meets the requirements for lower flammability limit, flammability limit range, flame projection, or flame propagation as specified in *C.F.R. Title 49, Sec.173.300(b)*. Examples: acetylene, butane, hydrogen, LPG, and propane.

ROUTES OF EXPOSURE

Skin and eye contact
Inhalation

LIFE THREAT

Respiratory failure and arrest.

SIGNS AND SYMPTOMS BY SYSTEM

Cardiovascular: Circulatory collapse and arrhythmias.

Respiratory: Tachypnea and dyspnea. Some act as asphyxiants or cause respiratory failure and pulmonary edema.

CNS: Headache, confusion, dizziness, progressive stupor, coma, and seizures may be present.

Gastrointestinal: Irritant to mucous membranes. Can cause nausea and vomiting.

Eye: Chemical conjunctivitis and corneal damage.

Skin: Skin irritation and frostbite from the freezing effect of the expanding gas.

DECONTAMINATION

- Wear positive-pressure SCBA and protective equipment specified by references such as the *North American Emergency Response Guidebook.* If special chemical protective clothing is required, consult the chemical manufacturer or specific protective clothing compatibility charts. Flash protection may be necessary. A qualified, experienced person should make decisions regarding the type of personal protective equipment necessary.
- Delay entry until trained personnel and proper protective equipment are available.
- Remove patient from contaminated area.
- If there are signs and symptoms of skin contamination or concomitant liquid/solid exposure:
  - Quickly remove and isolate patient's clothing, jewelry, and shoes.
  - Gently brush away dry particles and blot excess liquids with absorbent material.
  - Rinse patient with warm water, 32° C to 35° C (90° F to 95° F), if possible.
  - Wash patient with a mild liquid soap and large quantities of water.
  - Refer to decontamination protocol in Section Three.

IMMEDIATE FIRST AID

- Ensure that adequate decontamination has been carried out.

- If patient is not breathing, start artificial respiration, preferably with a demand-valve resuscitator, bag-valve-mask device, or pocket mask as trained. Perform CPR as necessary.
- Immediately flush contaminated eyes with gently flowing water.
- Do not induce vomiting. If vomiting occurs, lean patient forward or place on left side (head-down position, if possible) to maintain an open airway and prevent aspiration.
- Keep patient quiet and maintain normal body temperature.
- Obtain medical attention.

BASIC TREATMENT

- Establish a patent airway (oropharyngeal or nasopharyngeal airway, if needed). Suction if necessary.
- Watch for signs of respiratory insufficiency and assist ventilations as necessary.
- Administer oxygen by nonrebreather mask at 10 to 15 L/min.
- Monitor for pulmonary edema and treat if necessary (refer to pulmonary edema protocol in Section Three).
- Monitor for shock and treat if necessary (refer to shock protocol in Section Three).
- Anticipate seizures and treat if necessary (refer to seizure protocol in Section Three).
- For eye contamination, flush eyes immediately with water. Irrigate each eye continuously with 0.9% saline (NS) during transport (refer to eye irrigation protocol in Section Three).
- Treat frostbite with rapid rewarming (refer to frostbite protocol in Section Three).

ADVANCED TREATMENT

- Consider orotracheal or nasotracheal intubation for airway control in the patient who is unconscious, has severe pulmonary edema, or is in severe respiratory distress.
- Positive-pressure ventilation techniques with a bag-valve-mask device may be beneficial.
- Consider drug therapy for pulmonary edema (refer to pulmonary edema protocol in Section Three).
- Monitor cardiac rhythm and treat arrhythmias as necessary (refer to cardiac protocol in Section Three).
- Start IV administration of D_5W TKO. Use 0.9% saline (NS) or lactated Ringer's (LR) if signs of hypovolemia are present. For hypotension with signs of hypovolemia, administer fluid cautiously. Watch for signs of fluid overload (refer to shock protocol in Section Three).
- Treat seizures with diazepam (Valium) or lorazepam (Ativan) (refer to diazepam and lorazepam protocols in Section Four and seizure protocol in Section Three).
- Use proparacaine hydrochloride to assist eye irrigation (refer to proparacaine hydrochloride protocol in Section Four).

SPECIAL CONSIDERATIONS

- Be aware of fire and explosion hazard. Liquefied gas products have boiling liquid expanding vapor explosion (BLEVE) potential.

Nonflammable Gases

UN Class 2.2

SUBSTANCE IDENTIFICATION

Any nonflammable, nonpoisonous compressed gas that exerts in the container an absolute pressure of 280 kPa (41 psi) or greater at 20° C (68° F). May be compressed, liquefied, pressurized cryogenic, or compressed gas in solution. Examples: helium, xenon, argon, nitrogen, carbon dioxide.

ROUTES OF EXPOSURE

Skin and eye contact
Inhalation

LIFE THREAT

Pulmonary edema and respiratory failure. Many products may act as simple asphyxiants.

SIGNS AND SYMPTOMS BY SYSTEM

Cardiovascular: Circulatory collapse and arrhythmias.

Respiratory: Tachypnea, hypoxia, and dyspnea. Irritation to the respiratory tract. Signs of pulmonary edema.

CNS: Headache, confusion, dizziness, progressive stupor, coma, and seizures.

Gastrointestinal: Irritant to mucous membranes. Can cause nausea and vomiting.

Eye: Chemical conjunctivitis and corneal damage.

Skin: Skin irritation and frostbite from the freezing effect of the expanding gas.

DECONTAMINATION

- Wear positive-pressure SCBA and protective equipment specified by references such as the *North American Emergency Response Guidebook.* If special chemical protective clothing is required, consult the chemical manufacturer or specific protective clothing compatibility charts. A qualified, experienced person should make decisions regarding the type of personal protective equipment necessary.
- Delay entry until trained personnel and proper protective equipment are available.
- Remove patient from contaminated area.
- Quickly remove and isolate patient's clothing, jewelry, and shoes.
- *If there are signs and symptoms of skin contamination or concomitant liquid/solid exposure:*
  - Gently brush away dry particles and blot excess liquids with absorbent material.
  - Rinse patient with warm water, 32° C to 35° C (90° F to 95° F), if possible.
  - Wash patient with a mild liquid soap and large quantities of water.
  - Refer to decontamination protocol in Section Three.

IMMEDIATE FIRST AID

- Ensure that adequate decontamination has been carried out.
- If patient is not breathing, start artificial respiration, preferably with a demand-valve resuscitator, bag-valve-mask device, or pocket mask, as trained. Perform CPR as necessary.

- Immediately flush contaminated eyes with gently flowing water.
- Do not induce vomiting. If vomiting occurs, lean patient forward or place on left side (head-down position, if possible) to maintain an open airway and prevent aspiration.
- Keep patient quiet and maintain normal body temperature.
- Obtain medical attention.

BASIC TREATMENT

- Establish a patent airway (oropharyngeal or nasopharyngeal airway, if needed). Suction if necessary.
- Watch for signs of respiratory insufficiency and assist ventilations if necessary.
- Administer oxygen by nonrebreather mask at 10 to 15 L/min.
- Monitor for pulmonary edema and treat if necessary (refer to pulmonary edema protocol in Section Three).
- Monitor for shock and treat if necessary (refer to shock protocol in Section Three).
- Anticipate seizures and treat if necessary (refer to seizure protocol in Section Three).
- For eye contamination, flush eyes immediately with water. Irrigate each eye continuously with 0.9% saline (NS) during transport (refer to eye irrigation protocol in Section Three).
- Treat frostbite with rapid rewarming (refer to frostbite protocol in Section Three).

ADVANCED TREATMENT

- Consider orotracheal or nasotracheal intubation for airway control in the patient who is unconscious, has severe pulmonary edema, or is in severe respiratory distress.
- Positive-pressure ventilation techniques with a bag-valve-mask device may be beneficial.
- Consider drug therapy for pulmonary edema (refer to pulmonary edema protocol in Section Three).
- Monitor cardiac rhythm and treat arrhythmias as necessary (refer to cardiac protocol in Section Three).
- Start IV administration of D_5W TKO. Use 0.9% saline (NS) or lactated Ringer's (LR) if signs of hypovolemia are present. For hypotension with signs of hypovolemia, administer fluid cautiously. Watch for signs of fluid overload (refer to shock protocol in Section Three).
- Treat seizures with diazepam (Valium) or lorazepam (Ativan) (refer to diazepam and lorazepam protocols in Section Four and seizure protocol in Section Three).
- Use proparacaine hydrochloride to assist eye irrigation (refer to proparacaine hydrochloride protocol in Section Four).

SPECIAL CONSIDERATIONS

- Liquefied products may present boiling liquid expanding vapor explosion (BLEVE) hazard.

4

Combustible Liquids

UN Class 3

SUBSTANCE IDENTIFICATION

Any liquid having a flash point above 60° C (140° F) and below 93° C (200° F). Examples: brake fluid, glycol ethers, and camphor oil.

ROUTES OF EXPOSURE

Skin and eye contact
Inhalation
Ingestion
Skin absorption

LIFE THREAT

CNS depression may lead to respiratory arrest or may cause convulsions, cardiac arrhythmias, and pulmonary edema.

SIGNS AND SYMPTOMS BY SYSTEM

Cardiovascular: Cardiac arrhythmias, tachycardia, and hypotension.

Respiratory: Upper respiratory tract irritation. Dyspnea, tachypnea, and rales that may progress rapidly to massive pulmonary edema. Burning sensation in the chest.

CNS: CNS depression to coma. Confusion, disorientation, headache, drowsiness, weakness, and seizures.

Gastrointestinal: Pain and irritation of the mucous membranes. Nausea, vomiting, and diarrhea.

Eye: Chemical conjunctivitis and corneal damage.

Skin: Irritation and dermatitis. Cyanosis of the extremities.

DECONTAMINATION

- Wear positive-pressure SCBA and protective equipment specified by references such as the *North American Emergency Response Guidebook*. If special chemical protective clothing is required, consult the chemical manufacturer or specific protective clothing compatibility charts. Flash protection may be necessary. A qualified, experienced person should make decisions regarding the type of personal protective equipment necessary.
- Delay entry until trained personnel and proper protective equipment are available.
- Remove patient from contaminated area.
- Quickly remove and isolate patient's clothing, jewelry, and shoes.
- Gently blot excess liquids with absorbent material.
- Rinse patient with warm water, 32° C to 35° C (90° F to 95° F), if possible.
- Wash patient with a mild liquid soap and large quantities of water.
- Refer to decontamination protocol in Section Three.

IMMEDIATE FIRST AID

- Ensure that adequate decontamination has been carried out.

- If patient is not breathing, start artificial respiration, preferably with a demand-valve resuscitator, bag-valve-mask device, or pocket mask, as trained. Perform CPR as necessary.
- Immediately flush contaminated eyes with gently flowing water.
- Do not induce vomiting. If vomiting occurs, lean patient forward or place on left side (head-down position, if possible) to maintain an open airway and prevent aspiration.
- Keep patient quiet and maintain normal body temperature.
- Obtain medical attention.

BASIC TREATMENT

- Establish a patent airway (oropharyngeal or nasopharyngeal airway, if needed). Suction if necessary.
- Watch for signs of respiratory insufficiency and assist ventilations if necessary.
- Administer oxygen by nonrebreather mask at 10 to 15 L/min.
- Monitor for shock and treat if necessary (refer to shock protocol in Section Three).
- Monitor for pulmonary edema and treat if necessary (refer to pulmonary edema protocol in Section Three).
- Anticipate seizures and treat if necessary (refer to seizure protocol in Section Three).
- For eye contamination, flush eyes immediately with water. Irrigate each eye continuously with 0.9% saline (NS) during transport (refer to eye irrigation protocol in Section Three).
- Do not use emetics. For ingestion, rinse mouth and administer 5 ml/kg up to 200 ml of water for dilution if product was ingested and the patient can swallow, has a strong gag reflex, and does not drool (refer to ingestion protocol in Section Three).

ADVANCED TREATMENT

- Consider orotracheal or nasotracheal intubation for airway control in the patient who is unconscious, has severe pulmonary edema, or is in severe respiratory distress.
- Positive-pressure ventilation techniques with a bag-valve-mask device may be beneficial.
- Consider drug therapy for pulmonary edema (refer to pulmonary edema protocol in Section Three).
- Monitor cardiac rhythm and treat arrhythmias as necessary (refer to cardiac protocol in Section Three).
- Start IV administration of D_5W TKO. Use 0.9% saline (NS) or lactated Ringer's (LR) if signs of hypovolemia are present. For hypotension with signs of hypovolemia, administer fluid cautiously. Watch for signs of fluid overload (refer to shock protocol in Section Three).
- Treat seizures with diazepam (Valium) or lorazepam (Ativan) (refer to diazepam and lorazepam protocols in Section Four and seizure protocol in Section Three).
- Use proparacaine hydrochloride to assist eye irrigation (refer to proparacaine hydrochloride protocol in Section Four).

SPECIAL CONSIDERATIONS

- Avoid epinephrine and related beta agonists (unless patient is in cardiac arrest or has reactive airways disease refractory to other treatment) because of the possible irritable condition of the myocardium. Use of these medications may lead to ventricular fibrillation.
- Be prepared to treat thermal injuries.

Flammable Liquids

UN Class 3

SUBSTANCE IDENTIFICATION

Any liquid having a flash point of not more than 60.5° C (141° F). Examples: benzene, gasoline, toluene, trichlorethylene, and acetone.

ROUTES OF EXPOSURE

Skin and eye contact
Inhalation
Ingestion
Skin absorption

LIFE THREAT

CNS depression may lead to respiratory arrest or may cause seizures, cardiac arrhythmias, and pulmonary edema.

SIGNS AND SYMPTOMS BY SYSTEM

Cardiovascular: Cardiac arrhythmias, tachycardia, and hypotension.

Respiratory: Upper respiratory tract irritation. Dyspnea, tachypnea, and rales that may progress rapidly to massive pulmonary edema. Burning sensation in the chest.

CNS: CNS depression to coma. Confusion, disorientation, headache, drowsiness, weakness, and seizures.

Gastrointestinal: Pain and irritation of the mucous membranes, nausea, vomiting, and diarrhea.

Eye: Chemical conjunctivitis and corneal damage.

Skin: Irritation and dermatitis. Cyanosis of the extremities.

DECONTAMINATION

- Wear positive-pressure SCBA and protective equipment specified by references such as the *North American Emergency Response Guidebook*. If special chemical protective clothing is required, consult the chemical manufacturer or specific protective clothing compatibility charts. Flash protection may be required. A qualified, experienced person should make decisions regarding the type of personal protective equipment necessary.
- Delay entry until trained personnel and proper protective equipment are available.
- Remove patient from contaminated area.
- Quickly remove and isolate patient's clothing, jewelry, and shoes.
- Gently blot excess liquids with absorbent material.
- Rinse patient with warm water, 32° C to 35° C (90° F to 95° F), if possible.
- Wash patient with a mild liquid soap and large quantities of water.
- Refer to decontamination protocol in Section Three.

IMMEDIATE FIRST AID

- Ensure that adequate decontamination has been carried out.

- If patient is not breathing, start artificial respiration, preferably with a demand-valve resuscitator, bag-valve-mask device, or pocket mask, as trained. Perform CPR if necessary.
- Immediately flush contaminated eyes with gently flowing water.
- Do not induce vomiting. If vomiting occurs, lean patient forward or place on left side (head-down position, if possible) to maintain an open airway and prevent aspiration.
- Keep patient quiet and maintain normal body temperature.
- Obtain medical attention.

BASIC TREATMENT

- Establish a patent airway (oropharyngeal or nasopharyngeal airway, if needed). Suction if necessary.
- Watch for signs of respiratory insufficiency and assist ventilations if necessary.
- Administer oxygen by nonrebreather mask at 10 to 15 L/min.
- Monitor for shock and treat if necessary (refer to shock protocol in Section Three).
- Monitor for pulmonary edema and treat if necessary (refer to pulmonary edema protocol in Section Three).
- Anticipate seizures and treat if necessary (refer to seizure protocol in Section Three).
- For eye contamination, flush eyes immediately with water. Irrigate each eye continuously with 0.9% saline (NS) during transport (refer to eye irrigation protocol in Section Three).
- Do not use emetics. For ingestion, rinse mouth and administer 5 ml/kg up to 200 ml of water for dilution if the patient can swallow, has a strong gag reflex, and does not drool (refer to ingestion protocol in Section Three).

ADVANCED TREATMENT

- Consider orotracheal or nasotracheal intubation for airway control in the patient who is unconscious, has severe pulmonary edema, or is in severe respiratory distress.
- Positive-pressure ventilation techniques with a bag-valve-mask device may be beneficial.
- Consider drug therapy for pulmonary edema (refer to pulmonary edema protocol in Section Three).
- Monitor cardiac rhythm and treat arrhythmias if necessary (refer to cardiac protocol in Section Three).
- Start IV administration of D_5W TKO. Use 0.9% saline (NS) or lactated Ringer's (LR) if signs of hypovolemia are present. For hypotension with signs of hypovolemia, administer fluid cautiously. Watch for signs of fluid overload (refer to shock protocol in Section Three).
- Treat seizures with diazepam (Valium) or lorazepam (Ativan) (refer to diazepam and lorazepam protocols in Section Four and seizure protocol in Section Three).
- Use proparacaine hydrochloride to assist eye irrigation (refer to proparacaine hydrochloride protocol in Section Four).

SPECIAL CONSIDERATIONS

- Avoid epinephrine and related beta agonists (unless in cardiac arrest or reactive airway disease refractory to other treatment) because of the possible irritable condition of the myocardium. Use of these medications may lead to ventricular fibrillation.
- Be prepared to treat thermal injuries.

Flammable Solids

UN Class 4

SUBSTANCE IDENTIFICATION

A solid material, other than an explosive, that is liable to cause fires through friction, retained heat from manufacturing, or processing or that can be ignited readily. When these substances are ignited, they burn so vigorously and persistently that they create a serious hazard. Some products may be water reactive, whereas others may react in air. Examples: phosphorus, lithium, potassium, magnesium, titanium, and calcium resinate.

ROUTES OF EXPOSURE

Skin and eye contact
Inhalation
Ingestion
Skin absorption

LIFE THREAT

Shock and severe tissue burns. Severe respiratory irritant that can cause pulmonary edema and respiratory arrest. Electrocardiogram changes and sudden death have also been observed with some products.

SIGNS AND SYMPTOMS BY SYSTEM

Cardiovascular: Cardiac arrhythmias and shock.

Respiratory: Acute pulmonary edema, dyspnea, tachypnea, and irritation of the respiratory tract.

CNS: Headache, dizziness, fatigue, photophobia, and seizures.

Gastrointestinal: Nausea, vomiting, abdominal pain, and excessive salivation.

Eye: Lacrimation, conjunctivitis, and severe corneal injury.

Skin: Severe chemical and thermal burns and jaundice.

Other: Hypoglycemia. Symptoms, especially pulmonary edema, may be delayed. The ability to detect the product by smell may be lost after a short exposure time (olfactory nerve fatigue).

DECONTAMINATION

- Wear positive-pressure SCBA and protective equipment specified by references such as the *North American Emergency Response Guidebook*. If special chemical protective clothing is required, consult the chemical manufacturer or specific protective clothing compatibility charts. A qualified, experienced person should make decisions regarding the type of personal protective equipment necessary.
- Delay entry until trained personnel and proper protective equipment are available.
- Remove patient from contaminated area.
- Quickly remove and isolate patient's clothing, jewelry, and shoes.
- Gently brush away dry particles and blot excess liquids with absorbent material.
- If water-reactive products are embedded in the skin, no water should be applied. The embedded products should be covered with a light oil (mineral or cooking

oil), and the patient transported for surgical debridement. If products are not embedded, gently brush away as many as possible and flush with copious amounts of water to rapidly remove any residual product.

- If phosphorus particles are embedded in the skin, continuous water irrigation, water emersion, or sterile water-soaked dressings should be applied during transport to hospital for surgical debridement. Do not use oil for phosphorus exposure, since this may promote dermal absorption.
- Rinse patient with cool water unless contraindicated as above.
- Wash patient with a mild liquid soap and large quantities of water.
- Refer to decontamination protocol in Section Three.

IMMEDIATE FIRST AID

- Ensure that adequate decontamination has been carried out.
- If patient is not breathing, start artificial respiration, preferably with a demand-valve resuscitator, bag-valve-mask device, or pocket mask, as trained. Perform CPR if necessary.
- Immediately flush contaminated eyes with gently flowing water.
- Do not induce vomiting. If vomiting occurs, lean patient forward or place on left side (head-down position, if possible) to maintain an open airway and prevent aspiration.
- Keep patient quiet and maintain normal body temperature.
- Obtain medical attention.

BASIC TREATMENT

- Establish a patent airway (oropharyngeal or nasopharyngeal airway, if needed). Suction if necessary.
- Watch for signs of respiratory insufficiency and assist ventilations if necessary.
- Administer oxygen by nonrebreather mask at 10 to 15 L/min.
- Monitor for pulmonary edema and treat if necessary (refer to pulmonary edema protocol in Section Three).
- Monitor for shock and treat if necessary (refer to shock protocol in Section Three).
- Anticipate seizures and treat if necessary (refer to seizure protocol in Section Three).
- For eye contamination, flush eyes immediately with water. Irrigate each eye continuously with 0.9% saline (NS) during transport (refer to eye irrigation protocol in Section Three).
- Do not use emetics. For ingestion, rinse mouth and administer 5 ml/kg up to 200 ml of water for dilution if the patient can swallow, has a strong gag reflex, and does not drool (refer to ingestion protocol in Section Three).
- If product was ingested, protect yourself from contact with vomitus, since it may cause burns.

ADVANCED TREATMENT

- Consider orotracheal or nasotracheal intubation for airway control in the patient who is unconscious, has severe pulmonary edema, or is in severe respiratory distress.
- Positive-pressure ventilation techniques with a bag-valve-mask device may be beneficial.
- Consider drug therapy for pulmonary edema (refer to pulmonary edema protocol in Section Three).

- Monitor cardiac rhythm and treat arrhythmias as necessary (refer to cardiac protocol in Section Three).
- Start IV administration of D_5W TKO. Use 0.9% saline (NS) or lactated Ringer's (LR) if signs of hypovolemia are present. For hypotension with signs of hypovolemia, administer fluid cautiously. Watch for signs of fluid overload (refer to shock protocol in Section Three).
- Monitor for signs of hypoglycemia (decreased level of consciousness, tachycardia, pallor, dilated pupils, diaphoresis, and/or readings below 50 mg/dl on dextrose strip or glucometer) and administer 50% dextrose if necessary. Draw blood sample before administration (refer to 50% dextrose protocol in Section Four).
- Treat seizures with diazepam (Valium) or lorazepam (Ativan) (refer to diazepam and lorazepam protocols in Section Four and seizure protocol in Section Three).
- Use proparacaine hydrochloride to assist eye irrigation (refer to proparacaine hydrochloride protocol in Section Four).

7

Oxidizers

UN Class 5.1

SUBSTANCE IDENTIFICATION

A substance that yields oxygen readily to stimulate the combustion of matter. Examples: lithium peroxide and calcium chloride. Many products have corrosive properties. Products may be explosively sensitive to heat and shock.

ROUTES OF EXPOSURE

Skin and eye contact
Inhalation
Ingestion

LIFE THREAT

Pulmonary edema, circulatory collapse, laryngeal edema. Corrosive to skin, mucous membranes, and internal organs.

SIGNS AND SYMPTOMS BY SYSTEM

Cardiovascular: Hypovolemic shock and circulatory collapse. Tachycardia with weak pulse.

Respiratory: Acute pulmonary edema, asphyxia, chemical pneumonitis, and upper airway obstruction caused by edema.

CNS: Symptoms of hypoxia, stupor, lethargy, and coma.

Gastrointestinal: Acute toxicity from ingestion results in burns to the GI tract. Nausea, vomiting, and diarrhea, possibly with blood.

Eye: Conjunctivitis, opacification of the cornea, and possibly blindness.

Skin: Full- and partial-thickness burns.

DECONTAMINATION

- Wear positive-pressure SCBA and protective equipment specified by references such as the *North American Emergency Response Guidebook.* If special chemical protective clothing is required, consult the chemical manufacturer or specific protective clothing compatibility charts. A qualified, experienced person should make decisions regarding the type of personal protective equipment necessary.
- Delay entry until trained personnel and proper protective equipment are available.
- Remove patient from contaminated area.
- Quickly remove and isolate patient's clothing, jewelry, and shoes.
- Gently brush away dry particles and blot excess liquids with absorbent material.
- Rinse patient with warm water, 32° C to 35° C (90° F to 95° F), if possible.
- Wash patient with a mild liquid soap and large quantities of water.
- Refer to decontamination protocol in Section Three.

IMMEDIATE FIRST AID

- Ensure that adequate decontamination has been carried out.
- If patient is not breathing, start artificial respiration, preferably with a demand-valve resuscitator, bag-valve-mask device, or pocket mask, as trained. Perform CPR if necessary.

- Immediately flush contaminated eyes with gently flowing water.
- Do not induce vomiting. If vomiting occurs, lean patient forward or place on left side (head-down position, if possible) to maintain an open airway and prevent aspiration.
- Keep patient quiet and maintain normal body temperature.
- Obtain medical attention.

BASIC TREATMENT

- Establish a patent airway (oropharyngeal or nasopharyngeal airway, if needed). Suction if necessary.
- Watch for signs of respiratory insufficiency and assist ventilations if necessary.
- Administer oxygen by nonrebreather mask at 10 to 15 L/min.
- Monitor for pulmonary edema and treat if necessary (refer to pulmonary edema protocol in Section Three).
- Monitor for shock and treat if necessary (refer to shock protocol in Section Three).
- For eye contamination, flush eyes immediately with water. Irrigate each eye continuously with 0.9% saline (NS) during transport (refer to eye irrigation protocol in Section Three).
- Do not use emetics. For ingestion, rinse mouth and administer 5 ml/kg up to 200 ml of water for dilution if the patient can swallow, has a strong gag reflex, and does not drool (refer to ingestion protocol in Section Three).
- Do not attempt to neutralize because of exothermic reaction.
- Cover skin burns with dry, sterile dressings after decontamination (refer to chemical burn protocol in Section Three).

ADVANCED TREATMENT

- Consider orotracheal or nasotracheal intubation for airway control in the patient who is unconscious, has severe pulmonary edema, or is in severe respiratory distress. Early intubation, at the first sign of upper airway obstruction, may be necessary.
- Positive-pressure ventilation techniques with a bag-valve-mask device may be beneficial.
- Consider drug therapy for pulmonary edema (refer to pulmonary edema protocol in Section Three).
- Monitor cardiac rhythm and treat arrhythmias as necessary (refer to cardiac protocol in Section Three).
- Start IV administration of D_5W TKO. Use 0.9% saline (NS) or lactated Ringer's (LR) if signs of hypovolemia are present. For hypotension with signs of hypovolemia, administer fluid cautiously. Watch for signs of fluid overload (refer to shock protocol in Section Three).
- Use proparacaine hydrochloride to assist eye irrigation (refer to proparacaine hydrochloride protocol in Section Four).

Organic Peroxides

UN Class 5.2

SUBSTANCE IDENTIFICATION

An organic compound containing oxygen (O) in the bivalent -0-0 structure. It may be considered a derivative of hydrogen peroxide, in which one or more of the hydrogen atoms have been replaced by organic radicals. Many products are corrosive. Products also supply oxygen to support combustion of other materials. These agents may be explosively sensitive to shock and heat. Examples: benzoyl peroxide, peracetic acid, and methyl ethyl ketone peroxide.

ROUTES OF EXPOSURE

Skin and eye contact
Inhalation
Ingestion

LIFE THREAT

Pulmonary edema, circulatory collapse, laryngeal edema. Corrosive to skin, mucous membranes, and internal organs.

SIGNS AND SYMPTOMS BY SYSTEM

Cardiovascular: Hypovolemic shock and circulatory collapse. Tachycardia with weak pulse.

Respiratory: Acute pulmonary edema, asphyxia, chemical pneumonitis, and upper airway obstruction with stridor caused by edema.

CNS: Symptoms of hypoxia, stupor, lethargy, and coma.

Gastrointestinal: Acute toxicity from ingestion results in burns to the GI tract. Nausea, vomiting, and diarrhea, possibly with blood.

Eye: Conjunctivitis, opacification of the cornea, and possibly blindness.

Skin: Partial- and full-thickness burns.

DECONTAMINATION

- Wear positive-pressure SCBA and protective equipment specified by references such as the *North American Emergency Response Guidebook*. If special chemical protective clothing is required, consult the chemical manufacturer or specific protective clothing compatibility charts. A qualified, experienced person should make decisions regarding the type of personal protective equipment necessary.
- Delay entry until trained personnel and proper protective equipment are available.
- Remove patient from contaminated area.
- Quickly remove and isolate patient's clothing, jewelry, and shoes.
- Gently brush away dry particles and blot excess liquids with absorbent material.
- Rinse patient with warm water, 32° C to 35° C (90° F to 95° F), if possible.
- Wash patient with a mild liquid soap and large quantities of water.
- Refer to decontamination protocol in Section Three.

IMMEDIATE FIRST AID

- Ensure that adequate decontamination has been carried out.

- If patient is not breathing, start artificial respiration, preferably with a demand-valve resuscitator, bag-valve-mask device, or pocket mask, as trained. Perform CPR if necessary.
- Immediately flush contaminated eyes with gently flowing water.
- Do not induce vomiting. If vomiting occurs, lean patient forward or place on left side (head-down position, if possible) to maintain an open airway and prevent aspiration.
- Keep patient quiet and maintain normal body temperature.
- Obtain medical attention.

BASIC TREATMENT

- Establish a patent airway (oropharyngeal or nasopharyngeal airway, if needed). Suction if necessary.
- Watch for signs of respiratory insufficiency and assist ventilations if necessary.
- Administer oxygen by nonrebreather mask at 10 to 15 L/min.
- Monitor for pulmonary edema and treat if necessary (refer to pulmonary edema protocol in Section Three).
- Monitor for shock and treat if necessary (refer to shock protocol in Section Three).
- Anticipate seizures and treat if necessary (refer to seizure protocol in Section Three).
- For eye contamination, flush eyes immediately with water. Irrigate each eye continuously with 0.9% saline (NS) during transport (refer to eye irrigation protocol in Section Three).
- Do not use emetics. For ingestion, rinse mouth and administer 5 ml/kg up to 200 ml of water for dilution if the patient can swallow, has a strong gag reflex, and does not drool (refer to ingestion protocol in Section Three).
- Do not attempt to neutralize because of exothermic reaction.
- Cover skin burns with dry, sterile dressings after decontamination (refer to chemical burn protocol in Section Three).

ADVANCED TREATMENT

- Consider orotracheal or nasotracheal intubation for airway control in the patient who is unconscious, has severe pulmonary edema, or is in severe respiratory distress. Early intubation, at the first sign of upper airway obstruction, may be necessary.
- Positive-pressure ventilation techniques with a bag-valve-mask device may be beneficial.
- Consider drug therapy for pulmonary edema (refer to pulmonary edema protocol in Section Three).
- Monitor cardiac rhythm and treat arrhythmias if necessary (refer to cardiac protocol in Section Three).
- Start IV administration of D_5W TKO. Use 0.9% saline (NS) or lactated Ringer's (LR) if signs of hypovolemia are present. For hypotension with signs of hypovolemia, administer fluid cautiously. Watch for signs of fluid overload (refer to shock protocol in Section Three).
- Treat seizures with diazepam (Valium) or lorazepam (Ativan) (refer to diazepam and lorazepam protocols in Section Four and seizure protocol in Section Three).
- Use proparacaine hydrochloride to assist eye irrigation (refer to proparacaine hydrochloride protocol in Section Four).

Irritating Materials

UN Class 6

SUBSTANCE IDENTIFICATION

A liquid or solid substance that, on contact with fire or when exposed to air, gives off dangerous or intensely irritating fumes, but no poisonous material.

ROUTES OF EXPOSURE

Skin and eye contact
Inhalation
Ingestion

LIFE THREAT

Respiratory tract irritants can cause a severe, delayed pulmonary edema or immediate upper airway irritation and edema.

SIGNS AND SYMPTOMS BY SYSTEM

Cardiovascular: Cardiovascular collapse with a rapid and weak pulse. Can show a reflex bradycardia.

Respiratory: With most agents, a mild and transient cough is the only symptom at the time of exposure. Symptoms may be self-limited in mild exposures. A delayed onset of dyspnea, rapid respirations, violent coughing, and pulmonary edema may follow. Some agents work immediately on the upper airway, resulting in pain and choking and spasm of the glottis (resulting in a temporary reflex arrest of breathing). Severe exposures may cause upper airway obstruction from glottic spasm.

CNS: Fatigue, restlessness, and decreasing LOC are usually delayed signs.

Gastrointestinal: Burning of the mucous membranes, nausea, vomiting, and abdominal pain.

Eye: Chemical conjunctivitis.

Skin: Irritation of the skin, especially mucous membranes, and pallor and cyanosis.

Other: With most products, symptoms will be immediate. Some respiratory symptoms may be delayed for 5 to 72 hours.

DECONTAMINATION

- Wear positive-pressure SCBA and protective equipment specified by references such as the *North American Emergency Response Guidebook*. If special chemical protective clothing is required, consult the chemical manufacturer or specific protective clothing compatibility charts. A qualified, experienced person should make decisions regarding the type of personal protective equipment necessary.
- Delay entry until trained personnel and proper protective equipment are available.
- Remove patient from contaminated area.
- Quickly remove and isolate patient's clothing, jewelry, and shoes.
- Gently brush away dry particles and blot excess liquids with absorbent material.
- Rinse patient with warm water, 32° C to 35° C (90° F to 95° F), if possible.
- Wash patient with a mild liquid soap and large quantities of water.
- Refer to decontamination protocol in Section Three.

IMMEDIATE FIRST AID

- Ensure that adequate decontamination has been carried out.
- If patient is not breathing, start artificial respiration, preferably with a demand-valve resuscitator, bag-valve-mask device, or pocket mask, as trained. Perform CPR as necessary.
- Immediately flush contaminated eyes with gently flowing water.
- Do not induce vomiting. If vomiting occurs, lean patient forward or place on left side (head-down position, if possible) to maintain an open airway and prevent aspiration.
- Keep patient quiet and maintain normal body temperature.
- Obtain medical attention.

BASIC TREATMENT

- Establish a patent airway (oropharyngeal or nasopharyngeal airway, if needed). Suction if necessary.
- Encourage patient to take deep breaths.
- Watch for signs of respiratory insufficiency and assist ventilations if necessary.
- Administer oxygen by nonrebreather mask at 10 to 15 L/min.
- Monitor for pulmonary edema and treat if necessary (refer to pulmonary edema protocol in Section Three).
- Monitor for shock and treat if necessary (refer to shock protocol in Section Three).
- Anticipate seizures and treat if necessary (refer to seizure protocol in Section Three).
- For eye contamination, flush eyes immediately with water. Irrigate each eye continuously with 0.9% saline (NS) during transport (refer to eye irrigation protocol in Section Three).
- Do not use emetics. For ingestion, rinse mouth and administer 5 ml/kg up to 200 ml of water for dilution if the patient can swallow, has a strong gag reflex, and does not drool (refer to ingestion protocol in Section Three).

ADVANCED TREATMENT

- Consider orotracheal or nasotracheal intubation for airway control in the patient who is unconscious, has severe pulmonary edema, or is in severe respiratory distress. Early intubation at the first sign of upper airway obstruction may be necessary.
- Positive-pressure ventilation techniques with a bag-valve mask device may be beneficial.
- Consider drug therapy for pulmonary edema (refer to pulmonary edema protocol in Section Three).
- Monitor cardiac rhythm and treat arrhythmias if necessary (refer to cardiac protocol in Section Three).
- Start IV administration of D_5W TKO. Use 0.9% saline (NS) or lactated Ringer's (LR) if signs of hypovolemia are present. For hypotension with signs of hypovolemia, administer fluid cautiously. Watch for signs of fluid overload (refer to shock protocol in Section Three).
- Treat seizures with diazepam (Valium) or lorazepam (Ativan) (refer to diazepam and lorazepam protocols in Section Four and seizure protocol in Section Three).
- Use proparacaine hydrochloride to assist eye irrigation (refer to proparacaine hydrochloride protocol in Section Four).

SPECIAL CONSIDERATIONS

- In most cases of mild exposure, symptoms are self-limited and require supportive management only. Use of medications such as atropine, epinephrine, expectorants, and sedatives are not indicated and may cause further damage.
- Treat severe symptomatic exposures as required.

Poisons A and B

UN Class 2 and 6

SUBSTANCE IDENTIFICATION

Poisonous gases, liquids, or other substances of such nature that exposure to a very small amount of the gas, vapor, liquid, or solid is dangerous to life or presents a health hazard. Examples: cyanide, arsenic, phosgene, aniline, methyl bromide, and various insecticides/pesticides. Products may be very toxic.

ROUTES OF EXPOSURE

Skin and eye contact
Inhalation
Ingestion
Skin absorption

LIFE THREAT

Cardiovascular collapse, pulmonary edema, CNS depression, and cardiopulmonary arrest. These poisons have a variety of actions and life threats. Generalized symptoms are listed, but symptoms may vary markedly from product to product.

SIGNS AND SYMPTOMS BY SYSTEM

Cardiovascular: Cardiovascular collapse, arrhythmias, and cardiac arrest.

Respiratory: Acute pulmonary edema, dyspnea, stridor, tachypnea, bronchospasm with wheezing and other reactive airway symptoms, and respiratory arrest.

CNS: CNS depression, coma, and seizures.

Gastrointestinal: Nausea, vomiting, diarrhea (sometimes bloody), and abdominal pain.

Eye: Chemical conjunctivitis, corneal burns and opacification. Profuse lacrimation may occur.

Skin: Irritation and chemical burns.

Other: Some products may result in a syndrome of *s*alivation, *l*acrimation, *u*rination, *d*efecation, *g*astrointestinal pain, and *e*mesis (SLUDGE syndrome). Others may cause methemoglobinemia or interfere with cellular respiration (oxidative phosphorylation).

DECONTAMINATION

- Wear positive-pressure SCBA and protective equipment specified by references such as the *North American Emergency Response Guidebook*. If special chemical protective clothing is required, consult the chemical manufacturer or specific protective clothing compatibility charts. A qualified, experienced person should make decisions regarding the type of personal protective equipment necessary.
- Delay entry until trained personnel and proper protective equipment are available.
- Remove patient from contaminated area.
- Quickly remove and isolate patient's clothing, jewelry, and shoes.
- Gently brush away dry particles and blot excess liquids with absorbent material.
- Rinse patient with warm water, 32° C to 35° C (90° F to 95° F), if possible.

- Wash patient with a mild liquid soap and large quantities of water.
- Refer to decontamination protocol in Section Three.

IMMEDIATE FIRST AID

- Ensure that adequate decontamination has been carried out.
- If patient is not breathing, start artificial respiration, preferably with a demand valve resuscitator, bag-valve-mask device, or pocket mask, as trained. Perform CPR if necessary.
- Immediately flush contaminated eyes with gently flowing water.
- Do not induce vomiting. If vomiting occurs, lean patient forward or place on left side (head-down position, if possible) to maintain an open airway and prevent aspiration.
- Keep patient quiet and maintain normal body temperature.
- Obtain medical attention.

BASIC TREATMENT

- Establish a patent airway (oropharyngeal or nasopharyngeal airway, if needed). Suction if necessary.
- Watch for signs of respiratory insufficiency and assist ventilations if needed.
- Administer oxygen by nonrebreather mask at 10 to 15 L/min.
- Monitor for pulmonary edema and treat if necessary (refer to pulmonary edema protocol in Section Three).
- Monitor for shock and treat if necessary (refer to shock protocol in Section Three).
- Anticipate seizures and treat if necessary (refer to seizure protocol in Section Three).
- For eye contamination, flush eyes immediately with water. Irrigate each eye continuously with 0.9% saline (NS) during transport (refer to eye irrigation protocol in Section Three).
- Do not use emetics. For ingestion, rinse mouth and administer 5 ml/kg up to 200 ml of water for dilution if the patient can swallow, has a strong gag reflex, and does not drool (refer to ingestion protocol in Section Three).
- Cover skin burns with dry sterile dressings after decontamination (refer to chemical burn protocol in Section Three).

ADVANCED TREATMENT

- Consider orotracheal or nasotracheal intubation for airway control in the patient who is unconscious, has severe pulmonary edema, or is in severe respiratory distress.
- Positive-pressure ventilation techniques with a bag-valve-mask device may be beneficial.
- Consider drug therapy for pulmonary edema (refer to pulmonary edema protocol in Section Three).
- Consider administering a beta agonist such as albuterol for severe bronchospasm (refer to albuterol protocol in Section Four).
- Monitor cardiac rhythm and treat arrhythmias as necessary (refer to cardiac protocol in Section Three).
- Start IV administration of D_5W TKO. Use 0.9% saline (NS) or lactated Ringer's (LR) if signs of hypovolemia are present. For hypotension with signs of hypovolemia, administer fluid cautiously. Watch for signs of fluid overload (refer to shock protocol in Section Three).

- Treat seizures with diazepam (Valium) or lorazepam (Ativan) (refer to diazepam and lorazepam protocols in Section Four and seizure protocol in Section Three).
- Use proparacaine hydrochloride to assist eye irrigation (refer to proparacaine hydrochloride protocol in Section Four).

11

Etiological Agents

UN Class 6

SUBSTANCE IDENTIFICATION

Viable microorganisms or their toxins that may cause disease in humans or animals. Examples: anthrax, rabies, tetanus, botulism, polio, and HIV specimens.

ROUTES OF EXPOSURE

Inhalation
Ingestion
Skin absorption

LIFE THREAT

These etiological agents have a variety of actions and life threats. Most have an incubation period and no acute symptoms. Identification of the agent/organism is essential to determine severity of expected symptoms.

DECONTAMINATION

- Wear positive-pressure SCBA or air-purifying respirator with appropriate cartridge/filter and protective equipment specified by references such as the *North American Emergency Response Guidebook.* If special chemical protective clothing is required, consult the chemical manufacturer or specific protective clothing compatibility charts. A qualified, experienced person should make decisions regarding the type of personal protective equipment necessary.
- Delay entry until trained personnel and proper protective equipment are available.
- Remove patient from contaminated area.
- Quickly remove and isolate patient's clothing, jewelry, and shoes.
- Gently brush away dry particles and blot excess liquids with absorbent material.
- Rinse patient with warm water, 32° C to 35° C (90° F to 95° F), if possible.
- Wash patient with a mild liquid soap and large quantities of water.
- Refer to decontamination protocol in Section Three.

IMMEDIATE FIRST AID

- Ensure that adequate decontamination has been carried out.
- If patient is not breathing, start artificial respiration, preferably with a demand-valve resuscitator, bag-valve-mask device, or pocket mask, as trained. Perform CPR as necessary.
- Immediately flush contaminated eyes with gently flowing water.
- Do not induce vomiting. If vomiting occurs, lean patient forward or place on left side (head-down position, if possible) to maintain an open airway and prevent aspiration.
- Keep patient quiet and maintain normal body temperature.
- Obtain medical attention.

BASIC TREATMENT

- Establish a patent airway (oropharyngeal or nasopharyngeal airway, if needed). Suction if necessary.

- Watch for signs of respiratory insufficiency and assist ventilations if needed.
- Administer oxygen by nonrebreather mask at 10 to 15 L/min.
- For eye contamination, flush eyes immediately with water. Irrigate each eye continuously with 0.9% saline (NS) during transport (refer to eye irrigation protocol in Section Three).

ADVANCED TREATMENT

- Consider orotracheal or nasotracheal intubation for airway control in the patient who is unconscious or is in severe respiratory distress.
- Monitor cardiac rhythm and treat arrhythmias if necessary (refer to cardiac protocol in Section Three).
- Start IV administration of D_5W TKO.
- Proparacaine hydrochloride should be used to assist eye irrigation (refer to proparacaine hydrochloride protocol in Section Four).

SPECIAL CONSIDERATIONS

- Symptomatic and supportive care should be started immediately.
- Product identification is essential for specific therapy. Most toxins have incubation periods of varying length with no or few acute symptoms.
- Most exposures require little or no immediate treatment.
- Transport to hospital. Observe universal precautions.

12

Radioactives I, II, and III

UN Class 7

SUBSTANCE IDENTIFICATION

Any material or combination of materials that spontaneously emit ionizing radiation and have a specific activity greater than 0.002 μCi/g. Examples: plutonium, cobalt, uranium 235, and radioactive waste. There are three types of radiation-induced injuries: external irradiation, contamination with radioactive materials, and incorporation of radioactive materials into body cells, tissues, or organs. External irradiation occurs when patients are exposed to electromagnetic radiation sources emitting gamma rays. These patients are irradiated. They are not contaminated and do not pose a secondary contamination risk. Contamination can occur when patients come into direct contact with particle radiation sources (alpha and beta particles, neutrons, protons, and positrons) in the form of dusts, liquids, or gases. These patients will present a secondary contamination risk unless properly handled. Incorporation can occur following a contamination and an uptake of radioactive materials by body cells, tissues, or organs. For incidents involving nuclear detonation or when radiological materials have been used as a weapon, see Guidelines 110, 111, and 112.

ROUTES OF EXPOSURE

Skin and eye contact
Inhalation
Ingestion
Skin absorption
Proximity exposure risk with certain products

LIFE THREAT

Radiation ionizes atoms, resulting in intracellular formation of free radicals that damage DNA and RNA. Cells with high metabolic turnover rates such as those in the GI tract and hematopoietic system are affected the most. Massive radiation exposures may result in extensive neurological and GI damage. Loss of bone marrow function may also occur with resulting immunocompromise and systemic infection. Soluble radioactive compounds may cause local symptoms as well. Products may act as carcinogens.

SIGNS AND SYMPTOMS BY SYSTEM

Cardiovascular: Tachycardia and cardiovascular collapse.

Respiratory: Dyspnea, cough with irritation and edema to the upper airway, and pneumonitis.

CNS: Decreased level of consciousness and coma, ataxia, headache, lethargy, weakness, tremors, and convulsions.

Gastrointestinal: Nausea, vomiting, and diarrhea.

Eye: Lacrimation, conjunctivitis, and corneal damage.

Skin: Symptoms range from mild irritation to burns. Hair loss.

Blood: Bone marrow suppression.
Other: In most cases symptoms are delayed for hours to days.

DECONTAMINATION

- Wear positive-pressure SCBA and protective equipment specified by references such as the *North American Emergency Response Guidebook.* If special chemical protective clothing is required, consult the chemical manufacturer or specific protective clothing compatibility charts. A qualified, experienced person should make decisions regarding the type of personal protective equipment necessary.
- In a transportation accident, if a small quantity of radioactive material (such as a medical imaging isotope) is the only significant hazardous materials threat involved, immediate rescue and lifesaving care may be carried out, taking all reasonable precautions to avoid contact with the radioactive materials or their containers. The time responders spend in any potentially contaminated area should be kept to a minimum. Although some risk is present from the release of radioactive materials, history has shown that transportation accidents involving releases usually are small-quantity shipments unlikely to pose a life-threatening health hazard to responders. Patient risk caused by trauma is much greater.
- Remove patient from contaminated area.
- **Patients with electromagnetic radiation (gamma) exposure require no further decontamination. For patients with life-threatening injuries (from incidents involving small-quantity releases) and particle or liquid exposure:**
  - Quickly remove and isolate patient's clothing, jewelry, and shoes.
  - Package the patient, using reverse isolation procedures, such as transportation bags, plastic, or blankets. This helps prevent the spread of contamination during transport.
  - Provide adequate ambulance ventilation (intake and exhaust fans of proper size).
  - Use adequate personal protective equipment. See EMS/Hazardous Materials Equipment Procedure in Section Five.
  - Notify the emergency department that a potentially contaminated patient is en route and supply all available information concerning the identity and nature of the contaminant.
- **If it is known or highly suspected that a high-level radiation exposure (such as a large-quantity shipment with a container breech or a large release in a fixed facility) would be incurred, responders should delay entry until properly trained and equipped personnel are on scene.**
- **If high levels of radioactive contamination are present, other chemical contaminants are suspected, or large numbers of patients are involved (as in a terrorist use of a radiological dispersion device or weapon), complete patient decontamination procedures should be instituted:**
  - Gently brush away dry particles and blot excess liquids with absorbent material.
  - Rinse patient with warm water, 32° C to 35° C (90° F to 95° F), if possible. Use caution not to rinse contamination to areas of tissue damage or body cavity openings.
  - Wash patient with a mild liquid soap and large quantities of water.
  - Refer to decontamination protocol in Section Three.

IMMEDIATE FIRST AID

- Ensure that adequate decontamination has been carried out as needed.
- If patient is not breathing, start artificial respiration, preferably with a demand-valve resuscitator, bag-valve-mask device, or pocket mask, as trained. Perform CPR if necessary.
- Immediately flush contaminated eyes with gently flowing water.
- Do not induce vomiting. If vomiting occurs, lean patient forward or place on left side (head-down position, if possible) to maintain an open airway and prevent aspiration.
- Keep patient quiet and maintain normal body temperature.
- Obtain medical attention.

BASIC TREATMENT

- Establish a patent airway (oropharyngeal or nasopharyngeal airway, if needed). Suction if necessary.
- Watch for signs of respiratory insufficiency and assist ventilations if necessary.
- Administer oxygen by nonrebreather mask at 10 to 15 L/min.
- Monitor for shock and treat if necessary (refer to shock protocol in Section Three).
- Anticipate seizures and treat if necessary (refer to seizure protocol in Section Three).
- Perform routine emergency care for associated injuries.
- For eye contamination, flush eyes immediately with water. Irrigate each eye continuously during transport (refer to eye irrigation protocol in Section Three).
- Do not use emetics. For ingestion, rinse mouth and administer 5 ml/kg up to 200 ml of water for dilution if the patent can swallow, has a good gag reflex, and does not drool (refer to ingestion protocol in Section Three).
- Perform routine BLS care as necessary.

ADVANCED TREATMENT

- Consider orotracheal or nasotracheal intubation for airway control in the patient who is unconscious or is in severe respiratory distress.
- Monitor cardiac rhythm and treat arrhythmias as necessary (refer to cardiac protocol in Section Three).
- Start IV administration of 0.9% saline (NS) or lactated Ringer's (LR) TKO. For hypotension with signs of hypovolemia, administer fluid cautiously. Watch for signs of fluid overload (refer to shock protocol in Section Three).
- Treat seizures with diazepam (Valium) or lorazepam (Ativan) (refer to diazepam and lorazepam protocols in Section Four and seizure protocol in Section Three).
- Perform routine advanced life support care as needed.
- Use proparacaine hydrochloride to assist eye irrigation (refer to proparacaine hydrochloride protocol in Section Four).

INITIAL EMERGENCY DEPARTMENT CONSIDERATIONS

- Chelating agents or pharmacologic blocking drugs (potassium iodine, DTPA, BAL, bicarbonate, Prussian blue, calcium gluconate, ammonium chloride, barium sulfate, sodium alginate, D-penicillamine) may be useful if given before or immediately after exposure. The Oak Ridge number listed at the end of this guideline can be contacted for specific treatment advice.

SPECIAL CONSIDERATIONS

- For incidents involving nuclear detonation or when radiological materials have been used as a weapon, see Guidelines 110, 111, and 112.
- Most symptoms from radioactive product exposure are delayed; treat other medical or trauma problems according to normal protocols.
- An accurate history of the exposure is essential to determine risk and proper treatment modalities.
- The dose of radiation determines the type and clinical course of exposure:
    - *100 rads:* GI symptoms (nausea, vomiting, abdominal cramps, diarrhea). Symptom onset within a few hours.
    - *600 rads:* Severe GI symptoms (necrotic gastroenteritis) may result in dehydration and death within a few days.
    - *Several thousand rads:* neurological/cardiovascular symptoms (confusion, lethargy, ataxia, seizures, coma, cardiovascular collapse) within minutes to hours. Bone marrow depression, leukopenia, and infections usually follow severe exposures.
- Assistance and advice on patient care concerns may be obtained from the Oak Ridge Radiation Emergency Assistance Center and Training Site 24 hours a day by calling (615) 576-3131 or (615) 481-1000, ext. 1502 or beeper 241.

13

Corrosives

UN Class 8

SUBSTANCE IDENTIFICATION

Any liquid or solid that causes visible destruction of human skin tissue or has a severe corrosion rate on steel or aluminum. The Environmental Protection Agency (EPA) defines a corrosive product as having a pH of 2 or less or 12.5 or more. This group includes both acids and bases. Some products may cause systemic toxicity. Examples: hydrochloric acid, sulfuric acid, hydrofluoric acid, sodium hydroxide (lye), and caustic potash.

ROUTES OF EXPOSURE

Skin and eye contact
Inhalation
Ingestion

LIFE THREAT

Severe irritant to tissue that can cause upper airway burns and edema, circulatory collapse, and severe skin burns. May cause GI perforation, hemorrhage, and peritonitis. Absorption of some products may cause toxic systemic effects.

SIGNS AND SYMPTOMS BY SYSTEM

Cardiovascular: Tachycardia and shock.

Respiratory: Dyspnea, tachypnea, burns and edema in the upper airway, sneezing, coughing, stridor, and pulmonary edema.

CNS: Apathy, mental confusion, blurred vision, and tremors.

Gastrointestinal: Nausea; vomiting; hemorrhage; abdominal pain; painful swallowing; profuse salivation; and burns to the mouth, esophagus, stomach, and lower GI tract.

Eye: Chemical conjunctivitis to severe eye damage.

Skin: Chemical burns, skin rash (in milder cases), and cold and clammy skin with cyanosis or pale color.

DECONTAMINATION

- Wear positive-pressure SCBA and protective equipment specified by references such as the *North American Emergency Response Guidebook.* If special chemical protective clothing is required, consult the chemical manufacturer or specific protective clothing compatibility charts. A qualified, experienced person should make decisions regarding the type of personal protective equipment necessary.
- Delay entry until trained personnel and proper protective equipment are available.
- Remove patient from contaminated area.
- Quickly remove and isolate patient's clothing, jewelry, and shoes.
- Gently brush away dry particles and blot excess liquids with absorbent material.
- Rinse patient with warm water, 32° C to 35° C (90° F to 95° F), if possible.
- Wash patient with a mild liquid soap and large quantities of water.
- Refer to decontamination protocol in Section Three.

IMMEDIATE FIRST AID

- Ensure that adequate decontamination has been carried out.
- If patient is not breathing, start artificial respiration, preferably with a demand-valve resuscitator, bag-valve-mask device, or pocket mask, as trained. Perform CPR as necessary.
- Immediately flush contaminated eyes with gently flowing water.
- Do not induce vomiting. If vomiting occurs, lean patient forward or place on left side (head-down position, if possible) to maintain an open airway and prevent aspiration.
- Keep patient quiet and maintain normal body temperature.
- Obtain medical attention.

BASIC TREATMENT

- Establish a patent airway (oropharyngeal or nasopharyngeal airway, if needed). Suction if necessary.
- Watch for signs of respiratory insufficiency and assist ventilations if necessary.
- Administer oxygen by nonrebreather mask at 10 to 15 L/min.
- Monitor for pulmonary edema and treat if necessary (refer to pulmonary edema protocol in Section Three).
- Monitor for shock and treat if necessary (refer to shock protocol in Section Three).
- Anticipate seizures and treat if necessary (refer to seizure protocol in Section Three).
- For eye contamination, flush eyes immediately with water. Irrigate each eye continuously with 0.9% saline (NS) during transport (refer to eye irrigation protocol in Section Three).
- Do not use emetics. For ingestion, rinse mouth and administer 5 ml/kg up to 200 ml of water for dilution if the patient can swallow, has a strong gag reflex, and does not drool (refer to ingestion protocol in Section Three).
- Cover skin burns with dry sterile dressings after decontamination (refer to chemical burn protocol in Section Three).

ADVANCED TREATMENT

- Consider orotracheal or nasotracheal intubation for airway control in the patient who is unconscious, has severe pulmonary edema, or is in severe respiratory distress. Early intubation, at the first sign of upper airway obstruction, may be necessary.
- Positive-pressure ventilation techniques with a bag-valve mask device may be beneficial.
- Consider drug therapy for pulmonary edema (refer to pulmonary edema protocol in Section Three).
- Monitor cardiac rhythm and treat arrhythmias if necessary (refer to cardiac protocol in Section Three).
- Start IV administration of D_5W TKO. Use 0.9% saline (NS) or lactated Ringer's (LR) if signs of hypovolemia are present. For hypotension with signs of hypovolemia, administer fluid cautiously. Watch for signs of fluid overload (refer to shock protocol in Section Three).
- Treat seizures with diazepam (Valium) or lorazepam (Ativan) (refer to diazepam and lorazepam protocols in Section Four and seizure protocol in Section Three).

- Use proparacaine hydrochloride to assist eye irrigation (refer to proparacaine hydrochloride protocol in Section Four).

SPECIAL CONSIDERATIONS

- Do not attempt to neutralize products, because of exothermic reaction.

Inorganic Acids and Related Compounds

SUBSTANCE IDENTIFICATION

Found as crystalline solids or colorless to yellow liquids. Some products may fume in air. Products range from odorless to strongly irritating odors. Used in batteries, as cleaners, in many chemical reactions, and in numerous manufacturing processes. Products are highly corrosive to tissue and metals. Reactions with most metals may generate hydrogen gas. Reaction with water may generate heat (exothermic reaction) or in the case of sulfuric acid, violent reaction and spattering.

ROUTES OF EXPOSURE

Skin and eye contact
Inhalation
Ingestion

TARGET ORGANS

Primary
Skin
Eyes
Respiratory system
Gastrointestinal system
Metabolism
Secondary
Central nervous system
Cardiovascular system
Renal system
Blood

LIFE THREAT

Pulmonary edema, bronchospasm, circulatory collapse, laryngeal spasm and edema, GI tract perforation, hemorrhage, and peritonitis. Corrosive to skin, mucous membranes, and internal organs.

SIGNS AND SYMPTOMS BY SYSTEM

Cardiovascular: Hypovolemic shock, tachycardia with weak pulse, and circulatory collapse.

Respiratory: Coughing, chest pain, sneezing, rhinitis, dyspnea, bronchospasm, asphyxia, chemical pneumonitis, acute pulmonary fibrosis, reactive airways disease syndrome (RADS), acute pulmonary edema, upper airway obstruction from laryngeal spasm or glottic edema with stridor and pain, and aspiration pneumonia.

CNS: Symptoms of hypoxia, weakness, dizziness, stupor, lethargy, and coma.

Gastrointestinal: Acute toxicity results in burns to the mouth, esophagus, stomach, and lower GI tract. Nausea, vomiting, dysphagia, and diarrhea, possibly hemorrhagic.

Eye: Conjunctivitis, spasm of eyelids (blepharospasm), photophobia, opacification of the corneas, corneal perforation, and blindness.
Skin: Irritant dermatitis, hypersensitivity, and skin discoloration, full- and partial-thickness burns with coagulation necrosis, eschar formation, and scarring. Concomitant exothermic reaction may produce thermal burns.
Renal: Kidney damage.
Metabolism: Metabolic acidosis and hyponatremia.
Blood: Hemolysis, coagulopathy.
Other: Refer to Guideline 16 for hydrofluoric acid and related compounds.

SYMPTOM ONSET FOR ACUTE EXPOSURE

Immediate
Respiratory symptoms may be delayed
Water solubility determines whether initial symptoms are directed at upper or lower airways; highly water-soluble products affect the upper airway; less water-soluble agents are more likely to cause lower airway symptoms; systemic effects may be seen.

CO-EXPOSURE CONCERNS

Other acids
Alkalies (exothermic reactions possible)

THERMAL DECOMPOSITION PRODUCTS INCLUDE

Arsenic: Arsenic acid
Bromine: Hydrobromic acid
Chromium: Chromic acid
Hydrogen chloride/hydrogen/chlorine: Hydrochloric and hypochlorous acid
Nitrogen oxides: Nitric and nitrous acid
Sulfur oxides: Sulfuric and sulfurous acid

MEDICAL CONDITIONS POSSIBLY AGGRAVATED BY EXPOSURE

Respiratory disorders
Skin disorders

DECONTAMINATION

- Wear positive-pressure SCBA and protective equipment specified by references such as the *North American Emergency Response Guidebook*. If special chemical protective clothing is required, consult the chemical manufacturer or specific protective clothing compatibility charts. A qualified, experienced person should make decisions regarding the type of personal protective equipment necessary.
- Delay entry until trained personnel and proper protective equipment are available.
- Remove patient from contaminated area.
- Quickly remove and isolate patient's clothing, jewelry, and shoes.
- Gently brush away dry particles and blot excess liquids with absorbent material.
- Rinse patient with copious amounts of warm water, 32° C to 35° C (90° F to 95° F), if possible.
- Wash patient with a mild liquid soap and large quantities of water.
- Speed in removing product from skin is essential in limiting tissue damage.
- Refer to decontamination protocol in Section Three.

IMMEDIATE FIRST AID

- Ensure that adequate decontamination has been carried out.

- If patient is not breathing, start artificial respiration, preferably with a demand-valve resuscitator, bag-valve-mask device, or pocket mask, as trained. Perform CPR as necessary.
- Immediately flush contaminated eyes with gently flowing water.
- Do not induce vomiting. If vomiting occurs, lean patient forward or place on left side (head-down position, if possible) to maintain an open airway and prevent aspiration.
- Keep patient quiet and maintain normal body temperature.
- Obtain medical attention.

BASIC TREATMENT

- Establish a patent airway (oropharyngeal or nasopharyngeal airway, if needed). Suction if necessary.
- Watch for signs of respiratory insufficiency and assist respirations if needed.
- Administer oxygen by nonrebreather mask at 10 to 15 L/min.
- Monitor for pulmonary edema and treat if necessary (refer to pulmonary edema protocol in Section Three).
- Monitor for shock and treat if necessary (refer to shock protocol in Section Three).
- For eye contamination, flush eyes immediately with water. Irrigate each eye continuously with 0.9% saline (NS) during transport (refer to eye irrigation protocol in Section Three).
- Do not use emetics. Activated charcoal is not effective. For ingestion, rinse mouth and administer 5 ml/kg up to 200 ml of water for dilution if the patient can swallow, has a strong gag reflex, and does not drool (refer to ingestion protocol in Section Three).
- Do not attempt to neutralize, because of exothermic reaction.
- Cover skin burns with dry, sterile dressings after decontamination (refer to chemical burn protocol in Section Three).

ADVANCED TREATMENT

- Consider orotracheal or nasotracheal intubation for airway control in the patient who is unconscious, has severe pulmonary edema, or is in severe respiratory distress. Early intubation, at the first sign of upper airway obstruction, may be necessary.
- Positive-pressure ventilation techniques with a bag-valve-mask device may be beneficial.
- Consider drug therapy for pulmonary edema (refer to pulmonary edema protocol in Section Three).
- Consider administering a beta agonist such as albuterol for severe bronchospasm (refer to albuterol protocol in Section Four).
- Monitor cardiac rhythm and treat arrhythmias as necessary (refer to cardiac protocol in Section Three).
- Start IV administration of D_5W TKO. Use 0.9% saline (NS) or lactated Ringer's (LR) if signs of hypovolemia are present. For hypotension with signs of hypovolemia, administer fluid cautiously. Consider vasopressors if patient is hypotensive with a normal fluid volume. Watch for signs of fluid overload (refer to shock protocol in Section Three).
- Use proparacaine hydrochloride to assist eye irrigation (refer to proparacaine hydrochloride protocol in Section Four).

INITIAL EMERGENCY DEPARTMENT CONSIDERATIONS

- Useful initial laboratory studies include complete blood count, platelet count, coagulation profile, serum electrolytes, blood urea nitrogen (BUN), creatinine, glucose, urinalysis, and baseline biochemical profile, including serum aminotransferases (ALT and AST), calcium, phosphorus, and magnesium. Determination of anion and osmolar gaps may be helpful. Arterial blood gases (ABGs), chest radiograph, and electrocardiogram may be required.
- Products may cause acidosis; hyperventilation and sodium bicarbonate may be beneficial. Bicarbonate therapy should be guided by clinical presentation, ABG determinations, and serum electrolyte considerations.
- Positive end-expiratory pressure (PEEP)–assisted ventilation may be necessary in patients with acute parenchymal injury who develop pulmonary edema or acute respiratory distress syndrome.
- Bronchospastic symptoms should be treated with an inhalation medication regimen similar to that used for reactive airways disease. Inhaled corticosteroids may be of value in severe bronchospasm.
- Oral exposures may require endoscopy.
- Obtain toxicological consultation as necessary.

Organic Acids and Related Compounds

SUBSTANCE IDENTIFICATION

Short-chained organic acids are usually found as colorless liquids. Some products may fume in air, presenting an increased inhalation exposure hazard. Most products have pungent, penetrating odors. Longer-chained organic acids tend to be waxy solids. Used in food preservatives, dyes, insecticides, photographic chemicals, fumigants, leather tanning processes, and in the manufacture of pharmaceuticals, rubber, and plastics. Products are highly corrosive to tissue and reactive with metals.

ROUTES OF EXPOSURE

Skin and eye contact
Inhalation
Ingestion
Skin absorption

TARGET ORGANS

Primary
Skin
Eyes
Respiratory system
Gastrointestinal system
Metabolism
Secondary
Central nervous system
Cardiovascular system

LIFE THREAT

Pulmonary edema, circulatory collapse, laryngeal edema, spasm, GI tract perforation, hemorrhage, and peritonitis. Corrosive to skin, mucous membranes, and internal organs.

SIGNS AND SYMPTOMS BY SYSTEM

Cardiovascular: Hypovolemic shock, circulatory collapse, and tachycardia with weak pulse.

Respiratory: Mucosal edema, erythema, coughing, sneezing, dyspnea, upper airway obstruction from laryngeal spasm or glottic edema with stridor and pain, acute pulmonary edema, asphyxia, and chemical pneumonitis.

CNS: Symptoms of hypoxia, stupor, lethargy, and coma.

Gastrointestinal: Ingestion can result in burns to the mouth, esophagus, stomach, and lower GI tract. Salivation, nausea, vomiting, and diarrhea, hematemesis, melena, and abdominal muscle spasm.

Eye: Conjunctivitis, spasm of the eyelid (blepharospasm), blurred vision, corneal destruction, and possibly blindness.

Skin: Full- or partial-thickness burns with blistering and tissue damage. Dermal ulceration with eschar formation secondary to coagulation of superficial tissue proteins. This coagulation necrosis generally limits further tissue destruction and acid penetration.

Metabolism: Metabolic acidosis.

SYMPTOM ONSET FOR ACUTE EXPOSURE

Immediate; respiratory symptoms may be delayed.

CO-EXPOSURE CONCERNS

Other acids

Alkalies (exothermic reaction possible)

THERMAL DECOMPOSITION PRODUCTS INCLUDE

Carbon dioxide

Carbon monoxide

MEDICAL CONDITIONS POSSIBLY AGGRAVATED BY EXPOSURE

Respiratory system disorders

DECONTAMINATION

- Wear positive-pressure SCBA and protective equipment specified by references such as the *North American Emergency Response Guidebook*. If special chemical protective clothing is required, consult the chemical manufacturer or specific protective clothing compatibility charts. A qualified, experienced person should make decisions regarding the type of personal protective equipment necessary.
- Delay entry until trained personnel and proper protective equipment are available.
- Remove patient from contaminated area.
- Quickly remove and isolate patient's clothing, jewelry, and shoes.
- Gently brush away dry particles and blot excess liquids with absorbent material.
- Rinse patient with warm water, 32° C to 35° C (90° F to 95° F), if possible.
- Wash patient with a mild liquid soap and large quantities of water.
- Speed in removing product from skin is essential in limiting tissue damage.
- Refer to decontamination protocol in Section Three.

IMMEDIATE FIRST AID

- Ensure that adequate decontamination has been carried out.
- If patient is not breathing, start artificial respiration, preferably with a demand-valve resuscitator, bag-valve-mask device, or pocket mask, as trained. Perform CPR if necessary.
- Immediately flush contaminated eyes with gently flowing water.
- Do not induce vomiting. If vomiting occurs, lean patient forward or place on left side (head-down position, if possible) to maintain an open airway and prevent aspiration.
- Keep patient quiet and maintain normal body temperature.
- Obtain medical attention.

BASIC TREATMENT

- Establish a patent airway (oropharyngeal or nasopharyngeal airway, if needed). Suction if necessary.
- Watch for signs of respiratory insufficiency and assist respirations if necessary.
- Administer oxygen by nonrebreather mask at 10 to 15 L/min.
- Monitor for pulmonary edema and treat if necessary (refer to pulmonary edema protocol in Section Three).

- Monitor for shock and treat if necessary (refer to shock protocol in Section Three).
- For eye contamination, flush eyes immediately with water. Irrigate each eye continuously with 0.9% saline (NS) during transport (refer to eye irrigation protocol in Section Three).
- Do not use emetics. For ingestion, rinse mouth and administer 5 ml/kg up to 200 ml of water for dilution if the patient can swallow, has a strong gag reflex, and does not drool. Activated charcoal is not effective (refer to ingestion protocol in Section Three).
- Do not attempt to neutralize, because of exothermic reaction.
- Cover skin burns with dry, sterile dressings after decontamination (refer to chemical burn protocol in Section Three).

ADVANCED TREATMENT

- Consider orotracheal or nasotracheal intubation for airway control in the patient who is unconscious, has severe pulmonary edema, or is in severe respiratory distress. Early intubation, at the first sign of upper airway obstruction, may be necessary.
- Positive-pressure ventilation techniques with a bag-valve-mask device may be beneficial.
- Consider drug therapy for pulmonary edema (refer to pulmonary edema protocol in Section Three).
- Consider administering a beta agonist such as albuterol for severe bronchospasm (refer to albuterol protocol in Section Four).
- Monitor cardiac rhythm and treat arrhythmias as necessary (refer to cardiac protocol in Section Three).
- Start IV administration of D_5W TKO. Use 0.9% saline (NS) or lactated Ringer's (LR) if signs of hypovolemia are present. For hypotension with signs of hypovolemia, administer fluid cautiously. Consider vasopressors if patient is hypotensive with a normal fluid volume. Watch for signs of fluid overload (refer to shock protocol in Section Three).
- Use proparacaine hydrochloride to assist eye irrigation (refer to proparacaine hydrochloride protocol in Section Four).

INITIAL EMERGENCY DEPARTMENT CONSIDERATIONS

- Useful initial laboratory studies include complete blood count, serum electrolytes, blood urea nitrogen (BUN), creatinine, glucose, urinalysis, baseline biochemical profile, including serum aminotransferases (ALT and AST), calcium, phosphorus, magnesium, determination of anion and osmolar gaps, arterial blood gases (ABGs), chest radiograph, and electrocardiogram.
- Products may cause acidosis; hyperventilation and sodium bicarbonate may be beneficial. Bicarbonate therapy should be guided by clinical presentation, ABG determinations, and serum electrolyte considerations.
- Positive end-expiratory pressure (PEEP)–assisted ventilation may be necessary in patients with acute parenchymal injury who develop pulmonary edema or acute respiratory distress syndrome.
- Bronchospastic symptoms should be treated with an inhalation medication regimen similar to that used for reactive airways disease. Inhaled corticosteroids may be of value in severe bronchospasm.

- Oral exposures may require endoscopy.
- Obtain toxicological consultation as necessary.

SPECIAL CONSIDERATIONS

- Formic acid is a toxic metabolite of methanol. Formic acid and formaldehyde are the agents responsible for the anion gap acidosis and ocular toxicity of methanol poisoning. Refer to methanol (Guideline 31).

Hydrofluoric Acid (HF) and Related Compounds

SUBSTANCE IDENTIFICATION

An extremely volatile, colorless corrosive liquid or a colorless gas with a sharp, irritating odor. Used in etching, manufacturing of fluorinated chemicals, electropolishing of metals, and the semiconductor industry. May react with metal to generate hydrogen gas. The liquid product evaporates and produces large amounts of vapors and white fumes.

ROUTES OF EXPOSURE

Skin and eye contact
Inhalation
Ingestion
Skin absorption

TARGET ORGANS

Primary
Eyes
Skin
Respiratory system
Gastrointestinal system
Metabolism
Secondary
Central nervous system
Cardiovascular system

LIFE THREAT

Pulmonary edema, laryngeal edema, circulatory collapse, and severe skin burns. May cause perforation of GI tract. Systemic fluoride poisoning may result.

SIGNS AND SYMPTOMS BY SYSTEM

Cardiovascular: Cardiac arrhythmias, tachycardia with weak pulse, asystole, hypovolemic shock, and circulatory collapse.

Respiratory: Acute pulmonary edema, asphyxia, chemical pneumonitis. Upper airway obstruction with stridor, pain, and cough secondary to airway edema.

CNS: Symptoms of hypoxia, stupor, lethargy, altered sensorium, and coma.

Gastrointestinal: Acute toxicity results in burns to the mouth, esophagus, stomach, lower GI tract; nausea, vomiting, diarrhea, and possibly hemorrhage.

Eye: Conjunctivitis, opacification of the cornea, blindness.

Skin: Severe pain and normal-looking skin with small, total surface area burns. As concentration and surface area of burn increase, skin may look whitish (blanched). Burn is in lower skin layers. Damage may be severe with no outward signs or symptoms, except intense pain. In severe cases, demineralization of bone may occur.

Metabolism: Hypocalcemia and hypomagnesemia may occur. Even dilute solutions (less than 3% hydrofluoric acid) may cause serious or fatal injury in cases of large skin surface area involvement or oral ingestion.

Other: Hydrofluoric acid is a systemic poison, as well as a primary irritant. Burns over 20% of body surface may have a fatal outcome as a result of systemic fluoride poisoning. Any skin contamination in a hydrofluoric acid use area should be considered a hydrofluoric acid exposure.

SYMPTOM ONSET FOR ACUTE EXPOSURE

Immediate

Skin and systemic effects possibly delayed; onset depends on product concentration, route, and duration of exposure

THERMAL DECOMPOSITION PRODUCTS INCLUDE

Hydrogen

Hydrogen fluoride

MEDICAL CONDITIONS POSSIBLY AGGRAVATED BY EXPOSURE

Respiratory system disorders

Cardiac disorders

Kidney disorders

DECONTAMINATION

- Wear positive-pressure SCBA and protective equipment specified by references such as the *North American Emergency Response Guidebook*. If special chemical protective clothing is required, consult the chemical manufacturer or specific protective clothing compatibility charts. A qualified, experienced person should make decisions regarding the type of personal protective equipment necessary.
- Delay entry until trained personnel and proper protective equipment are available.
- Remove patient from contaminated area.
- Quickly remove and isolate patient's clothing, jewelry, and shoes.
- Gently brush away dry particles and blot excess liquids with absorbent material.
- Rinse patient with warm water, 32° C to 35° C (90° F to 95° F), if possible.
- Wash patient with a mild liquid soap and large quantities of water.
- A 0.13% benzalkonium chloride (Zephiran chloride) solution may be used for decontamination, if available. Do not delay decontamination to obtain benzalkonium chloride solution.
- Refer to decontamination protocol in Section Three.

IMMEDIATE FIRST AID

- Ensure that adequate decontamination has been carried out.
- If patient is not breathing, start artificial respiration, preferably with a demand-valve resuscitator, bag-valve-mask device, or pocket mask, as trained. Perform CPR if necessary.
- Immediately flush contaminated eyes with gently flowing water.
- Do not induce vomiting. If vomiting occurs, lean patient forward or place on left side (head-down position, if possible) to maintain an open airway and prevent aspiration.
- Keep patient quiet and maintain normal body temperature.
- Effects may be delayed. Obtain medical attention for any exposure.

BASIC TREATMENT

- Establish a patent airway (oropharyngeal or nasopharyngeal airway, if needed). Suction if necessary.
- Watch for signs of respiratory insufficiency and assist ventilations if necessary.
- Administer oxygen by nonrebreather mask at 10 to 15 L/min.
- Monitor for pulmonary edema and treat if necessary (refer to pulmonary edema protocol in Section Three).
- Monitor for shock and treat if necessary (refer to shock protocol in Section Three).
- For eye contamination, flush eyes immediately with water. Irrigate each eye continuously with 0.9% saline (NS) during transport (refer to ingestion protocol in Section Three).
- Do not use emetics. For ingestion, rinse mouth and administer 5 ml/kg up to 200 ml of water if the patient can swallow, has a strong gag reflex, and does not drool (refer to ingestion protocol in Section Three).
- Do not attempt to neutralize because of exothermic reaction.
- Cover skin burns with dry, sterile dressings after decontamination (refer to chemical burn protocol in Section Three).

ADVANCED TREATMENT

- Consider orotracheal or nasotracheal intubation for airway control in the patient who is unconscious, has severe pulmonary edema, or is in severe respiratory distress. Early intubation at the first sign of upper airway obstruction may be necessary.
- Positive-pressure ventilation with a bag-valve-mask device may be beneficial.
- Consider drug therapy for pulmonary edema (refer to pulmonary edema protocol in Section Three).
- Monitor cardiac rhythm and treat arrhythmias as necessary.
- Development of QT interval prolongation may signal hypocalcemia and need for IV calcium gluconate administration (refer to cardiac protocol in Section Three and calcium gluconate protocol in Section Four).
- Start IV administration of D_5W TKO. Use 0.9% saline (NS) or lactated Ringer's (LR) if signs of hypovolemia are present. For hypotension with signs of hypovolemia, administer fluid cautiously. Consider vasopressors if patient is hypotensive with a normal fluid volume. Watch for signs of fluid overload (refer to shock protocol in Section Three).
- Use 2.5% calcium gluconate gel for skin burns over painful areas after thorough decontamination (refer to calcium gluconate gel protocol in Section Four). Iced 0.13% benzalkonium chloride (Zephiran chloride) solution soak or compresses may be used with careful monitoring of body temperature. Compresses should be changed every 2 min.
- Use proparacaine hydrochloride to assist eye irrigation (refer to proparacaine hydrochloride protocol in Section Four).

INITIAL EMERGENCY DEPARTMENT CONSIDERATIONS

- Useful initial laboratory studies include complete blood count, serum electrolytes, blood urea nitrogen (BUN), glucose, creatinine, urinalysis and baseline biochemical profile, including serum aminotransferases (ALT and AST), calcium, phosphorus, and magnesium. Determination of anion and osmolar gaps may be helpful. Arterial blood gases (ABGs), chest radiograph, and electrocardiogram may be required.

- Positive end-expiratory pressure (PEEP)–assisted ventilation may be necessary in patients with acute parenchymal injury who develop pulmonary edema or acute respiratory distress syndrome.
- Subcutaneous or intraarterial 5% calcium gluconate may be needed for dermal exposure.
- IV calcium gluconate may be needed for severe systemic hypocalcemia (refer to calcium gluconate protocol in Section Three).
- Massive hypocalcemia/hypomagnesemia from concentrated hydrofluoric acid exposure demonstrates high morbidity/mortality. Rapid, aggressive treatment is required, with close monitoring of electrocardiogram, serum electrolytes, calcium, and magnesium.
- Monitor and treat for hyperkalemia as necessary.
- Obtain toxicological consultation as necessary.

SPECIAL CONSIDERATIONS

- Dermal injury is proportional to the concentration, duration of skin contact, and release of hydrogen and fluoride ions into soft tissue, blood, and bones. Fluoride ions bind with calcium and magnesium, forming insoluble salts. This reaction produces liquefaction necrosis in deep tissue/bone and interferes with cellular metabolism, such as in myocardial tissue, producing cell death.

Oxalate and Related Compounds

SUBSTANCE IDENTIFICATION

Found as a colorless, odorless solid or liquid. Used as a metal cleaner/polisher in textile cleaning, flameproofing, rust removal, anti-corrosion coating, and as a chemical intermediate/catalyst in the photography, ceramics, and rubber industries. Can be found in certain plants such as rhubarb leaves and dieffenbachia.

ROUTES OF EXPOSURE

Skin and eye contact
Inhalation
Ingestion
Slow skin absorption

TARGET ORGANS

Primary
Skin
Eyes
Respiratory system
Gastrointestinal tract
Renal system
Metabolism
Secondary
Central nervous system
Cardiovascular system

LIFE THREAT

Cardiovascular collapse, arrhythmias, and seizures.

SIGNS AND SYMPTOMS BY SYSTEM

Cardiovascular: Cardiovascular collapse, hypotension, and arrhythmias.
Respiratory: Irritation of respiratory tract.
CNS: Headache, muscle cramps, tetany, fasciculations, seizures, CNS depression, coma, increased deep tendon reflexes.
Gastrointestinal: Nausea, vomiting (hematemesis) and burning pain in mouth, esophagus, and stomach. Exposed mucous membranes turn white in color.
Eye: Chemical conjunctivitis, corneal damage, and burns.
Skin: Irritant dermatitis, full- or partial-thickness burns.
Renal: Kidney damage and oxaluria.
Metabolism: Hypocalcemia.

SYMPTOM ONSET FOR ACUTE EXPOSURE

Immediate
Systemic symptoms possibly delayed

THERMAL DECOMPOSITION PRODUCTS INCLUDE

Carbon dioxide

Carbon monoxide
Depending on product, may release:
Ammonia
Nitrogen oxides
Oxalic acid

MEDICAL CONDITIONS POSSIBLY AGGRAVATED BY EXPOSURE

Respiratory system disorders
Kidney disorders
Dermatitis

DECONTAMINATION

- Wear positive-pressure SCBA and protective equipment specified by references such as the *North American Emergency Response Guidebook*. If special chemical protective clothing is required, consult the chemical manufacturer or specific protective clothing compatibility charts. A qualified, experienced person should make decisions regarding the type of personal protective equipment necessary.
- Delay entry until trained personnel and proper protective equipment are available.
- Remove patient from contaminated area.
- Quickly remove and isolate patient's clothing, jewelry, and shoes.
- Gently brush away dry particles and blot excess liquids with absorbent material.
- Rinse patient with warm water, 32° C to 35° C (90° F to 95° F), if possible.
- Wash patient with a mild liquid soap and large quantities of water.
- Refer to decontamination protocol in Section Three.

IMMEDIATE FIRST AID

- Ensure that adequate decontamination has been carried out.
- If patient is not breathing, start artificial respiration, preferably with a demand-valve resuscitator, bag-valve-mask device, or pocket mask, as trained. Perform CPR if necessary.
- Immediately flush contaminated eyes with gently flowing water.
- Do not induce vomiting. If vomiting occurs, lean patient forward or place on left side (head-down position, if possible) to maintain an open airway and prevent aspiration.
- Keep patient quiet and maintain normal body temperature.
- Obtain medical attention.

BASIC TREATMENT

- Establish a patent airway (oropharyngeal or nasopharyngeal airway, if needed). Suction if necessary.
- Watch for signs of respiratory insufficiency and assist ventilations as needed.
- Administer oxygen by nonrebreather mask at 10 to 15 L/min.
- Monitor for shock and treat if necessary (refer to shock protocol in Section Three).
- Anticipate seizures and treat if necessary (refer to seizure protocol in Section Three).
- For eye contamination, flush eyes immediately with water. Irrigate each eye continuously with 0.9% saline (NS) during transport (refer to eye irrigation protocol in Section Three).
- Do not use emetics. For ingestion, rinse mouth and administer 5 ml/kg up to 200 ml of water for dilution if the patient can swallow, has a strong gag reflex, and does not drool (refer to ingestion protocol in Section Three).

- Cover chemical burns with dry, sterile dressings after decontamination (refer to chemical burn protocol in Section Three).

ADVANCED TREATMENT

- Consider orotracheal or nasotracheal intubation for airway control in the patient who is unconscious or is in severe respiratory distress.
- Monitor cardiac rhythm and treat arrhythmias as necessary (refer to cardiac protocol in Section Three).
- Start IV administration of 0.9% saline (NS) or lactated Ringer's (LR) TKO. For hypotension with signs of hypovolemia, administer fluid cautiously. Watch for signs of fluid overload (refer to shock protocol in Section Three).
- Treat seizures with diazepam (Valium) or lorazepam (Ativan) (refer to diazepam and lorazepam protocols in Section Four and seizure protocol in Section Three).
- Use proparacaine hydrochloride to assist eye irrigation (refer to proparacaine hydrochloride protocol in Section Four).

INITIAL EMERGENCY DEPARTMENT CONSIDERATIONS

- Useful initial laboratory studies include complete blood count, serum electrolytes, blood urea nitrogen (BUN), creatinine, glucose, urinalysis, and baseline biochemical profile, including serum aminotransferases (ALT and AST), calcium, phosphorus, and magnesium. Determination of anion and osmolar gaps may be helpful. Arterial blood gases (ABGs), chest radiograph, and electrocardiogram may be required.
- Hemodialysis may be indicated in the presence of renal failure.
- IV calcium gluconate may be needed for hypocalcemia. Treatment should be guided by clinical presentation and laboratory values.
- Obtain toxicological consultation as necessary.

SPECIAL CONSIDERATIONS

- Oxalic acid is produced by the metabolism of ethylene glycol. Refer to ethylene glycol, glycols, and related compounds (Guideline 40).

18

Sodium Azide (NaN_3) and Related Compounds

SUBSTANCE IDENTIFICATION

Found as a white, odorless crystalline solid. Used in the manufacture of explosives and pharmaceuticals; as a laboratory reagent; as a herbicide, fungicide, nematocide, and soil fumigant; in the preparation of hydrazolic acid (HN_3), lead azide, and pure sodium; and as an intermediate in organic synthesis. Sodium azide is also used as a propellant for inflating automobile air bags. The hermetically sealed gas generator in the air bag unit may contain 400 to 600 g of propellant that usually contains only 30% to 40% of sodium azide. On ignition, nitrogen gas, trace amounts of sodium metal, and sodium hydroxide are produced. The nitrogen gas inflates the air bag. Automobile manufacturer data show that there is complete combustion of the sodium azide on air bag inflation. Therefore sodium azide exposure risk after inflation is not expected. Skin or eye irritation, if present, may be the result of sodium hydroxide or direct trauma from air bag contact.

ROUTES OF EXPOSURE

Skin and eye contact
Inhalation
Ingestion
Skin absorption

TARGET ORGANS

Primary
Skin
Eyes
Central nervous system
Cardiovascular system
Respiratory system
Blood
Secondary
Gastrointestinal system
Metabolism

LIFE THREAT

Hypotension, cardiac arrhythmias, asystole, seizures, and coma.

SIGNS AND SYMPTOMS BY SYSTEM

Cardiovascular: Bradycardia and hypotension are common. Tachycardia, ventricular arrhythmias, asystole, and vasodilation are possible.

Respiratory: Irritation of respiratory tract, chest pain, pulmonary edema, and respiratory failure.

CNS: Headache, apprehension, dizziness, muscle weakness, blurred vision, hyperreflexia, decreased level of consciousness, syncope, coma, and seizures.

Gastrointestinal: Irritation of the GI tract, nausea, vomiting, diarrhea, and polydipsia.

Eye: Conjunctivitis.
Skin: Irritation and cyanosis.
Metabolism: Metabolic acidosis.
Blood: Increased white blood cell count (leukocytosis) and platelet aggregation inhibition.
Other: Body temperature regulation disturbances.

SYMPTOM ONSET FOR ACUTE EXPOSURE

Immediate
Some symptoms possibly delayed

CO-EXPOSURE CONCERNS

When mixed with acids, hydrazolic acid is produced.
Nitrites/nitrates

THERMAL DECOMPOSITION PRODUCTS INCLUDE

Hydrazolic acid fumes (explosion hazard)
Nitrogen oxides
Sodium
Sodium hydroxide

MEDICAL CONDITIONS POSSIBLY AGGRAVATED BY EXPOSURE

Hypertensive cardiac disease

DECONTAMINATION

- Wear positive-pressure SCBA and protective equipment specified by references such as the *North American Emergency Response Guidebook.* If special chemical protective clothing is required, consult the chemical manufacturer or specific protective clothing compatibility charts. A qualified, experienced person should make decisions regarding the type of personal protective equipment necessary.
- Delay entry until trained personnel and proper protective equipment are available.
- Remove patient from contaminated area.
- Quickly remove and isolate patient's clothing, jewelry, and shoes.
- Gently brush away dry particles and blot excess liquids with absorbent material.
- Rinse patient with warm water, 32° C to 35° C (90° F to 95° F), if possible.
- Wash patient with a mild liquid soap and large quantities of water.
- Refer to decontamination protocol in Section Three.

IMMEDIATE FIRST AID

- Ensure that adequate decontamination has been carried out.
- If patient is not breathing, start artificial respiration, preferably with a demand-valve resuscitator, bag-valve-mask device, or pocket mask, as trained. Perform CPR if necessary.
- Immediately flush contaminated eyes with gently flowing water.
- Do not induce vomiting. If vomiting occurs, lean patient forward or place on left side (head-down position, if possible) to maintain an open airway and prevent aspiration.
- Keep patient quiet and maintain normal body temperature.
- Obtain medical attention.

BASIC TREATMENT

- Establish a patent airway (oropharyngeal or nasopharyngeal airway, if needed). Suction if necessary.
- Watch for signs of respiratory insufficiency and assist respirations if necessary.

- Administer oxygen by nonrebreather mask at 10 to 15 L/min.
- Monitor for pulmonary edema and treat if necessary (refer to pulmonary edema protocol in Section Three).
- Monitor for shock and treat if necessary (refer to shock protocol in Section Three).
- Anticipate seizures and treat if necessary (refer to seizure protocol in Section Three).
- For eye contamination, flush eyes immediately with water. Irrigate each eye continuously with 0.9% saline (NS) during transport (refer to eye irrigation protocol in Section Three).
- Do not use emetics. For ingestion, rinse mouth and administer 5 ml/kg up to 200 ml of water for dilution if the patient can swallow, has a strong gag reflex, and does not drool. Administer activated charcoal (refer to ingestion protocol in Section Three and activated charcoal protocol in Section Four).

ADVANCED TREATMENT

- Consider orotracheal or nasotracheal intubation for airway control in the patient who is unconscious, has severe pulmonary edema, or is in severe respiratory distress. Early intubation, at the first sign of upper airway obstruction, may be necessary.
- Positive-pressure ventilation techniques with a bag-valve-mask device may be beneficial.
- Consider drug therapy for pulmonary edema (refer to pulmonary edema protocol in Section Three).
- Monitor cardiac rhythm and treat arrhythmias as necessary (refer to cardiac protocol in Section Three).
- Start IV administration of D_5W TKO. Use 0.9% saline (NS) or lactated Ringer's (LR) if signs of hypovolemia are present. For hypotension with signs of hypovolemia, administer fluid cautiously. Consider vasopressors if patient is hypotensive with a normal fluid volume. Watch for signs of fluid overload (refer to shock protocol in Section Three).
- Treat seizures with diazepam (Valium) or lorazepam (Ativan) (refer to diazepam and lorazepam protocols in Section Four and seizure protocol in Section Three).
- Use proparacaine hydrochloride to assist eye irrigation (refer to proparacaine hydrochloride protocol in Section Four).

INITIAL EMERGENCY DEPARTMENT CONSIDERATIONS

- Useful initial laboratory studies include complete blood count, serum electrolytes, blood urea nitrogen (BUN), creatinine, glucose, urinalysis, and baseline biochemical profile, including serum aminotransferases (ALT and AST), calcium, phosphorus, magnesium, and coagulation profiles. Arterial blood gases (ABGs), chest radiograph, and electrocardiogram may be required.
- Positive end-expiratory pressure (PEEP)–assisted ventilation may be necessary in patients with acute parenchymal injury who develop pulmonary edema or acute respiratory distress syndrome.
- Products may cause acidosis; hyperventilation and sodium bicarbonate may be beneficial. Bicarbonate therapy should be guided by patient presentation, ABG determination and serum electrolyte considerations.
- Obtain toxicological consultation as necessary.

SPECIAL CONSIDERATIONS

- Sodium azide may block oxidative phosphorylation and the cytochrome oxidase system. Symptoms may mimic cyanide poisoning. The use of the cyanide antidote kit has been recommended for sodium azide exposure. This treatment is controversial. There are not sufficient data at this time to recommend it.

19

Inorganic Bases/Alkaline Corrosives and Related Compounds

SUBSTANCE IDENTIFICATION

Found as solids in pellets, flakes, lumps, or sticks and liquids. Used as acid neutralizers; in petroleum refining; in cleaning agents, paint removers, solvents; and in water treatment processes. Part of the manufacturing process of cellulose, paper, textiles, and plastics.

ROUTES OF EXPOSURE

Skin and eye contact
Inhalation
Ingestion

TARGET ORGANS

Primary
Skin
Eyes
Respiratory system
Gastrointestinal system
Secondary
Central nervous system
Cardiovascular system

LIFE THREAT

Severe tissue irritant that may cause upper airway burns and edema, pulmonary edema, and skin burns. May cause GI perforation, hemorrhage, and peritonitis leading to circulatory collapse.

SIGNS AND SYMPTOMS BY SYSTEM

Cardiovascular: Tachycardia, hypotension, and shock.

Respiratory: Dyspnea, tachypnea, sneezing, coughing, stridor, burns, upper airway edema, and pulmonary edema.

CNS: Apathy, mental confusion, blurred vision, and tremors.

Gastrointestinal: Nausea; vomiting; hemorrhage; perforation; abdominal pain; painful swallowing; profuse salivation; and burns to the mouth, esophagus, stomach, and gastrointestinal tract may occur.

Eye: Chemical conjunctivitis, corneal ulceration, severe scarring, permanent blindness.

Skin: Deep tissue chemical burns, skin rash (in milder cases), cold and clammy skin with cyanosis or pale color.

SYMPTOM ONSET FOR ACUTE EXPOSURE

Immediate

Some symptoms such as pulmonary edema, GI perforation, and cardiovascular collapse possibly delayed

CO-EXPOSURE CONCERNS

Other alkalies
Acids (exothermic reaction)

MEDICAL CONDITIONS POSSIBLY AGGRAVATED BY EXPOSURE

Respiratory system disorders
Gastrointestinal disorders

DECONTAMINATION

- Wear positive-pressure SCBA and protective equipment specified by references such as the *North American Emergency Response Guidebook*. If special chemical protective clothing is required, consult the chemical manufacturer or specific protective clothing compatibility charts. A qualified, experienced person should make decisions regarding the type of personal protective equipment necessary.
- Delay entry until trained personnel and proper protective equipment are available.
- Remove patient from contaminated area.
- Quickly remove and isolate patient's clothing, jewelry, and shoes.
- Gently brush away dry particles and blot excess liquids with absorbent material.
- Rinse patient with warm water, 32° C to 35° C (90° F to 95° F), if possible.
- Wash patient with a mild liquid soap and large quantities of water.
- Speed in removing product from skin is essential in limiting tissue damage.
- Refer to decontamination protocol in Section Three.

IMMEDIATE FIRST AID

- Remove patient from contact with the material.
- Ensure that adequate decontamination has been carried out.
- If patient is not breathing, start artificial respiration, preferably with a demand-valve resuscitator, bag-valve-mask device, or pocket mask, as trained. Perform CPR if necessary.
- Immediately flush contaminated eyes with gently flowing water.
- Do not induce vomiting. If vomiting occurs, lean patient forward or place on left side (head-down position, if possible) to maintain an open airway and prevent aspiration.
- Keep patient quiet and maintain normal body temperature.
- Obtain medical attention.

BASIC TREATMENT

- Establish a patent airway (oropharyngeal or nasopharyngeal airway, if needed). Suction if necessary.
- Watch for signs of respiratory insufficiency and assist ventilations if necessary.
- Administer oxygen by nonrebreather mask at 6 to 12 L/min.
- Monitor for pulmonary edema and treat if necessary (refer to pulmonary edema protocol in Section Three).
- Monitor for shock and treat if necessary (refer to shock protocol in Section Three).
- For eye contamination, flush eyes immediately with water. Irrigate each eye continuously with 0.9% saline (NS) during transport (refer to eye irrigation protocol in Section Three).
- Do not use emetics. For ingestion, rinse mouth and administer 5 ml/kg up to 200 ml of water for dilution if the patent can swallow, has a strong gag reflex, and does not drool (refer to ingestion protocol in Section Three).

- Do not attempt to neutralize.
- Cover skin burns with dry sterile dressings after decontamination (refer to chemical burn protocol in Section Three).

ADVANCED TREATMENT

- Consider orotracheal or nasotracheal intubation for airway control in the patient who is unconscious, has severe pulmonary edema, or is in severe respiratory distress. Early intubation, at the first signs of upper airway obstruction, may be necessary.
- Positive-pressure ventilation techniques with a bag-valve-mask device may be beneficial.
- Consider drug therapy for pulmonary edema (refer to pulmonary edema protocol in Section Three).
- Monitor cardiac rhythm and treat arrhythmias as necessary (refer to cardiac protocol in Section Three).
- Start IV administration of D_5W TKO. Use 0.9% saline (NS) or lactated Ringer's (LR) if signs of hypovolemia are present. For hypotension with signs of hypovolemia, administer fluid cautiously. Watch for signs of fluid overload (refer to shock protocol in Section Three).
- Use proparacaine hydrochloride to assist eye irrigation (refer to proparacaine hydrochloride protocol in Section Four).

INITIAL EMERGENCY DEPARTMENT CONSIDERATIONS

- Useful initial laboratory studies include complete blood count, serum electrolytes, blood urea nitrogen (BUN), creatinine, glucose, urinalysis, and baseline biochemical profile, including serum aminotransferases (ALT and AST), calcium, phosphorus, and magnesium. Arterial blood gases (ABGs), chest radiograph, and electrocardiogram may be required.
- Positive end-expiratory pressure (PEEP)–assisted ventilation may be necessary in patients with acute parenchymal injury who develop pulmonary edema or acute respiratory distress syndrome.
- Endoscopy may be required for evaluation of oral ingestion.
- Obtain toxicological consultation as necessary.

SPECIAL CONSIDERATIONS

- Do not attempt to neutralize products, because of exothermic reaction risk.
- Alkalies on contact with skin, mucous membranes, or conjunctival tissue produce a liquefaction necrosis that allows the substance to penetrate into deep tissue structures.

Organic Bases/Amines and Related Compounds

SUBSTANCE IDENTIFICATION

Found as a colorless gas or colorless to yellow liquids with an odor of fish or ammonia. Used in the manufacture of explosives, detergents, dyes, pharmaceuticals, stabilizers, surfactants, soaps and detergents, pesticides, plastics, and paints. Also used as solvents and photographic chemicals. By-products of rubber manufacturing processes.

ROUTES OF EXPOSURE

Skin and eye contact
Inhalation
Ingestion
Skin absorption

TARGET ORGANS

Primary
Skin
Eyes
Cardiovascular system
Respiratory system
Gastrointestinal system
Hepatic system
Blood
Secondary
Central nervous system
Renal system

LIFE THREAT

Pulmonary edema, cardiac depression, and seizures.

SIGNS AND SYMPTOMS BY SYSTEM

Cardiovascular: Cardiac depression resulting in arrhythmias and cardiovascular collapse. Direct damage to the myocardium. Hemorrhagic shock.

Respiratory: Irritation of the respiratory tract. Dyspnea, coughing, sneezing, noncardiac chest pain, hemorrhagic pulmonary lesions, and pulmonary edema. Some products may cause respiratory tract sensitization.

CNS: CNS depression, coma, and seizures.

Gastrointestinal: Irritation and burns of the mucous membranes, nausea, vomiting, and excessive salivation may be present.

Eye: Visual disturbances, chemical conjunctivitis, corneal burns.

Skin: Irritant dermatitis, chemical burns, and ecchymosis.

Hepatic: Liver damage.

Renal: Kidney damage.

Blood: Coagulation problems manifested by decreased platelet count (thrombocytopenia) have been reported with nitrosamines. Methemoglobinemia secondary to NO_x thermal degradation production possible.

Other: Human carcinogen risk (nitrosamines).

SYMPTOM ONSET FOR ACUTE EXPOSURE

Immediate

Some symptoms (pulmonary edema) possibly delayed

CO-EXPOSURE CONCERNS

Methemoglobin formers

Nitrogen oxides

THERMAL DECOMPOSITION PRODUCTS INCLUDE

Carbon dioxide

Carbon monoxide

Nitrogen oxides

MEDICAL CONDITIONS POSSIBLY AGGRAVATED BY EXPOSURE

Respiratory disorders (COPD, asthma, bronchitis)

Liver disorders

Bleeding disorders

DECONTAMINATION

- Wear positive-pressure SCBA and protective equipment specified by references such as the *North American Emergency Response Guidebook*. If special chemical protective clothing is required, consult the chemical manufacturer or specific protective clothing compatibility charts. A qualified, experienced person should make decisions regarding the type of personal protective equipment necessary.
- Delay entry until trained personnel and proper protective equipment are available.
- Remove patient from contaminated area.
- Quickly remove and isolate patient's clothing, jewelry, and shoes.
- Gently brush away dry particles and blot excess liquids with absorbent material.
- Rinse patient with warm water, 32° C to 35° C (90° F to 95° F), if possible.
- Wash patient with a mild liquid soap and large quantities of water.
- Speed in removing product from skin is essential in limiting tissue damage.
- Refer to decontamination protocol in Section Three.

IMMEDIATE FIRST AID

- Ensure that adequate decontamination has been carried out.
- If patient is not breathing, start artificial respiration, preferably with a demand-valve resuscitator, bag-valve-mask device, or pocket mask, as trained. Perform CPR as necessary.
- Immediately flush contaminated eyes with gently flowing water.
- Do not induce vomiting. If vomiting occurs, lean patient forward or place on left side (head-down position, if possible) to maintain an open airway and prevent aspiration.
- Keep patient quiet and maintain normal body temperature.
- Obtain medical attention.

BASIC TREATMENT

- Establish a patent airway (oropharyngeal or nasopharyngeal airway, if needed). Suction if necessary.
- Watch for signs of respiratory insufficiency and assist ventilations if necessary.

- Administer oxygen by nonrebreather mask at 10 to 15 L/min.
- Monitor for pulmonary edema and treat if necessary (refer to pulmonary edema protocol in Section Three).
- Monitor for shock and treat if necessary (refer to shock protocol in Section Three).
- Anticipate seizures and treat if necessary (refer to seizure protocol in Section Three).
- For eye contamination, flush eyes immediately with water. Irrigate each eye continuously with 0.9% saline (NS) during transport (refer to eye irrigation protocol in Section Three).
- Do not use emetics. For ingestion, rinse mouth and administer 5 ml/kg up to 200 ml of water for dilution if the patent can swallow, has a strong gag reflex, and does not drool. Administer activated charcoal (refer to ingestion protocol in Section Three and activated charcoal protocol in Section Four).
- Cover skin burns with dry sterile dressings after decontamination (refer to chemical burn protocol in Section Three).

ADVANCED TREATMENT

- Consider orotracheal or nasotracheal intubation for airway control in the patient who is unconscious, has severe pulmonary edema, or is in severe respiratory distress.
- Positive-pressure ventilation techniques with a bag-valve-mask device may be beneficial.
- Consider drug therapy for pulmonary edema (refer to pulmonary edema protocol in Section Three).
- Monitor cardiac rhythm and treat arrhythmias as necessary (refer to cardiac protocol in Section Three).
- Start IV administration of D_5W TKO. Use 0.9% saline (NS) or lactated Ringer's (LR) if signs of hypovolemia are present For hypotension with signs of hypovolemia, administer fluid cautiously. If patient is unresponsive to these measures, vasopressors may be helpful. Watch for signs of fluid overload (refer to shock protocol in Section Three).
- Administer 1% solution methylene blue if patient is symptomatic with severe hypoxia, cyanosis, and cardiac compromise not responding to oxygen. DIRECT PHYSICIAN ORDER ONLY (refer to methylene blue protocol in Section Four).
- Treat seizures with diazepam (Valium) or lorazepam (Ativan) (refer to diazepam and lorazepam protocols in Section Four and seizure protocol in Section Three).
- Use proparacaine hydrochloride to assist eye irrigation (refer to proparacaine hydrochloride protocol in Section Four).

INITIAL EMERGENCY DEPARTMENT CONSIDERATIONS

- Useful initial laboratory studies include complete blood count, platelet count, coagulation profile, serum electrolytes, blood urea nitrogen (BUN), creatinine, glucose, urinalysis and baseline biochemical profile, including serum aminotransferases (ALT and AST), calcium, phosphorus, and magnesium. Arterial blood gases (ABGs), chest radiograph, and electrocardiogram may be required.
- Monitor blood methemoglobin levels and treat with methylene blue if patient is symptomatic and/or has a blood methemoglobin level greater than 30%. DIRECT PHYSICIAN ORDER ONLY (refer to methylene blue protocol in Section Four).

- Positive end-expiratory pressure (PEEP)–assisted ventilation may be necessary in patients with acute parenchymal injury who develop pulmonary edema or acute respiratory distress syndrome.
- Obtain toxicological consultation as necessary.

SPECIAL CONSIDERATIONS

Pulse oximetry readings may not be accurate in these exposures.

Ammonia and Related Compounds

SUBSTANCE IDENTIFICATION

Found as ammonia in solution and as a colorless, water-soluble alkaline gas. Used as cleaning agents, fertilizers, industrial refrigerants; intermediate in the manufacture of inorganic and organic nitrogen-containing compounds; used in dyeing, synthetic fibers, and as a neutralizing agent. Reacts with water to form ammonium hydroxide. On skin contact, liquefied ammonia may cause frostbite.

ROUTES OF EXPOSURE

Skin and eye contact
Inhalation
Ingestion

TARGET ORGANS

Primary
Skin
Eyes
Respiratory system
Gastrointestinal system
Secondary
Central nervous system
Cardiovascular system

LIFE THREAT

Pulmonary edema and hypotension.

SIGNS AND SYMPTOMS BY SYSTEM

Cardiovascular: Ventricular arrhythmias and hypotension.

Respiratory: Respiratory tract irritation with possible laryngeal edema, pulmonary edema, bronchospasm, stridor, cough, dyspnea, and chest pain.

CNS: Stupor, lethargy, and coma.

Gastrointestinal: Hemorrhage caused by liquefaction necrosis of the GI tract mucosa.

Eye: Chemical conjunctivitis with vapor exposure, conjunctivitis, corneal damage, and blindness with liquid and anhydrous gas exposures.

Skin: Full- and partial-thickness burns with liquefaction necrosis and/or frostbite with skin contact.

SYMPTOM ONSET FOR ACUTE EXPOSURE

Immediate
Respiratory symptoms possibly delayed

CO-EXPOSURE CONCERNS

Other alkalies

THERMAL DECOMPOSITION PRODUCTS INCLUDE

Ammonia

Hydrogen
Nitrogen oxides

MEDICAL CONDITIONS POSSIBLY AGGRAVATED BY EXPOSURE

Respiratory system disorders
Liver disorders
Skin disorders

DECONTAMINATION

- Wear positive-pressure SCBA and protective equipment specified by references such as the *North American Emergency Response Guidebook.* If special chemical protective clothing is required, consult the chemical manufacturer or specific protective clothing compatibility charts. A qualified, experienced person should make decisions regarding the type of personal protective equipment necessary.
- Delay entry until trained personnel and proper protective equipment are available.
- Remove patient from contaminated area.
- Quickly remove and isolate patient's clothing, jewelry, and shoes. If clothing is frozen (adherent) to skin, rinse with water before removal to prevent additional tissue damage.
- Gently brush away dry particles and blot excess liquids with absorbent material.
- Rinse patient with warm water, 32° C to 35° C (90° F to 95° F), if possible.
- Wash patient with a mild liquid soap and large quantities of water.
- Refer to decontamination protocol in Section Three.

IMMEDIATE FIRST AID

- Ensure that adequate decontamination has been carried out.
- If patient is not breathing, start artificial respiration, preferably with a demand-valve resuscitator, bag-valve-mask device, or pocket mask, as trained. Perform CPR as necessary.
- Immediately flush contaminated eyes with gently flowing water.
- Do not induce vomiting. If vomiting occurs, lean patient forward or place on left side (head-down position, if possible) to maintain an open airway and prevent aspiration.
- Keep patient quiet and maintain normal body temperature.
- Obtain medical attention.

BASIC TREATMENT

- Establish a patent airway (oropharyngeal or nasopharyngeal airway, if needed). Suction if necessary.
- Watch for signs of respiratory insufficiency and assist ventilations if necessary.
- Administer oxygen by nonrebreather mask at 10 to 15 L/min.
- Monitor for signs of pulmonary edema and treat if necessary (refer to pulmonary edema protocol in Section Three).
- Monitor for shock and treat if necessary (refer to shock protocol in Section Three).
- For eye contamination, flush eyes immediately with water. Irrigate each eye continuously with 0.9% saline (NS) during transport (refer to eye irrigation protocol in Section Three).
- Do not use emetics. For ingestion, rinse mouth and administer 5 ml/kg up to 200 ml of water for dilution if the patient can swallow, has a strong gag reflex, and does not drool (refer to ingestion protocol in Section Three).
- Do not attempt to neutralize.

ADVANCED TREATMENT

- Consider orotracheal or nasotracheal intubation for airway control if signs of upper airway obstruction are present or if the patient is unconscious, has severe pulmonary edema, or is in severe respiratory distress.
- Positive-pressure ventilation techniques with a bag-valve-mask device may be beneficial.
- Consider drug therapy for pulmonary edema (refer to pulmonary edema protocol in Section Three).
- Consider administering a beta agonist such as albuterol for severe bronchospasm (refer to albuterol protocol in Section Four).
- Monitor cardiac rhythm and treat arrhythmias if necessary (refer to cardiac protocol in Section Three).
- Start IV administration of D_5W TKO. Use 0.9% saline (NS) or lactated Ringer's (LR) if signs of hypovolemia are present. For hypotension with signs of hypovolemia, administer fluid cautiously. Consider vasopressors if patient is hypotensive with a normal fluid volume. Watch for signs of fluid overload (refer to shock protocol in Section Three).
- Use proparacaine hydrochloride to assist eye irrigation (refer to proparacaine hydrochloride protocol in Section Four).

INITIAL EMERGENCY DEPARTMENT CONSIDERATIONS

- Useful initial laboratory studies include complete blood count, serum electrolytes, blood urea nitrogen (BUN), creatinine, glucose, urinalysis, and baseline biochemical profile, including serum aminotransferases (ALT and AST), calcium, phosphorus, and magnesium. Arterial blood gases (ABGs), chest radiograph, and electrocardiogram may be required.
- Positive end-expiratory pressure (PEEP)–assisted ventilation may be necessary in patients with acute parenchymal injury who develop pulmonary edema or acute respiratory distress syndrome.
- Bronchospastic symptoms should be treated with an inhalation medication regimen similar to that used for reactive airway disease. Inhaled corticosteroids may be of value in severe bronchospasm.
- Exposure patients with inhalation exposure and respiratory symptoms should be observed in hospital for 24 hours.
- Endoscopy may be required for evaluation of oral ingestion.
- Obtain toxicological consultation as necessary.

SPECIAL CONSIDERATIONS

- Mixing ammonia and hypochlorite bleaches produces chloramine gas.
- Mixing ammonia and chlorine cleaners may result in the release of hydrochloric acid, nitrogen oxides, and chlorine active compounds.

22

Hypochlorite and Related Compounds

SUBSTANCE IDENTIFICATION

Found as a solid in white crystal form. Also found in solution. Used as bleaches, fungicides, chlorinating agents, disinfectants, and deodorants and in water purification processes. Severity of symptoms depends on concentration, type, and volume of product.

ROUTES OF EXPOSURE

Skin and eye contact
Inhalation
Ingestion

TARGET ORGANS

Primary
Skin
Eyes
Respiratory system
Gastrointestinal tract
Secondary
Central nervous system
Cardiovascular system
Metabolism

LIFE THREAT

Circulatory collapse, respiratory tract irritation with possible upper airway obstruction, and pulmonary edema.

SIGNS AND SYMPTOMS BY SYSTEM

Cardiovascular: Cardiovascular collapse and tachycardia.

Respiratory: Respiratory tract irritation that may lead to upper airway (glottic) edema and obstruction. Stridor, wheezing, pulmonary edema with dyspnea, tachypnea.

CNS: CNS confusion, delirium, depression, coma, and, rarely, seizures.

Gastrointestinal: Pain and irritation of the mucous membranes, nausea, vomiting (hematemesis), diarrhea, and abdominal pain.

Eye: Chemical conjunctivitis and corneal damage.

Skin: Irritant dermatitis and burns.

Metabolism: Hyperchloremia acidosis or hypernatremia is possible with concentrated product ingestion.

Other: If mixed with acids or heated, some products may release chlorine gas and other chlorine active compounds. When hypochlorites are mixed with ammonia, chloramine gas may be released.

SYMPTOM ONSET FOR ACUTE EXPOSURE

Immediate

CO-EXPOSURE CONCERNS

Acids
Ammonia
Other alkalies

THERMAL DECOMPOSITION PRODUCTS INCLUDE

Chlorine
Oxygen

MEDICAL CONDITIONS POSSIBLY AGGRAVATED BY EXPOSURE

Respiratory disorders
Gastrointestinal disorders
Skin disorders

DECONTAMINATION

- Wear positive-pressure SCBA and protective equipment specified by references such as the *North American Emergency Response Guidebook*. If special chemical protective clothing is required, consult the chemical manufacturer or specific protective clothing compatibility charts. A qualified, experienced person should make decisions regarding the type of personal protective equipment necessary.
- Delay entry until trained personnel and proper protective equipment are available.
- Remove patient from contaminated area.
- Quickly remove and isolate patient's clothing, jewelry, and shoes.
- Gently brush away dry particles and blot excess liquids with absorbent material.
- Rinse patient with warm water, 32° C to 35° C (90° F to 95° F), if possible.
- Wash patient with a mild liquid soap and large quantities of water.
- Refer to decontamination protocol in Section Three.

IMMEDIATE FIRST AID

- Ensure that adequate decontamination has been carried out.
- If patient is not breathing, start artificial respiration, preferably with a demand-valve resuscitator, bag-valve-mask device, or pocket mask, as trained. Perform CPR if necessary.
- Immediately flush contaminated eyes with gently flowing water.
- Do not induce vomiting. If vomiting occurs, lean patient forward or place on left side (head-down position, if possible) to maintain an open airway and prevent aspiration.
- Keep patient quiet and maintain normal body temperature.
- Obtain medical attention.

BASIC TREATMENT

- Establish a patent airway (oropharyngeal or nasopharyngeal airway, if needed). Suction if necessary.
- Watch for signs of respiratory insufficiency and assist ventilations if necessary.
- Administer oxygen by nonrebreather mask at 10 to 15 L/min.
- Monitor for pulmonary edema and treat if necessary (refer to pulmonary edema protocol in Section Three).
- Monitor for shock and treat if necessary (refer to shock protocol in Section Three).
- Anticipate seizures and treat if necessary (refer to seizure protocol in Section Three).

- For eye contamination, flush eyes immediately with water. Irrigate each eye continuously with 0.9% saline (NS) during transport (refer to eye irrigation protocol in Section Three).
- Do not use emetics. For ingestion, rinse mouth and administer 5 ml/kg up to 200 ml of water for dilution if the patient can swallow, has a strong gag reflex, and does not drool (refer to ingestion protocol in Section Three).
- Do not attempt to neutralize.

ADVANCED TREATMENT

- Consider orotracheal or nasotracheal intubation for airway control in the patient who is unconscious, has severe pulmonary edema, or is in severe respiratory distress. Early intubation, at the first signs of upper airway obstruction, may be necessary.
- Positive-pressure ventilation techniques with a bag-valve-mask device may be beneficial.
- Consider drug therapy for pulmonary edema (refer to pulmonary edema protocol in Section Three).
- Consider administering a beta agonist such as albuterol for severe bronchospasm (refer to albuterol protocol in Section Four).
- Monitor cardiac rhythm and treat arrhythmias if necessary (refer to cardiac protocol in Section Three).
- Start IV administration of D_5W TKO. Use 0.9% saline (NS) or lactated Ringer's (LR) if signs of hypovolemia are present. For hypotension with signs of hypovolemia, administer fluid cautiously. Consider vasopressors if patient is hypotensive with a normal fluid volume. Watch for signs of fluid overload (refer to shock protocol in Section Three).
- Treat seizures with diazepam (Valium) or lorazepam (Ativan) (refer to diazepam and lorazepam protocols in Section Four and seizure protocol in Section Three).
- Use proparacaine hydrochloride to assist eye irrigation (refer to proparacaine hydrochloride protocol in Section Four).

INITIAL EMERGENCY DEPARTMENT CONSIDERATIONS

- Useful initial laboratory studies include complete blood count, serum electrolytes, blood urea nitrogen (BUN), creatinine, glucose, urinalysis, and baseline biochemical profile, including serum aminotransferases (ALT and AST), calcium, phosphorus, and magnesium. Determination of the anion gap may be helpful. Arterial blood gases (ABGs), chest radiograph, and electrocardiogram may be required.
- Positive end-expiratory pressure (PEEP)–assisted ventilation may be necessary in patients with acute parenchymal injury who develop pulmonary edema or acute respiratory distress syndrome.
- Products may cause acidosis; hyperventilation and sodium bicarbonate may be beneficial. Bicarbonate therapy should be guided by clinical presentation, ABG determination, and serum electrolyte considerations.
- Bronchospastic symptoms should be treated with an inhalation medication regimen similar to that used for reactive airways disease. Inhaled corticosteroids may be of value in severe bronchospasm.
- Endoscopy may be required for evaluation of oral ingestion.
- Obtain toxicological consultation as necessary.

SPECIAL CONSIDERATIONS

- Sodium hypochlorite preparations (less than 5% concentration) rarely cause problems (dermal and mucosal burns or metabolic acidosis). More concentrated (15% to 20%) sodium hypochlorite products may cause severe burns and hyperchloremia metabolic acidosis. Calcium hypochlorite (5% concentration) is more than twice as toxic as the equivalent concentration of sodium hypochlorite solution.

23

Hydrazine and Related Compounds

SUBSTANCE IDENTIFICATION

A clear, colorless, fuming, oily liquid or white crystalline solid with an ammonia-like odor. Used as a rocket fuel, in chemical and pharmaceutical production, as a catalyst, as an inorganic solvent, and in plastic synthesis. The hydrate form is used as a reducing agent and is a strong base.

ROUTES OF EXPOSURE

Skin and eye contact
Inhalation
Ingestion
Skin absorption

TARGET ORGANS

Primary
Skin
Eyes
Central nervous system
Respiratory system
Blood

Secondary
Cardiovascular system
Gastrointestinal system
Hepatic system
Renal system
Metabolism

LIFE THREAT

Seizures, red blood cell destruction, pulmonary edema.

SIGNS AND SYMPTOMS BY SYSTEM

Cardiovascular: Hypotension.

Respiratory: Irritation of respiratory mucosa, coughing, dyspnea, pulmonary edema, and respiratory failure.

CNS: Headache, dizziness, narcosis (CNS depression), muscle tremors, and seizures.

Gastrointestinal: Irritation of the GI tract, nausea, and vomiting (possibly with blood).

Eye: Conjunctivitis, corneal damage, and chemical burns.

Skin: Irritant dermatitis and chemical burns. Facial edema may be noted. Prolonged contact may result in allergic sensitization.

Renal: Kidney damage.

Hepatic: Liver damage.

Metabolism: Hyperglycemia or hypoglycemia.

Blood: Red blood cell hemolysis, methemoglobinemia from exposure to monomethylhydrazine.

Other: Some products present a human carcinogenic risk.

SYMPTOM ONSET FOR ACUTE EXPOSURE

Immediate

Some symptoms such as methemoglobinemia and pulmonary edema possibly delayed

CO-EXPOSURE CONCERNS

Corrosives

Methemoglobin formers

THERMAL DECOMPOSITION PRODUCTS INCLUDE

Ammonia

Carbon dioxide

Carbon monoxide

Hydrogen

Nitrogen oxide

MEDICAL CONDITIONS POSSIBLY AGGRAVATED BY EXPOSURE

Nervous system disorders

Respiratory system disorders

Anemia

DECONTAMINATION

- Wear positive-pressure SCBA and protective equipment specified by references such as the *North American Emergency Response Guidebook*. If special chemical protective clothing is required, consult the chemical manufacturer or specific protective clothing compatibility charts. A qualified, experienced person should make decisions regarding the type of personal protective equipment necessary.
- Delay entry until trained personnel and proper protective equipment are available.
- Remove patient from contaminated area.
- Quickly remove and isolate patient's clothing, jewelry, and shoes.
- Gently brush away dry particles and blot excess liquids with absorbent material.
- Rinse patient with warm water, 32° C to 35° C (90° F to 95° F), if possible.
- Wash patient with a mild liquid soap and large quantities of water.
- Refer to decontamination protocol in Section Three.

IMMEDIATE FIRST AID

- Ensure that adequate decontamination has been carried out.
- If patient is not breathing, start artificial respiration, preferably with a demand-valve resuscitator, bag-valve-mask device, or pocket mask, as trained. Perform CPR if necessary.
- Immediately flush contaminated eyes with gently flowing water.
- Do not induce vomiting. If vomiting occurs, lean patient forward or place on left side (head-down position, if possible) in order to maintain an open airway and prevent aspiration.
- Keep patient quiet and maintain normal body temperature.
- Obtain medical attention.

BASIC TREATMENT

- Establish a patent airway (oropharyngeal or nasopharyngeal airway, if needed). Suction if necessary.

- Watch for signs of respiratory insufficiency and assist ventilations if necessary.
- Administer oxygen by nonrebreather mask at 10 to 15 L/min.
- Monitor for pulmonary edema and treat if necessary (refer to pulmonary edema protocol in Section Three).
- Monitor for shock and treat if necessary (refer to shock protocol in Section Three).
- Anticipate seizures and treat if necessary (refer to seizure protocol in Section Three).
- For eye contamination, flush eyes immediately with water. Irrigate each eye continuously with 0.9% saline (NS) during transport (refer to eye irrigation protocol in Section Three).
- Do not use emetics. For ingestion, rinse mouth and administer 5 ml/kg up to 200 mL of water for dilution if the patient can swallow, has a strong gag reflex, and does not drool. Administer activated charcoal (refer to ingestion protocol in Section Three and activated charcoal protocol in Section Four).
- Cover skin burns with dry, sterile dressings after decontamination (refer to chemical burn protocol in Section Three).

ADVANCED TREATMENT

- Consider orotracheal or nasotracheal intubation for airway control in the patient who is unconscious, has severe pulmonary edema, or is in severe respiratory distress.
- Positive-pressure ventilation techniques with a bag-valve-mask device may be beneficial.
- Consider drug therapy for pulmonary edema (refer to pulmonary edema protocol in Section Three).
- Monitor cardiac rhythm and treat arrhythmias if necessary (refer to cardiac protocol in Section Three).
- Start IV administration of D_5W TKO. Use 0.9% saline (NS) or lactated Ringer's (LR) if signs of hypovolemia are present. For hypotension with signs of hypovolemia, administer fluid cautiously. Consider vasopressors if patient is hypotensive with a normal fluid volume. Watch for signs of fluid overload (refer to shock protocol in Section Three).
- Administer 1% solution methylene blue if patient is symptomatic with severe hypoxia, cyanosis, and cardiac compromise not responding to oxygen. DIRECT PHYSICIAN ORDER ONLY (refer to methylene blue protocol in Section Four).
- Treat seizures with diazepam (Valium) or lorazepam (Ativan) (refer to diazepam and lorazepam protocols in Section Four and seizure protocol in Section Three).
- Monitor for signs of hypoglycemia (decreased level of consciousness, tachycardia, pallor, dilated pupils, diaphoresis, and/or a dextrose strip or glucometer reading less than 50 mg/dl) and administer 50% dextrose if necessary. Draw blood sample before administration (refer to 50% dextrose protocol in Section Four).
- Use proparacaine hydrochloride to assist eye irrigation (refer to proparacaine hydrochloride protocol in Section Four).

INITIAL EMERGENCY DEPARTMENT CONSIDERATIONS

- Useful initial laboratory studies include complete blood count, serum electrolytes, blood urea nitrogen (BUN), creatinine, bilirubin, glucose, urinalysis and baseline biochemical profile, including serum aminotransferases (ALT and AST), calcium, phosphorus, and magnesium. Arterial blood gases (ABGs), chest radiograph, and electrocardiogram may be required.

- Monitor methemoglobin levels in patients exposed to monomethylhydrazine. Treat with methylene blue if patient is symptomatic and/or has a blood methemoglobin level greater than 30%. DIRECT PHYSICIAN ORDER ONLY (refer to methylene blue protocol in Section Four).
- Positive end-expiratory pressure (PEEP)–assisted ventilation may be necessary in patients with acute parenchymal injury who develop pulmonary edema or acute respiratory distress syndrome.
- Pyridoxine (vitamin B_6) has been used to treat intractable seizures associated with monomethylhydrazine poisoning. Adult intravenous pyridoxine dosage: 25 mg/kg. If symptoms do not remit or recur, this dose may be repeated one time. Maximum total dosage not to exceed 5 g.
- Obtain toxicological consultation as necessary.

SPECIAL CONSIDERATIONS

Pulse oximetry readings may not be accurate in these exposures.

Aromatic Hydrocarbons and Related Compounds

SUBSTANCE IDENTIFICATION

Colorless, clear liquids with a faint etherlike or pleasant odor. Found in solvents, degreasers, wetting agents, agricultural chemicals, laboratory reagents, and antifreezes. Also used in the application and manufacture of varnishes, lacquers, paints, and detergents. May be an ingredient in gasoline and aviation fuel. Refer to Guideline 25 for benzene management.

ROUTES OF EXPOSURE

Skin and eye contact
Inhalation
Ingestion
Skin absorption

TARGET ORGANS

Primary
Skin
Eyes
Central nervous system
Renal system
Hepatic system
Secondary
Cardiovascular system
Respiratory system
Metabolism

LIFE THREAT

Arrhythmias, respiratory failure, pulmonary edema, and paralysis. May also cause brain and kidney damage.

SIGNS AND SYMPTOMS BY SYSTEM

Cardiovascular: Cardiovascular collapse, tachyarrhythmias, especially ventricular fibrillation. Bradycardia has also been reported.

Respiratory: Upper respiratory tract irritation, acute pulmonary edema, bronchospasm, dyspnea, tachypnea, respiratory failure, cough, hoarseness, and substernal chest pain.

CNS: Headache, drowsiness, dizziness, confusion, weakness, tremors, poor coordination, ataxia, seizures, CNS depression, coma, and disturbances in hearing and tinnitus. Patients may develop a transient euphoria after exposure.

Gastrointestinal: Nausea, vomiting, stomach pain, and excessive salivation.

Eye: Chemical conjunctivitis, corneal burns, and photophobia.

Skin: Drying and cracking of the skin, irritant dermatitis.

Renal: Hematuria, proteinuria, renal tubular acidosis, and renal failure.

Hepatic: Liver damage.

Metabolism: Metabolic acidosis.

Other: Human teratogenic risk: toluene. Refer to Guideline 25 for benzene management.

SYMPTOM ONSET FOR ACUTE EXPOSURE

Immediate

Pulmonary edema possibly delayed

CO-EXPOSURE CONCERNS

Ethanol

Other organic solvents

THERMAL DECOMPOSITION PRODUCTS INCLUDE

Carbon dioxide

Carbon monoxide

Organic compounds

MEDICAL CONDITIONS POSSIBLY AGGRAVATED BY EXPOSURE

Central nervous system disorders

Respiratory disorders

Skin and eye disorders

Liver disorders

Kidney disorders

DECONTAMINATION

- Wear positive-pressure SCBA and protective equipment specified by references such as the *North American Emergency Response Guidebook.* If special chemical protective clothing is required, consult the chemical manufacturer or specific protective clothing compatibility charts. A qualified, experienced person should make decisions regarding the type of personal protective equipment necessary.
- Delay entry until trained personnel and proper protective equipment are available.
- Remove patient from contaminated area.
- Quickly remove and isolate patient's clothing, jewelry, and shoes.
- Gently brush away dry particles and blot excess liquids with absorbent material.
- Rinse patient with warm water, 32° C to 35° C (90° F to 95° F), if possible.
- Wash patient with a mild liquid soap and large quantities of water.
- Refer to decontamination protocol in Section Three.

IMMEDIATE FIRST AID

- Ensure that adequate decontamination has been carried out.
- If patient is not breathing, start artificial respiration, preferably with a demand-valve resuscitator, bag-valve-mask device, or pocket mask, as trained. Perform CPR if necessary.
- Immediately flush contaminated eyes with gently flowing water.
- Do not induce vomiting. If vomiting occurs, lean patient forward or place on left side (head-down position, if possible) to maintain an open airway and prevent aspiration.
- Keep patient quiet and maintain normal body temperature.
- Obtain medical attention.

BASIC TREATMENT

- Establish a patent airway (oropharyngeal or nasopharyngeal airway, if needed). Suction if necessary.
- Watch for signs of respiratory insufficiency and assist ventilations if necessary.

- Administer oxygen by nonrebreather mask at 10 to 15 L/min.
- Monitor for pulmonary edema and treat if necessary (refer to pulmonary edema protocol in Section Three).
- Monitor for shock and treat if necessary (refer to shock protocol in Section Three).
- Anticipate seizures and treat if necessary (refer to seizure protocol in Section Three).
- For eye contamination, flush eyes immediately with water. Irrigate each eye continuously with 0.9% saline (NS) during transport (refer to eye irrigation protocol in Section Three).
- Do not use emetics. For ingestion, rinse mouth and administer 5 ml/kg up to 200 ml of water for dilution if the patient can swallow, has a strong gag reflex, and does not drool. Administer activated charcoal (refer to ingestion protocol in Section Three and activated charcoal protocol in Section Four).

ADVANCED TREATMENT

- Consider orotracheal or nasotracheal intubation for airway control in the patient who is unconscious, has severe pulmonary edema, or is in severe respiratory distress.
- Positive-pressure ventilation techniques with a bag-valve-mask device may be beneficial.
- Consider drug therapy for pulmonary edema (refer to pulmonary edema protocol in Section Three).
- Consider administering a beta agonist such as albuterol for severe bronchospasm (refer to albuterol protocol in Section Four) (see caution in Special Considerations below).
- Monitor cardiac rhythm and treat arrhythmias if necessary (refer to cardiac protocol in Section Three).
- Start IV administration of D_5W TKO. Use 0.9% saline (NS) or lactated Ringer's (LR) if signs of hypovolemia are present. For hypotension with signs of hypovolemia, administer fluid cautiously. Watch for signs of fluid overload (refer to shock protocol in Section Three).
- Treat seizures with diazepam (Valium) or lorazepam (Ativan) (refer to diazepam and lorazepam protocols in Section Four and seizure protocol in Section Three).
- Use proparacaine hydrochloride to assist eye irrigation (refer to proparacaine hydrochloride protocol in Section Four).

INITIAL EMERGENCY DEPARTMENT CONSIDERATIONS

- Useful initial laboratory studies include complete blood count, serum electrolytes, blood urea nitrogen (BUN), creatinine, glucose, urinalysis, and baseline biochemical profile, including serum aminotransferases (ALT and AST), calcium, phosphorus, and magnesium. Determination of the anion gap may be helpful. Arterial blood gases (ABGs), chest radiograph, and electrocardiogram may be required.
- Positive end-expiratory pressure (PEEP)–assisted ventilation may be necessary in patients with acute parenchymal injury who develop pulmonary edema or acute respiratory distress syndrome.
- Bronchospastic symptoms should be treated with an inhalation medication regimen similar to that used for reactive airways disease. Inhaled corticosteroids

may be of value in severe bronchospasm (see caution in Special Considerations below).

- Severe exposure may cause acidosis; hyperventilation and sodium bicarbonate may be beneficial. Bicarbonate therapy should be guided by patient presentation, ABG determination, and serum electrolyte considerations.
- Obtain toxicological consultation as necessary.

SPECIAL CONSIDERATIONS

- Avoid epinephrine and related beta agonists (unless patient is in cardiac arrest or has reactive airways disease refractory to other treatment) because of the possible irritable condition of the myocardium. Use of these medications may lead to ventricular fibrillation.
- Chronic exposure/inhalation abuse such as glue (toluene) sniffing produces CNS excitation followed by depression and visual and auditory disturbances. Decreased visual and color perception accuracy may be observed.
- Organic brain dysfunction known as the psycho-organic syndrome of solvents has been described in cases of chronic exposure. Neuroencephalopathy (dementia) may occur as a sequela of severe exposures. Permanent neurobehavioral changes may result.

25
Benzene and Related Compounds

SUBSTANCE IDENTIFICATION

Colorless liquids with an aromatic odor. Used in the manufacture of pharmaceuticals, dyes, textiles, varnishes, lacquers, solvents, degreasers, and many other compounds. Found in gasoline (0.8%), coal tar distillates, cigarette smoke, and petroleum naphtha.

ROUTES OF EXPOSURE

Skin and eye contact
Inhalation
Ingestion
Skin absorption

TARGET ORGANS

Primary
Skin
Eyes
Central nervous system
Cardiovascular system
Respiratory system
Hepatic system
Renal system
Blood
Secondary
Gastrointestinal system

LIFE THREAT

Arrhythmias, respiratory failure, pulmonary edema, CNS depression, liver and kidney damage.

SIGNS AND SYMPTOMS BY SYSTEM

Cardiovascular: Tachyarrhythmias, especially ventricular fibrillation and cardiovascular collapse.

Respiratory: Upper respiratory tract irritation, cough, hoarseness, dyspnea, tachypnea, substernal chest pain, bronchospasm, acute pulmonary edema, and respiratory failure.

CNS: Headache, drowsiness, dizziness, depression, decreased judgment, loss of balance, tinnitus, confusion, weakness, tremors, poor coordination, neurobehavioral changes, seizures, initial transient euphoria followed by CNS depression, and visual disturbances.

Gastrointestinal: Nausea, vomiting, stomach pain, and excessive salivation may be present.

Eye: Chemical conjunctivitis and corneal damage.

Skin: Drying and cracking of the skin (defatting, irritant dermatitis).

Renal: Kidney failure.
Hepatic: Liver toxicity.
Blood: Bone marrow suppression, aplastic anemia, and leukemia (acute myelogenous leukemia (AML).
Other: Human carcinogenic risk with benzene (AML).

SYMPTOM ONSET FOR ACUTE EXPOSURE

Immediate
Pulmonary edema possibly delayed
Bone marrow symptoms delayed

CO-EXPOSURE CONCERNS

Other hydrocarbon solvents
Other bone marrow poisons

THERMAL DECOMPOSITION PRODUCTS INCLUDE

Carbon dioxide
Carbon monoxide

MEDICAL CONDITIONS POSSIBLY AGGRAVATED BY EXPOSURE

Blood disorders
Kidney disorders
Liver disorders
Skin disorders

DECONTAMINATION

- Wear positive-pressure SCBA and protective equipment specified by references such as the *North American Emergency Response Guidebook*. If special chemical protective clothing is required, consult the chemical manufacturer or specific protective clothing compatibility charts. A qualified, experienced person should make decisions regarding the type of personal protective equipment necessary.
- Delay entry until trained personnel and proper protective equipment are available.
- Remove patient from contaminated area.
- Quickly remove and isolate patient's clothing, jewelry, and shoes.
- Gently brush away dry particles and blot excess liquids with absorbent material.
- Rinse patient with warm water, 32° C to 35° C (90° F to 95° F), if possible.
- Wash patient with a mild liquid soap and large quantities of water.
- Refer to decontamination protocol in Section Three.

IMMEDIATE FIRST AID

- Ensure that adequate decontamination has been carried out.
- If patient is not breathing, start artificial respiration, preferably with a demand-valve resuscitator, bag-valve-mask device, or pocket mask, as trained. Perform CPR if necessary.
- Immediately flush contaminated eyes with gently flowing water.
- Do not induce vomiting. If vomiting occurs, lean patient forward or place on left side (head-down position, if possible) to maintain an open airway and prevent aspiration.
- Keep patient quiet and maintain normal body temperature.
- Obtain medical attention.

BASIC TREATMENT

- Establish a patent airway (oropharyngeal or nasopharyngeal airway, if needed). Suction if necessary.

- Watch for signs of respiratory insufficiency and assist ventilations if necessary.
- Administer oxygen by nonrebreather mask at 10 to 15 L/min.
- Monitor for pulmonary edema and treat if necessary (refer to pulmonary edema protocol in Section Three).
- Monitor for shock and treat if necessary (refer to shock protocol in Section Three).
- Anticipate seizures and treat if necessary (refer to seizure protocol in Section Three).
- For eye contamination, flush eyes immediately with water. Irrigate each eye continuously with 0.9% saline (NS) during transport (refer to eye irrigation protocol in Section Three).
- Do not use emetics. For ingestion, rinse mouth and administer 5 ml/kg up to 200 ml of water for dilution if the patient can swallow, has a strong gag reflex, and does not drool. Administer activated charcoal (refer to ingestion protocol in Section Three and activated charcoal protocol in Section Four).

ADVANCED TREATMENT

- Consider orotracheal or nasotracheal intubation for airway control in the patient who is unconscious, has severe pulmonary edema, or is in severe respiratory distress.
- Positive-pressure ventilation techniques with a bag-valve-mask device may be beneficial.
- Consider drug therapy for pulmonary edema (refer to pulmonary edema protocol in Section Three).
- Consider administering a beta agonist such as albuterol for severe bronchospasm (refer to albuterol protocol in Section Four) (see caution in Special Considerations below).
- Monitor cardiac rhythm and treat arrhythmias as necessary (refer to cardiac protocol in Section Three).
- Start IV administration of D_5W TKO. Use 0.9% saline (NS) or lactated Ringer's (LR) if signs of hypovolemia are present For hypotension with signs of hypovolemia, administer fluid cautiously. Watch for signs of fluid overload (refer to shock protocol in Section Three).
- Treat seizures with diazepam (Valium) or lorazepam (Ativan) (refer to diazepam and lorazepam protocols in Section Four and seizure protocol in Section Three).
- Use proparacaine hydrochloride to assist eye irrigation (refer to proparacaine hydrochloride protocol in Section Four).

INITIAL EMERGENCY DEPARTMENT CONSIDERATIONS

- Useful initial laboratory studies include complete blood count, reticulocyte count, serum electrolytes, blood urea nitrogen (BUN), creatinine, glucose, urinalysis, and baseline biochemical profile, including serum aminotransferases (ALT and AST), calcium, phosphorus, and magnesium. Arterial blood gases (ABGs), chest radiograph, and electrocardiogram may be required.
- Positive end-expiratory pressure (PEEP)–assisted ventilation may be necessary in patients with acute parenchymal injury who develop pulmonary edema or acute respiratory distress syndrome.
- Bronchospastic symptoms should be treated with an inhalation medication regimen similar to that used for reactive airways disease. Inhaled corticosteroids

may be of value in severe bronchospasm (see caution in Special Considerations below).

- Obtain toxicological consultation as necessary.

SPECIAL CONSIDERATIONS

- Avoid epinephrine and related beta agonists (unless patient is in cardiac arrest or has reactive airways disease refractory to other treatment) because of the possible irritable condition of the myocardium. Use of these medications may lead to ventricular fibrillation.
- Chronic or high-dose, acute exposure patients require participation in a medical surveillance program.

26

Halogenated Aliphatic Hydrocarbons and Related Compounds

SUBSTANCE IDENTIFICATION

Waxy, amber-colored solids with a mild turpentine odor. Colorless or white volatile liquids, with a penetrating odor, that yield heavy vapors. Used as solvents, cleaners, degreasing agents, paint removers, fumigants, and refrigerants.

ROUTES OF EXPOSURE

Skin and eye contact
Inhalation
Ingestion
Skin absorption

TARGET ORGANS

Primary
Skin
Eyes
Central nervous system
Cardiovascular system
Respiratory system
Secondary
Gastrointestinal system
Hepatic system
Renal system

LIFE THREAT

CNS depression, respiratory arrest, and circulatory collapse.

SIGNS AND SYMPTOMS BY SYSTEM

Cardiovascular: Vasodilation (centrally mediated) leading to hypotension. Cardiovascular collapse, ventricular arrhythmias, and fibrillation.

Respiratory: Lung and mucous membrane irritation, dyspnea, tachypnea, signs of pulmonary edema, hypoxia, and respiratory arrest.

CNS: Headache, CNS depression, drowsiness, dizziness, confusion, vertigo, fatigue, lethargy, seizures, coma, visual disturbances, and numbness in hands and feet (paresthesias).

Gastrointestinal: Nausea, vomiting, diarrhea, and abdominal cramps.

Eye: Chemical conjunctivitis and corneal damage.

Skin: Irritant dermatitis and chemical burns.

Renal: Kidney damage may occur.

Hepatic: Liver damage (hepatotoxicity) and hepatorenal syndrome.

Other: Methylene chloride is metabolized in the body to carbon monoxide. Prolonged exposure in nonsmokers may produce carboxyhemoglobin concentrations in the 3% to 10% range. These concentrations may produce cardiovascular compromise in individuals with preexisting lung and/or cardiovascular disease. Some products can cross the placental membrane. Trichloroethylene, tetrachloroethylene, 1,2 dichloroethane, dichloromethane, tetrachloroethylene, and trichloromethane are suspected human carcinogens (other compounds may be added or deleted as further research data become available).

SYMPTOM ONSET FOR ACUTE EXPOSURE

Immediate
Pulmonary edema possibly delayed
Neurobehavioral changes possibly delayed

CO-EXPOSURE CONCERNS

Ethanol
Other organic solvents

THERMAL DECOMPOSITION PRODUCTS INCLUDE

Carbon dioxide
Carbon monoxide
Chlorine
Hydrogen bromide
Hydrogen chloride
Hydrogen iodide
Hydrogen fluoride
Phosgene

MEDICAL CONDITIONS POSSIBLY AGGRAVATED BY EXPOSURE

Central nervous system disorders
Liver disorders
Cardiovascular disorders

DECONTAMINATION

- Wear positive-pressure SCBA and protective equipment specified by references such as the *North American Emergency Response Guidebook.* If special chemical protective clothing is required, consult the chemical manufacturer or specific protective clothing compatibility charts. A qualified, experienced person should make decisions regarding the type of personal protective equipment necessary.
- Delay entry until trained personnel and proper protective equipment are available.
- Remove patient from contaminated area.
- Quickly remove and isolate patient's clothing, jewelry, and shoes.
- Gently brush away dry particles and blot excess liquids with absorbent material.
- Rinse patient with warm water, 32° C to 35° C (90° F to 95° F), if possible.
- Wash patient with a mild liquid soap and large quantities of water.
- Refer to decontamination protocol in Section Three.

IMMEDIATE FIRST AID

- Ensure that adequate decontamination has been carried out.
- If patient is not breathing, start artificial respiration, preferably with a demand-valve resuscitator, bag-valve-mask device, or pocket mask. as trained. Perform CPR if necessary.
- Immediately flush contaminated eyes with gently flowing water.

- Do not induce vomiting. If vomiting occurs, lean patient forward or place on left side (head-down position, if possible) to maintain an open airway and prevent aspiration.
- Keep patient quiet and maintain normal body temperature.
- Obtain medical attention.

BASIC TREATMENT

- Establish a patent airway (oropharyngeal or nasopharyngeal airway, if needed). Suction if necessary.
- Watch for signs of respiratory insufficiency and assist ventilations if necessary.
- Administer oxygen by nonrebreather mask at 10 to 15 L/min.
- Monitor for pulmonary edema and treat if necessary (refer to pulmonary edema protocol in Section Three).
- Monitor for shock and treat if necessary (refer to shock protocol in Section Three).
- Anticipate seizures and treat if necessary (refer to seizure protocol in Section Three).
- For eye contamination, flush eyes immediately with water. Irrigate each eye continuously with 0.9% saline (NS) during transport (refer to eye irrigation protocol in Section Three).
- Do not use emetics. For ingestion, rinse mouth and administer 5 ml/kg up to 200 ml of water for dilution if the patient can swallow, has a strong gag reflex, and does not drool. Administer activated charcoal (refer to ingestion protocol in Section Three and activated charcoal protocol in Section Four).
- Cover skin burns with sterile dressings after decontamination (refer to chemical burn protocol in Section Three).

ADVANCED TREATMENT

- Consider orotracheal or nasotracheal intubation for airway control in the patient who is unconscious, has severe pulmonary edema, or is in severe respiratory distress.
- Positive-pressure ventilation techniques with a bag-valve-mask device may be beneficial.
- Consider drug therapy for pulmonary edema (refer to pulmonary edema protocol in Section Three).
- Monitor cardiac rhythm and treat arrhythmias as necessary (refer to cardiac protocol in Section Three).
- Start IV administration of D_5W TKO. Use 0.9% saline (NS) or lactated Ringer's (LR) if signs of hypovolemia are present. For hypotension with signs of hypovolemia, administer fluid cautiously. Consider vasopressors if patient is hypotensive with a normal fluid volume. Watch for signs of cardiac irritability and fluid overload (refer to shock protocol in Section Three).
- Treat seizures with diazepam (Valium) or lorazepam (Ativan) (refer to diazepam and lorazepam protocols in Section Four and seizure protocol in Section Three).
- Use proparacaine hydrochloride to assist eye irrigation (refer to proparacaine hydrochloride protocol in Section Four).

INITIAL EMERGENCY DEPARTMENT CONSIDERATIONS

- Useful initial laboratory studies include complete blood count, serum electrolytes, blood urea nitrogen (BUN), creatinine, glucose, urinalysis, and

baseline biochemical profile, including serum aminotransferases (ALT and AST), calcium, phosphorus, and magnesium. Arterial blood gases (ABGs), chest radiograph, and electrocardiogram may be required.

- Monitor carboxyhemoglobin (CO) blood concentrations in cases of methylene chloride (refer to carbon monoxide, Guideline 89).
- Positive end-expiratory pressure (PEEP)–assisted ventilation may be necessary in patients with acute parenchymal injury who develop pulmonary edema or acute respiratory distress syndrome.
- Obtain toxicological consultation as necessary.

SPECIAL CONSIDERATIONS

- Dichloromethane (synonyms: methylene chloride and methylene dichloride) is decomposed by heat to phosgene and is metabolized in the body to carbon monoxide (example of lethal synthesis). Refer to appropriate guidelines (carbon monoxide, 89; phosgene, 101) for additional information.
- Avoid epinephrine and related beta agonists (unless patient is in cardiac arrest or has reactive airways disease refractory to other treatment) because of the possible irritable condition of the myocardium. Use of these medications may lead to ventricular fibrillation.
- Organic brain dysfunction known as the psycho-organic syndrome of solvents has been described in cases of chronic exposure. Neuroencephalopathy (dementia) may occur as a sequela of severe exposures. Permanent neurobehavioral changes may result. This syndrome is usually documented with neurobehavioral testing.

27 Chlorinated Fluorocarbons (CFCs) and Related Compounds

SUBSTANCE IDENTIFICATION

Colorless liquids or gases with fruitlike or etherlike odor. Some gases are odorless and an odorant is occasionally added. Used as propellants, solvents, polymer intermediates for dechlorination of chemicals, refrigerants (Freons), and fire-extinguishing agents (Halons), and in the manufacturing processes of many products. When heated, many of these products decompose to phosgene.

ROUTES OF EXPOSURE

Skin and eye contact
Inhalation
Ingestion
Skin absorption

TARGET ORGANS

Primary
Skin
Eyes
Central nervous system
Cardiovascular system
Secondary
Respiratory system
Gastrointestinal system

LIFE THREAT

Asphyxiation. Products demonstrate anesthetic properties at high concentrations. Cardiac arrhythmias.

SIGNS AND SYMPTOMS BY SYSTEM

Cardiovascular: Cardiovascular collapse and arrhythmias. May aggravate preexisting cardiac problem. May increase myocardial effects of catecholamines.

Respiratory: Narcotic effect may depress respirations. Irritation of the respiratory tract and, possibly, pulmonary edema.

CNS: Excitation, headache, disorientation, dizziness, weakness, and seizures. CNS depression and coma due to anesthetic effect or hypoxia. Neurobehavioral changes.

Gastrointestinal: Nausea, vomiting, excessive salivation, and abdominal cramps.

Eye: Irritation and lacrimation.

Skin: Mild skin irritation and possible frostbite as a result of freezing effect of gas expansion.

SYMPTOM ONSET FOR ACUTE EXPOSURE

Immediate

Respiratory and cardiovascular symptoms possibly delayed
Neurobehavioral changes possibly delayed

CO-EXPOSURE CONCERNS

Other halogenated hydrocarbons
Other chlorinated fluorocarbons
Hydrocarbon solvents

THERMAL DECOMPOSITION PRODUCTS INCLUDE

Halon
Carbonyl halides
Hydrogen bromide
Hydrogen fluoride
Halogen acids
Free halogens
Freon
Carbon dioxide
Carbon monoxide
Carbonyl halides
Chlorine
Phosgene
Hydrochloric acid
Hydrofluoric acid

MEDICAL CONDITIONS POSSIBLY AGGRAVATED BY EXPOSURE

CNS disorders
Cardiovascular disorders

DECONTAMINATION

- Wear positive-pressure SCBA and protective equipment specified by references such as the *North American Emergency Response Guidebook*. If special chemical protective clothing is required, consult the chemical manufacturer or specific protective clothing compatibility charts. A qualified, experienced person should make decisions regarding the type of personal protective equipment necessary.
- Delay entry until trained personnel and proper protective equipment are available.
- Remove patient from contaminated area.
- Quickly remove and isolate patient's clothing, jewelry, and shoes.
- Gently brush away dry particles and blot excess liquids with absorbent material.
- Rinse patient with warm water, 32° C to 35° C (90° F to 95° F), if possible.
- Wash patient with a mild liquid soap and large quantities of water.
- Refer to decontamination protocol in Section Three.

IMMEDIATE FIRST AID

- Ensure that adequate decontamination has been carried out.
- If patient is not breathing, start artificial respiration, preferably with a demand-valve resuscitator, bag-valve-mask device, or pocket mask, as trained. Perform CPR if necessary.
- Immediately flush contaminated eyes with gently flowing water.
- Do not induce vomiting. If vomiting occurs, lean patient forward or place on left side (head-down position, if possible) to maintain an open airway and prevent aspiration.

- Keep patient quiet and maintain normal body temperature.
- Obtain medical attention.

BASIC TREATMENT

- Establish a patent airway (oropharyngeal or nasopharyngeal airway, if needed). Suction if necessary.
- Watch for signs of respiratory insufficiency and assist ventilations as needed.
- Administer oxygen by nonrebreather mask at 10 to 15 L/min.
- Minimize physical activity and provide a quiet atmosphere.
- Monitor for pulmonary edema and treat if necessary (refer to pulmonary edema protocol in Section Three).
- Anticipate seizures and treat if necessary (refer to seizure protocol in Section Three).
- For eye contamination, flush eyes immediately with water. Irrigate each eye continuously with 0.9% saline (NS) during transport (refer to eye irrigation protocol in Section Three).
- Do not use emetics. Rinse mouth and administer 5 ml/kg up to 200 ml of water for dilution if the patient can swallow, has a strong gag reflex, and does not drool. Administer activated charcoal (refer to ingestion protocol in Section Three and activated charcoal protocol in Section Four).
- Treat frostbite with rapid rewarming techniques (refer to frostbite protocol in Section Three).

ADVANCED TREATMENT

- Consider orotracheal or nasotracheal intubation for airway control in the patient who is unconscious, has severe pulmonary edema, or is in severe respiratory distress.
- Positive-pressure ventilation techniques with a bag-valve-mask device may be beneficial.
- Consider drug therapy for pulmonary edema (refer to pulmonary edema protocol in Section Three).
- Monitor cardiac rhythm and treat arrhythmias if necessary (refer to cardiac protocol in Section Three).
- Start IV administration of D_5W TKO. Use 0.9% saline (NS) or lactated Ringer's (LR) if signs of hypovolemia are present. For hypotension with signs of hypovolemia, administer fluid cautiously. Watch for signs of fluid overload (refer to shock protocol in Section Three).
- Treat seizures with diazepam (Valium) or lorazepam (Ativan) (refer to diazepam and lorazepam protocols in Section Four and seizure protocol in Section Three).
- Use proparacaine hydrochloride to assist eye irrigation (refer to proparacaine hydrochloride protocol in Section Four).

INITIAL EMERGENCY DEPARTMENT CONSIDERATIONS

- Useful initial laboratory studies include complete blood count, serum electrolytes, blood urea nitrogen (BUN), creatinine, glucose, urinalysis, and baseline biochemical profile, including serum aminotransferases (ALT and AST), calcium, phosphorus, and magnesium. Determination of anion and osmolar gaps may be helpful. Arterial blood gases (ABGs), chest radiograph, and electrocardiogram may be required.

- Positive end-expiratory pressure (PEEP)–assisted ventilation may be necessary in patients with acute parenchymal injury who develop pulmonary edema or acute respiratory distress syndrome.
- Obtain toxicological consultation if necessary.

SPECIAL CONSIDERATIONS

- Avoid epinephrine and related beta agonists (unless patient is in cardiac arrest or has reactive airways disease refractory to other treatment) because of the possible irritable condition of the myocardium. Use of these medications may lead to ventricular fibrillation.

28

Carbon Tetrachloride and Related Compounds

SUBSTANCE IDENTIFICATION

Waxy, amber-colored solid with a mild turpentine odor. Colorless or white volatile liquid that yields heavy vapors. Sweet, aromatic odor resembling that of chloroform. Used in solvents, cleaners, and fumigants, refrigerants, metal degreasers, and semiconductor production.

ROUTES OF EXPOSURE

Skin and eye contact
Inhalation
Ingestion
Skin absorption

TARGET ORGANS

Primary
Skin
Eyes
Central nervous system
Cardiovascular system
Respiratory system
Secondary
Gastrointestinal system
Hepatic system
Renal system
Metabolism

LIFE THREAT

CNS depression, respiratory arrest, and circulatory collapse.

SIGNS AND SYMPTOMS BY SYSTEM

Cardiovascular: Cardiovascular collapse, hypotension, ventricular arrhythmias, and ventricular fibrillation. Possible hypertension.

Respiratory: Dyspnea, tachypnea, irritation to the lungs and mucous membranes, epistaxis, pulmonary edema, and respiratory arrest.

CNS: CNS depression, coma, headache, drowsiness, dizziness, confusion, and seizures, visual disturbances, and neurobehavioral changes.

Gastrointestinal: Nausea, vomiting, anorexia, diarrhea, and abdominal cramps.

Eye: Chemical conjunctivitis.

Skin: Irritant dermatitis, flushing, and chemical burns.

Renal: Kidney damage.

Hepatic: Jaundice and liver damage, including hepatitis.

Metabolism: Metabolic acidosis.

Other: Some products present a human carcinogenic risk.

SYMPTOM ONSET FOR ACUTE EXPOSURE

Immediate
Pulmonary edema possibly delayed
Hepatotoxicity possibly delayed

CO-EXPOSURE CONCERNS

Alcohols
Acetone
Chlorinated solvents
Sympathomimetic agents

THERMAL DECOMPOSITION PRODUCTS INCLUDE

Carbon dioxide
Carbon monoxide
Chlorine
Hydrogen chloride
Phosgene

MEDICAL CONDITIONS POSSIBLY AGGRAVATED BY EXPOSURE

Central nervous system disorders
Alcoholism
Liver disorders
Kidney disorders

DECONTAMINATION

- Wear positive-pressure SCBA and protective equipment specified by references such as the *North American Emergency Response Guidebook.* If special chemical protective clothing is required, consult the chemical manufacturer or specific protective clothing compatibility charts. A qualified, experienced person should make decisions regarding the type of personal protective equipment necessary.
- Delay entry until trained personnel and proper protective equipment are available.
- Remove patient from contaminated area.
- Quickly remove and isolate patient's clothing, jewelry, and shoes.
- Gently brush away dry particles and blot excess liquids with absorbent material.
- Rinse patient with warm water, 32° C to 35° C (90° F to 95° F), if possible.
- Wash patient with a mild liquid soap and large quantities of water.
- Refer to decontamination protocol in Section Three.

IMMEDIATE FIRST AID

- Ensure that adequate decontamination has been carried out.
- If patient is not breathing, start artificial respiration, preferably with a demand-valve resuscitator, bag-valve-mask device, or pocket mask, as trained. Perform CPR if necessary.
- Immediately flush contaminated eyes with gently flowing water.
- Do not induce vomiting. If vomiting occurs, lean patient forward or place on left side (head-down position, if possible) to maintain an open airway and prevent aspiration.
- Keep patient quiet and maintain normal body temperature.
- Obtain medical attention.

BASIC TREATMENT

- Establish a patent airway (oropharyngeal or nasopharyngeal airway, if needed). Suction if necessary.

- Watch for signs of respiratory insufficiency and assist ventilations if necessary.
- Administer oxygen by nonrebreather mask at 10 to 15 L/min.
- Monitor for pulmonary edema and treat if necessary (refer to pulmonary edema protocol in Section Three).
- Monitor for shock and treat if necessary (refer to shock protocol in Section Three).
- Anticipate seizures and treat if necessary (refer to seizure protocol in Section Three).
- For eye contamination, flush eyes immediately with water. Irrigate each eye continuously with 0.9% saline (NS) during transport (refer to eye irrigation protocol in Section Three).
- Do not use emetics. For ingestion, rinse mouth and administer 5 ml/kg up to 200 ml of water for dilution if the patient can swallow, has a strong gag reflex, and does not drool. Administer activated charcoal (refer to ingestion protocol in Section Three and activated charcoal protocol in Section Four).
- Cover skin burns with sterile dressings after decontamination (refer to chemical burn protocol in Section Three).

ADVANCED TREATMENT

- Consider orotracheal or nasotracheal intubation for airway control in the patient who is unconscious, has severe pulmonary edema, or is in severe respiratory distress.
- Positive-pressure ventilation techniques with a bag-valve-mask device may be beneficial.
- Consider drug therapy for pulmonary edema (refer to pulmonary edema protocol in Section Three).
- Monitor cardiac rhythm and treat arrhythmias if necessary (refer to cardiac protocol in Section Three).
- Start IV administration of D_5W TKO. Use 0.9% saline (NS) or lactated Ringer's (LR) if signs of hypovolemia are present. For hypotension with signs of hypovolemia, administer fluid cautiously. Consider vasopressors if patient is hypotensive with a normal fluid volume. Watch for signs of myocardial irritability and fluid overload (refer to shock protocol in Section Three).
- Treat seizures with diazepam (Valium) or lorazepam (Ativan) (refer to diazepam and lorazepam protocols in Section Four and seizure protocol in Section Three).
- Use proparacaine hydrochloride to assist eye irrigation (refer to proparacaine hydrochloride protocol in Section Four).

INITIAL EMERGENCY DEPARTMENT CONSIDERATIONS

- Useful initial laboratory studies include complete blood count, platelet count, coagulation profile, serum electrolytes, blood urea nitrogen (BUN), creatinine, glucose, urinalysis, and baseline biochemical profile, including serum aminotransferases (ALT and AST), calcium, phosphorus, and magnesium. Determination of the anion gap may be helpful. Arterial blood gases (ABGs), chest radiograph, and electrocardiogram may be required.
- Positive end-expiratory pressure (PEEP)–assisted ventilation may be necessary in patients with acute parenchymal injury who develop pulmonary edema or acute respiratory distress syndrome.

- Products may cause acidosis; hyperventilation and sodium bicarbonate may be beneficial. Bicarbonate therapy should be guided by patient presentation, ABG determination, and serum electrolyte considerations.
- Hyperbaric oxygen therapy may be beneficial in treating hepatotoxicity.
- *N*-acetylcysteine (NAC) therapy has been suggested as a possible therapeutic agent to prevent hepatotoxicity.
- Obtain toxicological consultation as necessary.

SPECIAL CONSIDERATIONS

- Avoid epinephrine and related beta agonists (unless patient is in cardiac arrest or has reactive airways disease refractory to other treatment) because of the possible irritable condition of the myocardium. Use of these medications may lead to ventricular fibrillation.

29

Lower Alcohols (1-3 Carbons) and Related Compounds

SUBSTANCE IDENTIFICATION

Found as colorless liquids with the odor of rubbing alcohol. Used as solvents, disinfectants, and sanitizers. Chemical intermediates in the manufacturing process of cleaning and degreasing agents, rubber products, adhesives, and cosmetics. Also found in rubbing alcohol, skin lotions, and antifreeze preparations.

ROUTES OF EXPOSURE

Skin and eye contact
Inhalation
Ingestion

TARGET ORGANS

Primary
Skin
Eyes
Central nervous system
Cardiovascular system
Respiratory system
Hepatic system
Metabolism
Secondary
Gastrointestinal system
Renal system

LIFE THREAT

CNS depression leading to coma and respiratory arrest. Cardiac arrhythmias.

SIGNS AND SYMPTOMS BY SYSTEM

Cardiovascular: Cardiovascular collapse, hypotension, arrhythmias, and bradycardia.

Respiratory: Upper airway mucosa irritation, respiratory depression and arrest, and risk of aspiration pneumonia.

CNS: Headache, dizziness, drowsiness, confusion, incoordination, CNS depression, and coma. CNS depression with isopropanol may be more profound and long-lasting than that seen with ethanol.

Gastrointestinal: Nausea, vomiting (hematemesis), gastritis, diarrhea, and stomach pain.

Eye: Chemical conjunctivitis.

Skin: Contact dermatitis.

Renal: Kidney damage.

Hepatic: Liver damage.

Metabolism: Anion gap metabolic acidosis and hypoglycemia.

Other: Hypothermia may be associated with coma.

SYMPTOM ONSET FOR ACUTE EXPOSURE

Immediate
Hypoglycemia possibly delayed

CO-EXPOSURE CONCERNS

Acetone and other ketones
Aromatic hydrocarbons
Other hydrocarbon solvents
Other alcohols

THERMAL DECOMPOSITION PRODUCTS INCLUDE

Carbon dioxide
Carbon monoxide

MEDICAL CONDITIONS POSSIBLY AGGRAVATED BY EXPOSURE

Respiratory system disorders
Eye disorders
Liver disorders
Blood disorders
Skin disorders

DECONTAMINATION

- Wear positive-pressure SCBA and protective equipment specified by references such as the *North American Emergency Response Guidebook*. If special chemical protective clothing is required, consult the chemical manufacturer or specific protective clothing compatibility charts. A qualified, experienced person should make decisions regarding the type of personal protective equipment necessary.
- Delay entry until trained personnel and proper protective equipment are available.
- Remove patient from contaminated area.
- Quickly remove and isolate patient's clothing, jewelry, and shoes.
- Gently brush away dry particles and blot excess liquids with absorbent material.
- Rinse patient with warm water, 32° C to 35° C (90° F to 95° F), if possible.
- Wash patient with a mild liquid soap and large quantities of water.
- Refer to decontamination protocol in Section Three.

IMMEDIATE FIRST AID

- Ensure that adequate decontamination has been carried out.
- If patient is not breathing, start artificial respiration, preferably with a demand-valve resuscitator, bag-valve-mask device, or pocket mask, as trained. Perform CPR if necessary.
- Immediately flush contaminated eyes with gently flowing water.
- Do not induce vomiting. If vomiting occurs, lean patient forward or place on left side (head-down position, if possible) to maintain an open airway and prevent aspiration.
- Keep patient quiet and maintain normal body temperature.
- Obtain medical attention.

BASIC TREATMENT

- Establish a patent airway (oropharyngeal or nasopharyngeal airway, if needed). Suction if necessary.
- Watch for signs of respiratory insufficiency and assist ventilations if necessary.
- Administer oxygen by nonrebreather mask at 10 to 15 L/min.
- Monitor for shock and treat if necessary (refer to shock protocol in Section Three).

- For eye contamination, flush eyes immediately with water. Irrigate each eye continuously with 0.9% saline (NS) during transport (refer to eye irrigation protocol in Section Three).
- Do not use emetics. For ingestion, rinse mouth and administer 5 ml/kg up to 200 ml of water for dilution if the patient can swallow, has a strong gag reflex, and does not drool. Administer activated charcoal (refer to ingestion protocol in Section Three and activated charcoal protocol in Section Four).

ADVANCED TREATMENT

- Consider orotracheal or nasotracheal intubation for airway control in the patient who is unconscious, has severe pulmonary edema, or is in severe respiratory distress.
- Monitor cardiac rhythm and treat arrhythmias if necessary (refer to cardiac protocol in Section Three).
- Start IV administration of 0.9% saline (NS) or lactated Ringer's (LR) TKO. For hypotension with signs of hypovolemia, administer fluid cautiously. Consider vasopressors if patient is hypotensive with a normal fluid volume. Watch for signs of fluid overload (refer to shock protocol in Section Three).
- Monitor for signs of hypoglycemia (decreased LOC, tachycardia, pallor, dilated pupils, diaphoresis, and/or a reading on a dextrose strip or glucometer of less than 50 mg/dl) and administer 50% dextrose if necessary (refer to 50% dextrose protocol in Section Four).
- Use proparacaine hydrochloride to assist eye irrigation (refer to proparacaine hydrochloride protocol in Section Four).

INITIAL EMERGENCY DEPARTMENT MANAGEMENT

- Useful initial laboratory studies include complete blood count, serum electrolytes, blood urea nitrogen (BUN), creatinine, glucose, urinalysis and baseline biochemical profile, including serum aminotransferases (ALT and AST), calcium, phosphorus, and magnesium. Determination of anion and osmolar gaps may be helpful. Arterial blood gases (ABGs), chest radiograph, and electrocardiogram may be required.
- Determine methanol, ethanol, or isopropanol serum concentrations.
- Products may cause acidosis; hyperventilation and sodium bicarbonate may be beneficial. Bicarbonate therapy should be guided by patient presentation, ABG determination, and serum electrolyte considerations.
- Hemodialysis may be beneficial in cases of severe poisoning.
- Obtain toxicological consultation as necessary.

SPECIAL CONSIDERATIONS

- Refer to Guideline 31 for methanol poisoning.

Higher Alcohols (>3 Carbons) and Related Compounds

SUBSTANCE IDENTIFICATION

Found as colorless liquids, singly or in mixtures, with sweet musty odors. Used in additives, paint strippers, hydraulic fluids, emulsifiers, and emollients. Found as solvents in paints, lacquers, coatings, and resins. Chemical intermediate in the manufacture of perfumes and esters. Also used in production of ceramics, latex, textiles, and paper coatings.

ROUTES OF EXPOSURE

Skin and eye contact
Inhalation
Ingestion
Skin absorption

TARGET ORGANS

Primary
Skin
Eyes
Central nervous system
Cardiovascular system
Respiratory system
Hepatic system
Metabolism
Secondary
Gastrointestinal system
Renal system

LIFE THREAT

CNS depression, respiratory failure, and cardiac arrhythmias.

SIGNS AND SYMPTOMS BY SYSTEM

Cardiovascular: Arrhythmias and hypotension.

Respiratory: Respiratory insufficiency. Respiratory depression secondary to CNS depression. Pulmonary edema, chemical pneumonitis, and bronchitis. Irritation of respiratory tract mucosa.

CNS: Headache, dizziness, drowsiness, muscle weakness, delirium, CNS depression, coma, seizures, and neurobehavioral changes. Symptoms are more acute with the higher alcohols.

Gastrointestinal: Hemorrhage, nausea, vomiting, and diarrhea.

Eye: Chemical conjunctivitis, corneal damage, lacrimation, blurred vision, and photophobia.

Skin: Symptoms range from irritant dermatitis to partial- or full-thickness burns.

Renal: Kidney damage.

Hepatic: Liver damage.

Metabolism: Anion gap metabolic acidosis.
Other: Early symptoms may mimic ethanol intoxication. Hypoglycemia.

SYMPTOM ONSET FOR ACUTE EXPOSURE

Immediate
Pulmonary edema possibly delayed

CO-EXPOSURE CONCERNS

Acetone and other ketones
Aromatic hydrocarbons
Other hydrocarbon solvents
Other alcohols

THERMAL DECOMPOSITION PRODUCTS INCLUDE

Carbon dioxide
Carbon monoxide

MEDICAL CONDITIONS POSSIBLY AGGRAVATED BY EXPOSURE

Liver disorders
Blood disorders
Skin disorders

DECONTAMINATION

- Wear positive-pressure SCBA and protective equipment specified by references such as the *North American Emergency Response Guidebook*. If special chemical protective clothing is required, consult the chemical manufacturer or specific protective clothing compatibility charts. A qualified, experienced person should make decisions regarding the type of personal protective equipment necessary.
- Delay entry until trained personnel and proper protective equipment are available.
- Remove patient from contaminated area.
- Quickly remove and isolate patient's clothing, jewelry, and shoes.
- Gently brush away dry particles and blot excess liquids with absorbent material.
- Rinse patient with warm water, 32° C to 35° C (90° F to 95° F), if possible.
- Wash patient with a mild liquid soap and large quantities of water.
- Refer to decontamination protocol in Section Three.

IMMEDIATE FIRST AID

- Ensure that adequate decontamination has been carried out.
- If patient is not breathing, start artificial respiration, preferably with a demand-valve resuscitator, bag-valve-mask device, or pocket mask, as trained. Perform CPR if necessary.
- Immediately flush contaminated eyes with gently flowing water.
- Do not induce vomiting. If vomiting occurs, lean patient forward or place on left side (head-down position, if possible), maintain an open airway, and prevent aspiration.
- Keep patient quiet and maintain normal body temperature.
- Obtain medical attention.

BASIC TREATMENT

- Establish a patent airway (oropharyngeal or nasopharyngeal airway, if needed). Suction if necessary.
- Watch for signs of respiratory insufficiency and assist ventilations if necessary.
- Administer oxygen by nonrebreather mask at 10 to 15 L/min.
- Monitor for shock and treat if necessary (refer to shock protocol in Section Three).

- Monitor for pulmonary edema and treat if necessary (refer to pulmonary edema protocol, Section Three).
- Anticipate seizures and treat if necessary (refer to seizure protocol in Section Three).
- For eye contamination, flush eyes immediately with water. Irrigate each eye continuously with 0.9% saline (NS) during transport (refer to eye irrigation protocol in Section Three).
- Do not use emetics. For ingestion, rinse mouth and administer 5 ml/kg up to 200 ml of water for dilution if the patient can swallow, has a strong gag reflex, and does not drool. Administer activated charcoal (refer to ingestion protocol in Section Three and activated charcoal protocol in Section Four).

ADVANCED TREATMENT

- Consider orotracheal or nasotracheal intubation for airway control in the patient who is unconscious, has severe pulmonary edema, or is in severe respiratory distress.
- Positive-pressure ventilation techniques, with a bag-valve-mask device, may be beneficial.
- Consider drug therapy for pulmonary edema (refer to pulmonary edema protocol in Section Three).
- Monitor cardiac rhythm and treat arrhythmias as necessary (refer to cardiac protocol in Section Three).
- Start IV administration of D_5W TKO. Use 0.9% saline (NS) or lactated Ringer's (LR) if signs of hypovolemia are present. For hypotension with signs of hypovolemia, administer fluid cautiously. Consider vasopressors if patient is hypotensive with a normal fluid volume. Watch for signs of fluid overload (refer to shock protocol in Section Three).
- Monitor for signs of hypoglycemia (decreased LOC, tachycardia, pallor, dilated pupils, diaphoresis, and/or dextrose strip or glucometer readings below 50 mg) and administer 50% dextrose if necessary (refer to 50% dextrose protocol in Section Four).
- Treat seizures with diazepam (Valium) or lorazepam (Ativan) (refer to diazepam and lorazepam protocols in Section Four and seizure protocol in Section Three).
- Use proparacaine hydrochloride to assist eye irrigation (refer to proparacaine hydrochloride protocol in Section Three).

INITIAL EMERGENCY DEPARTMENT CONSIDERATIONS

- Useful initial laboratory studies include complete blood count, serum electrolytes, blood urea nitrogen (BUN), creatinine, glucose, urinalysis, and baseline biochemical profile, including serum aminotransferases (ALT and AST), calcium, phosphorus, and magnesium. Determination of anion and osmolar gaps may be helpful. Arterial blood gases (ABGs), chest radiograph, and electrocardiogram may be required.
- Positive end-expiratory pressure (PEEP)–assisted ventilation may be necessary in patients with acute parenchymal injury who develop pulmonary edema or acute respiratory distress syndrome.
- Products may cause acidosis; hyperventilation and sodium bicarbonate may be beneficial. Bicarbonate therapy should be guided by patient presentation, ABG determination, and serum electrolyte consideration.
- Hemodialysis may be beneficial in severe exposures.
- Obtain toxicological consultation as necessary.

31

Methyl Alcohol and Related Compounds

SUBSTANCE IDENTIFICATION

Found as a colorless liquid with a characteristic pungent odor. Used as a solvent, cleaning agent, antifreeze, denatured alcohol, and fuel. Also used in the production of formaldehyde, methyl esters, plasticizers, paints, varnishes, adhesives, inks, dyes, plastics, pharmaceuticals, and softening agents. Chemical agent used in dehydration process of natural gas.

ROUTES OF EXPOSURE

Skin and eye contact
Inhalation
Ingestion
Skin absorption

TARGET ORGANS

Primary
Skin
Eyes
Central nervous system
Gastrointestinal system
Secondary
Cardiovascular system
Respiratory system
Renal system
Metabolism

LIFE THREAT

Respiratory failure and circulatory collapse.

SIGNS AND SYMPTOMS BY SYSTEM

Cardiovascular: Mild tachycardia, occasional bradycardia, and cardiovascular collapse.

Respiratory: Rapid and shallow respirations and respiratory failure.

CNS: CNS depression to coma, headache, drowsiness, weakness, vertigo, fatigue, leg cramps, seizures, and chronic neurobehavioral symptoms. Initial symptoms may be those of inebriation.

Gastrointestinal: Nausea, vomiting, and diarrhea. Severe back and abdominal pain.

Eye: Chemical conjunctivitis, blindness secondary to metabolism of methanol to formic acid (formate) toxicity, blurred vision, dilated pupils, photophobia, nystagmus, and sensitivity to tactile pressure on globes and eye movement.

Skin: Irritant dermatitis.

Renal: Kidney damage.

Metabolism: Anion gap metabolic acidosis.

SYMPTOM ONSET FOR ACUTE EXPOSURE

Immediate
Visual impairment possibly delayed for 12 to 18 hours
Signs and symptoms of acidosis possibly delayed for 24 hours

CO-EXPOSURE CONCERNS

Hydrocarbon solvents
Carbon tetrachloride
Other alcohols
Ethylene glycol

THERMAL DECOMPOSITION PRODUCTS INCLUDE

Carbon dioxide
Carbon monoxide

MEDICAL CONDITIONS POSSIBLY AGGRAVATED BY EXPOSURE

Preexisting retinal disease
CNS disorders
Liver disorders

DECONTAMINATION

- Wear positive-pressure SCBA and protective equipment specified by references such as the *North American Emergency Response Guidebook*. If special chemical protective clothing is required, consult the chemical manufacturer or specific protective clothing compatibility charts. A qualified, experienced person should make decisions regarding the type of personal protective equipment necessary.
- Delay entry until trained personnel and proper protective equipment are available.
- Remove patient from contaminated area.
- Quickly remove and isolate patient's clothing, jewelry, and shoes.
- Gently blot excess liquids with absorbent material.
- Rinse patient with warm water, 32° C to 35° C (90° F to 95° F), if possible.
- Wash patient with a mild liquid soap and large quantities of water.
- Refer to decontamination protocol in Section Three.

IMMEDIATE FIRST AID

- Ensure that adequate decontamination has been carried out.
- If patient is not breathing, start artificial respiration, preferably with a demand-valve resuscitator, bag-valve-mask device, or pocket mask, as trained. Perform CPR as necessary.
- Immediately flush contaminated eyes with gently flowing water.
- Do not induce vomiting. If vomiting occurs, lean patient forward or place on left side (head-down position, if possible) to maintain an open airway and prevent aspiration.
- Keep patient quiet and maintain normal body temperature.
- Obtain medical attention.

BASIC TREATMENT

- Establish a patent airway (oropharyngeal or nasopharyngeal airway, if needed). Suction if necessary.
- Watch for signs of respiratory insufficiency and assist ventilations if necessary.
- Administer oxygen by nonrebreather mask at 10 to 15 L/min.
- Monitor for shock and treat if necessary (refer to shock protocol in Section Three).

- Anticipate seizures and minimize all external stimuli. Treat seizures if necessary (refer to seizure protocol in Section Three).
- For eye contamination, flush eyes immediately with water. Irrigate each eye continuously with 0.9% saline (NS) during transport (refer to eye irrigation protocol in Section Three).
- Do not use emetics. For ingestion, rinse mouth and administer 5 ml/kg up to 200 ml of water for dilution if the patient can swallow, has a strong gag reflex, and does not drool. Administer activated charcoal (refer to ingestion protocol in Section Three and activated charcoal protocol in Section Four).

ADVANCED TREATMENT

- Consider orotracheal or nasotracheal intubation for airway control in the patient who is unconscious, has severe pulmonary edema, or is in severe respiratory distress.
- Hyperventilation may be beneficial for treating acidosis.
- Start IV administration of 0.9% saline (NS) or lactated Ringer's (LR) TKO. For hypotension with signs of hypovolemia, administer fluid cautiously. Watch for signs of fluid overload (refer to shock protocol in Section Three).
- Treat seizures with diazepam (Valium) or lorazepam (Ativan) (refer to diazepam and lorazepam protocols in Section Four and seizure protocol in Section Three).
- Use proparacaine hydrochloride to assist eye irrigation (refer to proparacaine hydrochloride protocol in Section Four).

INITIAL EMERGENCY DEPARTMENT CONSIDERATIONS

- Useful initial laboratory studies include complete blood count, serum electrolytes, blood urea nitrogen (BUN), creatinine, glucose, urinalysis, and baseline biochemical profile, including serum aminotransferases (ALT and AST), calcium, phosphorus, and magnesium. Determination of anion and osmolar gaps may be helpful. Arterial blood gases (ABGs), chest radiograph, and electrocardiogram may be required.
- Determine methanol and ethanol (ethyl alcohol) blood concentrations.
- Products may cause anion gap acidosis; hyperventilation and sodium bicarbonate may be beneficial. Bicarbonate therapy should be guided by patient presentation, ABG determination, and serum electrolyte considerations.
- Ethanol and fomepizole are antagonists of methanol metabolism. Antagonist therapy is beneficial as a primary treatment measure, depending on clinical symptoms, acidosis, and methanol blood concentration. Do not delay antagonist administration in symptomatic patients pending blood methanol results. Hemodialysis is necessary for definitive treatment. Patients with blood methanol concentrations >20 mg/dl usually require treatment and hemodialysis (refer to ethanol and fomepizole protocols in Section Four).
- Obtain toxicological consultation as necessary.

SPECIAL CONSIDERATIONS

- If ethanol is co-ingested with methanol, symptoms may be delayed.
- Example of lethal synthesis: methanol is metabolized in the liver by the enzyme alcohol dehydrogenase to the toxic metabolites formic acid and formaldehyde. These agents cause the blindness and anion gap metabolic acidosis seen in methanol poisoning.

Aniline and Related Compounds

SUBSTANCE IDENTIFICATION

Found as a colorless to brown, oily liquid with a characteristic (fishy) odor. Used as an intermediate in a variety of chemical processes including production of pharmaceuticals, explosives, herbicides, and fungicides. Also found in paints, inks, polishes, dyes, and varnishes.

ROUTES OF EXPOSURE

Skin and eye contact
Inhalation
Ingestion
Skin absorption

TARGET ORGANS

Primary
Skin
Eyes
Cardiovascular system
Blood
Secondary
Central nervous system
Respiratory system
Gastrointestinal system
Hepatic system
Renal system

LIFE THREAT

Causes methemoglobinemia (i.e., state of relative hypoxia resulting from inability of the red blood cells to carry oxygen). Condition is additive with carbon monoxide, simple asphyxiants, or other cellular metabolic poisons (oxygen "excluder").

SIGNS AND SYMPTOMS BY SYSTEM

Cardiovascular: Cardiovascular collapse, hypotension, ventricular arrhythmias, and heart block.
Respiratory: Dyspnea and irritation of the respiratory tract.
CNS: CNS depression and coma. Headache, ataxia, vertigo, confusion, lethargy, disorientation, and tinnitus. Seizures are rare.
Gastrointestinal: Corrosive to the GI tract, causing gastritis and hemorrhage.
Eye: Chemical conjunctivitis and corneal damage.
Skin: Severe, bluish-gray to black cyanosis secondary to methemoglobinemia.
Renal: Kidney damage.
Hepatic: Liver damage.
Blood: Methemoglobinemia and Heinz body hemolytic anemia.

Other: The fetus may be at high risk from methemoglobinemia and resultant hypoxia. Some products may present a human mutagenic risk.

SYMPTOM ONSET FOR ACUTE EXPOSURE

Immediate

Symptoms of methemoglobinemia possibly delayed up to 4 hours (particularly when skin exposure has occurred)

CO-EXPOSURE CONCERNS

Trauma

Simple asphyxiants

Carbon monoxide

Cellular metabolic poisons

THERMAL DECOMPOSITION PRODUCTS INCLUDE

Ammonia

Carbon dioxide

Carbon monoxide

Nitrogen oxides

Sulfur dioxide

MEDICAL CONDITIONS POSSIBLY AGGRAVATED BY EXPOSURE

Central nervous system disorders

Cardiovascular disorders

Liver disorders

Kidney disorders

Bone marrow diseases

DECONTAMINATION

- Wear positive-pressure SCBA and protective equipment specified by references such as the *North American Emergency Response Guidebook*. If special chemical protective clothing is required, consult the chemical manufacturer or specific protective clothing compatibility charts. A qualified, experienced person should make decisions regarding the type of personal protective equipment necessary.
- Delay entry until trained personnel and proper protective equipment are available.
- Remove patient from contaminated area.
- Quickly remove and isolate patient's clothing, jewelry, and shoes.
- Gently blot excess liquids with absorbent material.
- Rinse patient with warm water, 32° C to 35° C (90° F to 95° F), if possible.
- Wash patient with a mild liquid soap and large quantities of water.
- Refer to decontamination protocol in Section Three.

IMMEDIATE FIRST AID

- Ensure that adequate decontamination has been carried out.
- If patient is not breathing, start artificial respiration, preferably with a demand-valve resuscitator, bag-valve-mask device, or pocket mask, as trained. Perform CPR if necessary.
- Immediately flush contaminated eyes with gently flowing water.
- Do not induce vomiting. If vomiting occurs, lean patient forward or place on left side (head-down position, if possible) to maintain an open airway and prevent aspiration.
- Keep patient quiet and maintain normal body temperature.
- Obtain medical attention.

BASIC TREATMENT

- Establish a patent airway (oropharyngeal or nasopharyngeal airway, if needed). Suction if necessary.
- Watch for signs of respiratory insufficiency and assist ventilations if necessary.
- Administer oxygen by nonrebreather mask at 10 to 15 L/min.
- Monitor for shock and treat if necessary (refer to shock protocol in Section Three).
- Anticipate seizures and treat if necessary (refer to seizure protocol in Section Three).
- For eye contamination, flush eyes immediately with water. Irrigate each eye continuously with 0.9% saline (NS) during transport (refer to eye irrigation protocol in Section Three).
- Do not use emetics. For ingestion, rinse mouth and administer 5 ml/kg up to 200 ml of water for dilution if the patent can swallow, has a strong gag reflex, and does not drool. Administer activated charcoal (refer to ingestion protocol in Section Three and activated charcoal protocol in Section Four).

ADVANCED TREATMENT

- Consider orotracheal or nasotracheal intubation for airway control in the patient who is unconscious or is in severe respiratory distress.
- Monitor cardiac rhythm and treat arrhythmias as necessary (refer to cardiac protocol in Section Three).
- Start IV administration of D_5W TKO. Use 0.9% saline (NS) or lactated Ringer's (LR) if signs of hypovolemia are present. For hypotension with signs of hypovolemia, administer fluid cautiously. Consider vasopressors if patient is hypotensive with a normal fluid volume. Watch for signs of fluid overload (refer to shock protocol in Section Three).
- Administer 1% solution methylene blue if patient is symptomatic with severe hypoxia, cyanosis, and cardiac compromise not responding to oxygen. DIRECT PHYSICIAN ORDER ONLY (refer to methylene blue protocol in Section Four).
- Treat seizures with diazepam (Valium) or lorazepam (Ativan) (refer to diazepam and lorazepam protocols in Section Four and seizure protocol in Section Three).
- Use proparacaine hydrochloride to assist eye irrigation (refer to proparacaine hydrochloride protocol in Section Four).

INITIAL EMERGENCY DEPARTMENT CONSIDERATIONS

- Useful initial laboratory studies include complete blood count, serum electrolytes, blood urea nitrogen (BUN), creatinine, glucose, urinalysis, and baseline biochemical profile, including serum aminotransferases (ALT and AST), calcium, phosphorus, and magnesium. Arterial blood gases (ABGs), chest radiograph, and electrocardiogram may be required.
- Monitor blood methemoglobin levels and treat with methylene blue if patient is symptomatic and/or has a blood methemoglobin level greater than 30%. DIRECT PHYSICIAN ORDER ONLY (refer to methylene blue protocol in Section Four).
- Hyperbaric oxygen may be beneficial in severe exposures as an adjunct to methylene blue treatment as necessary.
- Obtain toxicological consultation if necessary.

SPECIAL CONSIDERATIONS

Pulse oximetry readings may not be accurate in these exposures.

33 Aliphatic Hydrocarbons and Related Compounds

SUBSTANCE IDENTIFICATION

Colorless liquids or gases with fruitlike or etherlike odor. Some gases are odorless, and an odorant is occasionally added. Used as fuels, solvents, anesthetics, refrigerants, and in the manufacturing process of many products.

ROUTES OF EXPOSURE

Skin and eye contact
Inhalation
Ingestion
Skin absorption

TARGET ORGANS

Primary
Skin
Eyes
Central nervous system
Respiratory system
Secondary
Cardiovascular system
Gastrointestinal system
Hepatic system
Renal system

LIFE THREAT

Cardiac arrhythmias. Asphyxiation or anesthetic properties at high concentrations.

SIGNS AND SYMPTOMS BY SYSTEM

Cardiovascular: Cardiovascular collapse and arrhythmias. May aggravate preexisting cardiac problem.

Respiratory: Narcotic-like effect may depress respirations. Irritation of the respiratory tract and mucous membranes, chemical pneumonitis, and/or pulmonary edema. Low-molecular aliphatic chains (methane through butane) may act as simple asphyxiants.

CNS: Excitation, headache, disorientation, dizziness, incoordination, weakness, muscle spasms, paresthesias, seizures, CNS depression and coma due to anesthetic effect or hypoxia, and neurobehavioral changes.

Gastrointestinal: Nausea, excessive salivation, vomiting, and abdominal cramps.

Eye: Irritation, lacrimation, and blurred vision.

Skin: Mild skin irritation, dermatitis, and frostbite.

Renal: Kidney damage and hematuria.

Hepatic: Liver damage.

SYMPTOM ONSET FOR ACUTE EXPOSURE

Immediate
Pulmonary edema possibly delayed

CO-EXPOSURE CONCERNS

Other hydrocarbons
Sympathomimetic agents

THERMAL DECOMPOSITION PRODUCTS INCLUDE

Carbon dioxide
Carbon monoxide

MEDICAL CONDITIONS POSSIBLY AGGRAVATED BY EXPOSURE

Central nervous system disorders
Cardiovascular disorders
Liver disorders
Kidney disorders

DECONTAMINATION

- Wear positive-pressure SCBA and protective equipment specified by references such as the *North American Emergency Response Guidebook*. If special chemical protective clothing is required, consult the chemical manufacturer or specific protective clothing compatibility charts. A qualified, experienced person should make decisions regarding the type of personal protective equipment necessary.
- Delay entry until trained personnel and proper protective equipment are available.
- Remove patient from contaminated area.
- Quickly remove and isolate patient's clothing, jewelry, and shoes.
- Gently blot any excess liquids with absorbent material.
- Rinse patient with warm water, 32° C to 35° C (90° F to 95° F), if possible.
- Wash patient with a mild liquid soap and large quantities of water.
- Refer to decontamination protocol in Section Three.

IMMEDIATE FIRST AID

- Ensure that adequate decontamination has been carried out.
- If patient is not breathing, start artificial respiration, preferably with a demand-valve resuscitator, bag-valve-mask device, or pocket mask, as trained. Perform CPR if necessary.
- Immediately flush contaminated eyes with gently flowing water.
- Do not induce vomiting. If vomiting occurs, lean patient forward or place on left side (head-down position, if possible) o maintain an open airway and prevent aspiration.
- Keep patient quiet and maintain normal body temperature.
- Obtain medical attention.

BASIC TREATMENT

- Establish a patent airway (oropharyngeal or nasopharyngeal airway, if needed). Suction if necessary.
- Watch for signs of respiratory insufficiency and assist ventilations if necessary.
- Administer oxygen by nonrebreather mask at 10 to 15 L/min.
- Monitor for pulmonary edema and treat if necessary (refer to pulmonary edema protocol in Section Three).
- Anticipate seizures and treat as necessary (refer to seizure protocol in Section Three).
- For eye contamination, flush eyes immediately with water. Irrigate each eye continuously with 0.9% saline (NS) during transport (refer to eye irrigation protocol in Section Three).

- Do not use emetics. For ingestion, rinse mouth and administer 5 ml/kg up to 200 ml of water for dilution if the patient can swallow, has a strong gag reflex, and does not drool. Administer activated charcoal (refer to ingestion protocol in Section Three and activated charcoal protocol in Section Four).
- Treat frostbite with rapid rewarming techniques (refer to frostbite protocol in Section Three).

ADVANCED TREATMENT

- Consider orotracheal or nasotracheal intubation for airway control in the patient who is unconscious, has severe pulmonary edema, or is in severe respiratory distress.
- Positive-pressure ventilation techniques with a bag-valve-mask device may be beneficial.
- Consider drug therapy for pulmonary edema (refer to pulmonary edema protocol in Section Three).
- Monitor cardiac rhythm and treat arrhythmias as necessary (refer to cardiac protocol in Section Three).
- Start IV administration of D_5W TKO. Use 0.9% saline (NS) or lactated Ringer's (LR) if signs of hypovolemia are present. For hypotension with signs of hypovolemia, administer fluid cautiously. Watch for signs of fluid overload (refer to shock protocol in Section Three).
- Treat seizures with diazepam (Valium) or lorazepam (Ativan) (refer to diazepam and lorazepam protocols in Section Four and seizure protocol in Section Three).
- Use proparacaine hydrochloride to assist eye irrigation (refer to proparacaine hydrochloride protocol in Section Four).

INITIAL EMERGENCY DEPARTMENT CONSIDERATIONS

- Useful initial laboratory studies include complete blood count, serum electrolytes, blood urea nitrogen (BUN), creatinine, glucose, urinalysis, and baseline biochemical profile, including serum aminotransferases (ALT and AST), calcium, phosphorus, and magnesium. Arterial blood gases (ABGs), chest radiograph, and electrocardiogram may be required.
- Positive end-expiratory pressure (PEEP)–assisted ventilation may be necessary in patients with acute parenchymal injury who develop pulmonary edema or acute respiratory distress syndrome.
- Obtain toxicological consultation as necessary.

SPECIAL CONSIDERATIONS

- Avoid epinephrine and related beta agonists (unless patient is in cardiac arrest or has reactive airways disease refractory to other treatment) because of the possible irritable condition of the myocardium. Use of these medications may lead to ventricular fibrillation.

Turpentine, Terpenes, and Related Compounds

SUBSTANCE IDENTIFICATION

Found as a colorless liquid with an unpleasant odor. Used as a solvent and in the manufacture of insecticides, polishes, cleaners, inks, putty, cutting fluids, and paint thinners.

ROUTES OF EXPOSURE

Skin and eye contact
Inhalation
Ingestion
Skin absorption

TARGET ORGANS

Primary
Skin
Eyes
Central nervous system
Cardiovascular system
Respiratory system
Secondary
Gastrointestinal system
Renal system

LIFE THREAT

Respiratory failure, pulmonary edema, and tachycardia.

SIGNS AND SYMPTOMS BY SYSTEM

Cardiovascular: Tachycardia and arrhythmias.

Respiratory: Respiratory tract irritant that can cause coughing, choking, and dyspnea. Aspiration pneumonia and pulmonary edema possible from direct pulmonary effect or absorption after systemic poisoning.

CNS: Headache, confusion, excitement, hyperreflexia, and ataxia, followed by decreased level of consciousness and coma. Seizures.

Gastrointestinal: Mucous membrane irritation with burning pain, nausea, vomiting, diarrhea, and abdominal pain.

Eye: Chemical conjunctivitis and corneal burns.

Skin: Irritant dermatitis and cyanosis (if respiratory complications are present).

Renal: Kidney damage.

SYMPTOM ONSET FOR ACUTE EXPOSURE

Immediate
Pulmonary edema symptoms possibly delayed

CO-EXPOSURE CONCERNS

Other hydrocarbon solvents

THERMAL DECOMPOSITION PRODUCTS INCLUDE

Acrid fumes and irritating smoke
Carbon dioxide
Carbon monoxide

MEDICAL CONDITIONS POSSIBLY AGGRAVATED BY EXPOSURE

Respiratory system disorders
Skin disorders

DECONTAMINATION

- Wear positive-pressure SCBA and protective equipment specified by references such as the *North American Emergency Response Guidebook*. If special chemical protective clothing is required, consult the chemical manufacturer or specific protective clothing compatibility charts. A qualified, experienced person should make decisions regarding the type of personal protective equipment necessary.
- Delay entry until trained personnel and proper protective equipment are available.
- Remove patient from contaminated area.
- Quickly remove and isolate patient's clothing, jewelry, and shoes.
- Gently blot excess liquids with absorbent material.
- Rinse patient with warm water, 32° C to 35° C (90° F to 95° F), if possible.
- Wash patient with a mild liquid soap and large quantities of water.
- Refer to decontamination protocol in Section Three.

IMMEDIATE FIRST AID

- Ensure that adequate decontamination has been carried out.
- If patient is not breathing, start artificial respiration, preferably with a demand-valve resuscitator, bag-valve-mask device, or pocket mask, as trained. Perform CPR if necessary.
- Immediately flush contaminated eyes with gently flowing water.
- Do not induce vomiting. If vomiting occurs, lean patient forward or place on left side (head-down position, if possible) to maintain an open airway and prevent aspiration.
- Keep patient quiet and maintain normal body temperature.
- Obtain medical attention.

BASIC TREATMENT

- Establish a patent airway (oropharyngeal or nasopharyngeal airway, if needed). Suction if necessary.
- Watch for signs of respiratory insufficiency and assist ventilations if necessary.
- Administer oxygen by nonrebreather mask at 10 to 15 L/min.
- Monitor for pulmonary edema and treat if necessary (refer to pulmonary edema protocol in Section Three).
- Anticipate seizures and treat if necessary (refer to seizure protocol in Section Three).
- For eye contamination, flush eyes immediately with water. Irrigate each eye continuously with 0.9% saline (NS) during transport (refer to eye irrigation protocol in Section Three).
- Do not use emetics. For ingestion, rinse mouth and administer 5 ml/kg up to 200 ml of water for dilution if the patient can swallow, has a strong gag reflex, and does not drool (refer to ingestion protocol in Section Three).

ADVANCED TREATMENT

- Consider orotracheal or nasotracheal intubation for airway control in the patient who is unconscious, has severe pulmonary edema, or is in severe respiratory distress.
- Positive-pressure ventilation techniques with a bag-valve-mask device may be beneficial.
- Consider drug therapy for pulmonary edema (refer to pulmonary edema protocol in Section Three).
- Monitor cardiac rhythm and treat arrhythmias if necessary (refer to cardiac protocol in Section Three).
- Start IV administration of D_5W TKO. Use 0.9% saline (NS) or lactated Ringer's (LR) if signs of hypovolemia are present. For hypotension with signs of hypovolemia, administer fluid cautiously. Watch for signs of fluid overload (refer to shock protocol in Section Three).
- Treat seizures with diazepam (Valium) or lorazepam (Ativan) (refer to diazepam and lorazepam protocols in Section Four and seizure protocol in Section Three).
- Use proparacaine hydrochloride to assist eye irrigation (refer to proparacaine hydrochloride protocol in Section Four).

INITIAL EMERGENCY DEPARTMENT CONSIDERATIONS

- Useful initial laboratory studies include complete blood count, serum electrolytes, blood urea nitrogen (BUN), creatinine, glucose, urinalysis, and baseline biochemical profile including serum aminotransferases (ALT and AST), calcium, phosphorus, and magnesium. Arterial blood gases (ABGs), chest radiograph, and electrocardiogram may be required.
- Positive end-expiratory pressure (PEEP)–assisted ventilation may be necessary in patients with acute parenchymal injury who develop pulmonary edema or acute respiratory distress syndrome.
- Obtain toxicological consultation as necessary.

SPECIAL CONSIDERATIONS

- Avoid epinephrine and related beta agonists (unless patient is in cardiac arrest or has reactive airways disease refractory to other treatment) because of the possible irritable condition of the myocardium. Use of these medications may lead to ventricular fibrillation.

35

Hydrocarbon Blends, Mixtures, and Related Compounds

SUBSTANCE IDENTIFICATION

Liquid hydrocarbons that are colorless or pale yellow, with a gasoline-type odor. Used as cleaners and degreasers; fuels; solvents; vehicle for paints, thinners, enamels, and varnishes; and aerosol propellants. Components of various manufacturing processes.

ROUTES OF EXPOSURE

Skin and eye contact
Inhalation
Ingestion
Skin absorption

TARGET ORGANS

Primary
Skin
Eyes
Central nervous system
Cardiovascular system
Hepatic system
Secondary
Respiratory system
Gastrointestinal system
Renal system

LIFE THREAT

CNS depression may lead to respiratory arrest. Seizures, cardiac arrhythmias, and pulmonary edema.

SIGNS AND SYMPTOMS BY SYSTEM

Cardiovascular: Cardiac arrhythmias, tachycardia, hypotension, shock, and cardiovascular collapse.

Respiratory: Upper respiratory tract irritation and a burning sensation in the chest, dyspnea, tachypnea, and rales, which may progress rapidly to massive pulmonary edema.

CNS: Confusion, tinnitus, disorientation, headache, drowsiness, weakness, CNS depression, coma, and seizures.

Gastrointestinal: Pain and irritation of the GI mucous membranes; nausea, vomiting, and diarrhea.

Eye: Chemical conjunctivitis.

Skin: Minor erythema to irritant dermatitis. Cyanosis of the extremities in hypoperfusion states.

Renal: Kidney failure.
Hepatic: Liver injury.

SYMPTOM ONSET FOR ACUTE EXPOSURE

Immediate
Pulmonary edema symptoms possibly delayed

CO-EXPOSURE CONCERNS

Chlorinated hydrocarbons
Other hydrocarbon products

THERMAL DECOMPOSITION PRODUCTS INCLUDE

Carbon dioxide
Carbon monoxide

MEDICAL CONDITIONS POSSIBLY AGGRAVATED BY EXPOSURE

Respiratory system disorders
Cardiovascular disorders

DECONTAMINATION

- Wear positive-pressure SCBA and protective equipment specified by references such as the *North American Emergency Response Guidebook*. If special chemical protective clothing is required, consult the chemical manufacturer or specific protective clothing compatibility charts. A qualified, experienced person should make decisions regarding the type of personal protective equipment necessary.
- Delay entry until trained personnel and proper protective equipment are available.
- Remove patient from contaminated area.
- Quickly remove and isolate patient's clothing, jewelry, and shoes.
- Gently blot excess liquids with absorbent material.
- Rinse patient with warm water, 32° C to 35° C (90° F to 95° F), if possible.
- Wash patient with a mild liquid soap and large quantities of water.
- Refer to decontamination protocol in Section Three.

IMMEDIATE FIRST AID

- Ensure that adequate decontamination has been carried out.
- If patient is not breathing, start artificial respiration, preferably with a demand-valve resuscitator, bag-valve-mask device, or pocket mask, as trained. Perform CPR if necessary.
- Immediately flush contaminated eyes with gently flowing water.
- Do not induce vomiting. If vomiting occurs, lean patient forward or place on left side (head-down position, if possible) to maintain an open airway and prevent aspiration.
- Keep patient quiet and maintain normal body temperature.
- Obtain medical attention.

BASIC TREATMENT

- Establish a patent airway (oropharyngeal or nasopharyngeal airway, if needed). Suction if necessary.
- Watch for signs of respiratory insufficiency and assist ventilations if necessary.
- Administer oxygen by nonrebreather mask at 10 to 15 L/min.
- Monitor for pulmonary edema and treat if necessary (refer to pulmonary edema protocol in Section Three).
- Anticipate seizures and treat if necessary (refer to seizure protocol in Section Three).

- For eye contamination, flush eyes immediately with water. Irrigate each eye continuously with 0.9% saline (NS) during transport (refer to eye irrigation protocol in Section Three).
- Do not use emetics. For ingestion, rinse mouth and administer 5 m/kg up to 200 ml of water for dilution if the patient can swallow, has a strong gag reflex, and does not drool (refer to ingestion protocol in Section Three).

ADVANCED TREATMENT

- Consider orotracheal or nasotracheal intubation for airway control in the patient who is unconscious, has severe pulmonary edema, or is in respiratory distress.
- Positive-pressure ventilation techniques with a bag-valve-mask device may be beneficial.
- Consider drug therapy for pulmonary edema (refer to pulmonary edema protocol in Section Three).
- Monitor cardiac rhythm and treat arrhythmias as necessary (refer to cardiac protocol in Section Three).
- Start IV administration of D_5W TKO. Use 0.9% saline (NS) or lactated Ringer's (LR) if signs of hypovolemia are present. For hypotension with signs of hypovolemia, administer fluid cautiously. Watch for signs of pulmonary edema (refer to shock protocol in Section Three).
- Treat seizures with diazepam (Valium) or lorazepam (Ativan) (refer to diazepam and lorazepam protocols in Section Four and seizure protocol in Section Three).
- Use proparacaine hydrochloride to assist eye irrigation (refer to proparacaine hydrochloride protocol in Section Four).

INITIAL EMERGENCY DEPARTMENT CONSIDERATIONS

- Useful initial laboratory studies include complete blood count, serum electrolytes, blood urea nitrogen (BUN), creatinine, glucose, urinalysis, and baseline biochemical profile, including serum aminotransferases (ALT and AST), calcium, phosphorus, and magnesium. Arterial blood gases (ABGs), chest radiograph, and electrocardiogram may be required.
- Positive end-expiratory pressure (PEEP)–assisted ventilation may be necessary in patients with acute parenchymal injury who develop pulmonary edema or acute respiratory distress syndrome.
- Obtain toxicological consultation as necessary.

SPECIAL CONSIDERATIONS

- Avoid epinephrine and related beta agonists (unless patient is in cardiac arrest or has reactive airways disease refractory to other treatment) because of the possible irritable condition of the myocardium. Use of these medications may lead to ventricular fibrillation.

Camphor and Related Compounds

SUBSTANCE IDENTIFICATION

Found in solid and liquid form. Extracted from the wood of the *Cinnamomum camphora* tree or synthesized from turpentine oil. Solids are usually a colorless, glassy, or white color with a penetrating, characteristic odor. Liquids usually have an oily consistency with a colorless to brown color. Products are commonly used in the manufacture of film, explosives, disinfectants, lacquers, and varnishes. Also used as moth and insect repellents and found in a variety of over-the-counter medicinal preparations.

ROUTES OF EXPOSURE

Skin and eye contact
Inhalation
Ingestion
Skin absorption

TARGET ORGANS

Primary
Skin
Eyes
Central nervous system
Respiratory system
Secondary
Cardiovascular system
Gastrointestinal system
Hepatic system
Metabolism

LIFE THREAT

Status epilepticus and respiratory failure.

SIGNS AND SYMPTOMS BY SYSTEM

Cardiovascular: Cardiovascular collapse, hypotension, arrhythmias, and asystole.

Respiratory: Feeling of coolness in respiratory tract and sore throat. Periods of apnea may follow seizures.

CNS: Headache, dizziness, confusion, irrational behavior, and excitement, coma, seizures, possibly becoming status epilepticus, and generalized CNS depression.

Gastrointestinal: Nausea, vomiting, diarrhea, and abdominal pain. Vomiting is sometimes projectile in nature. With ingestion a warm feeling is present in the stomach and breath will smell strongly of camphor.

Eye: Chemical conjunctivitis and pupillary dilation.

Skin: Paleness with cyanosis.

Hepatic: Liver damage.

Metabolism: Fever.

SYMPTOM ONSET FOR ACUTE EXPOSURE

Immediate

Some symptoms possibly minimally delayed

THERMAL DECOMPOSITION PRODUCTS INCLUDE

Carbon dioxide

Carbon monoxide

MEDICAL CONDITIONS POSSIBLY AGGRAVATED BY EXPOSURE

Cardiovascular disorders

Seizure disorders

Kidney disorders

Liver disorders

DECONTAMINATION

- Wear positive-pressure SCBA and protective equipment specified by references such as the *North American Emergency Response Guidebook*. If special chemical protective clothing is required, consult the chemical manufacturer or specific protective clothing compatibility charts. A qualified, experienced person should make decisions regarding the type of personal protective equipment necessary.
- Delay entry until trained personnel and proper protective equipment are available.
- Remove patient from contaminated area.
- Quickly remove and isolate patient's clothing, jewelry, and shoes.
- Gently brush away dry particles and blot excess liquids with absorbent material.
- Rinse patient with warm water, 32° C to 35° C (90° F to 95° F), if possible.
- Wash patient with a mild liquid soap and large quantities of water.
- Refer to decontamination protocol in Section Three.

IMMEDIATE FIRST AID

- Ensure that adequate decontamination has been carried out.
- If patient is not breathing, start artificial respiration, preferably with a demand-valve resuscitator, bag-valve-mask device, or pocket mask, as trained. Perform CPR as necessary.
- Immediately flush contaminated eyes with gently flowing water.
- Do not induce vomiting. If vomiting occurs, lean patient forward or place on left side (head-down position, if possible) to maintain an open airway and prevent aspiration.
- Keep patient quiet and maintain normal body temperature.
- Obtain medical attention.

BASIC TREATMENT

- Establish a patent airway (oropharyngeal or nasopharyngeal airway, if needed). Suction if necessary.
- Watch for signs of respiratory insufficiency and assist ventilations if necessary.
- Administer oxygen by nonrebreather mask at 10 to 15 L/min.
- Anticipate seizures and minimize all external stimuli. Treat seizures as necessary (refer to seizure protocol in Section Three).
- Monitor for shock and treat as necessary (refer to shock protocol in Section Three).
- For eye contamination, flush eyes immediately with water. Irrigate each eye continuously with 0.9% saline (NS) during transport (refer to eye irrigation protocol in Section Three).

- Do not use emetics. For ingestion, rinse mouth and administer 5 ml/kg up to 200 ml of water for dilution if the patient can swallow, has a strong gag reflex, and does not drool. Administer activated charcoal (refer to ingestion protocol in Section Three and activated charcoal protocol in Section Four).

ADVANCED TREATMENT

- Consider orotracheal or nasotracheal intubation for airway control in the patient who is unconscious or is in respiratory distress.
- Monitor and treat cardiac arrhythmias as necessary (refer to cardiac protocol in Section Three).
- Start IV administration of D_5W TKO. Use 0.9% saline (NS) or lactated Ringer's (LR) if signs of hypovolemia are present. For hypotension with signs of hypovolemia, administer fluid cautiously. Consider vasopressors if patient is hypotensive with a normal fluid volume. Watch for signs of fluid overload (refer to shock protocol in Section Three).
- Treat seizures with diazepam (Valium) or lorazepam (Ativan) (refer to diazepam and lorazepam protocols in Section Four and seizure protocol in Section Three).
- Use proparacaine hydrochloride to assist eye irrigation (refer to proparacaine hydrochloride protocol in Section Four).

INITIAL EMERGENCY DEPARTMENT CONSIDERATIONS

- Useful initial laboratory studies include complete blood count, serum electrolytes, blood urea nitrogen (BUN), creatinine, glucose, urinalysis, and baseline biochemical profile including serum aminotransferases (ALT and AST), calcium, phosphorus, and magnesium. Determination of anion and osmolar gaps may be helpful. Arterial blood gases (ABGs), chest radiograph, and electrocardiogram may be required.
- Observe for seizure activity.
- Obtain toxicological consultation as necessary.

SPECIAL CONSIDERATIONS

- Chronic ingestion in children may mimic Reye's syndrome with hepatic and neurological toxicity.

37

Esters and Related Compounds

SUBSTANCE IDENTIFICATION

Clear, colorless liquids with a fruity odor. Used as solvents, flavoring agents, fragrance additives, and chemical intermediates in the manufacture of pharmaceuticals and many other products. Produced by the reaction of an alcohol or phenol with organic acids.

ROUTES OF EXPOSURE

Skin and eye contact
Inhalation
Ingestion
Skin absorption

TARGET ORGANS

Primary
Skin
Eyes
Central nervous system
Cardiovascular system
Respiratory system
Secondary
Hepatic system

LIFE THREAT

CNS depression, respiratory tract irritation, bronchitis, and pneumonitis.

SIGNS AND SYMPTOMS BY SYSTEM

Cardiovascular: Cardiovascular collapse, hypotension, and ventricular arrhythmias.

Respiratory: Mucous membrane irritation, dyspnea, and tachypnea, pharyngitis, bronchitis, pneumonitis, and pulmonary edema in massive exposures.

CNS: Headache, drowsiness, dizziness, CNS depression, coma, neurobehavioral changes.

Gastrointestinal: Nausea, vomiting, diarrhea, and abdominal cramps.

Eye: Chemical conjunctivitis, lacrimation, and corneal damage.

Skin: Erythema, irritant dermatitis, or allergic dermatitis.

Hepatic: Liver damage.

Other: Some products are rapidly broken down to ethanol and acetic acid in the body.

SYMPTOM ONSET FOR ACUTE EXPOSURE

Immediate
Pulmonary edema symptoms possibly delayed

CO-EXPOSURE CONCERNS

Other petroleum products

THERMAL DECOMPOSITION PRODUCTS INCLUDE

Carbon dioxide
Carbon monoxide

MEDICAL CONDITIONS POSSIBLY AGGRAVATED BY EXPOSURE

Respiratory disorders
Skin disorders

DECONTAMINATION

- Wear positive-pressure SCBA and protective equipment specified by references such as the *North American Emergency Response Guidebook.* If special chemical protective clothing is required, consult the chemical manufacturer or specific protective clothing compatibility charts. A qualified, experienced person should make decisions regarding the type of personal protective equipment necessary.
- Delay entry until trained personnel and proper protective equipment are available.
- Remove patient from contaminated area.
- Quickly remove and isolate patient's clothing, jewelry, and shoes.
- Gently blot excess liquids with absorbent material.
- Rinse patient with warm water, 32° C to 35° C (90° F to 95° F), if possible.
- Wash patient with a mild liquid soap and large quantities of water.
- Refer to decontamination protocol in Section Three.

IMMEDIATE FIRST AID

- Ensure that adequate decontamination has been carried out.
- If patient is not breathing, start artificial respiration, preferably with a demand-valve resuscitator, bag-valve-mask device, or pocket mask, as trained. Perform CPR as necessary.
- Immediately flush contaminated eyes with gently flowing water.
- Do not induce vomiting. If vomiting occurs, lean patient forward or place on left side (head-down position, if possible) to maintain an open airway and prevent aspiration.
- Keep patient quiet and maintain normal body temperature.
- Obtain medical attention.

BASIC TREATMENT

- Establish a patent airway (oropharyngeal or nasopharyngeal airway, if needed). Suction if necessary.
- Watch for signs of respiratory insufficiency and assist ventilations if necessary.
- Administer oxygen by nonrebreather mask at 10 to 15 L/min.
- Monitor for pulmonary edema and treat if necessary (refer to pulmonary edema protocol in Section Three).
- Monitor for shock and treat if necessary (refer to shock protocol in Section Three).
- For eye contamination, flush eyes immediately with water. Irrigate each eye continuously with 0.9% saline (NS) during transport (refer to eye irrigation protocol in Section Three).
- Do not use emetics. For ingestion, rinse mouth and administer 5 ml/kg up to 200 ml of water for dilution if the patient can swallow, has a strong gag reflex, and does not drool. Administer activated charcoal (refer to ingestion protocol in Section Three and activated charcoal protocol in Section Four).

ADVANCED TREATMENT

- Consider orotracheal or nasotracheal intubation for airway control in the patient who is unconscious, has severe pulmonary edema, or is in severe respiratory distress.
- Positive-pressure ventilation techniques with a bag-valve-mask device may be beneficial.
- Consider drug therapy for pulmonary edema (refer to pulmonary edema protocol in Section Three).
- Monitor cardiac rhythm and treat arrhythmias if necessary (refer to cardiac protocol in Section Three).
- Start IV administration of D_5W TKO. Use 0.9% saline (NS) or lactated Ringer's (LR) if signs of hypovolemia are present. For hypotension with signs of hypovolemia, administer fluid cautiously. Consider vasopressors if patient is hypotensive with a normal fluid volume. Watch for signs of fluid overload (refer to shock protocol in Section Three).
- Use proparacaine hydrochloride to assist eye irrigation (refer to proparacaine hydrochloride protocol in Section Four).

INITIAL EMERGENCY DEPARTMENT CONSIDERATIONS

- Useful initial laboratory studies include complete blood count, serum electrolytes, blood urea nitrogen (BUN), creatinine, glucose, urinalysis, and baseline biochemical profile including serum aminotransferases (ALT and AST), calcium, phosphorus, and magnesium. Arterial blood gases (ABGs), chest radiograph, and electrocardiogram may be required.
- Positive end-expiratory pressure (PEEP)–assisted ventilation may be necessary in patients with acute parenchymal injury who develop pulmonary edema or acute respiratory distress syndrome.
- Obtain toxicological consultation as necessary.

Ethers and Related Compounds

SUBSTANCE IDENTIFICATION

Colorless liquids or colorless, highly flammable gases with a sweet odor. Used as solvents for fats, oils, perfumes, alkaloids, and gums. Also found as starter fluid for gasoline and diesel engines, as additives, and as anesthetics. Used in a variety of manufacturing processes, including plastics and dyes.

ROUTES OF EXPOSURE

Skin and eye contact
Inhalation
Ingestion

TARGET ORGANS

Primary
Skin
Eyes
Central nervous system
Cardiovascular system
Respiratory system
Blood
Secondary
Gastrointestinal system
Renal system
Hepatic system
Metabolism

LIFE THREAT

Predominant narcotic properties leading to anesthesia and respiratory arrest.

SIGNS AND SYMPTOMS BY SYSTEM

Cardiovascular: Hypotension, bradycardia, and cardiovascular collapse.

Respiratory: Respiratory tract irritation, cough, laryngeal spasms, irregular respirations, depression, pulmonary edema, and respiratory arrest.

CNS: Depression or excitation, headache, dizziness, weakness, seizures, and possible coma.

Gastrointestinal: Nausea, vomiting, and salivation.

Eye: Chemical conjunctivitis and possible corneal damage with blurred vision.

Skin: Mild skin irritation and irritant dermatitis. Expanding gases may cause frostbite.

Renal: Kidney damage and interstitial cystitis.

Hepatic: Increased chance of liver damage when patient has preexisting liver disease.

Metabolism: Hyperglycemia and anion-gap metabolic acidosis.

Blood: Bone marrow toxicity. Certain products may easily cross the placental membrane.

SYMPTOM ONSET FOR ACUTE EXPOSURE
Immediate
Acidosis possibly delayed
Central nervous system depression possibly delayed

CO-EXPOSURE CONCERNS
Hydrocarbon solvents
Glycol ethers

THERMAL DECOMPOSITION PRODUCTS INCLUDE
Carbon dioxide
Carbon monoxide
Peroxides may form on contact with air

MEDICAL CONDITIONS POSSIBLY AGGRAVATED BY EXPOSURE
Dermatitis

DECONTAMINATION
- Wear positive-pressure SCBA and protective equipment specified by references such as the *North American Emergency Response Guidebook*. If special chemical protective clothing is required, consult the chemical manufacturer or specific protective clothing compatibility charts. A qualified, experienced person should make decisions regarding the type of personal protective equipment necessary.
- Delay entry until trained personnel and proper protective equipment are available.
- Remove patient from contaminated area.
- Quickly remove and isolate patient's clothing, jewelry, and shoes.
- Gently blot excess liquids with absorbent material.
- Rinse patient with warm water, 32° C to 35° C (90° F to 95° F), if possible.
- Wash patient with a mild liquid soap and large quantities of water.
- Refer to decontamination protocol in Section Three.

IMMEDIATE FIRST AID
- Ensure that adequate decontamination has been carried out.
- If patient is not breathing, start artificial respiration, preferably with a demand-valve resuscitator, bag-valve-mask device, or pocket mask, as trained. Perform CPR if necessary.
- Immediately flush contaminated eyes with gently flowing water.
- Do not induce vomiting. If vomiting occurs, lean patient forward or place on left side (head-down position, if possible) to maintain an open airway and prevent aspiration.
- Keep patient quiet and maintain normal body temperature.
- Obtain medical attention.

BASIC TREATMENT
- Establish a patent airway (oropharyngeal or nasopharyngeal airway, if needed). Suction if necessary.
- Watch for signs of respiratory insufficiency and assist ventilations if necessary.
- Administer oxygen by nonrebreather mask at 10 to 15 L/min.
- Provide a low-stimulus environment.
- Monitor for shock and treat if necessary (refer to shock protocol in Section Three).
- Anticipate seizures and treat if necessary (refer to seizure protocol in Section Three).

- For eye contamination, flush eyes immediately with water. Irrigate each eye continuously with 0.9% saline (NS) during transport (refer to eye irrigation protocol in Section Three).
- Do not use emetics. For ingestion, rinse mouth and administer 5 ml/kg up to 200 ml of water for dilution if the patient can swallow, has a strong gag reflex, and does not drool (refer to ingestion protocol in Section Three).
- Treat frostbite by rapid rewarming (refer to frostbite protocol in Section Three).

ADVANCED TREATMENT

- Consider orotracheal or nasotracheal intubation for airway control in the patient who is unconscious or is in severe respiratory distress.
- Monitor cardiac rhythm and treat arrhythmias if necessary (refer to cardiac protocol in Section Three).
- Start IV administration of D_5W TKO. Use 0.9% saline (NS) or lactated Ringer's (LR) if signs of hypovolemia are present. For hypotension with signs of hypovolemia, administer fluid cautiously. Consider vasopressors if patient is hypotensive with a normal fluid volume. Watch for signs of fluid overload (refer to shock protocol in Section Three).
- Treat seizures with diazepam (Valium) or lorazepam (Ativan) (refer to diazepam and lorazepam protocols in Section Four and seizure protocol in Section Three).
- Use proparacaine hydrochloride to assist eye irrigation (refer to proparacaine hydrochloride protocol in Section Four).

INITIAL EMERGENCY DEPARTMENT CONSIDERATIONS

- Useful initial laboratory studies include complete blood count, serum electrolytes, blood urea nitrogen (BUN), creatinine, glucose, urinalysis, and baseline biochemical profile including serum aminotransferases (ALT and AST), calcium, phosphorus, and magnesium. Determination of anion and osmolar gaps may be helpful. Arterial blood gases (ABGs), chest radiograph, and electrocardiogram may be required.
- Products may cause anion gap acidosis; hyperventilation and sodium bicarbonate may be beneficial. Bicarbonate therapy should be guided by patient presentation, ABG determination, and serum electrolyte considerations.
- Hemodialysis may be beneficial in the severely poisoned patient with renal failure.
- Obtain toxicological consultation as necessary.

39

Dioxane and Related Compounds

SUBSTANCE IDENTIFICATION

Colorless liquids with a pleasant alcohol-like odor. Used as stabilizers for chlorinated solvents, as wetting and dispersing agents in textile processing, and as solvents for resins and oils. Found in dyes, cleaning agents, stains and printing chemicals. Also used in the manufacture of adhesives, cosmetics, deodorants, fumigants, and polishing compositions.

ROUTES OF EXPOSURE

Skin and eye contact
Inhalation
Ingestion
Skin absorption

TARGET ORGANS

Primary
Skin
Eyes
Renal system
Hepatic system
Secondary
Central nervous system
Cardiovascular system
Respiratory system
Gastrointestinal system

LIFE THREAT

Pulmonary irritant. Respiratory failure, pulmonary edema, and CNS depression.

SIGNS AND SYMPTOMS BY SYSTEM

Cardiovascular: Tachyarrhythmias.

Respiratory: Mucous membrane irritation, acute pulmonary edema, dyspnea, hyperpnea, coughing, tachypnea, and respiratory failure.

CNS: Headache, drowsiness, poor sense of balance (ataxia), seizures, CNS depression, and coma.

Gastrointestinal: Nausea, vomiting, loss of appetite, and stomach pain.

Eye: Conjunctival irritation and lacrimation.

Skin: Mild irritation and irritant dermatitis.

Renal: Kidney damage.

Hepatic: Liver damage.

Other: These products may cause olfactory fatigue and therefore may not demonstrate adequate warning properties. Some products present a human carcinogenic and mutagenic risk.

SYMPTOM ONSET FOR ACUTE EXPOSURE

Immediate
Pulmonary edema symptoms possibly delayed

CO-EXPOSURE CONCERNS

Air (may form explosive peroxides on contact with air)

THERMAL DECOMPOSITION PRODUCTS INCLUDE

Carbon dioxide
Carbon monoxide

MEDICAL PROBLEMS POSSIBLY AGGRAVATED BY EXPOSURE

Skin disorders
Asthma and other pulmonary disorders
Liver disorders
Kidney disorders

DECONTAMINATION

- Wear positive-pressure SCBA and protective equipment specified by references such as the *North American Emergency Response Guidebook.* If special chemical protective clothing is required, consult the chemical manufacturer or specific protective clothing compatibility charts. A qualified, experienced person should make decisions regarding the type of personal protective equipment necessary.
- Delay entry until trained personnel and proper protective equipment are available.
- Remove patient from contaminated area.
- Quickly remove and isolate patient's clothing, jewelry, and shoes.
- Gently blot excess liquids with absorbent material.
- Rinse patient with warm water, 32° C to 35° C (90° F to 95° F), if possible.
- Wash patient with a mild liquid soap and large quantities of water.
- Refer to decontamination protocol in Section Three.

IMMEDIATE FIRST AID

- Ensure that adequate decontamination has been carried out.
- If patient is not breathing, start artificial respiration, preferably with a demand-valve resuscitator, bag-valve-mask device, or pocket mask, as trained. Perform CPR if necessary.
- Immediately flush contaminated eyes with gently flowing water.
- Do not induce vomiting. If vomiting occurs, lean patient forward or place on left side (head-down position, if possible) to maintain an open airway and prevent aspiration.
- Keep patient quiet and maintain normal body temperature.
- Obtain medical attention.

BASIC TREATMENT

- Establish a patent airway (oropharyngeal or nasopharyngeal airway, if needed). Suction if necessary.
- Watch for signs of respiratory insufficiency and assist ventilations if necessary.
- Administer oxygen by nonrebreather mask at 10 to 15 L/min.
- Monitor for pulmonary edema and treat if necessary (refer to pulmonary edema protocol in Section Three).
- Anticipate seizures and treat if necessary (refer to seizure protocol in Section Three).

- For eye contamination, flush eyes immediately with water. Irrigate each eye continuously with 0.9% saline (NS) during transport (refer to eye irrigation protocol in Section Three).
- Do not use emetics. For ingestion, rinse mouth and administer 5 ml/kg up to 200 ml of water for dilution if the patient can swallow, has a strong gag reflex, and does not drool. Administer activated charcoal (refer to ingestion protocol in Section Three and activated charcoal protocol in Section Four).

ADVANCED TREATMENT

- Consider orotracheal or nasotracheal intubation for airway control in the patient who is unconscious, has severe pulmonary edema, or is in severe respiratory distress.
- Positive-pressure ventilation techniques with a bag-valve-mask device may be beneficial.
- Consider drug therapy for pulmonary edema (refer to pulmonary edema protocol in Section Three).
- Monitor cardiac rhythm and treat arrhythmias if necessary (refer to cardiac protocol in Section Three).
- Start IV administration of D_5W TKO. Consider vasopressors if patient is hypotensive with a normal fluid volume. Watch for signs of fluid overload (refer to shock protocol in Section Three).
- Treat seizures with diazepam (Valium) or lorazepam (Ativan) (refer to diazepam and lorazepam protocols in Section Four and seizure protocol in Section Three).
- Use proparacaine hydrochloride to assist eye irrigation (refer to proparacaine hydrochloride protocol in Section Four).

INITIAL EMERGENCY DEPARTMENT CONSIDERATIONS

- Useful initial laboratory studies include complete blood count, serum electrolytes, blood urea nitrogen (BUN), creatinine, glucose, urinalysis, and baseline biochemical profile including serum aminotransferases (ALT and AST), calcium, phosphorus, and magnesium. Arterial blood gases (ABGs), chest radiographs and electrocardiogram may be required.
- Positive end-expiratory pressure (PEEP)–assisted ventilation may be necessary in patients with acute parenchymal injury who develop pulmonary edema or acute respiratory distress syndrome.
- Obtain toxicological consultation as necessary.

Ethylene Glycol, Glycols, and Related Compounds

SUBSTANCE IDENTIFICATION

Syrupy, colorless liquids with a faint etherlike or pleasant odor. Ethylene glycol has a sweet taste. Found as solvents, degreasers, wetting agents, agricultural chemicals, hydraulic fluids, and antifreezes. Also used in the application and manufacture of varnishes, lacquers, paints, and detergents.

ROUTES OF EXPOSURE

Skin and eye contact
Inhalation
Ingestion
Skin absorption

TARGET ORGANS

Primary
Skin
Eyes
Central nervous system
Cardiovascular system
Respiratory system
Renal system
Metabolism
Secondary
Gastrointestinal system
Hepatic system

LIFE THREAT

Respiratory failure, pulmonary edema, paralysis, cardiovascular collapse, and severe acidosis.

SIGNS AND SYMPTOMS BY SYSTEM

Cardiovascular: Cardiovascular collapse and tachyarrhythmias.

Respiratory: Respiratory tract irritation with dyspnea, hyperpnea, and tachypnea. Acute pulmonary edema and respiratory failure.

CNS: Headache, drowsiness, dizziness, weakness, muscle tenderness, tremors, seizures, CNS depression, coma, paralysis, disturbances in vision and hearing.

Gastrointestinal: Nausea, vomiting, and stomach pain.

Eye: Chemical conjunctivitis, photophobia, and lacrimation.

Skin: Drying and cracking of the skin.

Renal: Nephropathy.

Hepatic: Liver damage.

Metabolism: Anion gap metabolic acidosis and hypocalcemia.

Other: Products may cause an inebriation-like effect similar to ethanol. Ethylene glycol symptoms show three stages of clinical effects:

Phase I: 30 minutes to 12 hours after exposure; CNS and metabolic effects.

Phase II: 12 to 36 hours after exposure; cardiopulmonary effects and metabolic acidosis; ethylene glycol metabolized to glycolic and oxalic acids.

Phase III: 2 to 3 days after exposure; nephropathy.

SYMPTOM ONSET FOR ACUTE EXPOSURE

Immediate

Some symptoms possibly delayed (see above)

CO-EXPOSURE CONCERNS

Other glycol ethers

Hydrocarbon solvents

THERMAL DECOMPOSITION PRODUCTS INCLUDE

Carbon dioxide

Carbon monoxide

MEDICAL CONDITIONS POSSIBLY AGGRAVATED BY EXPOSURE

Respiratory system disorders

Kidney disorders

Skin disorders

DECONTAMINATION

- Wear positive-pressure SCBA and protective equipment specified by references such as the *North American Emergency Response Guidebook*. If special chemical protective clothing is required, consult the chemical manufacturer or specific protective clothing compatibility charts. A qualified, experienced person should make decisions regarding the type of personal protective equipment necessary.
- Delay entry until trained personnel and proper protective equipment are available.
- Remove patient from contaminated area.
- Quickly remove and isolate patient's clothing, jewelry, and shoes.
- Gently blot excess liquids with absorbent material.
- Rinse patient with warm water, 32° C to 35° C (90° F to 95° F), if possible.
- Wash patient with a mild liquid soap and large quantities of water.
- Refer to decontamination protocol in Section Three.

IMMEDIATE FIRST AID

- Ensure that adequate decontamination has been carried out.
- If patient is not breathing, start artificial respiration, preferably with a demand-valve resuscitator, bag-valve-mask device, or pocket mask, as trained. Perform CPR if necessary.
- Immediately flush contaminated eyes with gently flowing water.
- Do not induce vomiting. If vomiting occurs, lean patient forward or place on left side (head-down position, if possible) to maintain an open airway and prevent aspiration.
- Keep patient quiet and maintain normal body temperature.
- Obtain medical attention.

BASIC TREATMENT

- Establish a patent airway (oropharyngeal or nasopharyngeal airway, if needed). Suction if necessary.
- Watch for signs of respiratory insufficiency and assist ventilations if necessary.

- Administer oxygen by nonrebreather mask at 10 to 15 L/min.
- Monitor for pulmonary edema and treat if necessary (refer to pulmonary edema protocol in Section Three).
- Monitor for shock and treat if necessary (refer to shock protocol in Section Three).
- Anticipate seizures and treat if necessary (refer to seizure protocol in Section Three).
- For eye contamination, flush eyes immediately with water. Irrigate each eye continuously with 0.9% saline (NS) during transport (refer to eye irrigation protocol in Section Three).
- Do not use emetics. For ingestion, rinse mouth and administer 5 ml/kg up to 200 ml of water for dilution if the patient can swallow, has a strong gag reflex, and does not drool. Administer activated charcoal (refer to ingestion protocol in Section Three and activated charcoal protocol in Section Four).

ADVANCED TREATMENT

- Consider orotracheal or nasotracheal intubation for airway control in the patient who is unconscious, has severe pulmonary edema, or is in severe respiratory distress.
- Positive-pressure ventilation techniques with a bag-valve-mask device may be beneficial.
- Consider drug therapy for pulmonary edema (refer to pulmonary edema protocol in Section Three).
- Monitor cardiac rhythm and treat arrhythmias if necessary (refer to cardiac protocol in Section Three).
- Start IV administration of D_5W TKO. Use 0.9% saline (NS) or lactated Ringer's (LR) if signs of hypovolemia are present. For hypotension with signs of hypovolemia, administer fluid cautiously. Consider vasopressors if patient is hypotensive with a normal fluid volume. Watch for signs of fluid overload (refer to shock protocol in Section Three).
- Treat seizures with diazepam (Valium) or lorazepam (Ativan) (refer to diazepam and lorazepam protocols in Section Four and seizure protocol in Section Three).
- Use proparacaine hydrochloride to assist eye irrigation (refer to proparacaine hydrochloride protocol in Section Four).

INITIAL EMERGENCY DEPARTMENT CONSIDERATIONS

- Useful initial laboratory studies include complete blood count, serum electrolytes, blood urea nitrogen (BUN), creatinine, glucose, urinalysis, and baseline biochemical profile including serum aminotransferases (ALT and AST), calcium, phosphorus, and magnesium. Determination of anion and osmolar gaps may be helpful. Arterial blood gases (ABGs), chest radiograph, and electrocardiogram may be required.
- Determine ethylene glycol blood concentration. Look for oxalate or hippurate crystals in the urine.
- Positive end-expiratory pressure (PEEP) assisted–ventilation may be necessary in patients with acute parenchymal injury who develop pulmonary edema or acute respiratory distress syndrome.
- Products may cause anion gap metabolic acidosis and osmolar gap; hyperventilation and sodium bicarbonate may be beneficial. Bicarbonate therapy

should be guided by patient presentation, ABG determination, and serum electrolyte considerations.

- Ethanol and fomepizole inhibition therapy of the alcohol dehydrogenase enzyme may be beneficial for severe poisoning with ethylene glycol. Therapy should be guided by severity of acidosis, patient presentation, and ethylene glycol serum concentrations. Do not delay administration in symptomatic patients pending blood ethylene glycol results (refer to ethanol and fomepizole protocols in Section Four).
- Hemodialysis is the treatment of choice in the severely poisoned patient with refractory acidosis, pulmonary edema, or cerebral edema.
- Obtain toxicological consultation as necessary.

SPECIAL CONSIDERATIONS

- Co-ingestion of ethanol will delay onset of metabolic symptoms in cases of ethylene glycol poisoning.

Aldehydes and Related Compounds

SUBSTANCE IDENTIFICATION

Colorless gases with an irritating odor, or colorless to light brown solutions with a faint almond odor. Used as fumigants, disinfectants, germicides, preservatives, embalming fluids, cleaning products, preservatives, and in the manufacture of various plastic and resin products. An important laboratory reagent and process chemical. Formalin is a 37% formaldehyde solution with 0.5% to 15% methanol added to prevent polymerization.

ROUTES OF EXPOSURE

Skin and eye contact
Inhalation
Ingestion
Skin absorption

TARGET ORGANS

Primary
Eyes
Skin
Respiratory system
Metabolism

Secondary
Central nervous system
Cardiovascular system
Gastrointestinal system
Hepatic system
Renal system

LIFE THREAT

Seizures, respiratory failure, and pulmonary edema.

SIGNS AND SYMPTOMS BY SYSTEM

Cardiovascular: Tachycardia, cardiovascular collapse, and hypotension.

Respiratory: Respiratory tract irritant. Upper airway edema and laryngospasm, cough, dysphagia, pulmonary edema, bronchial constriction, reactive airways disease (asthmalike) symptoms.

CNS: Headache, vertigo, seizures, CNS depression, and coma.

Gastrointestinal: Nausea, vomiting (hematemesis), diarrhea, severe mucosal necrosis, and abdominal pain.

Eye: Chemical conjunctivitis, lacrimation, and corneal damage.

Skin: Irritant dermatitis: tingling, drying, and reddening of the skin. Allergic (hypersensitization) dermatitis.

Renal: Kidney damage and hematuria.

Hepatic: Liver damage and jaundice.

Metabolism: Anion gap metabolic acidosis.

Other: These products may cause olfactory fatigue and therefore not demonstrate adequate warning properties. Formaldehyde may present a carcinogenic risk to humans. More data are needed on products in this group.

SYMPTOM ONSET FOR ACUTE EXPOSURE

Immediate

Respiratory symptoms possibly delayed

THERMAL DECOMPOSITION PRODUCTS INCLUDE

Carbon dioxide

Carbon monoxide

MEDICAL CONDITIONS POSSIBLY AGGRAVATED BY EXPOSURE

Skin or eye disorders

Respiratory system disorders

DECONTAMINATION

- Wear positive-pressure SCBA and protective equipment specified by references such as the *North American Emergency Response Guidebook*. If special chemical protective clothing is required, consult the chemical manufacturer or specific protective clothing compatibility charts. A qualified, experienced person should make decisions regarding the type of personal protective equipment necessary.
- Delay entry until trained personnel and proper protective equipment are available.
- Remove patient from contaminated area.
- Quickly remove and isolate patient's clothing, jewelry, and shoes.
- Gently blot excess liquids with absorbent material.
- Rinse patient with warm water, 32° C to 35° C (90° F to 95° F), if possible.
- Wash patient with a mild liquid soap and large quantities of water.
- Refer to decontamination protocol in Section Three.

IMMEDIATE FIRST AID

- Ensure that adequate decontamination has been carried out.
- If patient is not breathing, start artificial respiration, preferably with a demand-valve resuscitator, bag-valve-mask device, or pocket mask, as trained. Perform CPR if necessary.
- Immediately flush contaminated eyes with gently flowing water.
- Do not induce vomiting. If vomiting occurs, lean patient forward or place on left side (head-down position, if possible) to maintain an open airway and prevent aspiration.
- Keep patient quiet and maintain normal body temperature.
- Obtain medical attention.

BASIC TREATMENT

- Establish a patent airway (oropharyngeal or nasopharyngeal airway, if needed). Suction if necessary.
- Watch for signs of respiratory insufficiency and assist ventilations if necessary.
- Aggressive airway management may be necessary.
- Administer oxygen by nonrebreather mask at 10 to 15 L/min.
- Anticipate seizures and treat if necessary (refer to seizure protocol in Section Three).
- Monitor for shock and treat if necessary (refer to shock protocol in Section Three).

- Monitor for pulmonary edema and treat if necessary (refer to pulmonary edema protocol in Section Three).
- For eye contamination, flush eyes immediately with water. Irrigate each eye continuously with 0.9% saline (NS) during transport (refer to eye irrigation protocol in Section Three).
- Do not use emetics. For ingestion, rinse mouth and administer 5 ml/kg up to 200 ml of water for dilution if the patient can swallow, has a strong gag reflex, and does not drool. Administer activated charcoal (refer to ingestion protocol in Section Three and activated charcoal protocol in Section Four).

ADVANCED TREATMENT

- Consider orotracheal or nasotracheal intubation for airway control in the patient who is unconscious, has severe pulmonary edema, or is in severe respiratory distress. Intubation should be considered at the first sign of upper airway obstruction caused by edema.
- Positive-pressure ventilation techniques with a bag-valve-mask device may be beneficial.
- Consider drug therapy for pulmonary edema (refer to pulmonary edema protocol in Section Three).
- Consider administering a beta agonist such as albuterol for severe bronchospasm (refer to albuterol protocol in Section Four).
- Start IV administration of D_5W TKO. Use 0.9% saline (NS) or lactated Ringer's (LR) if signs of hypovolemia are present. For hypotension with signs of hypovolemia, administer fluid cautiously. Consider vasopressors if patient is hypotensive with a normal fluid volume. Watch for signs of fluid overload (refer to shock protocol in Section Three).
- Treat seizures with diazepam (Valium) or lorazepam (Ativan) (refer to diazepam and lorazepam protocols in Section Four and seizure protocol in Section Three).
- Use proparacaine hydrochloride to assist eye irrigation (refer to proparacaine hydrochloride protocol in Section Four).

INITIAL EMERGENCY DEPARTMENT CONSIDERATIONS

- Useful initial laboratory studies include complete blood count, serum electrolytes, blood urea nitrogen (BUN), creatinine, glucose, urinalysis, and baseline biochemical profile including serum aminotransferases (ALT and AST), calcium, phosphorus, and magnesium. Determination of anion and osmolar gaps may be helpful. Arterial blood gases (ABGs), chest radiographs, and electrocardiogram may be required.
- Positive end-expiratory pressure (PEEP)–assisted ventilation may be necessary in patients with acute parenchymal injury who develop pulmonary edema or acute respiratory distress syndrome.
- Bronchospastic symptoms should be treated with an inhalation medication regimen similar to that used for reactive airways disease. Inhaled corticosteroids may be of value in severe bronchospasm.
- Sodium bicarbonate may be needed to correct metabolic acidosis. Administration should be guided by patient presentation, ABG determination, and serum electrolyte considerations.
- Hemodialysis may be beneficial in the severely symptomatic patient. Treatment should be guided by patient presentation and laboratory values.

- Obtain toxicological consultation as necessary.

SPECIAL CONSIDERATIONS

- Formalin solutions may contain 0.5% to 15% methanol (refer to methanol, Guideline 31).

Ketones and Related Compounds

SUBSTANCE IDENTIFICATION

Colorless organic liquids with a sharp, fragrant, acetone-type or sweet odor. Used as intermediates and solvents for inks, resins, adhesives; components of cleaning agents and paint/varnish removers. Also used in the production of numerous products, including perfumes, pesticides, and petroleum oils.

ROUTES OF EXPOSURE

Skin and eye contact
Inhalation
Ingestion
Skin absorption

TARGET ORGANS

Primary
Skin
Eyes
Central nervous system
Cardiovascular system
Respiratory system
Metabolism
Secondary
Gastrointestinal system
Hepatic system

LIFE THREAT

Respiratory tract (mucous membrane) irritation, pulmonary edema, and depression of CNS. Certain products (ketone peroxides) can be extremely corrosive.

SIGNS AND SYMPTOMS BY SYSTEM

Cardiovascular: Tachycardia and arrhythmias.

Respiratory: Respiratory tract irritation, bronchospasm, dyspnea, pulmonary edema, and respiratory depression.

CNS: Headache, paresthesias, muscle weakness, drowsiness, dizziness, incoordination, CNS depression, coma, neurobehavioral changes, central and peripheral neuropathy.

Gastrointestinal: Nausea, vomiting, and abdominal pain.

Eye: Chemical conjunctivitis and temporary clouding of the cornea to serious, permanent damage, including blindness.

Skin: Drying of the skin, irritant dermatitis, and chemical burns.

Hepatic: Liver damage.

Metabolism: Metabolic acidosis with anion gap.

Other: Some products may cause olfactory fatigue and therefore not demonstrate adequate warning properties. Hypothermia has been reported.

SYMPTOM ONSET FOR ACUTE EXPOSURE

Immediate

Respiratory symptoms possibly delayed

Neuropathy symptoms possibly delayed

CO-EXPOSURE CONCERNS

Other hydrocarbon solvents

THERMAL DECOMPOSITION PRODUCTS INCLUDE

Carbon dioxide

Carbon monoxide

MEDICAL CONDITIONS POSSIBLY AGGRAVATED BY EXPOSURE

Eye disorders

Nervous system disorders

Respiratory system disorders

DECONTAMINATION

- Wear positive-pressure SCBA and protective equipment specified by references such as the *North American Emergency Response Guidebook*. If special chemical protective clothing is required, consult the chemical manufacturer or specific protective clothing compatibility charts. A qualified, experienced person should make decisions regarding the type of personal protective equipment necessary.
- Delay entry until trained personnel and proper protective equipment are available.
- Remove patient from contaminated area.
- Quickly remove and isolate patient's clothing, jewelry, and shoes.
- Gently blot excess liquids with absorbent material.
- Rinse patient with warm water, 32° C to 35° C (90° F to 95° F), if possible.
- Wash patient with a mild liquid soap and large quantities of water.
- Refer to decontamination protocol in Section Three.

IMMEDIATE FIRST AID

- Ensure that adequate decontamination has been carried out.
- If patient is not breathing, start artificial respiration, preferably with a demand-valve resuscitator, bag-valve-mask device, or pocket mask, as trained. Perform CPR if necessary.
- Immediately flush contaminated eyes with gently flowing water.
- Do not induce vomiting. If vomiting occurs, lean patient forward or place on left side (head-down position, if possible) to maintain an open airway and prevent aspiration.
- Keep patient quiet and maintain normal body temperature.
- Obtain medical attention.

BASIC TREATMENT

- Establish a patent airway (oropharyngeal or nasopharyngeal airway, if needed). Suction if necessary.
- Watch for signs of respiratory insufficiency and assist ventilations if necessary.
- Administer oxygen by nonrebreather mask at 10 to 15 L/min.
- Monitor for pulmonary edema and treat if necessary (refer to pulmonary edema protocol in Section Three).
- For contamination, flush eyes immediately with water. Irrigate each eye continuously with 0.9% saline (NS) during transport (refer to eye irrigation protocol in Section Three).

- Do not use emetics. For ingestion, rinse mouth and administer 5 ml/kg up to 200 ml of water for dilution if the patient can swallow, has a strong gag reflex, and does not drool. Administer activated charcoal (refer to ingestion protocol in Section Three and activated charcoal protocol in Section Four).

ADVANCED TREATMENT

- Consider orotracheal or nasotracheal intubation for airway control in the patient who is unconscious, has severe pulmonary edema, or is in severe respiratory distress.
- Positive-pressure ventilation techniques with a bag-valve-mask device may be beneficial.
- Consider drug therapy for pulmonary edema (refer to pulmonary edema protocol in Section Three).
- Consider administering a beta agonist such as albuterol for severe bronchospasm (refer to albuterol protocol in Section Four).
- Monitor cardiac rhythm and treat arrhythmias if necessary (refer to cardiac protocol in Section Three).
- Start IV administration of D_5W TKO. Use 0.9% saline (NS) or lactated Ringer's (LR) if signs of hypovolemia are present. For hypotension with signs of hypovolemia, administer fluid cautiously. Watch for signs of fluid overload (refer to shock protocol in Section Three).
- Use proparacaine hydrochloride to assist eye irrigation (refer to proparacaine hydrochloride protocol in Section Four).

INITIAL EMERGENCY DEPARTMENT CONSIDERATIONS

- Useful initial laboratory studies include complete blood count, serum electrolytes, blood urea nitrogen (BUN), creatinine, glucose, urinalysis, and baseline biochemical profile including serum aminotransferases (ALT and AST), calcium, phosphorus, and magnesium. Determination of anion and osmolar gaps may be helpful. Arterial blood gases (ABGs), chest radiograph, and electrocardiogram may be required.
- Positive end-expiratory pressure (PEEP)–assisted ventilation may be necessary in patients with acute parenchymal injury who develop pulmonary edema or acute respiratory distress syndrome.
- Bronchospastic symptoms should be treated with an inhalation medication regimen similar to that used for reactive airway disease. Inhaled corticosteroids may be of value in severe bronchospasm.
- Sodium bicarbonate may be needed to reduce metabolic acidosis. Bicarbonate therapy should be guided by patient presentation, ABG determination, and serum electrolyte considerations.
- Obtain toxicological consultation as necessary.

SPECIAL CONSIDERATIONS

- Methyl *n*-butyl ketone (MBK) is a known neurotoxin. The primary metabolite of MBK, 2,5-hexanedione, produces central and peripheral neurotoxicity characterized by the dying-back axonopathy. Symptoms are usually delayed.

43

Naphthalene and Related Compounds

SUBSTANCE IDENTIFICATION

Found as a colorless to brown solid with an odor of mothballs. Used as insecticides, moth repellents, fumigants, and toilet bowl deodorants. Also used in the manufacture of phthalic anhydride, solvents, insecticides, pigments, rubber chemicals, waxes, rodenticides, and numerous other products.

ROUTES OF EXPOSURE

Skin and eye contact
Inhalation
Ingestion
Skin absorption

TARGET ORGANS

Primary
Skin
Eyes
Central nervous system
Cardiovascular system
Respiratory system
Blood
Secondary
Gastrointestinal system
Hepatic system
Renal system

LIFE THREAT

Acute intravascular hemolysis that can be delayed for several days.

SIGNS AND SYMPTOMS BY SYSTEM

Cardiovascular: Tachycardia. Hemolysis and anemia often after the third day and subsequent hypovolemia.

Respiratory: Respiratory tract irritation and mild tachypnea.

CNS: Headache, confusion, excitement, occasional coma and seizures, and neurobehavioral changes.

Gastrointestinal: Nausea, vomiting, and abdominal pain.

Eye: Chemical conjunctivitis, corneal ulcerations, cataracts, and inflammation of the optic nerve.

Skin: Irritation, diaphoresis, dermatitis, hypersensitivity dermatitis, and jaundice secondary to hemolysis. Acneform rashes reported with chronic exposure.

Hepatic: Liver injury and jaundice.

Renal: Renal damage.

Blood: Mild methemoglobinemia. Increased white blood cell count (leukocytosis), Heinz bodies, free hemoglobin (hemoglobinemia). Acute red blood cell hemolysis and anemia may occur.

SYMPTOM ONSET FOR ACUTE EXPOSURE

Immediate

Symptoms of hemolysis possibly delayed

CO-EXPOSURE CONCERNS

Chlorinated hydrocarbon solvents

THERMAL DECOMPOSITION PRODUCTS INCLUDE

Carbon dioxide

Carbon monoxide

Chloride fumes

MEDICAL CONDITIONS POSSIBLY AGGRAVATED BY EXPOSURE

Chronic anemia

Glucose-6-phosphate dehydrogenase (G6PD) deficiency

DECONTAMINATION

- Wear positive-pressure SCBA and protective equipment specified by references such as the *North American Emergency Response Guidebook*. If special chemical protective clothing is required, consult the chemical manufacturer or specific protective clothing compatibility charts. A qualified, experienced person should make decisions regarding the type of personal protective equipment necessary.
- Delay entry until trained personnel and proper protective equipment are available.
- Remove patient from contaminated area.
- Quickly remove and isolate patient's clothing, jewelry, and shoes.
- Gently brush away dry particles and blot excess liquids with absorbent material.
- Rinse patient with warm water, 32° C to 35° C (90° F to 95° F), if possible.
- Wash patient with a mild liquid soap and large quantities of water.
- Refer to decontamination protocol in Section Three.

IMMEDIATE FIRST AID

- Ensure that adequate decontamination has been carried out.
- If patient is not breathing, start artificial respiration, preferably with a demand-valve resuscitator, bag-valve-mask device, or pocket mask, as trained. Perform CPR if necessary.
- Immediately flush contaminated eyes with gently flowing water.
- Do not induce vomiting. If vomiting occurs, lean patient forward or place on left side (head-down position, if possible) to maintain an open airway and prevent aspiration.
- Keep patient quiet and maintain normal body temperature.
- Obtain medical attention.

BASIC TREATMENT

- Establish a patent airway (oropharyngeal or nasopharyngeal airway, if needed). Suction if necessary.
- Watch for signs of respiratory insufficiency and assist ventilations if necessary.
- Administer oxygen by nonrebreather mask at 10 to 15 L/min.
- Monitor for shock and treat if necessary (refer to shock protocol in Section Three).
- Anticipate seizures and treat if necessary (refer to seizure protocol in Section Three).

- For eye contamination, flush eyes immediately with water. Irrigate each eye continuously with 0.9% saline (NS) during transport (refer to eye irrigation protocol in Section Three).
- Do not use emetics. For ingestion, rinse mouth and administer 5 ml/kg up to 200 ml of water for dilution if the patient can swallow, has a strong gag reflex, and does not drool. Administer activated charcoal (refer to ingestion protocol in Section Three and activated charcoal protocol in Section Four).

ADVANCED TREATMENT

- Consider orotracheal or nasotracheal intubation for airway control in the patient who is unconscious or is in severe respiratory distress.
- Start IV administration of 0.9% saline (NS) or lactated Ringer's (LR). Adequate hydration must be maintained to prevent renal failure secondary to myoglobinuria unless signs of cerebral or pulmonary edema are present.
- For hypotension with signs of hypovolemia, administer fluid cautiously. Watch for signs of fluid overload (refer to shock protocol in Section Three).
- Administer 1% solution methylene blue if patient is symptomatic with severe hypoxia, cyanosis, and cardiac compromise not responding to oxygen. DIRECT PHYSICIAN ORDER ONLY (refer to methylene blue protocol in Section Four).
- Treat seizures with diazepam (Valium) or lorazepam (Ativan) (refer to diazepam and lorazepam protocols in Section Four and seizure protocol in Section Three).
- Use proparacaine hydrochloride to assist eye irrigation (refer to proparacaine hydrochloride protocol in Section Four).

INITIAL EMERGENCY DEPARTMENT CONSIDERATIONS

- Useful initial laboratory studies include complete blood count, serum electrolytes, blood urea nitrogen (BUN), creatinine, glucose, urinalysis, and baseline biochemical profile including serum aminotransferases (ALT and AST), calcium, phosphorus, and magnesium. Arterial blood gases (ABGs), chest radiograph, and electrocardiogram may be required.
- Free hemoglobin, urine hemoglobin, haptoglobin, hematocrit, and bilirubin determinations are useful in assessing extent of hemolysis.
- Monitor blood methemoglobin levels and treat with methylene blue if patient is symptomatic and/or has a blood methemoglobin level greater than 30%. DIRECT PHYSICIAN ORDER ONLY (refer to methylene blue protocol in Section Four).
- Obtain toxicological consultation as necessary.

SPECIAL CONSIDERATIONS

- Naphthalene is metabolized to naphthol. This is an example of lethal synthesis, with the metabolite 1-naphthol responsible for the late symptoms of red blood cell hemolysis.
- Patients with glucose-6-phosphate dehydrogenase (G6PD) deficiency, a hereditary problem, are more susceptible to the hemolytic effects of 1-naphthol.
- Pulse oximetry readings may not be accurate in these exposures.

Phenols and Related Compounds

SUBSTANCE IDENTIFICATION

Colorless to pink solid or thick liquid. Laboratory reagents; disinfectants, sanitizers, fumigants, and barn deodorants; and photographic chemicals. Products used in the manufacturing of plywood, electrical appliances, and automotive parts. Sometimes used as an industrial coating of drums and cans.

ROUTES OF EXPOSURE

Skin and eye contact
Inhalation
Ingestion
Skin absorption

TARGET ORGANS

Primary
Skin
Eyes
Central nervous system
Cardiovascular system
Respiratory system
Gastrointestinal system
Metabolism
Secondary
Renal system
Hepatic system
Blood

LIFE THREAT

Coma, hypotension, cardiac arrhythmias, pulmonary edema, and respiratory arrest are common findings.

SIGNS AND SYMPTOMS BY SYSTEM

Cardiovascular: Cardiovascular collapse, hypotension, tachycardia, and arrhythmias (supraventricular and ventricular).

Respiratory: Snoring, tachypnea, shallow respirations, and pulmonary edema.

CNS: Headache, dizziness, tinnitus, weakness, confusion, and excitement, followed by coma. Seizures.

Gastrointestinal: Burns in mouth and throat, nausea, vomiting, diarrhea, hemorrhage, and abdominal pain.

Eye: Severe eye damage and blindness.

Skin: Strong corrosive effect on tissue. Pain from skin exposure is rapidly followed by numbness and blanching with severe burn. Cyanosis, pallor, sweating, hypothermia and irritant dermatitis possible.

Renal: Nephritis.

Hepatic: Liver damage, jaundice, and increases in serum aminotransferases.
Metabolism: Metabolic acidosis with anion gap.
Blood: Methemoglobinemia may be seen with some phenols.
Other: Possible mutagenic effects; may be a tumor promoter.

SYMPTOM ONSET FOR ACUTE EXPOSURE

Immediate
Some effects possibly delayed

THERMAL DECOMPOSITION PRODUCTS INCLUDE

Carbon dioxide
Carbon monoxide
Nitrogen oxides
Possibly hydrogen chloride gas

MEDICAL CONDITIONS POSSIBLY AGGRAVATED BY EXPOSURE

Respiratory disorders (asthma, bronchitis)
Skin disorders
Liver disorders
Kidney disorders

DECONTAMINATION

- Wear positive-pressure SCBA and protective equipment specified by references such as the *North American Emergency Response Guidebook*. If special chemical protective clothing is required, consult the chemical manufacturer or specific protective clothing compatibility charts. A qualified, experienced person should make decisions regarding the type of personal protective equipment necessary.
- Delay entry until trained personnel and proper protective equipment are available.
- Remove patient from contaminated area.
- Quickly remove and isolate patient's clothing, jewelry, and shoes.
- Gently brush away dry particles and blot excess liquids with absorbent material.
- Rinse patient with warm water, 32° C to 35° C (90° F to 95° F), if possible.
- Wash patient with a mild liquid soap and large quantities of water.
- Polyethylene glycol (PEG 300 or 400) may be an effective decontamination solution. Follow with soap and water wash.
- 70% Isopropanol may be an alternative decontamination solution for phenol skin contamination/burns less than 5% body surface area (BSA). For phenol burns greater than 5% BSA use PEG, since isopropanol may increase systemic absorption. Further studies are required to assess the efficacy of isopropanol for phenol dermal decontamination.
- Refer to decontamination protocol in Section Three.

IMMEDIATE FIRST AID

- Ensure that adequate decontamination has been carried out.
- If patient is not breathing, start artificial respiration, preferably with a demand valve resuscitator, bag-valve-mask, device or pocket mask, as trained. Perform CPR if necessary.
- Immediately flush contaminated eyes with gently flowing water.
- Do not induce vomiting. If vomiting occurs, lean patient forward or place on left side (head-down position, if possible) to maintain an open airway and prevent aspiration.

- Keep patient quiet and maintain normal body temperature.
- Obtain medical attention.

BASIC TREATMENT

- Establish a patent airway (oropharyngeal or nasopharyngeal airway, if needed). Suction if necessary.
- Watch for signs of respiratory insufficiency and assist ventilations if necessary.
- Administer oxygen by nonrebreather mask at 10 to 15 L/min.
- Monitor for pulmonary edema and treat if necessary (refer to pulmonary edema protocol in Section Three).
- Monitor for shock and treat if necessary (refer to shock protocol in Section Three).
- Anticipate seizures and treat if necessary (refer to seizure protocol in Section Three).
- For eye contamination, flush eyes immediately with water. Irrigate each eye continuously with 0.9% saline (NS) during transport (refer to eye irrigation protocol in Section Three).
- Administer activated charcoal (refer to activated charcoal protocol in Section Four). Dilution may be contraindicated because it may increase absorption.
- Do not use emetics (refer to ingestion protocol in Section Three).
- Cover skin burns with dry, sterile dressings after decontamination (refer to chemical burn protocol in Section Three).
- Maintain body temperature.

ADVANCED TREATMENT

- Consider orotracheal or nasotracheal intubation for airway control in the patient who is unconscious, has severe pulmonary edema, or is in severe respiratory distress.
- Positive-pressure ventilation techniques with a bag-valve-mask device may be beneficial.
- Consider drug therapy for pulmonary edema (refer to pulmonary edema protocol in Section Three).
- Monitor cardiac rhythm and treat arrhythmias if necessary (refer to cardiac protocol in Section Three).
- Start IV administration of D_5W TKO. Use 0.9% saline (NS) or lactated Ringer's (LR) if signs of hypovolemia are present. For hypotension with signs of hypovolemia, administer fluid cautiously. Consider vasopressors if patient is hypotensive with a normal fluid volume. Watch for signs of fluid overload (refer to shock protocol in Section Three).
- Administer 1% solution methylene blue if patient is symptomatic with severe hypoxia, cyanosis, and cardiac compromise not responding to oxygen. DIRECT PHYSICIAN ORDER ONLY (refer to methylene blue protocol in Section Four).
- Treat seizures with diazepam (Valium) or lorazepam (Ativan) (refer to diazepam and lorazepam protocols in Section Four and seizure protocol in Section Three).
- Use proparacaine hydrochloride to assist eye irrigation (refer to proparacaine hydrochloride protocol in Section Four).

INITIAL EMERGENCY DEPARTMENT CONSIDERATIONS

- Useful initial laboratory studies include complete blood count, serum electrolytes, blood urea nitrogen (BUN), creatinine, glucose, urinalysis, and

baseline biochemical profile, including serum aminotransferases (AST and ALT), calcium, phosphorus, and magnesium. Determination of anion and osmolar gaps may be helpful. Arterial blood gases (ABGs), chest radiograph, and electrocardiogram may be required.

- Certain products, especially dinitrophenol and hydroquinone, may cause methemoglobinemia. Monitor blood methemoglobin levels and treat with methylene blue if patient is symptomatic and/or has a blood methemoglobin level greater than 30%. DIRECT PHYSICIAN ORDER ONLY (refer to methylene blue protocol in Section Four).
- Positive end-expiratory pressure (PEEP)–assisted ventilation may be necessary in patients with acute parenchymal injury who develop pulmonary edema or acute respiratory distress syndrome.
- Obtain toxicological consultation as necessary.

SPECIAL CONSIDERATIONS

Pulse oximetry readings may not be accurate in these exposures.

Ethylene Oxide and Related Compounds

SUBSTANCE IDENTIFICATION

Colorless liquid or gas with a sweet or ether-type odor. High fire and explosion hazard. Used in the tobacco industry, in the manufacture of many industrial chemicals, as fumigants, and as rocket propellants. Widely used in hospital sterilizers. Poor warning property: olfactory fatigue may occur early.

ROUTES OF EXPOSURE

Skin and eye contact
Inhalation
Ingestion
Skin absorption

TARGET ORGANS

Primary
Eyes and skin
Respiratory system
Central nervous system
Hepatic system
Renal system
Secondary
Cardiovascular system
Gastrointestinal system

LIFE THREAT

Irritant to respiratory tract. Pulmonary edema.

SIGNS AND SYMPTOMS BY SYSTEM

Cardiovascular: Arrhythmias.

Respiratory: Respiratory tract and mucous membrane irritant. Cough, dyspnea, nasal burning, and chest pain. Acute pulmonary edema.

CNS: Headache, drowsiness, slurred speech, weakness, dizziness, incoordination, ataxia, nystagmus, loss of taste and smell, syncope, seizures, and peripheral neuropathy may be seen. Neurobehavioral changes possible.

Gastrointestinal: Nausea, protracted vomiting, and abdominal pain may be present.

Eye: Chemical conjunctivitis, corneal damage, cataract formation.

Skin: Irritation to contact dermatitis with vesicular eruptions, chemical burns, frostbite, and cyanosis may be seen.

Renal: Kidney damage.

Hepatic: Liver damage.

Other: Ethylene oxide may present a carcinogenic and mutagenic risk to humans. Allergic reactions.

SYMPTOM ONSET FOR ACUTE EXPOSURE

Immediate

Some symptoms, especially respiratory, possibly delayed

THERMAL DECOMPOSITION PRODUCTS INCLUDE

Carbon dioxide

Carbon monoxide

Irritating vapors

MEDICAL CONDITIONS POSSIBLY AGGRAVATED BY EXPOSURE

Respiratory disorders (asthma, bronchitis)

Nervous system disorders

Skin disorders

DECONTAMINATION

- Wear positive-pressure SCBA and protective equipment specified by references such as the *North American Emergency Response Guidebook*. If special chemical protective clothing is required, consult the chemical manufacturer or specific protective clothing compatibility charts. A qualified, experienced person should make decisions regarding the type of personal protective equipment necessary.
- Delay entry until trained personnel and proper protective equipment are available.
- Remove patient from contaminated area.
- Quickly remove and isolate patient's clothing, jewelry, and shoes.
- Gently blot excess liquids with absorbent material.
- Rinse patient with warm water, 32° C to 35° C (90° F to 95° F), if possible.
- Wash patient with a mild liquid soap and large quantities of water.
- Refer to decontamination protocol in Section Three.

IMMEDIATE FIRST AID

- Ensure that adequate decontamination has been carried out.
- If patient is not breathing, start artificial respiration, preferably with a demand-valve resuscitator, bag-valve-mask device, or pocket mask, as trained. Perform CPR if necessary.
- Immediately flush contaminated eyes with gently flowing water.
- Do not induce vomiting. If vomiting occurs, lean patient forward or place on left side (head-down position, if possible) to maintain an open airway and prevent aspiration.
- Keep patient quiet and maintain normal body temperature.
- Obtain medical attention.

BASIC TREATMENT

- Establish a patent airway (oropharyngeal or nasopharyngeal airway, if needed). Suction if necessary.
- Watch for signs of respiratory insufficiency and assist ventilations if necessary.
- Administer oxygen by nonrebreather mask at 10 to 15 L/min.
- Monitor for pulmonary edema and treat if necessary (refer to pulmonary edema protocol in Section Three).
- Anticipate seizures and treat if necessary (refer to seizure protocol in Section Three).
- For eye contamination, flush eyes immediately with water. Irrigate each eye continuously with 0.9% saline (NS) during transport (refer to eye irrigation protocol in Section Three).

- Do not use emetics. For ingestion, rinse mouth and administer 5 ml/kg up to 200 ml of water for dilution if the patient can swallow, has a strong gag reflex, and does not drool. Administer activated charcoal (refer to ingestion protocol in Section Three and activated charcoal protocol in Section Four).
- Cover skin burns with dry sterile dressings after decontamination (refer to chemical burn protocol in Section Three).
- Treat frostbite with rapid rewarming techniques (refer to frostbite protocol in Section Three).

ADVANCED TREATMENT

- Consider orotracheal or nasotracheal intubation for airway control in the patient who is unconscious, has severe pulmonary edema, or is in severe respiratory distress.
- Positive-pressure ventilation techniques with a bag-valve-mask device may be beneficial.
- Consider drug therapy for pulmonary edema (refer to pulmonary edema protocol in Section Three).
- Monitor cardiac rhythm and treat arrhythmias if necessary (refer to cardiac protocol in Section Three).
- Start IV administration of D_5W TKO. Use 0.9% saline (NS) or lactated Ringer's (LR) if signs of hypovolemia are present. For hypotension with signs of hypovolemia, administer fluid cautiously. Watch for signs of fluid overload (refer to shock protocol in Section Three).
- Treat seizures with diazepam (Valium) or lorazepam (Ativan) (refer to diazepam and lorazepam protocols in Section Four and seizure protocol in Section Three).
- Use proparacaine hydrochloride to assist eye irrigation (refer to proparacaine hydrochloride protocol in Section Four).

INITIAL EMERGENCY DEPARTMENT CONSIDERATIONS

- Useful initial laboratory studies include complete blood count, serum electrolytes, blood urea nitrogen (BUN), creatinine, glucose, urinalysis, and baseline biochemical profile, including serum aminotransferases (ALT and AST), calcium, phosphorus, and magnesium. Arterial blood gases (ABGs), chest radiograph, and electrocardiogram may be required.
- Positive end-expiratory pressure (PEEP)–assisted ventilation may be necessary in patients with acute parenchymal injury who develop pulmonary edema or acute respiratory distress syndrome.
- Obtain toxicological consultation as necessary.

SPECIAL CONSIDERATIONS

- Ethylene oxide has been reported to cause chromosomal changes and sister chromatid exchanges and increase the spontaneous abortion rate. Studies continue on these effects.
- Exposed individuals may require genetic/reproductive counseling. Ethylene oxide medical surveillance programs should be instituted for individuals who may have potential occupational exposure.

46

Polychlorinated Biphenyls (PCBs), Polybrominated Biphenyls (PBBs), Polychlorinated Dibenzofurans (PCDFs), and Related Compounds

SUBSTANCE IDENTIFICATION

Found as a straw-colored liquid. Used as petroleum additives; dielectric (cooling fluid) in capacitors/transformers, investment cast processes, and hydraulic and heat exchange fluids; ingredients in inks, adhesives, and paints. Also used in insulation for electric cables/wire, coatings for foundry use, fire retardants, and thermoplastic manufacture. Products are no longer produced in or imported into the United States. PCBs and PBBs may be found contaminated with PCDFs or polychlorinated dibenzodioxins (dioxin), which may be responsible for the carcinogenic and reproductive hazard.

ROUTES OF EXPOSURE

Skin and eye contact
Inhalation
Ingestion
Skin absorption

TARGET ORGANS

Primary
Skin
Eye
Central nervous system
Hepatic system
Secondary
Cardiovascular system
Respiratory system
Gastrointestinal system

LIFE THREAT

Acute and chronic exposure can cause liver and kidney damage.

SIGNS AND SYMPTOMS BY SYSTEM

Cardiovascular: Hypertension.
Respiratory: Irritation of the respiratory tract.
CNS: Transient visual disturbances, headache, and fatigue.

Gastrointestinal: Irritation of the mucous membranes, anorexia, abdominal pain, and nausea.
Eye: Chemical conjunctivitis, increased eye discharge, and swelling of the eyelids.
Skin: Acneform dermatitis (chloracne) and edema of the face and hands.
Hepatic: Liver damage with or without jaundice, hypercholesterolemia, and hypertriglyceridemia have been observed.
Other: Products may present a human carcinogenic and reproductive risk (controversial) in humans.

SYMPTOM ONSET FOR ACUTE EXPOSURE

Most symptoms delayed

CO-EXPOSURE CONCERNS

Carbon tetrachloride

THERMAL DECOMPOSITION PRODUCTS INCLUDE

Polychlorinated dibenzo-para-dioxins (PCDDs)
Polychlorinated dibenzofurans (PCDFs)
Chloride fumes

MEDICAL CONDITIONS POSSIBLY AGGRAVATED BY EXPOSURE

Central nervous system disorders
Liver disorders

DECONTAMINATION

- Wear positive-pressure SCBA and protective equipment specified by references such as the *North American Emergency Response Guidebook*. If special chemical protective clothing is required, consult the chemical manufacturer or specific protective clothing compatibility charts. A qualified, experienced person should make decisions regarding the type of personal protective equipment necessary.
- Delay entry until trained personnel and proper protective equipment are available.
- Remove patient from contaminated area.
- Quickly remove and isolate patient's clothing, jewelry, and shoes.
- Gently blot excess liquids with absorbent material.
- Rinse patient with warm water, 32° C to 35° C (90° F to 95° F), if possible.
- Wash patient with a mild liquid soap and large quantities of water.
- Products may be extremely difficult to remove from the skin. Multiple washes may be necessary.
- Refer to decontamination protocol in Section Three.

IMMEDIATE FIRST AID

- Ensure that adequate decontamination has been carried out.
- If patient is not breathing, start artificial respiration, preferably with a demand-valve resuscitator, bag-valve-mask device, or pocket mask, as trained. Perform CPR if necessary.
- Immediately flush contaminated eyes with gently flowing water.
- Do not induce vomiting. If vomiting occurs, lean patient forward or place on left side (head-down position, if possible) to maintain an open airway and prevent aspiration.
- Keep patient quiet and maintain normal body temperature.
- Obtain medical attention.

BASIC TREATMENT

- Establish a patent airway (oropharyngeal or nasopharyngeal airway, if needed). Suction if necessary.
- Watch for signs of respiratory insufficiency and assist ventilations if necessary.
- Administer oxygen by nonrebreather mask at 10 to 15 L/min.
- For eye contamination, flush eyes immediately with water. Irrigate each eye continuously with 0.9% saline (NS) during transport (refer to eye irrigation protocol in Section Three).
- Do not use emetics. For ingestion, rinse mouth and administer 5 ml/kg up to 200 ml of water for dilution if the patent can swallow, has a strong gag reflex, and does not drool. Administer activated charcoal (refer to ingestion protocol in Section Three and activated charcoal protocol in Section Four).
- Cover skin irritation with dry sterile dressings after decontamination.

ADVANCED TREATMENT

- Consider orotracheal or nasotracheal intubation for airway control in the patient who is unconscious or is in severe respiratory distress.
- Monitor cardiac rhythm and treat arrhythmias if necessary (refer to cardiac protocol in Section Three).
- Start IV administration of 0.9% saline (NS) or lactated Ringer's (LR) TKO. Watch for signs of fluid overload.
- Use proparacaine hydrochloride to assist eye irrigation (refer to proparacaine hydrochloride protocol in Section Four).

INITIAL EMERGENCY DEPARTMENT CONSIDERATIONS

- Useful initial laboratory studies include complete blood count, serum electrolytes, blood urea nitrogen (BUN), creatinine, glucose, urinalysis, and baseline biochemical profile, including serum aminotransferases (ALT and AST), calcium, phosphorus, and magnesium. Arterial blood gases (ABGs), chest radiograph, and electrocardiogram may be required.
- Following massive acute exposure, PCB serum concentrations may be helpful in assessing absorption. Adipose tissue biopsy measurements are more useful in evaluation of chronic exposures.
- Obtain toxicological consultation as necessary.

SPECIAL CONSIDERATIONS

- Since most signs and symptoms will be delayed, exposures will need little acute therapy. Treatment should be aimed at decontamination and emergency care of the eyes.
- Medical counseling for exposure patients concerning reproductive and carcinogenic risk is beneficial.

Nitrates, Nitrites, and Related Compounds

SUBSTANCE IDENTIFICATION

Colorless to pale yellow liquid or solid. Used as fertilizers, pharmaceuticals, food preservatives; in metal treatment and finishing; as anticorrosion inhibitors; and in the manufacturing process of a variety of products. When mixed with organic compounds, many of these products may create flammable or explosive compounds.

ROUTES OF EXPOSURE

Skin and eye contact
Inhalation
Ingestion
Skin absorption

TARGET ORGANS

Primary
Skin
Eyes
Central nervous system
Cardiovascular system
Blood
Secondary
Respiratory system
Gastrointestinal system

LIFE THREAT

Products may cause methemoglobinemia, hypotension, and/or circulatory collapse.

SIGNS AND SYMPTOMS BY SYSTEM

Cardiovascular: Cardiovascular collapse secondary to vasodilation and arrhythmias; tachycardia followed by bradycardia, rapid fall in blood pressure and orthostatic hypotension.

Respiratory: Tachypnea and dyspnea. A slowed respiratory rate may be observed in late stages of toxicity.

CNS: Headache, dizziness, visual disturbances, roaring in the ears, seizures, syncope, coma, and a generalized tingling sensation (paresthesia).

Gastrointestinal: Nausea, vomiting, diarrhea, and abdominal pain.

Eye: Chemical conjunctivitis.

Skin: Flushed or extreme cyanosis with profuse sweating.

Blood: Methemoglobinemia.

SYMPTOM ONSET FOR ACUTE EXPOSURE

Immediate

CO-EXPOSURE CONCERNS

Alcohols

Organophosphates/carbamates
Hydrocarbon solvents

THERMAL DECOMPOSITION PRODUCTS INCLUDE

Nitrites
Nitrogen oxides

MEDICAL CONDITIONS POSSIBLY AGGRAVATED BY EXPOSURE

Respiratory disorders
Cardiac arrhythmias
Trauma

DECONTAMINATION

- Wear positive-pressure SCBA and protective equipment specified by references such as the *North American Emergency Response Guidebook.* If special chemical protective clothing is required, consult the chemical manufacturer or specific protective clothing compatibility charts. A qualified, experienced person should make decisions regarding the type of personal protective equipment necessary.
- Delay entry until trained personnel and proper protective equipment are available.
- Remove patient from contaminated area.
- Quickly remove and isolate patient's clothing, jewelry, and shoes.
- Gently brush away any dry particles and blot excess liquids with absorbent material.
- Rinse patient with warm water, 32° C to 35° C (90° F to 95° F), if possible.
- Wash patient with a mild liquid soap and large quantities of water.
- Refer to decontamination protocol in Section Three.

IMMEDIATE FIRST AID

- Ensure that adequate decontamination has been carried out.
- If patient is not breathing, start artificial respiration, preferably with a demand-valve resuscitator, bag-valve-mask device, or pocket mask, as trained. Perform CPR as necessary.
- Immediately flush contaminated eyes with gently flowing water.
- Do not induce vomiting. If vomiting occurs, lean patient forward or place on left side (head-down position, if possible) to maintain an open airway and prevent aspiration.
- Keep patient quiet and maintain normal body temperature.
- Obtain medical attention.

BASIC TREATMENT

- Establish a patent airway (oropharyngeal or nasopharyngeal airway, if needed). Suction if necessary.
- Watch for signs of respiratory insufficiency and assist ventilations if necessary.
- Administer oxygen by nonrebreather mask at 10 to 15 L/min.
- Monitor for shock and treat if necessary (refer to shock protocol in Section Three).
- Anticipate seizures and treat as necessary (refer to seizure protocol in Section Three).
- For eye contamination, flush eyes immediately with water. Irrigate each eye continuously with 0.9% saline (NS) during transport (refer to eye irrigation protocol in Section Three).

- Do not use emetics. For ingestion, rinse mouth and administer 5 ml/kg up to 200 ml of water for dilution if the patient can swallow, has a strong gag reflex, and does not drool. Administer activated charcoal (refer to ingestion protocol in Section Three and activated charcoal protocol in Section Four).

ADVANCED TREATMENT

- Consider orotracheal or nasotracheal intubation for airway control in the patient who is unconscious or is in severe respiratory distress.
- Monitor cardiac rhythm and treat arrhythmias if necessary (refer to cardiac protocol in Section Three).
- Start IV administration of D_5W TKO. Use 0.9% saline (NS) or lactated Ringer's (LR) if signs of hypovolemia are present. For hypotension with signs of hypovolemia, administer fluid cautiously. If unresponsive to these measures, vasopressors may be helpful. Watch for signs of fluid overload (refer to shock protocol in Section Three).
- Treat seizures with diazepam (Valium) or lorazepam (Ativan) (refer to diazepam and lorazepam protocols in Section Four and seizure protocol in Section Three).
- Administer 1% solution methylene blue if patient is symptomatic with severe hypoxia, cyanosis, and cardiac compromise not responding to oxygen. DIRECT PHYSICIAN ORDER ONLY (refer to methylene blue protocol in Section Four).
- Use proparacaine hydrochloride to assist eye irrigation (refer to proparacaine hydrochloride protocol in Section Four).

INITIAL EMERGENCY DEPARTMENT CONSIDERATIONS

- Useful initial laboratory studies include complete blood count, serum electrolytes, blood urea nitrogen (BUN), creatinine, glucose, urinalysis, and baseline biochemical profile, including serum aminotransferases (ALT and AST), calcium, phosphorus, and magnesium. Arterial blood gases (ABGs), chest radiograph, and electrocardiogram may be required.
- Monitor blood methemoglobin levels and treat with methylene blue if patient is symptomatic and/or has a blood methemoglobin level greater than 30%. DIRECT PHYSICIAN ORDER ONLY (refer to methylene blue protocol in Section Four).
- Hyperbaric oxygen may be helpful.
- Obtain toxicological consultation as necessary.

SPECIAL CONSIDERATIONS

- Withdrawal from chronic occupational (usually longer than 1 year) nitrate/nitrite exposure may cause coronary vasospasm in the absence of atherosclerosis. This condition mimics ischemic heart disease. Therefore the use of epinephrine and other sympathomimetic compounds should be administered with caution.
- Pulse oximetry readings may not be accurate in these exposures.

48

Nitrogen Oxides (NO_x) and Related Compounds

SUBSTANCE IDENTIFICATION

Can be found in gas, liquid, or solid form. Most gases are colorless to brown with a sharp odor. Used as chemical warfare and personal protection agents, propellant fuels, and agricultural fumigants. Others are used in laboratory research and as solvents, bleaching agents, and refrigerants. They may be released from the combustion or decomposition of substances that contain nitrogen. Toxic exposure symptoms may result from working in grain silos ("silo filler's disease"). Some products may ignite other combustible materials. Nitrous oxide (N_2O) is used as an anesthetic gas.

ROUTES OF EXPOSURE

Skin and eye contact
Inhalation
Ingestion
Skin absorption (rare)

TARGET ORGANS

Primary
Skin
Eyes
Cardiovascular system
Respiratory system
Blood
Secondary
Central nervous system
Gastrointestinal system

LIFE THREAT

As a result of poor water solubility, lower respiratory tract symptoms predominate: pulmonary edema, laryngospasm, bronchospasm, and asphyxiation.

SIGNS AND SYMPTOMS BY SYSTEM

Cardiovascular: Cardiovascular collapse with a rapid and weak pulse, reflex bradycardia.

Respiratory: Dyspnea, cough, laryngospasm, bronchospasm, wheezing, chest pain, chemical pneumonitis, pulmonary edema, and upper airway obstruction from edema of the glottis. With most agents, a mild and transient cough is the only symptom at the time of exposure. Onset of dyspnea, rapid respirations, violent coughing, and pulmonary edema usually are delayed. Some agents work immediately on the upper airway, resulting in chest pain, choking, and spasm of the glottis, which may result in a temporary apneic period.

CNS: Fatigue, restlessness, and decreasing level of consciousness are usually delayed signs.

Gastrointestinal: Burning/irritation of the mucous membranes, nausea, vomiting, and abdominal pain.
Eye: Chemical conjunctivitis.
Skin: Irritation of moist skin areas, pallor, and cyanosis.
Blood: Methemoglobinemia (usually mild).
Other: Olfactory fatigue. Some products may present a human carcinogenic risk.

SYMPTOM ONSET FOR ACUTE EXPOSURE

Immediate
Pulmonary edema symptoms possibly delayed for 4 to 12 hours
Other respiratory symptoms possibly delayed
CNS symptoms possibly delayed

CO-EXPOSURE CONCERNS

Carbon monoxide
Simple asphyxiants
Nitrates/nitrites

THERMAL DECOMPOSITION PRODUCTS INCLUDE

Nitrogen oxides

MEDICAL CONDITIONS POSSIBLY AGGRAVATED BY EXPOSURE

Respiratory system disorders

DECONTAMINATION

- Wear positive-pressure SCBA and protective equipment specified by references such as the *North American Emergency Response Guidebook*. If special chemical protective clothing is required, consult the chemical manufacturer or specific protective clothing compatibility charts. A qualified, experienced person should make decisions regarding the type of personal protective equipment necessary.
- Delay entry until trained personnel and proper protective equipment are available.
- Remove patient from contaminated area.
- Quickly remove and isolate patient's clothing, jewelry, and shoes.
- Gently brush away any dry particles and blot excess liquids with absorbent material.
- Rinse patient with warm water, 32° C to 35° C (90° F to 95° F), if possible.
- Wash patient with a mild liquid soap and large quantities of water.
- Refer to decontamination protocol in Section Three.

IMMEDIATE FIRST AID

- Ensure that adequate decontamination has been carried out.
- If patient is not breathing, start artificial respiration, preferably with a demand-valve resuscitator, bag-valve-mask device, or pocket mask, as trained. Perform CPR if necessary.
- Immediately flush contaminated eyes with gently flowing water.
- Do not induce vomiting. If vomiting occurs, lean patient forward or place on left side (head-down position, if possible) to maintain an open airway and prevent aspiration.
- Keep patient quiet and maintain normal body temperature.
- Obtain medical attention.

BASIC TREATMENT

- Establish a patent airway (oropharyngeal or nasopharyngeal airway, if needed). Suction if necessary.

- Aggressive airway management may be needed.
- Encourage patient to take deep breaths.
- Watch for signs of respiratory insufficiency and assist ventilations if necessary.
- Administer oxygen by nonrebreather mask at 10 to 15 L/min.
- Monitor for pulmonary edema and treat if necessary (refer to pulmonary edema protocol in Section Three).
- Monitor for shock and treat if necessary (refer to shock protocol in Section Three).
- For eye contamination, flush eyes immediately with water. Irrigate each eye continuously with 0.9% saline (NS) during transport (refer to eye irrigation protocol in Section Three).
- Do not use emetics. For ingestion, rinse mouth and administer 5 ml/kg up to 200 ml of water for dilution if the patient can swallow, has a strong gag reflex, and does not drool. Administer activated charcoal (refer to ingestion protocol in Section Three and activated charcoal protocol in Section Four).

ADVANCED TREATMENT

- Consider orotracheal or nasotracheal intubation for airway control in the patient who is unconscious, has severe pulmonary edema, or is in severe respiratory distress. Early intubation at the first signs of upper airway obstruction may be necessary.
- Positive-pressure ventilation techniques with a bag-valve-mask device may be beneficial.
- Consider drug therapy for pulmonary edema (refer to pulmonary edema protocol in Section Three).
- Considering administering a beta agonist such as albuterol for severe bronchospasm (refer to albuterol protocol in Section Four).
- Monitor cardiac rhythm and treat arrhythmias as necessary (refer to cardiac protocol in Section Three).
- Start IV administration of D_5W TKO. Consider the use of vasopressors if patient is hypotensive with a normal fluid volume. Watch for signs of fluid overload (refer to shock protocol in Section Three).
- Administer 1% solution methylene blue if patient is symptomatic with severe hypoxia, cyanosis, and cardiac compromise not responding to oxygen. DIRECT PHYSICIAN ORDER ONLY (refer to methylene blue protocol in Section Four).
- Use proparacaine hydrochloride to assist eye irrigation (refer to proparacaine hydrochloride protocol in Section Four).

INITIAL EMERGENCY DEPARTMENT CONSIDERATIONS

- Useful initial laboratory studies include complete blood count, serum electrolytes, blood urea nitrogen (BUN), creatinine, glucose, urinalysis, and baseline biochemical profile including serum aminotransferases (ALT and AST), calcium, phosphorus, and magnesium. Arterial blood gases (ABGs), chest radiograph, and electrocardiogram may be required.
- Monitor blood methemoglobin levels and treat with methylene blue if patient is symptomatic and/or has a blood methemoglobin level greater than 30%. DIRECT PHYSICIAN ORDER ONLY (refer to methylene blue protocol in Section Four).

- Positive end-expiratory pressure (PEEP)–assisted ventilation may be necessary in patients with acute parenchymal injury who develop pulmonary edema or acute respiratory distress syndrome.
- Bronchospastic symptoms should be treated with an inhalation medication regimen similar to that used for reactive airway disease. Inhaled corticosteroids may be of value in severe bronchospasm.
- Obtain toxicological consultation as necessary.

SPECIAL CONSIDERATIONS

- In most cases of mild exposure, symptoms are self-limited and require supportive management only. Use of medications such as atropine, epinephrine, expectorants, and sedatives is not indicated and may cause further damage.
- Treat severe symptomatic exposures as required.
- Besides its role as an environmental poison, nitric oxide (NO) is also synthesized in the body by two enzyme systems to function as a physiologic messenger in the immune, cardiovascular, and neurological systems. It is metabolized to nitrite after its messenger function is complete. The exact role of nitric oxide in health and disease requires further study.
- Pulse oximetry readings may not be accurate in these exposures.

49

Organophosphates and Related Compounds

SUBSTANCE IDENTIFICATION

Found as liquids, dusts, wettable powders, concentrates, and aerosols with a garlic-type odor. Used as insecticides. Products are among the most poisonous commonly used for pest control. Related to chemical warfare agents soman, sarin, and tabun.

ROUTES OF EXPOSURE

Skin and eye contact
Inhalation
Ingestion
Skin absorption

TARGET ORGANS

Primary
Central nervous system
Cardiovascular system
Respiratory system

Secondary
Skin
Eyes
Gastrointestinal system
Hepatic system
Metabolism

LIFE THREAT

Respiratory failure caused by chemically mediated pulmonary edema and respiratory muscle paralysis. Inhibits acetylcholinesterase, causing over-stimulation of parasympathetic nervous system, striated muscle, sympathetic ganglia, and CNS. Causes bradycardia, hypotension, and pulmonary edema.

SIGNS AND SYMPTOMS BY SYSTEM

Cardiovascular: Bradycardia (tachycardia possible), ventricular arrhythmias, A-V blocks, and hypotension.

Respiratory: Respiratory failure, bronchoconstriction, profuse pulmonary secretions (bronchorrhea), acute pulmonary edema, dyspnea, and tightness of the chest.

CNS: CNS depression, coma, anxiety, headache, dizziness, weakness, loss of muscle coordination, muscle fasciculations, seizures, disorientation, confusion, drowsiness, and slurred speech.

Gastrointestinal: Nausea, vomiting, diarrhea, abdominal cramps; excessive salivation, urination, and defecation.

Eye: Lacrimation, blurred vision. Constricted pupils are common; however, dilated pupils may be present.

Skin: Pale, cyanotic skin with excessive diaphoresis.

Hepatic: Liver damage.

Metabolism: Hypoglycemia or hyperglycemia, and acidosis.

Other: Hypothermia may occur. Classic SLUDGE syndrome (*s*alivation, *l*acrimation, *u*rination, *d*efecation, GI pain, and *e*mesis). May range from flu-type symptoms to anxiety, seizures, and coma. Symptoms may be broken down into muscarinic effects (classic SLUDGE syndrome, cardiac effects, constricted pupils, bronchoconstriction, pulmonary edema) and nicotinic symptoms (muscle fasciculations, tachycardia, hypertension, respiratory paralysis). If dermal absorption and nicotinic receptors are the primary sites of stimulation, the SLUDGE syndrome may not be clinically present. Instead, cardiovascular collapse may be the primary clinical manifestation. Cholinesterase inhibitor exposures may be cumulative. Symptoms in children may differ from those found in adults. Pediatric signs and symptoms include CNS depression, flaccid muscle tone, dyspnea, and coma. Many of these products use a hydrocarbon as a solvent vehicle. Identify the solvent and consult the appropriate guideline for related toxic effects.

SYMPTOM ONSET FOR ACUTE EXPOSURE

Immediate

Some symptoms possibly delayed

After initial treatment, possible recurrence of symptoms several days to a week later

CO-EXPOSURE CONCERNS

Carbamates

Insecticide solvent

THERMAL DECOMPOSITION PRODUCTS INCLUDE

Carbon monoxide

Nitrogen oxides

Phosphorus oxides

Sulfur oxides

MEDICAL CONDITIONS POSSIBLY AGGRAVATED BY EXPOSURE

Respiratory disorders

Neurological disorders

DECONTAMINATION

- Wear positive-pressure SCBA and protective equipment specified by references such as the *North American Emergency Response Guidebook*. If special chemical protective clothing is required, consult the chemical manufacturer or specific protective clothing compatibility charts. A qualified, experienced person should make decisions regarding the type of personal protective equipment necessary.
- Delay entry until trained personnel and proper protective equipment are available.
- Remove patient from contaminated area.
- Quickly remove and isolate patient's clothing, jewelry, and shoes.
- Gently brush away any dry particles and blot any excess liquids with absorbent material.
- Rinse patient with warm water, 32° C to 35° C (90° F to 95° F), if possible.
- Wash patient with a mild liquid soap and large quantities of water.
- Products are highly absorbable, and decontamination is critical.
- Discard all exposed leather products.
- Refer to decontamination protocol in Section Three.

IMMEDIATE FIRST AID

- Ensure that adequate decontamination has been carried out.
- If patient is not breathing, start artificial respiration, preferably with a demand-valve resuscitator, bag-valve-mask device, or pocket mask, as trained. Perform CPR if necessary.
- Immediately flush contaminated eyes with gently flowing water.
- Do not induce vomiting. If vomiting occurs, lean patient forward or place on left side (head-down position, if possible) to maintain an open airway and prevent aspiration.
- Keep patient quiet and maintain normal body temperature.
- Obtain medical attention.

BASIC TREATMENT

- Establish a patent airway (oropharyngeal or nasopharyngeal airway, if needed). Suction if necessary.
- Aggressive airway control may be needed.
- Watch for signs of respiratory insufficiency and assist ventilations if necessary.
- Administer oxygen by nonrebreather mask at 10 to 15 L/min.
- Monitor for pulmonary edema and treat if necessary (refer to pulmonary edema protocol in Section Three).
- Monitor for shock and treat if necessary (refer to shock protocol in Section Three).
- Anticipate seizures and treat if necessary (refer to seizure protocol in Section Three).
- For eye contamination, flush eyes immediately with water. Irrigate each eye continuously with 0.9% saline (NS) during transport (refer to eye irrigation protocol in Section Three).
- Do not use emetics. For ingestion, rinse mouth and administer 5 ml/kg up to 200 ml of water for dilution if the patient can swallow, has a strong gag reflex, and does not drool. Administer activated charcoal (refer to ingestion protocol in Section Three and activated charcoal protocol in Section Four).

ADVANCED TREATMENT

- Consider orotracheal or nasotracheal intubation for airway control in the patient who is unconscious, has severe pulmonary edema, or is in severe respiratory distress.
- Positive-pressure ventilation techniques with a bag-valve-mask device may be beneficial.
- Monitor cardiac rhythm and treat arrhythmias if necessary (refer to cardiac protocol in Section Three).
- Start IV administration of D_5W TKO. Use 0.9% saline (NS) or lactated Ringer's (LR) if signs of hypovolemia are present. For hypotension with signs of hypovolemia, administer fluid cautiously and consider vasopressors if patient is hypotensive with a normal fluid volume. Watch for signs of fluid overload (refer to shock protocol in Section Three).
- Administer atropine. Correct hypoxia before giving atropine (refer to atropine protocol in Section Four).
- Administer pralidoxime chloride (2-PAM). UNDER DIRECT PHYSICIAN ORDERS ONLY (refer to pralidoxime chloride protocol in Section Four).

- Treat seizures with adequate atropinization and correction of hypoxia. In rare cases diazepam (Valium) or lorazepam (Ativan) may be necessary (refer to diazepam and lorazepam protocols in Section Four and seizure protocol in Section Three).
- Use proparacaine hydrochloride to assist eye irrigation (refer to proparacaine hydrochloride protocol in Section Four).

INITIAL EMERGENCY DEPARTMENT CONSIDERATIONS

- Useful initial laboratory studies include complete blood count, serum electrolytes, blood urea nitrogen (BUN), creatinine, glucose, urinalysis, and baseline biochemical profile, including serum aminotransferases (ALT and AST), calcium, phosphorus, and magnesium. Arterial blood gases (ABGs), chest radiograph, and electrocardiogram may be required.
- Both plasma and red blood cell acetylcholinesterase levels should be obtained. Do not delay therapeutic interventions pending laboratory results. Treat symptomatically.
- Positive end-expiratory pressure (PEEP)–assisted ventilation may be necessary in patients with acute parenchymal injury who develop pulmonary edema or acute respiratory distress syndrome.
- Products may cause acidosis; hyperventilation and sodium bicarbonate may be beneficial. Bicarbonate therapy should be guided by patient presentation, ABG determination, and serum electrolyte considerations.
- In cases of skin absorption and primary nicotinic stimulation, atropine may not reverse the respiratory paralysis. Be prepared to assist ventilations and administer 2-PAM. Initial symptoms may be diaphoresis, muscle fasciculations, and respiratory arrest.
- Depending on clinical symptoms, 2-PAM will be most effective if administered within 24 to 48 hours after exposure. After this time the organophosphate-acetylcholinesterase complex may "age" (develop an irreversible covalent bond) (refer to pralidoxime chloride protocol in Section Four).
- Obtain toxicological consultation as necessary.

SPECIAL CONSIDERATIONS

- Three clinical syndromes of organophosphate toxicity have been described: immediate, intermediate (1 to 4 days), and delayed (8 to 14 days) after exposure.
- Succinylcholine, other cholinergic agents, and aminophylline are contraindicated.
- Preservative-free atropine should be used to avoid toxicity from preservative agents.
- Mydriasis should not be used to determine the endpoint of atropine administration; the endpoint for atropine administration is the drying of pulmonary secretions.
- Immediate or delayed ascending paralysis (dying-back axonopathy) starting in the lower extremities may occur. This may be confused with Guillain-Barré syndrome.
- Parathion and possibly other organophosphate insecticide residues may persist in clothing, despite repeated laundering.

50

Carbamates and Related Compounds

SUBSTANCE IDENTIFICATION

Found in solid, powder, or liquid form with a white to gray color and a weak odor. Reversible cholinesterase inhibitors, found in insecticides and herbicides. Products may be dissolved in hydrocarbon solvents and have concomitant hydrocarbon exposure effects.

ROUTES OF EXPOSURE

Skin and eye contact
Inhalation
Ingestion
Skin absorption

TARGET ORGANS

Primary
Central nervous system
Cardiovascular system
Respiratory system
Secondary
Skin
Eyes
Gastrointestinal system

LIFE THREAT

Reversible inhibitor of acetylcholinesterase. Causes bradycardia, hypotension, paralysis of the respiratory muscles, respiratory arrest, and chemically mediated pulmonary edema.

SIGNS AND SYMPTOMS BY SYSTEM

Cardiovascular: Bradycardia, ventricular arrhythmias, hypotension. Tachycardia and disseminated intravascular coagulation may occur.

Respiratory: Bronchoconstriction, profuse bronchial secretions (bronchorrhea) with dyspnea, upper airway irritation, tightness of the chest, and paralysis of respiratory muscles. Chemically mediated pulmonary edema.

CNS: CNS depression and coma. Headache, slurred speech, dizziness, weakness, loss of muscle coordination, muscle fasciculations, and seizures.

Gastrointestinal: Nausea, vomiting, diarrhea, abdominal cramps; excessive salivation, urination, and defecation.

Eye: Lacrimation, blurred vision, and constricted pupils.

Skin: Pale, cyanotic skin with excessive diaphoresis.

Other: Classic SLUDGE syndrome (*s*alivation, *l*acrimation, *u*rination, *d*efecation, GI pain, and *e*mesis). May range from flu-type symptoms to anxiety, seizures, and coma. Symptoms may be broken down into muscarinic effects (classic SLUDGE syndrome, cardiac effects, constricted pupils, bronchoconstriction, pulmonary edema) and nicotinic symptoms (muscle fasciculations, tachycardia, hypertension, respiratory paralysis). If dermal absorption and nicotinic receptor sites are the primary site of stimulation, the SLUDGE syndrome may not be clinically present; instead, cardiovascular collapse may be the primary clinical manifestation. Cholinesterase inhibitor exposures may be accumulative. Symptoms in children may differ from those found in adults. Pediatric signs and symptoms include CNS depression, flaccid muscle tone, dyspnea, and coma. Many of these products use a hydrocarbon as a solvent vehicle. Identify the solvent and consult the appropriate guideline for related toxic effects.

SYMPTOM ONSET FOR ACUTE EXPOSURE

Immediate
Depending on absorption rate, some symptoms possibly delayed

CO-EXPOSURE CONCERNS

Organophosphates
Other carbamates
Insecticide solvent vehicle

THERMAL DECOMPOSITION PRODUCTS INCLUDE

Carbon monoxide
Methylamine
Methyl isocyanate
Nitrogen oxides

MEDICAL CONDITIONS POSSIBLY AGGRAVATED BY EXPOSURE

Respiratory disorders
Neurological disorders

DECONTAMINATION

- Wear positive-pressure SCBA and protective equipment specified by references such as the *North American Emergency Response Guidebook*. If special chemical protective clothing is required, consult the chemical manufacturer or specific protective clothing compatibility charts. A qualified, experienced person should make decisions regarding the type of personal protective equipment necessary.
- Delay entry until trained personnel and proper protective equipment are available.
- Remove patient from contaminated area.
- Quickly remove and isolate patient's clothing, jewelry, and shoes.
- Gently brush away dry particles and blot excess liquids with absorbent material.
- Rinse patient with warm water, 32° C to 35° C (90° F to 95° F), if possible.
- Wash patient with a mild liquid soap and large quantities of water.
- Products are highly absorbable; decontamination is critical.
- Discard all leather products.
- Refer to decontamination protocol in Section Three.

IMMEDIATE FIRST AID

- Ensure that adequate decontamination has been carried out.
- If patient is not breathing, start artificial respiration, preferably with a demand-valve resuscitator, bag-valve-mask device or pocket mask, as trained. Perform CPR if necessary.
- Immediately flush contaminated eyes with gently flowing water.

- Do not induce vomiting. If vomiting occurs, lean patient forward or place on left side (head-down position, if possible) to maintain an open airway and prevent aspiration.
- Keep patient quiet and maintain normal body temperature.
- Obtain medical attention.

BASIC TREATMENT

- Establish a patent airway (oropharyngeal or nasopharyngeal airway, if needed). Suction if necessary.
- Aggressive airway management may be needed.
- Watch for signs of respiratory insufficiency and assist ventilations if necessary.
- Administer oxygen by nonrebreather mask at 10 to 15 L/min.
- Monitor for shock and treat if necessary (refer to shock protocol in Section Three).
- Monitor for pulmonary edema and treat if necessary (refer to pulmonary edema protocol in Section Three).
- Anticipate seizures and treat if necessary (refer to seizure protocol in Section Three).
- For eye contamination, flush eyes immediately with water. Irrigate each eye continuously with 0.9% saline (NS) during transport (refer to eye irrigation protocol in Section Three).
- Do not use emetics. For ingestion, rinse mouth and administer 5 ml/kg up to 200 ml of water for dilution if the patient can swallow, has a strong gag reflex, and does not drool. Administer activated charcoal (refer to ingestion protocol in Section Three and activated charcoal protocol in Section Four).

ADVANCED TREATMENT

- Consider orotracheal or nasotracheal intubation for airway control in the patient who is unconscious, has severe pulmonary edema, or is in severe respiratory distress.
- Positive-pressure ventilation techniques with a bag-valve-mask device may be beneficial.
- Monitor cardiac rhythm and treat arrhythmias if necessary (refer to cardiac protocol in Section Three).
- Start IV administration of D_5W TKO. Use 0.9% saline (NS) or lactated Ringer's (LR) if signs of hypovolemia are present. For hypotension with signs of hypovolemia, administer fluid cautiously. Watch for signs of fluid overload (refer to shock protocol in Section Three).
- Administer atropine. Correct hypoxia before administration (refer to atropine protocol in Section Four).
- In severely poisoned patients, administer pralidoxime chloride (2-PAM). DIRECT PHYSICIAN ORDERS ONLY (refer to pralidoxime chloride protocol in Section Four).
- Treat seizures with adequate atropinization and correction of hypoxia. In rare cases diazepam (Valium) or lorazepam (Ativan) may be necessary (refer to diazepam and lorazepam protocols in Section Four and seizure protocol in Section Three).
- Use proparacaine hydrochloride to assist eye irrigation (refer to proparacaine hydrochloride protocol in Section Four).

INITIAL EMERGENCY DEPARTMENT CONSIDERATIONS

- Useful initial laboratory studies include complete blood count, serum electrolytes, blood urea nitrogen (BUN), creatinine, glucose, urinalysis, and baseline biochemical profile, including serum aminotransferases (ALT and AST), calcium, phosphorus, and magnesium. Arterial blood gases (ABGs), chest radiograph, and electrocardiogram may be required.
- Both plasma and red blood cell acetylcholinesterase levels should be obtained. Do not delay therapeutic interventions pending laboratory results.
- Positive end-expiratory pressure (PEEP)–assisted ventilation may be necessary in patients with acute parenchymal injury who develop pulmonary edema or acute respiratory distress syndrome.
- Products may cause acidosis; hyperventilation and sodium bicarbonate may be beneficial. Bicarbonate therapy should be guided by patient presentation, ABG determination, and serum electrolyte considerations.
- Depending on clinical symptoms, 2-PAM is most effective if administered within 24 to 48 hours after exposure. Use of 2-PAM is controversial because of self-release of carbamate-acetylcholinesterase bond within 48 hours of poisoning. (Refer to pralidoxime chloride protocol in Section Four).
- Obtain toxicological consultation as necessary.

SPECIAL CONSIDERATIONS

- Succinylcholine, other cholinergic agents, and aminophylline are contraindicated.
- Preservative-free atropine should be used to avoid toxicity from preservative agents.
- Mydriasis should not be used to determine the endpoint of atropine administration; the endpoint for atropine administration is the drying of pulmonary secretions.

51

Nicotine and Related Compounds

SUBSTANCE IDENTIFICATION

Found as a colorless to brown liquid plant alkaloid with a tobacco-like odor. Found in tobacco products, pesticides, and insecticides. Used in tanning processes.

ROUTES OF EXPOSURE

Skin and eye contact
Inhalation
Ingestion
Skin absorption

TARGET ORGANS

Primary
Skin
Eyes
Central nervous system
Cardiovascular system
Respiratory system
Gastrointestinal system
Secondary
Metabolism

LIFE THREAT

Respiratory arrest and cardiac standstill. The alkaloid demonstrates stimulant and depressive action effects.

SIGNS AND SYMPTOMS BY SYSTEM

Cardiovascular: Initial hypertension and bradycardia, followed by tachycardia and hypotension. Cardiac standstill and paroxysmal atrial fibrillation.

Respiratory: Rapid, deep respirations followed by dyspnea, increased bronchial secretions, and paralysis of the respiratory muscles leading to respiratory arrest.

CNS: Agitation followed by headache, dizziness, confusion, muscle tremors/weakness, fasciculations, hyporeflexia, incoordination, auditory and visual disturbances. Seizures.

Gastrointestinal: Nausea, vomiting, diarrhea, abdominal pain, salivation, and burning pain in the throat/mouth.

Eye: Chemical conjunctivitis and lacrimation. Pupils generally constricted (miotic) at first, then dilated (mydriatic).

Skin: Dermatitis and cyanosis.

Metabolism: Respiratory acidosis.

SYMPTOM ONSET FOR ACUTE EXPOSURE

Immediate
Initial stimulation followed by depression

CO-EXPOSURE CONCERNS

Chlorinated hydrocarbon insecticides
Other insecticides, pesticides

THERMAL DECOMPOSITION PRODUCTS INCLUDE

Carbon dioxide
Carbon monoxide
Nitrogen oxides

MEDICAL CONDITIONS POSSIBLY AGGRAVATED BY EXPOSURE

Central nervous system disorders
Cardiovascular system disorders

DECONTAMINATION

- Wear positive-pressure SCBA and protective equipment specified by references such as the *North American Emergency Response Guidebook*. If special chemical protective clothing is required, consult the chemical manufacturer or specific protective clothing compatibility charts. A qualified, experienced person should make decisions regarding the type of personal protective equipment necessary.
- Delay entry until trained personnel and proper protective equipment are available.
- Remove patient from contaminated area.
- Quickly remove and isolate patient's clothing, jewelry, and shoes.
- Gently brush away dry particles and blot excess liquids with absorbent material.
- Rinse patient with warm water, 32° C to 35° C (90° F to 95° F), if possible.
- Wash patient with a mild liquid soap and large quantities of water.
- Refer to decontamination protocol in Section Three.

IMMEDIATE FIRST AID

- Ensure that adequate decontamination has been carried out.
- If patient is not breathing, start artificial respiration, preferably with a demand-valve resuscitator, bag-valve-mask device, or pocket mask, as trained. Perform CPR if necessary.
- Immediately flush contaminated eyes with gently flowing water.
- Do not induce vomiting. If vomiting occurs, lean patient forward or place on left side (head-down position, if possible) to maintain an open airway and prevent aspiration.
- Keep patient quiet and maintain normal body temperature.
- Obtain medical attention.

BASIC TREATMENT

- Establish a patent airway (oropharyngeal or nasopharyngeal airway, if needed). Suction if necessary.
- Aggressive airway management may be needed.
- Watch for signs of respiratory insufficiency and assist ventilations if necessary.
- Administer oxygen by nonrebreather mask at 10 to 15 L/min.
- Anticipate seizures and treat if necessary (refer to seizure protocol in Section Three).
- For eye contamination, flush eyes immediately with water. Irrigate each eye continuously with 0.9% saline (NS) during transport (refer to eye irrigation protocol in Section Three).
- Do not use emetics. For ingestion, rinse mouth and administer 5 ml/kg up to 200 ml of water for dilution if the patient can swallow, has a strong gag reflex,

and does not drool. Administer activated charcoal (refer to ingestion protocol in Section Three and activated charcoal protocol in Section Four).

ADVANCED TREATMENT

- Consider orotracheal or nasotracheal intubation for airway control in the patient who is unconscious or is in severe respiratory distress.
- Monitor cardiac rhythm and treat arrhythmias if necessary (refer to cardiac protocol in Section Three).
- Start IV administration of D_5W TKO. Use 0.9% saline (NS) or lactated Ringer's (LR) if signs of hypovolemia are present. For hypotension with signs of hypovolemia, administer fluid cautiously. Watch for signs of fluid overload (refer to shock protocol in Section Three).
- Treat seizures with diazepam (Valium) or lorazepam (Ativan) (refer to diazepam and lorazepam protocols in Section Four and seizure protocol in Section Three).
- Use proparacaine hydrochloride to assist eye irrigation (refer to proparacaine hydrochloride protocol in Section Four).

INITIAL EMERGENCY DEPARTMENT CONSIDERATIONS

- Useful initial laboratory studies include complete blood count, serum electrolytes, blood urea nitrogen (BUN), creatinine, glucose, urinalysis, and baseline biochemical profile, including serum aminotransferases (ALT and AST), calcium, phosphorus, and magnesium. Determination of anion and osmolar gaps may be helpful. Arterial blood gases (ABGs), chest radiograph, and electrocardiogram may be required.
- Products may cause acidosis; hyperventilation and sodium bicarbonate may be beneficial. Bicarbonate therapy should be guided by patient presentation, ABG determination, and serum electrolyte considerations.
- Atropine may be administered for signs and symptoms of parasympathetic effects (respiratory tract secretions, bradycardia, bronchoconstriction). Adult dosage: 0.5 mg titrated to effect. Correct hypoxia before giving atropine (refer to atropine protocol in Section Four).
- Obtain toxicological consultation as necessary.

Pyrethrins, Pyrethroids, and Related Compounds

SUBSTANCE IDENTIFICATION

Found as a brown resin or solid or as a yellow to brown, viscous liquid. Can be found in powder or spray form. Hydrocarbon solvents are often used as vehicles for the chemical. Used as an insecticide. Most products have a low human toxicity potential. There are numerous natural (pyrethrins) and synthetic (pyrethroids) insecticides. Originally found as compounds extracted from the *Chrysanthemum cinerariaefolium* plant.

ROUTES OF EXPOSURE

Skin and eye contact
Inhalation
Ingestion

TARGET ORGANS

Primary
Skin
Eyes
Central nervous system
Respiratory system
Secondary
Cardiovascular system
Gastrointestinal system

LIFE THREAT

Respiratory paralysis and convulsions. Toxicity from the hydrocarbon solvent.

SIGNS AND SYMPTOMS BY SYSTEM

Cardiovascular: Mild tachycardia, hypotension, and arrhythmias caused by hypoxia.

Respiratory: Dyspnea, wheezing (reactive airway disease picture), sneezing, nasal stuffiness, and discharge. Respiratory failure caused by paralysis.

CNS: Headache, loss of coordination, tinnitus, decreased LOC, coma, seizures, tetanic paralysis, and paresthesias of the extremities may occur.

Gastrointestinal: Nausea, vomiting, and diarrhea.

Eye: Chemical conjunctivitis.

Skin: Contact dermatitis and facial swelling. May be exacerbated by sunlight exposure.

Other: Early symptoms may mimic hay fever symptoms. Toxicity from the solvent may be more acute than the product. Identify the solvent and consult the appropriate guideline. Synthetic pyrethroids with a cyano group are the most toxic compounds of this type.

SYMPTOM ONSET FOR ACUTE EXPOSURES

Immediate
Allergic symptoms possibly delayed

CO-EXPOSURE CONCERNS

Organophosphates
Hydrocarbon solvents

THERMAL DECOMPOSITION PRODUCTS INCLUDE

Carbon monoxide
Carbon dioxide
Acrid smoke and fumes

MEDICAL CONDITIONS POSSIBLY AGGRAVATED BY EXPOSURE

Respiratory system disorders (asthma, allergies)

DECONTAMINATION

- Wear positive-pressure SCBA and protective equipment specified by references such as the *North American Emergency Response Guidebook.* If special chemical protective clothing is required, consult the chemical manufacturer or specific protective clothing compatibility charts. A qualified, experienced person should make decisions regarding the type of personal protective equipment necessary.
- Delay entry until trained personnel and proper protective equipment are available.
- Remove patient from contaminated area.
- Quickly remove and isolate patient's clothing, jewelry, and shoes.
- Gently brush away dry particles and blot excess liquids with absorbent material.
- Rinse patient with warm water, 32° C to 35° C (90° F to 95° F), if possible.
- Wash patient with a mild liquid soap and large quantities of water.
- Refer to decontamination protocol in Section Three.

IMMEDIATE FIRST AID

- Ensure that adequate decontamination has been carried out.
- If patient is not breathing, start artificial respiration, preferably with a demand-valve resuscitator, bag-valve-mask device, or pocket mask, as trained. Perform CPR if necessary.
- Immediately flush contaminated eyes with gently flowing water.
- Do not induce vomiting. If vomiting occurs, lean patient forward or place on left side (head-down position, if possible) to maintain an open airway and prevent aspiration.
- Keep patient quiet and maintain normal body temperature.
- Obtain medical attention.

BASIC TREATMENT

- Establish a patent airway (oropharyngeal or nasopharyngeal airway, if needed). Suction if necessary.
- Watch for signs of respiratory insufficiency and assist ventilations if necessary.
- Administer oxygen by nonrebreather mask at 10 to 15 L/min.
- Anticipate seizures and treat if necessary (refer to seizure protocol in Section Three).
- For eye contamination, flush eyes immediately with water. Irrigate each eye continuously with 0.9% saline (NS) during transport (refer to eye irrigation protocol in Section Three).
- Do not use emetics. For ingestion, rinse mouth and administer 5 mL/kg up to 200 mL of water for dilution if the patient can swallow, has a strong gag reflex, and does not drool. Administer activated charcoal (refer to ingestion protocol in Section Three and activated charcoal protocol in Section Four).

ADVANCED TREATMENT

- Consider orotracheal or nasotracheal intubation for airway control in the patient who is unconscious or is in severe respiratory distress.
- Consider administering a beta agonist such as albuterol for severe bronchospasm (refer to albuterol protocol in Section Four).
- Monitor cardiac rhythm and treat arrhythmias if necessary (refer to cardiac protocol in Section Three).
- Start IV administration of D_5W TKO. Use 0.9% saline (NS) or lactated Ringer's (LR) if signs of hypovolemia are present. For hypotension with signs of hypovolemia, administer fluid cautiously. Watch for signs of fluid overload (refer to shock protocol in Section Three).
- Treat seizures with diazepam (Valium) or lorazepam (Ativan) (refer to diazepam and lorazepam protocols in Section Four and seizure protocol in Section Three).
- Use proparacaine hydrochloride to assist eye irrigation (refer to proparacaine hydrochloride protocol in Section Four).

INITIAL EMERGENCY DEPARTMENT CONSIDERATIONS

- Useful initial laboratory studies include complete blood count, serum electrolytes, blood urea nitrogen (BUN), creatinine, glucose, urinalysis, and baseline biochemical profile, including serum aminotransferases (ALT and AST), calcium, phosphorus, and magnesium. Determination of anion and osmolar gaps may be helpful. Arterial blood gases (ABGs), chest radiograph, and electrocardiogram may be required.
- Bronchospastic symptoms should be treated with an inhalation medication regimen similar to that used for reactive airway disease. Inhaled corticosteroids may be of value in severe bronchospasm.
- Obtain toxicological consultation if necessary.

SPECIAL CONSIDERATIONS

- Toxicity may result from the solvent that is used as a vehicle. Identify the solvent and consult the appropriate guideline.

53

Rotenone and Related Compounds

SUBSTANCE IDENTIFICATION

A colorless to red, odorless solid. May be found in dusts and sprays and as an insecticide and pesticide. Kerosene and naphtha are frequently used as vehicles and may be more hazardous than the product itself.

ROUTES OF EXPOSURE

Skin and eye contact
Inhalation
Ingestion

TARGET ORGANS

Primary
Skin
Eyes
Central nervous system
Respiratory system
Secondary
Cardiovascular system
Gastrointestinal system
Hepatic system
Renal system
Metabolism

LIFE THREAT

Asphyxia from respiratory arrest.

SIGNS AND SYMPTOMS BY SYSTEM

Cardiovascular: Mild tachycardia, congestive heart failure. Arrhythmias and bradycardia may occur.

Respiratory: Irritation of the respiratory tract, pharyngitis, rhinitis, and respiratory paralysis. At first, respiratory stimulation, followed by depression.

CNS: Incoordination, CNS depression, numbness of mouth and tongue, and seizures.

Gastrointestinal: Nausea, vomiting, and abdominal pain.

Eye: Chemical conjunctivitis.

Skin: Dermatitis and cyanosis.

Renal: Kidney damage.

Hepatic: Liver damage.

Metabolism: Acidosis and hypoglycemia.

Other: The chief hazard is found in the solvent used as a vehicle. Identify the solvent and consult the appropriate guideline.

SYMPTOM ONSET FOR ACUTE EXPOSURE

Immediate

CO-EXPOSURE CONCERNS

Kerosene
Naphtha

MEDICAL CONDITIONS POSSIBLY AGGRAVATED BY EXPOSURE

Central nervous system disorders
Liver disorders
Kidney disorders

DECONTAMINATION

- Wear positive-pressure SCBA and protective equipment specified by references such as the *North American Emergency Response Guidebook*. If special chemical protective clothing is required, consult the chemical manufacturer or specific protective clothing compatibility charts. A qualified, experienced person should make decisions regarding the type of personal protective equipment necessary.
- Delay entry until trained personnel and proper protective equipment are available.
- Remove patient from contaminated area.
- Quickly remove and isolate patient's clothing, jewelry, and shoes.
- Gently brush away dry particles and blot excess liquids with absorbent material.
- Rinse patient with warm water, 32° C to 35° C (90° F to 95° F), if possible.
- Wash patient with a mild liquid soap and large quantities of water.
- Refer to decontamination protocol in Section Three.

IMMEDIATE FIRST AID

- Ensure that adequate decontamination has been carried out.
- If patient is not breathing, start artificial respiration, preferably with a demand-valve resuscitator, bag-valve-mask device, or pocket mask, as trained. Perform CPR if necessary.
- Immediately flush contaminated eyes with gently flowing water.
- Do not induce vomiting. If vomiting occurs, lean patient forward or place on left side (head-down position, if possible) to maintain an open airway and prevent aspiration.
- Keep patient quiet and maintain normal body temperature.
- Obtain medical attention.

BASIC TREATMENT

- Establish a patent airway (oropharyngeal or nasopharyngeal airway, if needed). Suction if necessary.
- Watch for signs of respiratory insufficiency and assist ventilations if necessary.
- Administer oxygen by nonrebreather mask at 10 to 15 L/min.
- Anticipate seizures and treat if necessary (refer to seizure protocol in Section Three).
- For eye contamination, flush eyes immediately with water. Irrigate each eye continuously with 0.9% saline (NS) during transport (refer to eye irrigation protocol in Section Three).
- Do not use emetics. For ingestion, rinse mouth and administer 5 ml/kg up to 200 ml of water for dilution if the patient can swallow, has a strong gag reflex, and does not drool. Administer activated charcoal (refer to ingestion protocol in Section Three and activated charcoal protocol in Section Four).

ADVANCED TREATMENT

- Consider orotracheal or nasotracheal intubation for airway control in the patient who is unconscious or is in severe respiratory distress.

- Start IV administration of D_5W TKO. Use 0.9% saline (NS) or lactated Ringer's (LR) if signs of hypovolemia are present. For hypotension with signs of hypovolemia, administer fluid cautiously. Watch for signs of fluid overload (refer to shock protocol in Section Three).
- Treat seizures with diazepam (Valium) or lorazepam (Ativan) (refer to diazepam and lorazepam protocols in Section Four and seizure protocol in Section Three).
- Monitor for signs of hypoglycemia (decreased LOC, tachycardia, pallor, dilated pupils, diaphoresis, and/or dextrose strip or glucometer readings less than 50 mg/dL) and administer 50% dextrose if necessary. Draw blood sample before administration (refer to 50% dextrose protocol in Section Four).
- Use proparacaine hydrochloride to assist eye irrigation (refer to proparacaine hydrochloride protocol in Section Four).

INITIAL EMERGENCY DEPARTMENT CONSIDERATIONS

- Useful initial laboratory studies include complete blood count, serum electrolytes, blood urea nitrogen (BUN), creatinine, glucose, urinalysis, and baseline biochemical profile, including serum aminotransferases (ALT and AST), calcium, phosphorus, and magnesium. Determination of the anion gap may be helpful. Arterial blood gases (ABGs), chest radiograph, and electrocardiogram may be required.
- Products may cause acidosis; hyperventilation and sodium bicarbonate may be beneficial. Bicarbonate therapy should be guided by clinical presentation, ABG determination, and serum electrolyte considerations.
- Obtain toxicological consultation as necessary.

SPECIAL CONSIDERATIONS

- Because of the toxicity of the solvents used with these products, identify the solvent and consult the appropriate guideline.

Chlordane and Related Compounds

SUBSTANCE IDENTIFICATION

Found in solid form as a colorless to light tan waxy substance with a musty odor. In liquid form it can be found as a colorless-to-thick amber liquid with a mild or chlorine-like odor. Also found in dust, emulsifiable concentrate, and granular or wettable powder. Used as termiticides, fumigants, pesticides, and insecticides. The EPA revoked the registration for the commercial production, distribution, sale, and use of chlordane in April 1988.

ROUTES OF EXPOSURE

Skin and eye contact
Inhalation
Ingestion
Skin absorption

TARGET ORGANS

Primary
Skin
Eyes
Central nervous system
Blood
Secondary
Cardiovascular system
Respiratory system
Gastrointestinal system
Hepatic system
Renal system

LIFE THREAT

Death from respiratory failure and exhaustion secondary to seizures.

SIGNS AND SYMPTOMS BY SYSTEM

Cardiovascular: Circulatory collapse with tachycardia and hypotension.
Respiratory: Sudden onset of dyspnea, followed by respiratory failure. Upper respiratory tract irritation, sinusitis, and pneumonia.
CNS: Headache, confusion, fatigue, hyperexcitability, shivering, muscle tremors, spasms of leg/back muscles, and coma. Seizures that can be precipitated by external stimuli and tetanic muscular contractions. Neurobehavioral changes.
Gastrointestinal: Nausea, vomiting, and excessive salivation.
Eye: Chemical conjunctivitis and blurred vision.
Skin: Mild irritation, cyanosis, and dermatitis.
Hepatic: Liver damage.
Renal: Kidney damage.

Blood: Leukocytosis (elevation of white blood count), blood dyscrasias.
Other: Some products may present a human carcinogenic risk.

SYMPTOM ONSET FOR ACUTE EXPOSURES

Immediate
Some symptoms possibly delayed (up to 10 hours)

CO-EXPOSURE CONCERNS

Other organochlorine insecticides

THERMAL DECOMPOSITION PRODUCTS INCLUDE

Carbon monoxide
Chlorine
Hydrogen chloride
Phosgene

MEDICAL CONDITIONS POSSIBLY AGGRAVATED BY EXPOSURE

Central nervous system disorders
Liver disorders
Kidney disorders
Bone marrow disorders

DECONTAMINATION

- Wear positive-pressure SCBA and protective equipment specified by references such as the *North American Emergency Response Guidebook*. If special chemical protective clothing is required, consult the chemical manufacturer or specific protective clothing compatibility charts. A qualified, experienced person should make decisions regarding the type of personal protective equipment necessary.
- Delay entry until trained personnel and proper protective equipment are available.
- Remove patient from contaminated area.
- Quickly remove and isolate patient's clothing, jewelry, and shoes.
- Gently brush away dry particles and blot excess liquids with absorbent material.
- Rinse patient with warm water, 32° C to 35° C (90° F to 95° F), if possible.
- Wash patient with a mild liquid soap and large quantities of water.
- Leather absorbs pesticides and should be isolated and properly disposed of.
- Refer to decontamination protocol in Section Three.

IMMEDIATE FIRST AID

- Ensure that adequate decontamination has been carried out.
- If patient is not breathing, start artificial respiration, preferably with a demand-valve resuscitator, bag-valve-mask device, or pocket mask, as trained. Perform CPR if necessary.
- Immediately flush contaminated eyes with gently flowing water.
- Do not induce vomiting. If vomiting occurs, lean patient forward or place on left side (head-down position, if possible) to maintain an open airway and prevent aspiration.
- Keep patient quiet and maintain normal body temperature.
- Obtain medical attention.

BASIC TREATMENT

- Establish a patent airway (oropharyngeal or nasopharyngeal airway, if needed). Suction if necessary.
- Watch for signs of respiratory insufficiency and assist ventilations if necessary.
- Administer oxygen by nonrebreather mask at 10 to 15 L/min.

- Anticipate seizures, minimize external stimuli, and treat if necessary (refer to seizure protocol in Section Three).
- For eye contamination, flush eyes immediately with water. Irrigate each eye continuously with 0.9% saline (NS) during transport (refer to eye irrigation protocol in Section Three).
- Do not use emetics. For ingestion, rinse mouth and administer 5 ml/kg up to 200 ml of water for dilution if the patient can swallow, has a strong gag reflex, and does not drool. Administer activated charcoal (refer to ingestion protocol in Section Three and activated charcoal protocol in Section Four).

ADVANCED TREATMENT

- Consider orotracheal or nasotracheal intubation for airway control in the patient who is unconscious or is in severe respiratory distress.
- Monitor cardiac rhythm and treat arrhythmias if necessary (refer to cardiac protocol in Section Three).
- Start IV administration of D_5W TKO. Use 0.9% saline (NS) or lactated Ringer's (LR) if signs of hypovolemia are present. For hypotension with signs of hypovolemia, administer fluid cautiously. Watch for signs of fluid overload (refer to shock protocol in Section Three).
- Treat seizures with diazepam (Valium) or lorazepam (Ativan) (refer to diazepam and lorazepam protocols in Section Four and seizure protocol in Section Three).
- Proparacaine hydrochloride should be used to assist eye irrigation (refer to proparacaine hydrochloride protocol in Section Four).

INITIAL EMERGENCY DEPARTMENT CONSIDERATIONS

- Useful initial laboratory studies include complete blood count, serum electrolytes, blood urea nitrogen (BUN), creatinine, glucose, urinalysis, and baseline biochemical profile, including serum aminotransferases (ALT and AST), prothrombin time, calcium, phosphorus, and magnesium. Arterial blood gases (ABGs), chest radiograph, and electrocardiogram may be required.
- Obtain toxicological consultation as necessary.

SPECIAL CONSIDERATIONS

- Avoid epinephrine and related beta agonists (unless in cardiac arrest or reactive airways disease refractory to other treatment) because of the possible irritable condition of the myocardium. Use of these medications may lead to ventricular fibrillation.
- Chlordane and related cyclodiene organochlorine compounds are fat soluble and easily store and accumulate in adipose tissue. Adipose tissue biopsies are required for estimation of body pesticide burden.
- Chlordane has been detected in homes (air and soil) where it was used as a termiticide for up to 15 years after the original application.

55

DDT and Related Compounds

SUBSTANCE IDENTIFICATION

Found as a white to deep gray solid with a fruitlike odor. May be used as a wettable powder, emulsion, or suspension or in solvent or aerosol form. Except for special circumstances, the EPA has severely restricted the use of these products. DDT has an extremely long biological half-life. May have a hydrocarbon vehicle that can cause additional toxic effects.

ROUTES OF EXPOSURE

Skin and eye contact
Inhalation
Ingestion
Skin absorption

TARGET ORGANS

Primary
Skin
Eyes
Central nervous system
Peripheral nervous system
Hepatic system
Renal system
Secondary
Cardiovascular system
Respiratory system
Gastrointestinal system

LIFE THREAT

Ventricular fibrillation, seizures, and respiratory arrest caused by central nervous system disruption and paralysis of the respiratory control center.

SIGNS AND SYMPTOMS BY SYSTEM

Cardiovascular: Circulatory collapse with arrhythmias, tachycardia, hypotension, and, rarely, bradycardia.

Respiratory: Upper respiratory tract irritation. Sudden onset of dyspnea, followed by respiratory failure. Pulmonary edema.

CNS: Headache, anorexia, nausea, fatigue, hyperexcitability, shivering, paresthesias (face, lips, tongue, legs), muscle tremor, and spasms of leg and back muscles. Seizures may be precipitated by external stimuli. Tetanic muscular contractions and neurobehavioral changes.

Gastrointestinal: Nausea, vomiting, and excessive salivation.

Eye: Chemical conjunctivitis and blurred vision.

Skin: Mild irritation, cyanosis, and dermatitis.

Renal: Kidney damage.

Hepatic: Liver damage.

Other: Some products may present a human carcinogenic risk. Oil-based solutions or mixtures are absorbed faster than dusts or powders. Dermal absorption variable by compound. NOTE: Some of these products may be mixed with a hydrocarbon solvent as a vehicle. Toxicity may result from the solvent.

SYMPTOM ONSET FOR ACUTE EXPOSURES

Immediate
Pulmonary edema possibly delayed

CO-EXPOSURE CONCERNS

Other organochlorine compounds

THERMAL DECOMPOSITION PRODUCTS INCLUDE

Hydrogen chloride
Carbon monoxide

MEDICAL CONDITIONS POSSIBLY AGGRAVATED BY EXPOSURE

Nervous system disorders
Liver disorders
Kidney disorders
Skin disorders

DECONTAMINATION

- Wear positive-pressure SCBA and protective equipment specified by references such as the *North American Emergency Response Guidebook.* If special chemical protective clothing is required, consult the chemical manufacturer or specific protective clothing compatibility charts. A qualified, experienced person should make decisions regarding the type of personal protective equipment necessary.
- Delay entry until trained personnel and proper protective equipment are available.
- Remove patient from contaminated area.
- Quickly remove and isolate patient's clothing, jewelry, and shoes.
- Gently brush away dry particles and blot excess liquids with absorbent material.
- Rinse patient with warm water, 32° C to 35° C (90° F to 95° F), if possible.
- Wash patient with a mild liquid soap and large quantities of water.
- Leather absorbs pesticides and should be isolated and properly disposed of.
- Refer to decontamination protocol in Section Three.

IMMEDIATE FIRST AID

- Ensure that adequate decontamination has been carried out.
- If patient is not breathing, start artificial respiration, preferably with a demand-valve resuscitator, bag-valve-mask device, or pocket mask, as trained. Perform CPR if necessary.
- Immediately flush contaminated eyes with gently flowing water.
- Do not induce vomiting. If vomiting occurs, lean patient forward or place on left side (head-down position, if possible) to maintain an open airway and prevent aspiration.
- Keep patient quiet and maintain normal body temperature.
- Obtain medical attention.

BASIC TREATMENT

- Establish a patent airway (oropharyngeal or nasopharyngeal airway, if needed). Suction if necessary.
- Watch for signs of respiratory insufficiency and assist ventilations if necessary.
- Administer oxygen by nonrebreather mask at 10 to 15 L/min.

- Monitor for shock and treat if necessary (refer to shock protocol in Section Three).
- Monitor for signs of pulmonary edema and treat if necessary (refer to pulmonary edema protocol in Section Three).
- Anticipate seizures and treat if necessary (refer to seizure protocol in Section Three).
- For eye contamination, flush eyes immediately with water. Irrigate each eye continuously with 0.9% saline (NS) during transport (refer to eye irrigation protocol in Section Three).
- Do not use emetics. For ingestion, rinse mouth and administer 5 ml/kg up to 200 ml of water for dilution if the patient can swallow, has a strong gag reflex, and does not drool. Administer activated charcoal (refer to ingestion protocol in Section Three and activated charcoal protocol in Section Four).

ADVANCED TREATMENT

- Consider orotracheal or nasotracheal intubation for airway control in the patient who is unconscious or is in severe respiratory distress.
- Positive-pressure ventilation techniques with a bag-valve-mask device may be beneficial.
- Consider drug therapy for pulmonary edema (refer to pulmonary edema protocol in Section Three).
- Monitor and treat cardiac arrhythmias if necessary (refer to cardiac protocol in Section Three).
- Start IV administration of D_5W TKO. Use 0.9% saline (NS) or lactated Ringer's (LR) if signs of hypovolemia are present. For hypotension with signs of hypovolemia, administer fluid cautiously. Watch for signs of fluid overload (refer to shock protocol in Section Three).
- Treat seizures with diazepam (Valium) or lorazepam (Ativan) (refer to diazepam and lorazepam protocols in Section Four and seizure protocol in Section Three).
- Use proparacaine hydrochloride to assist eye irrigation (refer to proparacaine hydrochloride protocol in Section Four).

INITIAL EMERGENCY DEPARTMENT CONSIDERATIONS

- Useful initial laboratory studies include complete blood count, serum electrolytes, blood urea nitrogen (BUN), creatinine, glucose, urinalysis, and baseline biochemical profile, including serum aminotransferases (ALT and AST), calcium, phosphorus, and magnesium. Determination of anion and osmolar gaps may be helpful. Arterial blood gases (ABG), chest radiograph, and electrocardiogram may be required.
- Positive end-expiratory pressure (PEEP)–assisted ventilation may be necessary in patients with acute parenchymal injury who develop pulmonary edema or acute respiratory distress syndrome.
- Obtain toxicological consultation as necessary.

SPECIAL CONSIDERATIONS

- DDT (dichlorodiphenyl trichloroethane) and its primary metabolites DDD and DDE are extremely lipid soluble. These compounds rapidly bioaccumulate in adipose tissue, where they may remain for years.
- Products may have a hydrocarbon vehicle that may add to their toxicity. Identify the solvent and consult the appropriate guideline.

Aldrin, Dieldrin, Endrin, and Related Compounds

SUBSTANCE IDENTIFICATION

Cyclodiene pesticides, found in solid form as a colorless to light tan waxy substance with a musty odor. Used as wettable powders, emulsifiable concentrates, dusts, granules, seed dressings, and solutions. Used as pesticides and insecticides. Use of most products in the United States is allowed on a limited basis. Aldrin is environmentally converted to dieldrin.

ROUTES OF EXPOSURE

Skin and eye contact
Inhalation
Ingestion
Skin absorption

TARGET ORGANS

Primary
Skin
Eyes
Central nervous system
Hepatic system
Renal system
Metabolism
Secondary
Cardiovascular system
Respiratory system
Gastrointestinal system

LIFE THREAT

Seizures and respiratory failure.

SIGNS AND SYMPTOMS BY SYSTEM

Cardiovascular: Increased blood pressure followed by circulatory collapse with tachycardia and hypotension. Myocardial irritability and arrhythmias.

Respiratory: Sudden onset of dyspnea, followed by respiratory failure. Upper respiratory tract irritation and sinusitis.

CNS: Headache, fatigue, apprehension, hyperexcitability, shivering, muscle tremor, spasms of leg/back muscles, and ataxia. Seizures, usually without warning, that may be precipitated by external stimuli. Tetanic muscular contractions and neurobehavioral changes.

Gastrointestinal: Nausea, vomiting, and excessive salivation.

Eye: Chemical conjunctivitis and blurred vision.

Skin: Mild irritation and cyanosis. Dermatitis.

Renal: Kidney damage.

Hepatic: Liver damage.

Metabolism: Metabolic acidosis may occur.

Other: Oil-based solutions are absorbed faster than dusts or powders. NOTE: Some of these products may be mixed with a hydrocarbon solvent as a vehicle. Toxicity may result from the solvent. Some pesticides may present a human carcinogenic risk.

SYMPTOM ONSET FOR ACUTE EXPOSURE

Immediate

Symptoms may be delayed up to 1 hour

CO-EXPOSURE CONCERNS

Other organochlorine compounds

THERMAL DECOMPOSITION PRODUCTS INCLUDE

Chloride fumes

MEDICAL CONDITIONS POSSIBLY AGGRAVATED BY EXPOSURE

Central nervous system disorders

Liver disorders

Kidney disorders

DECONTAMINATION

- Wear positive-pressure SCBA and protective equipment specified by references such as the *North American Emergency Response Guidebook*. If special chemical protective clothing is required, consult the chemical manufacturer or specific protective clothing compatibility charts. A qualified, experienced person should make decisions regarding the type of personal protective equipment necessary.
- Delay entry until trained personnel and proper protective equipment are available.
- Remove patient from contaminated area.
- Quickly remove and isolate patient's clothing, jewelry, and shoes.
- Gently brush away dry particles and blot excess liquids with absorbent material.
- Rinse patient with warm water, 32° C to 35° C (90° F to 95° F), if possible.
- Wash patient with a mild liquid soap and large quantities of water.
- Leather absorbs pesticides and should be isolated and properly disposed of.
- Refer to decontamination protocol in Section Three.

IMMEDIATE FIRST AID

- Ensure that adequate decontamination has been carried out.
- If patient is not breathing, start artificial respiration, preferably with a demand-valve resuscitator, bag-valve-mask device, or pocket mask, as trained. Perform CPR if necessary.
- Immediately flush contaminated eyes with gently flowing water.
- Do not induce vomiting. If vomiting occurs, lean patient forward or place on left side (head-down position, if possible) to maintain an open airway and prevent aspiration.
- Keep patient quiet and maintain normal body temperature.
- Obtain medical attention.

BASIC TREATMENT

- Establish a patent airway (oropharyngeal or nasopharyngeal airway, if needed). Suction if necessary.
- Watch for signs of respiratory insufficiency and assist ventilations if necessary.
- Administer oxygen by nonrebreather mask at 10 to 15 L/min.

- Anticipate seizures, reduce all external stimuli, and treat if necessary (refer to seizure protocol in Section Three).
- For eye contamination, flush eyes immediately with water. Irrigate each eye continuously with 0.9% saline (NS) during transport (refer to eye irrigation protocol in Section Three).
- Do not use emetics. For ingestion, rinse mouth and administer 5 ml/kg up to 200 ml of water for dilution if the patient can swallow, has a strong gag reflex, and does not drool. Administer activated charcoal (refer to ingestion protocol in Section Three and activated charcoal protocol in Section Four).

ADVANCED TREATMENT

- Consider orotracheal or nasotracheal intubation for airway control in the patient who is unconscious or is in severe respiratory distress.
- Monitor cardiac rhythm and treat arrhythmias if necessary (refer to cardiac protocol in Section Three).
- Start IV administration of D_5W TKO. Use 0.9% saline (NS) or lactated Ringer's (LR) if signs of hypovolemia are present. For hypotension with signs of hypovolemia, administer fluid cautiously. Watch for signs of fluid overload (refer to shock protocol in Section Three).
- Treat seizures with diazepam (Valium) or lorazepam (Ativan) (refer to diazepam and lorazepam protocols in Section Four and seizure protocol in Section Three).
- Use proparacaine hydrochloride to assist eye irrigation (refer to proparacaine hydrochloride protocol in Section Four).

INITIAL EMERGENCY DEPARTMENT CONSIDERATIONS

- Useful initial laboratory studies include complete blood count, serum electrolytes, blood urea nitrogen (BUN), creatinine, glucose, urinalysis, and baseline biochemical profile, including serum aminotransferases (ALT and AST), calcium, phosphorus, and magnesium. Determination of anion and osmolar gaps may be helpful. Arterial blood gases (ABGs), chest radiograph, and electrocardiogram may be required.
- Obtain toxicological consultation if necessary.

SPECIAL CONSIDERATIONS

- Avoid epinephrine and related beta agonists (unless patient is in cardiac arrest or has reactive airways disease refractory to other treatment) because of the possible irritable condition of the myocardium. Use of these medications may lead to ventricular fibrillation.
- Identify the solvent involved and consult the appropriate guideline.
- These products are fat soluble. They are excreted in breast milk and may cross the placenta. Compounds persist for years in the environment and bioaccumulate in adipose tissue.

57

Lindane and Related Compounds

SUBSTANCE IDENTIFICATION

Found as a colorless solid. Formulated as emulsifiable concentrate, wettable powder, sprays, aerosols, dusts, granules, or crystal. Wettable forms are in water. Products have a musty or aromatic odor. Liquid forms have a hydrocarbon vehicle. Toxicity from the solvent should be considered. Used as insecticides, scabicides, pediculicides, and pesticides. Lindane has greater vapor activity than most organochlorine insecticides. Lindane (1%) is the active ingredient in the miticides Kwell, Kildane, Scabene, and Gammabenzene. Although some of these products use "benzene" in their names, they do not contain benzene.

ROUTES OF EXPOSURE

Skin and eye contact
Inhalation
Ingestion
Skin absorption

TARGET ORGANS

Primary
Skin
Eyes
Central nervous system
Cardiovascular system
Hepatic system
Renal system
Blood
Metabolism
Secondary
Respiratory system
Gastrointestinal system

LIFE THREAT

Causes central nervous system excitation leading to seizures and respiratory failure.

SIGNS AND SYMPTOMS BY SYSTEM

Cardiovascular: Arrhythmias caused by hypoxia. Products may sensitize the myocardium to catecholamines.

Respiratory: Irritation of the mucous membranes, throat, and upper airway. Respiratory failure secondary to seizures. Pulmonary edema has been seen in some fatal cases.

CNS: Headache, CNS stimulation, irritability, restlessness, memory disturbances, slurred speech, muscle tremors, ataxia, paresthesias, and spasms. Seizures.

Gastrointestinal: Nausea, vomiting, abdominal pain, and diarrhea.

Eye: Chemical conjunctivitis and corneal damage.

Skin: Dermatitis, pruritus, burns, and cyanosis.

Renal: Kidney damage.

Hepatic: Liver damage.

Metabolism: Rhabdomyolysis and myoglobinuria.

Blood: Aplastic anemia (bone marrow suppression) has been reported. Abnormalities in white blood cell count (leukopenia, granulocytopenia, granulocytosis, eosinophilia) have been reported. Decreased platelet count (thrombocytopenia).

Other: Some products may present a human carcinogenic risk. The hydrocarbon solvent may cause additional toxicity.

SYMPTOM ONSET FOR ACUTE EXPOSURE

Immediate

Some symptoms may be delayed up to 24 hours

CO-EXPOSURE CONCERNS

Other organochlorine compounds

THERMAL DECOMPOSITION PRODUCTS INCLUDE

Phosgene

Hydrogen chloride

Carbon monoxide

MEDICAL CONDITIONS POSSIBLY AGGRAVATED BY EXPOSURE

Central nervous system disorders

Seizure disorders

Liver disorders

Kidney disorders

Bone marrow disorders

DECONTAMINATION

- Wear positive-pressure SCBA and protective equipment specified by references such as the *North American Emergency Response Guidebook*. If special chemical protective clothing is required, consult the chemical manufacturer or specific protective clothing compatibility charts. A qualified, experienced person should make decisions regarding the type of personal protective equipment necessary.
- Delay entry until trained personnel and proper protective equipment are available.
- Remove patient from contaminated area.
- Quickly remove and isolate patient's clothing, jewelry, and shoes.
- Gently brush away dry particles and blot excess liquids with absorbent material.
- Rinse patient with warm water, 32° C to 35° C (90° F to 95° F), if possible.
- Wash patient with a mild liquid soap and large quantities of water.
- Leather absorbs pesticides and should be isolated and properly disposed of.
- Refer to decontamination protocol in Section Three.

IMMEDIATE FIRST AID

- Ensure that adequate decontamination has been carried out.
- If patient is not breathing, start artificial respiration, preferably with a demand-valve resuscitator, bag-valve-mask device, or pocket mask, as trained. Perform CPR if necessary.
- Immediately flush contaminated eyes with gently flowing water.
- Do not induce vomiting. If vomiting occurs, lean patient forward or place on left side (head-down position, if possible) to maintain an open airway and prevent aspiration.

- Keep patient quiet and maintain normal body temperature.
- Obtain medical attention.

BASIC TREATMENT

- Establish a patent airway (oropharyngeal or nasopharyngeal airway, if needed). Suction if necessary.
- Watch for signs of respiratory insufficiency and assist ventilations if necessary.
- Administer oxygen by nonrebreather mask at 10 to 15 L/min.
- Monitor for pulmonary edema and treat if necessary (refer to pulmonary edema protocol in Section Three).
- Anticipate seizures and treat if necessary (refer to seizure protocol in Section Three).
- For eye contamination, flush eyes immediately with water. Irrigate each eye continuously with 0.9% saline (NS) during transport (refer to eye irrigation protocol in Section Three).
- Do not use emetics. For ingestion, rinse mouth and administer 5 ml/kg up to 200 ml of water for dilution if the patient can swallow, has a strong gag reflex, and does not drool. Administer activated charcoal (refer to ingestion protocol in Section Three and activated charcoal protocol in Section Four).

ADVANCED TREATMENT

- Consider orotracheal or nasotracheal intubation for airway control in the patient who is unconscious, has severe pulmonary edema, or is in severe respiratory distress.
- Positive-pressure ventilation techniques with a bag-valve-mask device may be beneficial.
- Consider drug therapy for pulmonary edema (refer to pulmonary edema protocol in Section Three).
- Monitor cardiac rhythm and treat arrhythmias if necessary (refer to cardiac protocol in Section Three).
- Start IV administration of 0.9% saline (NS) or lactated Ringer's (LR) to maintain hydration and adequate urine flow. Watch for signs of fluid overload and pulmonary edema (refer to shock protocol in Section Three).
- Treat seizures with diazepam (Valium) or lorazepam (Ativan) (refer to diazepam and lorazepam protocols in Section Four and seizure protocol in Section Three).
- Use proparacaine hydrochloride to assist eye irrigation (refer to proparacaine hydrochloride protocol in Section Four).

INITIAL EMERGENCY DEPARTMENT CONSIDERATIONS

- Useful initial laboratory studies include complete blood count, serum electrolytes, blood urea nitrogen (BUN), creatinine, glucose, urinalysis, and baseline biochemical profile, including serum aminotransferases (ALT and AST), calcium, phosphorus, and magnesium. Determination of anion and osmolar gaps may be helpful. Arterial blood gases (ABGs), chest radiograph, and electrocardiogram may be required.
- If rhabdomyolysis is suspected, monitor urine for myoglobin. If myoglobinuria is present, maintain adequate hydration status and urine flow. Alkalinization of the urine may be indicated to prevent renal damage.
- Positive end-expiratory pressure (PEEP)–assisted ventilation may be necessary in patients with acute parenchymal injury who develop pulmonary edema or acute respiratory distress syndrome.
- Obtain toxicological consultation if necessary.

SPECIAL CONSIDERATIONS

- Avoid epinephrine and related beta agonists (unless patient is in cardiac arrest or has reactive airways disease refractory to other treatment) because of the possible irritable condition of the myocardium. Use of these medications may lead to ventricular fibrillation.
- These fat-soluble compounds accumulate in adipose tissue. They are excreted in breast milk and cross the placenta. Also found as contaminants in air and water.
- Additional toxicity may result from the hydrocarbon solvent. Identify the solvent and consult the appropriate guideline.

58

Toxaphene and Related Compounds

SUBSTANCE IDENTIFICATION

Found as a waxy, amber-colored solid with a mild pine odor. Also found in dusts, sprays, wettable powders, and liquid preparations with oil solvents. Used as insecticides.

ROUTES OF EXPOSURE

Skin and eyes
Inhalation
Ingestion
Skin absorption

TARGET ORGANS

Primary
Skin
Eyes
Central nervous system
Secondary
Cardiovascular system
Respiratory system
Gastrointestinal system
Hepatic system

LIFE THREAT

Death from respiratory failure and exhaustion secondary to seizures.

SIGNS AND SYMPTOMS BY SYSTEM

Cardiovascular: Circulatory collapse with tachycardia and hypotension.

Respiratory: Sudden onset of dyspnea, followed by respiratory failure. Upper respiratory tract irritation and sinusitis.

CNS: Headache, fatigue, hyperexcitability, shivering, muscle tremor, and spasms of leg and back muscles. Seizures that can be precipitated by external stimuli and tetanic muscular contractions may also be seen.

Gastrointestinal: Nausea, vomiting, and excessive salivation.

Eye: Chemical conjunctivitis and blurred vision.

Skin: Mild irritation, cyanosis, and dermatitis.

Hepatic: Liver damage.

Other: The onset of symptoms is usually abrupt. Oil-based solutions are absorbed faster than dusts or powders. NOTE: Some of these products may be mixed with a hydrocarbon solvent as a vehicle. Toxicity may result from the solvent. Identify the solvent and consult the appropriate guideline. Some products may present a human carcinogenic risk.

SYMPTOM ONSET FOR ACUTE EXPOSURES

Immediate
Symptoms may be delayed up to 1 hour

CO-EXPOSURE CONCERNS

Chlorinated hydrocarbon insecticides

THERMAL DECOMPOSITION PRODUCTS INCLUDE

Hydrogen chloride
Carbon monoxide

MEDICAL CONDITIONS POSSIBLY AGGRAVATED BY EXPOSURE

Respiratory system disorders
Cardiovascular system disorders
Central nervous system disorders

DECONTAMINATION

- Wear positive-pressure SCBA and protective equipment specified by references such as the *North American Emergency Response Guidebook*. If special chemical protective clothing is required, consult the chemical manufacturer or specific protective clothing compatibility charts. A qualified, experienced person should make decisions regarding the type of personal protective equipment necessary.
- Delay entry until trained personnel and proper protective equipment are available.
- Remove patient from contaminated area.
- Quickly remove and isolate patient's clothing, jewelry, and shoes.
- Gently brush away dry particles and blot excess liquids with absorbent material.
- Rinse patient with warm water, 32° C to 35° C (90° F to 95° F), if possible.
- Wash patient with a mild liquid soap and large quantities of water.
- Leather absorbs pesticides and should be isolated and properly disposed of.
- Refer to decontamination protocol in Section Three.

IMMEDIATE FIRST AID

- Ensure that adequate decontamination has been carried out.
- If patient is not breathing, start artificial respiration, preferably with a demand-valve resuscitator, bag-valve-mask device, or pocket mask, as trained. Perform CPR if necessary.
- Immediately flush contaminated eyes with gently flowing water.
- Do not induce vomiting. If vomiting occurs, lean patient forward or place on left side (head-down position, if possible) to maintain an open airway and prevent aspiration.
- Keep patient quiet and maintain normal body temperature.
- Obtain medical attention.

BASIC TREATMENT

- Establish a patent airway (oropharyngeal or nasopharyngeal airway, if needed). Suction if necessary.
- Watch for signs of respiratory insufficiency and assist ventilations if necessary.
- Administer oxygen by nonrebreather mask at 10 to 15 L/min.
- Monitor for shock and treat if necessary (refer to shock protocol in Section Three).
- Keep patient quiet, reduce external stimuli, and be prepared to treat seizures (refer to seizure protocol in Section Three).
- For eye contamination, flush eyes immediately with water. Irrigate each eye continuously with 0.9% saline (NS) during transport (refer to eye irrigation protocol in Section Three).

- Do not use emetics. For ingestion, rinse mouth and administer 5 ml/kg up to 200 ml of water for dilution if the patient can swallow, has a strong gag reflex, and does not drool. Administer activated charcoal (refer to ingestion protocol in Section Three and activated charcoal protocol in Section Four).

ADVANCED TREATMENT

- Consider orotracheal or nasotracheal intubation for airway control in the patient who is unconscious or is in severe respiratory distress.
- Monitor cardiac rhythm and treat arrhythmias if necessary (refer to cardiac protocol in Section Three).
- Start IV administration of D_5W TKO. Use 0.9% saline (NS) or lactated Ringer's (LR) if signs of hypovolemia are present. For hypotension with signs of hypovolemia, administer fluid cautiously. Watch for signs of fluid overload (refer to shock protocol in Section Three).
- Treat seizures with diazepam (Valium) or lorazepam (Ativan) (refer to diazepam and lorazepam protocols in Section Four and seizure protocol in Section Three).
- Use proparacaine hydrochloride to assist eye irrigation (refer to proparacaine hydrochloride protocol in Section Four).

INITIAL EMERGENCY DEPARTMENT CONSIDERATIONS

- Useful initial laboratory studies include complete blood count, serum electrolytes, blood urea nitrogen (BUN), creatinine, glucose, urinalysis, and baseline biochemical profile, including serum aminotransferases (ALT and AST), calcium, phosphorus, and magnesium. Arterial blood gases (ABGs), chest radiograph, and electrocardiogram may be required.
- Obtain toxicological consultation if necessary.

SPECIAL CONSIDERATIONS

- Avoid epinephrine and related beta agonists (unless patient is in cardiac arrest or has reactive airways disease refractory to other treatment) because of the possible irritable condition of the myocardium. Use of these medications may lead to ventricular fibrillation.
- Products may be dissolved in hydrocarbon solvents. The solvent may add to the toxicity. Identify the solvent and consult the appropriate guideline.

Acrolein and Related Compounds

SUBSTANCE IDENTIFICATION

Colorless to yellow liquid unsaturated aldehyde with a disagreeable, choking odor. Used as a herbicide and biocide to control weed and algae; as a warning agent in methyl chloride refrigerants; in the manufacture of perfumes, pharmaceuticals, plastics, glycerin, and resins as a chemical intermediate; as a tissue fixative; and in military poison gas mixtures. Acrolein is more irritating than formaldehyde.

ROUTES OF EXPOSURE

Skin and eye contact
Inhalation
Ingestion
Skin absorption

TARGET ORGANS

Primary
Skin
Eyes
Cardiovascular system
Respiratory system
Secondary
Central nervous system
Gastrointestinal system

LIFE THREAT

Severe respiratory tract irritation leading to pulmonary edema and respiratory failure.

SIGNS AND SYMPTOMS BY SYSTEM

Cardiovascular: Tachycardia, arrhythmias, and hypertension.

Respiratory: Upper airway irritation, cough, dyspnea, and pulmonary edema. Bronchoconstriction.

CNS: Dizziness, headache, coma.

Gastrointestinal: Nausea, vomiting, and diarrhea.

Eye: Conjunctivitis, burns and corneal damage. Intense lacrimation.

Skin: Irritant dermatitis, erythema, and chemical burns.

Other: Nitrogen is usually added to biocide preparations to exclude air and prevent polymerization reactions. Hydroquinone may be added to inhibit oxygen-mediated polymerizations. Some products may present a human mutagenic risk.

SYMPTOM ONSET FOR ACUTE EXPOSURE

Immediate
Possible delay of some symptoms, especially respiratory

THERMAL DECOMPOSITION PRODUCTS INCLUDE

Carbon dioxide

Carbon monoxide
Peroxides

MEDICAL CONDITIONS POSSIBLY AGGRAVATED BY EXPOSURE

Respiratory system disorders

DECONTAMINATION

- Wear positive-pressure SCBA and protective equipment specified by references such as the *North American Emergency Response Guidebook.* If special chemical protective clothing is required, consult the chemical manufacturer or specific protective clothing compatibility charts. A qualified, experienced person should make decisions regarding the type of personal protective equipment necessary.
- Delay entry until trained personnel and proper protective equipment are available.
- Remove patient from contaminated area.
- Quickly remove and isolate patient's clothing, jewelry, and shoes.
- Gently blot excess liquids with absorbent material.
- Rinse patient with warm water, 32° C to 35° C (90° F to 95° F), if possible.
- Wash patient with a mild liquid soap and large quantities of water.
- Refer to decontamination protocol in Section Three.

IMMEDIATE FIRST AID

- Ensure that adequate decontamination has been carried out.
- If patient is not breathing, start artificial respiration, preferably with a demand-valve resuscitator, bag-valve-mask device, or pocket mask, as trained. Perform CPR if necessary.
- Immediately flush contaminated eyes with gently flowing water.
- Do not induce vomiting. If vomiting occurs, lean patient forward or place on left side (head-down position, if possible) to maintain an open airway and prevent aspiration.
- Keep patient quiet and maintain normal body temperature.
- Obtain medical attention.

BASIC TREATMENT

- Establish a patent airway (oropharyngeal or nasopharyngeal airway, if needed). Suction if necessary.
- Watch for signs of respiratory insufficiency and assist ventilations if necessary.
- Administer oxygen by nonrebreather mask at 10 to 15 L/min.
- Monitor for pulmonary edema and treat if necessary (refer to pulmonary edema protocol in Section Three).
- For eye contamination, flush eyes immediately with water. Irrigate each eye continuously with 0.9% saline (NS) during transport (refer to eye irrigation protocol in Section Three).
- Do not use emetics. For ingestion, rinse mouth and administer 5 ml/kg up to 200 ml of water for dilution if the patient can swallow, has a strong gag reflex, and does not drool. Administer activated charcoal (refer to ingestion protocol in Section Three and activated charcoal protocol in Section Four).
- Cover skin burns with dry sterile dressings after decontamination (refer to chemical burn protocol in Section Three).

ADVANCED TREATMENT

- Consider orotracheal or nasotracheal intubation for airway control in the patient who is unconscious, has severe pulmonary edema, or is in severe respiratory distress.

- Positive-pressure ventilation techniques with a bag-valve-mask device may be beneficial.
- Consider drug therapy for pulmonary edema (refer to pulmonary edema protocol in Section Three).
- Monitor cardiac rhythm and treat arrhythmias if necessary (refer to cardiac protocol in Section Three).
- Start IV administration of D_5W TKO. Use 0.9% saline (NS) or lactated Ringer's (LR) if signs of hypovolemia are present. For hypotension with signs of hypovolemia, administer fluid cautiously. Watch for signs of fluid overload (refer to shock protocol in Section Three).
- Use proparacaine hydrochloride to assist eye irrigation (refer to proparacaine hydrochloride protocol in Section Four).

INITIAL EMERGENCY DEPARTMENT CONSIDERATIONS

- Useful initial laboratory studies include complete blood count, serum electrolytes, blood urea nitrogen (BUN), creatinine, glucose, urinalysis, and baseline biochemical profile, including serum aminotransferases (ALT and AST), calcium, phosphorus, and magnesium. Determination of anion and osmolar gaps may be helpful. Arterial blood gases (ABGs), chest radiograph, and electrocardiogram may be required.
- Positive end-expiratory pressure (PEEP)–assisted ventilation may be necessary in patients with acute parenchymal injury who develop pulmonary edema or acute respiratory distress syndrome.
- Obtain toxicological consultation as necessary.

SPECIAL CONSIDERATIONS

- Acrolein functions as a cellular poison by binding to sulfhydryl groups.

Chlorophenoxy Herbicides and Related Compounds

SUBSTANCE IDENTIFICATION

Colorless to white, yellow, or tan odorless solid. Formulated as an emulsifiable concentrate, granule, or liquid. Used as a broad-leaf herbicide, defoliant, and plant hormone (growth regulator). May be mixed with other herbicides before use. Over 60 million pounds of 2,4-D are used in the United States annually. 2,4,5-T was banned for use in the United States by the EPA in 1979. In Vietnam, from 1966 to 1971, United States military forces used a 50/50 mixture of 2,4-D and 2,4,5-T known as Agent Orange (named for the orange stripe on the 55-gallon drums). Agent White was 2,4-D, and Agent Blue was dimethylarsinic acid.

ROUTES OF EXPOSURE

Skin and eye contact
Inhalation
Ingestion
Skin absorption

TARGET ORGANS

Primary
Skin
Eyes
Central nervous system
Cardiovascular system
Secondary
Respiratory system
Gastrointestinal tract
Hepatic system
Renal system
Metabolism

LIFE THREAT

Hypoexcitation/hyperexcitation of the nervous system and respiratory failure. Ventricular fibrillation and seizures.

SIGNS AND SYMPTOMS BY SYSTEM

Cardiovascular: Electrocardiogram abnormalities, including inverted or flattened T waves. Ventricular arrhythmias, vasodilation, and cardiovascular collapse.

Respiratory: Tachypnea, respiratory failure, and pulmonary edema.

CNS: Stiffness of the extremities, paresthesias, ataxia, vertigo, incoordination, paralysis, stupor, CNS depression, and coma. Muscle twitching and weakness. May cause peripheral neuropathy with nerve conduction velocity and/or electromyogram (NCV/EMG) changes and seizures. Neurobehavioral changes.

Gastrointestinal: Nausea, vomiting, abdominal pain, diarrhea, or blood in the stool.

Eye: Chemical conjunctivitis. Constricted pupils.

Skin: Dermatitis, diaphoresis, and chloracne.
Renal: Kidney damage
Hepatic: Liver damage.
Metabolism: Metabolic acidosis and hyperkalemia.
Other: May cause disturbances in body temperature: reduction in cold climates and febrile responses on exertion in warm climates. Skeletal muscle myotonia, rhabdomyolysis, and myoglobinuria.

SYMPTOM ONSET FOR ACUTE EXPOSURES

Immediate
Some symptoms may be delayed

CO-EXPOSURE CONCERNS

Other chlorophenoxy herbicides

THERMAL DECOMPOSITION PRODUCTS INCLUDE

Carbon monoxide
Chlorine
Hydrogen chloride
Phosgene

MEDICAL CONDITIONS POSSIBLY AGGRAVATED BY EXPOSURE

Nervous system disorders

DECONTAMINATION

- Wear positive-pressure SCBA and protective equipment specified by references such as the *North American Emergency Response Guidebook*. If special chemical protective clothing is required, consult the chemical manufacturer or specific protective clothing compatibility charts. A qualified, experienced person should make decisions regarding the type of personal protective equipment necessary.
- Delay entry until trained personnel and proper protective equipment are available.
- Remove patient from contaminated area.
- Quickly remove and isolate patient's clothing, jewelry, and shoes.
- Gently brush away dry particles and blot excess liquids with absorbent material.
- Rinse patient with warm water, 32° C to 35° C (90° F to 95° F), if possible.
- Wash patient with a mild liquid soap and large quantities of water.
- Refer to decontamination protocol in Section Three.

IMMEDIATE FIRST AID

- Ensure that adequate decontamination has been carried out.
- If patient is not breathing, start artificial respiration, preferably with a demand-valve resuscitator, bag-valve-mask device, or pocket mask, as trained. Perform CPR if necessary.
- Immediately flush contaminated eyes with gently flowing water.
- Do not induce vomiting. If vomiting occurs, lean patient forward or place on left side (head-down position, if possible) to maintain an open airway and prevent aspiration.
- Keep patient quiet and maintain normal body temperature.
- Obtain medical attention.

BASIC TREATMENT

- Establish a patent airway (oropharyngeal or nasopharyngeal airway, if needed). Suction if necessary.
- Watch for signs of respiratory insufficiency and assist ventilations if necessary.

- Administer oxygen by nonrebreather mask at 10 to 15 L/min.
- Monitor for pulmonary edema and treat if necessary (refer to pulmonary edema protocol in Section Three).
- Monitor for shock and treat if necessary (refer to shock protocol in Section Three).
- Anticipate seizures and treat if necessary (refer to seizure protocol in Section Three).
- For eye contamination, flush eyes immediately with water. Irrigate each eye continuously with 0.9% saline (NS) during transport (refer to eye irrigation protocol in Section Three).
- Do not use emetics. For ingestion, rinse mouth and administer 5 ml/kg up to 200 ml of water for dilution if the patient can swallow, has a strong gag reflex, and does not drool. Administer activated charcoal (refer to ingestion protocol in Section Three and activated charcoal protocol in Section Four).
- Monitor body temperature and treat if necessary.

ADVANCED TREATMENT

- Consider orotracheal or nasotracheal intubation for airway control in the patient who is unconscious or is in severe respiratory distress.
- Positive-pressure ventilation techniques with a bag-valve-mask device may be beneficial.
- Consider drug therapy for pulmonary edema (refer to pulmonary edema protocol in Section Three).
- Monitor and treat cardiac arrhythmias if necessary (refer to cardiac protocol in Section Three).
- Start IV administration of 0.9% saline (NS) or lactated Ringer's TKO. Titrate to maintain adequate urine flow. For hypotension with signs of hypovolemia, administer fluid cautiously. Consider vasopressors if patient is hypotensive with a normal fluid volume (refer to shock protocol in Section Three).
- Treat seizures with diazepam (Valium) or lorazepam (Ativan) (refer to diazepam and lorazepam protocols in Section Four and seizure protocol in Section Three).
- Use proparacaine hydrochloride to assist eye irrigation (refer to proparacaine hydrochloride protocol in Section Four).

INITIAL EMERGENCY DEPARTMENT CONSIDERATIONS

- Useful initial laboratory studies include complete blood count, serum electrolytes, blood urea nitrogen (BUN), creatinine, glucose, urinalysis, and baseline biochemical profile, including serum aminotransferases (ALT and AST), calcium, phosphorus, and magnesium. Determination of anion and osmolar gaps may be helpful. Arterial blood gases (ABGs), chest radiograph, and electrocardiogram may be required.
- Chronically exposed individuals require CBC, biochemistry profile, thyroid, folate, and vitamin B_{12} determinations. Adipose tissue measurements of TCDD and neurobehavioral tests may be useful.
- Positive end-expiratory pressure (PEEP)–assisted ventilation may be necessary in patients with acute parenchymal injury who develop pulmonary edema or acute respiratory distress syndrome.
- Products may cause acidosis; hyperventilation and sodium bicarbonate may be beneficial. Bicarbonate therapy should be guided by patient presentation, ABG determination, and serum electrolyte considerations.

- If patient is comatose, exhibits severe metabolic acidosis, or myoglobinuria, forced alkaline diuresis with adequate potassium replacement may be beneficial to enhance elimination.
- Obtain toxicological consultation as necessary.

SPECIAL CONSIDERATIONS

- TCDD (dioxin) contamination, as well as the chlorophenoxy herbicides themselves, may be responsible for the chronic neurological effects observed. Products contaminated with TCDD may pose a human carcinogenic risk.
- Unlike TCDD, which bioaccumulates, there is no evidence that the chlorophenoxy herbicides behave similarly.

61

Dichloropropane, Dichloropropene, and Related Compounds

SUBSTANCE IDENTIFICATION

A colorless, yellow, or purple liquid with an unpleasant mustard or chloroform-like odor. Used as a preplant fumigant with nematocidal properties.

ROUTES OF EXPOSURE

Skin and eye contact
Inhalation
Ingestion
Skin absorption

TARGET ORGANS

Primary
Skin
Eyes
Respiratory system
Gastrointestinal system
Hepatic system
Renal system
Secondary
Cardiovascular system
Central nervous system

LIFE THREAT

Pulmonary edema, bronchospasm, and alveolar hemorrhage.

SIGNS AND SYMPTOMS BY SYSTEM

Cardiovascular: Arrhythmias caused by hypoxia.

Respiratory: Increased respiratory rate, coughing, dyspnea, substernal chest pain, bronchospasm, and pulmonary edema. Irritation to the upper airway.

CNS: Headache, dizziness, decreased level of consciousness, and coma.

Gastrointestinal: Nausea, vomiting, and diarrhea.

Eye: Chemical conjunctivitis, lacrimation, corneal damage, eye pain, and photophobia.

Skin: Dermatitis, irritation, and chemical burns with deep-seated pain in the area of absorption.

Renal: Kidney damage.

Hepatic: Liver damage.

Other: Some products may present a human carcinogenic risk. NOTE: Some of these products may be mixed with a hydrocarbon solvent as a vehicle. Toxicity may result from the solvent.

SYMPTOM ONSET FOR ACUTE EXPOSURE

Immediate
Possible delay of some symptoms

CO-EXPOSURE CONCERNS

Hydrocarbon solvents

THERMAL DECOMPOSITION PRODUCTS INCLUDE

Carbon dioxide
Carbon monoxide
Hydrogen chloride
Phosgene

MEDICAL CONDITIONS POSSIBLY AGGRAVATED BY EXPOSURE

Respiratory disorders (COPD, asthma)

DECONTAMINATION

- Wear positive-pressure SCBA and protective equipment specified by references such as the *North American Emergency Response Guidebook*. If special chemical protective clothing is required, consult the chemical manufacturer or specific protective clothing compatibility charts. A qualified, experienced person should make decisions regarding the type of personal protective equipment necessary.
- Delay entry until trained personnel and proper protective equipment are available.
- Remove patient from contaminated area.
- Quickly remove and isolate patient's clothing, jewelry, and shoes.
- Gently blot excess liquids with absorbent material.
- Rinse patient with warm water, 32° C to 35° C (90° F to 95° F), if possible.
- Wash patient with a mild liquid soap and large quantities of water.
- Refer to decontamination protocol in Section Three.

IMMEDIATE FIRST AID

- Remove patient from contact with the material.
- Ensure that adequate decontamination has been carried out.
- If patient is not breathing, start artificial respiration, preferably with a demand-valve resuscitator, bag-valve-mask device, or pocket mask, as trained. Perform CPR if necessary.
- Immediately flush contaminated eyes with gently flowing water.
- Do not induce vomiting. If vomiting occurs, lean patient forward or place on left side (head-down position, if possible) to maintain an open airway and prevent aspiration.
- Keep patient quiet and maintain normal body temperature.
- Obtain medical attention.

BASIC TREATMENT

- Establish a patent airway (oropharyngeal or nasopharyngeal airway, if needed). Suction if necessary.
- Watch for signs of respiratory insufficiency and assist ventilations if necessary.
- Administer oxygen by nonrebreather mask at 10 to 15 L/min.
- Monitor for pulmonary edema and treat if necessary (refer to pulmonary edema protocol in Section Three).
- For eye contamination, flush eyes immediately with water. Irrigate each eye continuously with 0.9% saline (NS) during transport (refer to eye irrigation protocol in Section Three).

- Do not use emetics. For ingestion, rinse mouth and administer 5 ml/kg up to 200 ml of water for dilution if the patient can swallow, has a strong gag reflex, and does not drool. Administer activated charcoal (refer to ingestion protocol in Section Three and activated charcoal protocol in Section Four).
- Cover skin burns with dry sterile dressings after decontamination (refer to chemical burn protocol in Section Three).

ADVANCED TREATMENT

- Consider orotracheal or nasotracheal intubation for airway control in the patient who is unconscious, has severe pulmonary edema, or is in severe respiratory distress.
- Positive-pressure ventilation techniques with a bag-valve-mask device may be beneficial.
- Consider drug therapy for pulmonary edema (refer to pulmonary edema protocol in Section Three).
- Consider administering a beta agonist such as albuterol for severe bronchospasm (refer to albuterol protocol in Section four).
- Monitor and treat cardiac arrhythmias if necessary (refer to cardiac protocol in Section Three).
- Start IV administration of D_5W TKO. Use 0.9% saline (NS) or lactated Ringer's (LR) if signs of hypovolemia are present. For hypotension with signs of hypovolemia, administer fluid cautiously. Watch for signs of fluid overload (refer to shock protocol in Section Three).
- Use proparacaine hydrochloride to assist eye irrigation (refer to proparacaine hydrochloride protocol in Section Four).

INITIAL EMERGENCY DEPARTMENT CONSIDERATIONS

- Useful initial laboratory studies include complete blood count, serum electrolytes, blood urea nitrogen (BUN), creatinine, glucose, urinalysis, and baseline biochemical profile, including serum aminotransferases (ALT and AST), calcium, phosphorus, and magnesium. Determination of anion and osmolar gaps may be helpful. Arterial blood gases (ABGs), chest radiograph, and electrocardiogram may be required.
- Positive end-expiratory pressure (PEEP)–assisted ventilation may be necessary in patients with acute parenchymal injury who develop pulmonary edema or acute respiratory distress syndrome.
- Bronchospastic symptoms should be treated with an inhalation medication regimen similar to that used for reactive airway disease. Inhaled corticosteroids may be of value in severe bronchospasm.
- Obtain toxicological consultation as necessary.

SPECIAL CONSIDERATIONS

- Identify the solvent involved and consult the appropriate guideline.

Dinitrophenol and Related Compounds

SUBSTANCE IDENTIFICATION

Found as a yellow solid with a musty, sweet odor. Used in solid, wettable powder and oil solution form. Formulated as fungicides, insecticides, and herbicides. Also used in wood preservatives, explosives, dyestuffs, photographic developers, and chemical intermediates.

ROUTES OF EXPOSURE

Skin and eye contact
Inhalation
Ingestion
Skin absorption

TARGET ORGANS

Primary
Skin
Eyes
Central nervous system
Cardiovascular system
Respiratory system
Hepatic system
Renal system
Metabolism
Blood
Secondary
Gastrointestinal system

LIFE THREAT

Respiratory and circulatory collapse. Pulmonary edema and marked elevation in body temperature.

SIGNS AND SYMPTOMS BY SYSTEM

Cardiovascular: Initially, blood pressure increase followed by hypotension. Ventricular arrhythmias and tachycardia.

Respiratory: Deep breathing followed by dyspnea, decreased rate, and respiratory arrest. Occasionally, pulmonary edema.

CNS: Extreme fatigue, headache, dizziness, weakness, and excitation, followed by mental status changes, depression, coma, and seizures.

Gastrointestinal: Nausea, vomiting, diarrhea, and abdominal pains. Extreme thirst.

Eye: Chemical conjunctivitis, corneal damage, dilated pupils, and nystagmus possible. *Secondary* glaucoma and/or cataracts.

Skin: Dermatitis and chemical burns. Cyanosis or flushed color with profuse sweating. Yellow staining of the skin seen with dinitrophenol poisoning.

Renal: Kidney damage.

Hepatic: Liver damage with jaundice.

Metabolism: Fever (hyperthermia). Compounds are uncouplers of oxidative phosphorylation. Metabolic acidosis. Thyroid damage.

Blood: Methemoglobinemia.

Other: Some products may present a human teratogenic risk. Exposure may alter metabolism and cause severe hyperthermia. Response personnel should be warned against overheating, since the toxicity of these products may be exaggerated by high temperature environments. NOTE: Some of these products may be mixed with a hydrocarbon solvent as a vehicle. Toxicity may also result from the solvent.

SYMPTOM ONSET FOR ACUTE EXPOSURE

Immediate

Possible delay of some symptoms

Possible delay of liver and kidney damage 12 to 72 hours

CO-EXPOSURE CONCERNS

High temperature environments

Hydrocarbon solvents

THERMAL DECOMPOSITION PRODUCTS INCLUDE

Carbon dioxide

Carbon monoxide

Nitrogen oxides

MEDICAL CONDITIONS POSSIBLY AGGRAVATED BY EXPOSURE

Cardiovascular disorders

DECONTAMINATION

- Wear positive-pressure SCBA and protective equipment specified by references such as the *North American Emergency Response Guidebook*. If special chemical protective clothing is required, consult the chemical manufacturer or specific protective clothing compatibility charts. A qualified, experienced person should make decisions regarding the type of personal protective equipment necessary.
- Delay entry until trained personnel and proper protective equipment are available.
- Remove patient from contaminated area.
- Quickly remove and isolate patient's clothing, jewelry, and shoes.
- Gently brush away dry particles and blot excess liquids with absorbent material.
- Rinse patient with warm water, 32° C to 35° C (90° F to 95° F), if possible.
- Wash patient with a mild liquid soap and large quantities of water.
- Refer to decontamination protocol in Section Three.

IMMEDIATE FIRST AID

- Ensure that adequate decontamination has been carried out.
- If patient is not breathing, start artificial respiration, preferably with a demand-valve resuscitator, bag-valve-mask device, or pocket mask, as trained. Perform CPR if necessary.
- Immediately flush contaminated eyes with gently flowing water.
- Do not induce vomiting. If vomiting occurs, lean patient forward or place on left side (head-down position, if possible) to maintain an open airway and prevent aspiration.
- Keep patient quiet and maintain normal body temperature.
- Obtain medical attention.

BASIC TREATMENT

- Establish a patent airway (oropharyngeal or nasopharyngeal airway, if needed). Suction if necessary.
- Watch for signs of respiratory insufficiency and assist ventilations if necessary.
- Administer oxygen by nonrebreather mask at 10 to 15 L/min.
- Monitor for shock and treat if necessary (refer to shock protocol in Section Three).
- Monitor for pulmonary edema and treat if necessary (refer to pulmonary edema protocol in Section Three).
- Anticipate seizures and treat if necessary (refer to seizure protocol in Section Three).
- For eye contamination, flush eyes immediately with water. Irrigate each eye continuously with 0.9% saline (NS) during transport (refer to eye irrigation protocol in Section Three).
- Do not use emetics. For ingestion, rinse mouth and administer 5 ml/kg up to 200 ml of water for dilution if the patient can swallow, has a strong gag reflex, and does not drool. Administer activated charcoal (refer to ingestion protocol in Section Three and activated charcoal protocol in Section Four).
- Cover skin burns with dry sterile dressings after decontamination (refer to chemical burn protocol in Section Three).
- Rapid body cooling may be necessary in case of hyperthermia. Salicylates are contraindicated.

ADVANCED TREATMENT

- Consider orotracheal or nasotracheal intubation for airway control in the patient who is unconscious, has severe pulmonary edema, or is in severe respiratory distress.
- Positive-pressure ventilation techniques with a bag-valve-mask device may be beneficial.
- Consider drug therapy for pulmonary edema (refer to pulmonary edema protocol in Section Three).
- Monitor cardiac rhythm and treat arrhythmias if necessary (refer to cardiac protocol in Section Three).
- Start IV administration of 0.9% saline (NS) or lactated Ringer's (LR) TKO. For dehydration and hypotension with signs of hypovolemia, administer fluid cautiously. Consider vasopressors if patient is hypotensive with a normal fluid volume. Watch for signs of fluid overload (refer to shock protocol in Section Three).
- Treat seizures with diazepam (Valium) or lorazepam (Ativan) (refer to diazepam and lorazepam protocols in Section Four and seizure protocol in Section Three).
- Administer 1% solution methylene blue if patient is symptomatic with severe hypoxia, cyanosis, and cardiac compromise not responding to oxygen. DIRECT PHYSICIAN ORDER ONLY (refer to methylene blue protocol in Section Four).
- Use proparacaine hydrochloride to assist eye irrigation (refer to proparacaine hydrochloride protocol in Section Four).

INITIAL EMERGENCY DEPARTMENT CONSIDERATIONS

- Useful initial laboratory studies include complete blood count, serum electrolytes, blood urea nitrogen (BUN), creatinine, glucose, urinalysis, and

baseline biochemical profile, including thyroid profile, serum aminotransferases (ALT and AST), bilirubin, calcium, phosphorus, and magnesium. Determination of anion and osmolar gaps may be helpful. Arterial blood gases (ABGs), chest radiograph, and electrocardiogram may be required.

- Monitor blood methemoglobin levels and treat with methylene blue if patient is symptomatic and/or has a blood methemoglobin level greater than 30%. DIRECT PHYSICIAN ORDER ONLY (refer to methylene blue protocol in Section Four).
- Positive end-expiratory pressure (PEEP)–assisted ventilation may be necessary in patients with acute parenchymal injury who develop pulmonary edema or acute respiratory distress syndrome.
- Products may cause acidosis; hyperventilation and sodium bicarbonate may be beneficial. Bicarbonate therapy should be guided by patient presentation, ABG determination, and serum electrolyte considerations.
- Use of atropine is contraindicated.
- Obtain toxicological consultation as necessary.

SPECIAL CONSIDERATIONS

- Identify the solvent involved and consult the appropriate guideline.
- Pulse oximetry readings may not be accurate in these exposures.

Dithiocarbamates and Related Compounds

SUBSTANCE IDENTIFICATION

White, yellowish, grayish, or black powder or crystals with a characteristic odor. Available as a wettable powder, dust, aqueous suspension. Also found in mixtures with other fungicides (mixtures, oil dispersable). Used as fungicides, seed disinfectants, insecticides, animal repellents, and soil sterilants and in soap and antiseptic sprays and rubber manufacturing.

ROUTES OF EXPOSURE

Skin and eye contact
Inhalation
Ingestion
Skin absorption

TARGET ORGANS

Primary
Skin
Eyes
Central nervous system
Hepatic system
Renal system
Secondary
Cardiovascular system
Respiratory system
Gastrointestinal system
Blood
Metabolism

LIFE THREAT

Hypotension and respiratory failure.

SIGNS AND SYMPTOMS BY SYSTEM

Cardiovascular: Cardiovascular collapse and hypotension.
Respiratory: Upper respiratory tract irritation with cough. Respiratory paralysis.
CNS: Headache, weakness, lethargy, dizziness, ataxia, confusion, drowsiness, and coma. Suppression of deep tendon reflexes, flaccid paralysis, and weakness/numbness of the extremities. Cerebral edema may occur with exposure to some products. Late development of peripheral neuropathy.
Gastrointestinal: Nausea, vomiting, diarrhea. Ingestion may cause GI tract necrosis.
Eye: Conjunctivitis, lacrimation, and corneal damage.
Skin: Allergic and contact dermatitis, pruritus, and photosensitivity.
Renal: Kidney damage.
Hepatic: Liver damage.

Blood: Low white count (leukopenia) and abnormality in red blood cell size (anisocytosis).

Metabolism: Thyroid dysfunction

Other: Some products may present human mutagenic or teratogenic risk. Some may present a carcinogenic risk from metabolites. Many of these products are carbamates; however, exposure does not lead to cholinergic findings (SLUDGE syndrome). NOTE: Some of these products may be mixed with a hydrocarbon solvent as a vehicle. Toxicity may result from the solvent.

SYMPTOM ONSET FOR ACUTE EXPOSURE

Immediate
Possible delay of cerebral edema
Peripheral neuropathy delayed

CO-EXPOSURE CONCERNS

Alcohol: May cause disulfiram (Antabuse)-like reaction

THERMAL DECOMPOSITION PRODUCTS INCLUDE

Carbon dioxide
Carbon disulfide
Carbon monoxide
Sulfur dioxide

MEDICAL PROBLEMS POSSIBLY AGGRAVATED BY EXPOSURE

Respiratory system disorders
Skin disorders
Thyroid disorders

DECONTAMINATION

- Wear positive-pressure SCBA and protective equipment specified by references such as the *North American Emergency Response Guidebook*. If special chemical protective clothing is required, consult the chemical manufacturer or specific protective clothing compatibility charts. A qualified, experienced person should make decisions regarding the type of personal protective equipment necessary.
- Delay entry until trained personnel and proper protective equipment are available.
- Remove patient from contaminated area.
- Quickly remove and isolate patient's clothing, jewelry, and shoes.
- Gently brush away dry particles and blot excess liquids with absorbent material.
- Rinse patient with warm water, 32° C to 35° C (90° F to 95° F), if possible.
- Wash patient with a mild liquid soap and large quantities of water.
- Refer to decontamination protocol in Section Three.

IMMEDIATE FIRST AID

- Remove patient from contact with the material.
- Ensure that adequate decontamination has been carried out.
- If patient is not breathing, start artificial respiration, preferably with a demand-valve resuscitator, bag-valve-mask device, or pocket mask, as trained. Perform CPR if necessary.
- Immediately flush contaminated eyes with gently flowing water.
- Do not induce vomiting. If vomiting occurs, lean patient forward or place on left side (head-down position, if possible) to maintain an open airway and prevent aspiration.

- Keep patient quiet and maintain normal body temperature.
- Obtain medical attention.

BASIC TREATMENT

- Establish a patent airway (oropharyngeal or nasopharyngeal airway, if needed). Suction if necessary.
- Watch for signs of respiratory insufficiency and assist ventilations if necessary.
- Administer oxygen by nonrebreather mask at 10 to 15 L/min.
- Monitor for shock and treat if necessary (refer to shock protocol in Section Three).
- Anticipate seizures and treat if necessary (refer to seizure protocol in Section Three).
- For eye contamination, flush eyes immediately with water. Irrigate each eye continuously with 0.9% saline (NS) during transport (refer to eye irrigation protocol in Section Three).
- Do not use emetics. For ingestion, rinse mouth and administer 5 ml/kg up to 200 ml of water for dilution if the patient can swallow, has a strong gag reflex, and does not drool. Administer activated charcoal (refer to ingestion protocol in Section Three and activated charcoal protocol in Section Four).

ADVANCED TREATMENT

- Consider orotracheal or nasotracheal intubation for airway control in the patient who is unconscious or is in severe respiratory distress.
- Use moderate hyperventilation (rate of 20 respirations per minute) if signs of cerebral edema are present.
- Monitor cardiac rhythm and treat arrhythmias if necessary (refer to cardiac protocol in Section Three).
- Start IV administration of D_5W TKO. Use 0.9% saline (NS) or lactated Ringer's (LR) if signs of hypovolemia are present. For hypotension with signs of hypovolemia, administer fluid cautiously. Consider vasopressors if patient is hypotensive with a normal fluid volume. Watch for signs of fluid overload (refer to shock protocol in Section Three).
- Treat seizures with diazepam (Valium) or lorazepam (Ativan) (refer to diazepam and lorazepam protocols in Section Four and seizure protocol in Section Three).
- Use proparacaine hydrochloride to assist eye irrigation (refer to proparacaine hydrochloride protocol in Section Four).

INITIAL EMERGENCY DEPARTMENT CONSIDERATIONS

- Useful initial laboratory studies include complete blood count, serum electrolytes, blood urea nitrogen (BUN), creatinine, glucose, urinalysis, and baseline biochemical profile, including thyroid profile, serum aminotransferases (ALT and AST), calcium, phosphorus, and magnesium. Determination of anion and osmolar gaps may be helpful. Arterial blood gases (ABGs), chest radiograph, and electrocardiogram may be required.
- Obtain toxicological consultation as necessary.

SPECIAL CONSIDERATIONS

- Identify the solvent involved and consult the appropriate guideline.
- These compounds may be metabolized to carbon disulfide, hydrogen sulfide, dimethylamine, methylisothiocyanate, and ethylene thiourea. These metabolites contribute to the clinical picture seen with these compounds.

- Fields treated with dithiocarbamate may demonstrate high air concentrations of carbon disulfide, hydrogen sulfide, and methylisocyanate.
- Disulfiram (Antabuse) is a dithiocarbamate. Consumption of alcohol may cause a disulfiram-like reaction.

Monofluoroacetate and Related Compounds

SUBSTANCE IDENTIFICATION

A white, water-soluble, odorless solid. Usually found in a water solution with a black warning color. Used as a rodenticide. Has been misused for predator elimination, or mixed with a black dye added to grain rodent baits.

ROUTES OF EXPOSURE

Skin and eye contact
Inhalation
Ingestion
Skin absorption

TARGET ORGANS

Primary
Skin
Eyes
Central nervous system
Cardiovascular system
Secondary
Respiratory system
Gastrointestinal system
Hepatic system
Renal system

LIFE THREAT

Ventricular arrhythmias and seizures.

SIGNS AND SYMPTOMS BY SYSTEM

Cardiovascular: Sinus bradycardia with frequent ventricular ectopy (may be multifocal in nature), ventricular tachycardia, ventricular fibrillation, hypotension, and cardiac arrest.

Respiratory: Respiratory depression.

CNS: Excitation, apprehension, auditory disturbances, carpopedal spasm, and paresthesia of the face and nose. Seizures with periods of CNS depression, coma, and death.

Gastrointestinal: Nausea, vomiting, diarrhea, excessive salivation.

Eye: Chemical conjunctivitis and blurred vision.

Skin: Irritation. Cyanosis.

Hepatic: Liver damage.

Renal: Kidney damage.

Other: Extremely toxic compounds that prevent the conversion of citrate to isocitrate in the Krebs cycle. Hypocalcemia.

SYMPTOM ONSET FOR ACUTE EXPOSURE

Immediate
Symptoms possibly delayed 30 minutes to 3 hours

THERMAL DECOMPOSITION PRODUCTS INCLUDE

Fluorides

Carbon oxides

MEDICAL CONDITIONS POSSIBLY AGGRAVATED BY EXPOSURE

Cardiovascular disorders

Neurological disorders

DECONTAMINATION

- Wear positive-pressure SCBA and protective equipment specified by references such as the *North American Emergency Response Guidebook*. If special chemical protective clothing is required, consult the chemical manufacturer or specific protective clothing compatibility charts. A qualified, experienced person should make decisions regarding the type of personal protective equipment necessary.
- Delay entry until trained personnel and proper protective equipment are available.
- Remove patient from contaminated area.
- Quickly remove and isolate patient's clothing, jewelry, and shoes.
- Gently brush away dry particles and blot excess liquids with absorbent material.
- Rinse patient with warm water, 32° C to 35° C (90° F to 95° F), if possible.
- Wash patient with a mild liquid soap and large quantities of water.
- Refer to decontamination protocol in Section Three.

IMMEDIATE FIRST AID

- Ensure that adequate decontamination has been carried out.
- If patient is not breathing, start artificial respiration, preferably with a demand-valve resuscitator, bag-valve-mask device, or pocket mask, as trained. Perform CPR if necessary.
- Immediately flush contaminated eyes with gently flowing water.
- Do not induce vomiting. If vomiting occurs, lean patient forward or place on left side (head-down position, if possible) to maintain an open airway and prevent aspiration.
- Keep patient quiet and maintain normal body temperature.
- Obtain medical attention.

BASIC TREATMENT

- Establish a patent airway (oropharyngeal or nasopharyngeal airway, if needed). Suction if necessary.
- Watch for signs of respiratory insufficiency and assist ventilations if necessary.
- Administer oxygen by nonrebreather mask at 10 to 15 L/min.
- Anticipate seizures and treat if necessary (refer to seizure protocol in Section Three).
- For eye contamination, flush eyes immediately with water. Irrigate each eye continuously with 0.9% saline (NS) during transport (refer to eye irrigation protocol in Section Three).
- Do not use emetics. For ingestion, rinse mouth and administer 5 ml/kg up to 200 ml of water for dilution if the patient can swallow, has a strong gag reflex, and does not drool. Administer activated charcoal (refer to ingestion protocol in Section Three and activated charcoal protocol in Section Four).

ADVANCED TREATMENT

- Consider orotracheal or nasotracheal intubation for airway control in the patient who is unconscious or is in severe respiratory distress.

- Monitor cardiac rhythm and treat arrhythmias if necessary (refer to cardiac protocol in Section Three).
- Start IV administration of D_5W TKO. Use 0.9% saline (NS) or lactated Ringer's (LR) if signs of hypovolemia are present. For hypotension with signs of hypovolemia, administer fluid cautiously. Watch for signs of fluid overload (refer to shock protocol in Section Three).
- Treat seizures with diazepam (Valium) or lorazepam (Ativan) (refer to diazepam and lorazepam protocols in Section Four and seizure protocol in Section Three).
- Use proparacaine hydrochloride to assist eye irrigation (refer to proparacaine hydrochloride protocol in Section Four).

INITIAL EMERGENCY DEPARTMENT CONSIDERATIONS

- Useful initial laboratory studies include complete blood count, serum electrolytes, blood urea nitrogen (BUN), creatinine, glucose, urinalysis, and baseline biochemical profile, including thyroid profile, serum aminotransferases (ALT and AST), calcium, phosphorus, and magnesium. Determination of anion and osmolar gaps may be helpful. Arterial blood gases (ABGs), chest radiograph, and electrocardiogram may be required.
- If hypocalcemia is present, calcium gluconate should be administered. Therapy should be guided by patient presentation and serum calcium levels.
- Obtain toxicological consultation as necessary.

65

Organotins and Related Compounds

SUBSTANCE IDENTIFICATION

Colorless to yellow liquids or solids with a weak odor. Used as fungicides, bactericides, pesticides, wood preservatives, and corrosion inhibitors.

ROUTES OF EXPOSURE

Skin and eye contact
Inhalation
Ingestion

TARGET ORGANS

Primary
Skin
Eyes
Central nervous system
Respiratory system
Gastrointestinal system
Secondary
Cardiovascular system
Hepatic system
Renal system
Metabolism

LIFE THREAT

Respiratory failure, pulmonary edema, and cerebral edema.

SIGNS AND SYMPTOMS BY SYSTEM

Cardiovascular: Cardiovascular collapse and arrhythmias.

Respiratory: Respiratory tract irritation, respiratory failure, and pulmonary edema.

CNS: Headache, dizziness, visual disturbances, tinnitus, cerebral edema, muscle weakness, flaccid muscle paralysis, seizures, and coma. Neurobehavioral changes.

Gastrointestinal: Nausea, vomiting, diarrhea, GI tract hemorrhage, and peritonitis may occur.

Eye: Conjunctivitis, lacrimation, corneal damage, conjunctival edema, and photophobia.

Skin: Irritation, dermatitis, and chemical burns.

Hepatic: Liver damage.

Renal: Glucose in the urine (glycosuria).

Metabolism: Inhibitors of oxidative phosphorylation. Hyperglycemia.

Other: Some of these products may be mixed with a hydrocarbon solvent as a vehicle. Toxicity may result from the solvent. Trialkytin compounds have the highest toxicity.

SYMPTOM ONSET FOR ACUTE EXPOSURE
Immediate
Cerebral and pulmonary edema possibly delayed

CO-EXPOSURE CONCERNS
Hydrocarbon solvents

THERMAL DECOMPOSITION PRODUCTS INCLUDE
Irritating fumes
Organic acid vapors
Tin oxides

MEDICAL CONDITIONS POSSIBLY AGGRAVATED BY EXPOSURE
Respiratory system disorders

DECONTAMINATION
- Wear positive-pressure SCBA and protective equipment specified by references such as the *North American Emergency Response Guidebook*. If special chemical protective clothing is required, consult the chemical manufacturer or specific protective clothing compatibility charts. A qualified, experienced person should make decisions regarding the type of personal protective equipment necessary.
- Delay entry until trained personnel and proper protective equipment are available.
- Remove patient from contaminated area.
- Quickly remove and isolate patient's clothing, jewelry, and shoes.
- Gently brush away dry particles and blot excess liquids with absorbent materials.
- Rinse patient with warm water, 32° C to 35° C (90° F to 95° F), if possible.
- Wash patient with a mild liquid soap and large quantities of water.
- Refer to decontamination protocol in Section Three.

IMMEDIATE FIRST AID
- Remove patient from contact with the material.
- Ensure that adequate decontamination has been carried out.
- If patient is not breathing, start artificial respiration, preferably with a demand-valve resuscitator, bag-valve-mask device, or pocket mask, as trained. Perform CPR if necessary.
- Immediately flush contaminated eyes with gently flowing water.
- Do not induce vomiting. If vomiting occurs, lean patient forward or place on left side (head-down position, if possible) to maintain an open airway and prevent aspiration.
- Keep patient quiet and maintain normal body temperature.
- Obtain medical attention.

BASIC TREATMENT
- Establish a patent airway (oropharyngeal or nasopharyngeal airway, if needed). Suction if necessary.
- Watch for signs of respiratory insufficiency and assist ventilations if necessary.
- Administer oxygen by nonrebreather mask at 10 to 15 L/min.
- Monitor for pulmonary edema and treat if necessary (refer to pulmonary edema protocol in Section Three).
- Monitor for shock and treat if necessary (refer to shock protocol in Section Three).
- Anticipate seizures and treat if necessary (refer to seizure protocol in Section Three).

- For eye contamination, flush eyes immediately with water. Irrigate each eye continuously with 0.9% saline (NS) during transport (refer to eye irrigation protocol in Section Three).
- Do not use emetics. For ingestion, rinse mouth and administer 5 ml/kg up to 200 ml of water for dilution if the patient can swallow, has a strong gag reflex, and does not drool. Administer activated charcoal (refer to ingestion protocol in Section Three and activated charcoal protocol in Section Four).
- Cover skin burns with dry sterile dressings after decontamination (refer to chemical burn protocol in Section Three).

ADVANCED TREATMENT

- Consider orotracheal or nasotracheal intubation for airway control in the patient who is unconscious, has severe pulmonary edema, or is in severe respiratory distress.
- Positive-pressure ventilation techniques with a bag-valve-mask device may be beneficial.
- Consider drug therapy for pulmonary edema (refer to pulmonary edema protocol in Section Three).
- Moderate hyperventilation (20 respirations per minute) may be beneficial for intracranial pressure.
- Monitor cardiac rhythm and treat arrhythmias if necessary (refer to cardiac protocol in Section Three).
- Start IV administration of 0.9% saline (NS) or lactated Ringer's (LR) TKO. For hypotension with signs of hypovolemia, administer fluid cautiously. Consider vasopressors if patient is hypotensive with a normal fluid volume. Watch for signs of fluid overload (refer to shock protocol in Section Three).
- Treat seizures with diazepam (Valium) or lorazepam (Ativan) (refer to diazepam and lorazepam protocols in Section Four and seizure protocol in Section Three).
- Use proparacaine hydrochloride to assist eye irrigation (refer to proparacaine hydrochloride protocol in Section Four).

INITIAL EMERGENCY DEPARTMENT CONSIDERATION

- Useful initial laboratory studies include complete blood count, serum electrolytes, blood urea nitrogen (BUN), creatinine, glucose, urinalysis, and baseline biochemical profile, including serum aminotransferases (ALT and AST), calcium, phosphorus, and magnesium. Determination of anion and osmolar gaps may be helpful. Arterial blood gases (ABGs), chest radiograph, and electrocardiogram may be required.
- Positive end-expiratory pressure (PEEP)–assisted ventilation may be necessary in patients with acute parenchymal injury who develop pulmonary edema or acute respiratory distress syndrome.
- Osmotic diuretics and/or hyperventilation may be useful in treating cerebral edema.
- In animal studies, chelators such as BAL or D-penicillamine have demonstrated no therapeutic benefit in removing organotin compounds.
- Obtain toxicological consultation as necessary.

SPECIAL CONSIDERATIONS

- Identify the solvent involved and consult the appropriate guideline.
- Oral exposures result in relatively more severe toxicity.

Paraquat and Related Compounds

SUBSTANCE IDENTIFICATION

Paraquat is a colorless to yellow solid with a mild, ammonia-like odor, but may be found in (0.5% to 20%) solutions and sprays. Used as a herbicide, desiccant, defoliation agent, and redox indicator. Products are extremely toxic.

ROUTES OF EXPOSURE

Skin and eye contact
Inhalation
Ingestion
Skin absorption

TARGET ORGANS

Primary
Skin
Eyes
Cardiovascular system
Respiratory system
Gastrointestinal system
Hepatic system
Renal system
Secondary
Central nervous system

LIFE THREAT

Paraquat and diquat are poisons that target multiple organ systems. Death results from pulmonary edema, cardiac damage, circulatory collapse, and cerebral hemorrhages/infarctions.

SIGNS AND SYMPTOMS BY SYSTEM

Cardiovascular: Cardiovascular collapse, hypotension, and arrhythmias.

Respiratory: Irritation of the mucous membranes. Coughing, dyspnea, epistaxis, and pulmonary edema followed by a late development of pulmonary fibrosis. Diquat does not cause fibrosis.

CNS: Headache, lethargy, CNS depression, and coma. Diquat may cause brain stem hemorrhage and infarction.

Gastrointestinal: Burning pain in mouth, pharynx, esophagus, and abdomen. Likely to produce burns or ulceration of the mouth, pharynx, esophagus, and stomach. Nausea, profuse, bloody vomiting (hematemesis), paralytic ileus, and diarrhea with bloody stools. Pancreatic damage.

Eye: Chemical conjunctivitis and severe eye injury resembling corrosive injuries. Corneal scarring possible.

Skin: Irritation, dryness, erythema, blistering, ulceration, and nail changes (transverse ridging, furrowing). Irritant or contact dermatitis. Exposure to paraquat solutions may cause skin burns. Cyanosis and sometimes jaundice.

Renal: Renal failure.
Hepatic: Liver damage.
Other: Fever.

SYMPTOM ONSET FOR ACUTE EXPOSURE

Immediate
Some symptoms possibly delayed
Pulmonary fibrosis may occur 2 to 14 days after exposure

THERMAL DECOMPOSITION PRODUCTS INCLUDE

Carbon monoxide
Hydrogen chloride
Nitrogen oxides
Sulfur oxides

MEDICAL CONDITIONS POSSIBLY AGGRAVATED BY EXPOSURE

Eye disorders
Respiratory system disorders
Cardiovascular system disorders
Liver disorders
Kidney disorders

DECONTAMINATION

- Wear positive-pressure SCBA and protective equipment specified by references such as the *North American Emergency Response Guidebook.* If special chemical protective clothing is required, consult the chemical manufacturer or specific protective clothing compatibility charts. A qualified, experienced person should make decisions regarding the type of personal protective equipment necessary.
- Delay entry until trained personnel and proper protective equipment are available.
- Remove patient from contaminated area.
- Quickly remove and isolate patient's clothing, jewelry, and shoes.
- Gently brush away dry particles and blot excess liquids with absorbent material.
- Rinse patient with warm water, 32° C to 35° C (90° F to 95° F), if possible.
- Wash patient with a mild liquid soap and large quantities of water.
- Refer to decontamination protocol in Section Three.

IMMEDIATE FIRST AID

- Remove patient from contact with the material.
- Ensure that adequate decontamination has been carried out.
- If patient is not breathing, start artificial respiration, preferably with a demand-valve resuscitator, bag-valve-mask device, or a pocket mask, as trained. Perform CPR if necessary.
- Immediately flush contaminated eyes with gently flowing water.
- Do not induce vomiting. If vomiting occurs, lean patient forward or place on left side (head: down position, if possible) to maintain an open airway and prevent aspiration.
- Keep patient quiet and maintain normal body temperature.
- Obtain medical attention.

BASIC TREATMENT

- Establish a patent airway (oropharyngeal or nasopharyngeal airway, if needed). Suction if necessary.

- Watch for signs of respiratory insufficiency and assist ventilations if necessary. Do not use supplemental oxygen in cases of paraquat or diquat exposure.
- Monitor for pulmonary edema and treat if necessary (refer to pulmonary edema protocol in Section Three).
- Monitor for shock and treat if necessary (refer to shock protocol in Section Three).
- For eye contamination, flush eyes immediately with water. Irrigate each eye continuously with 0.9% saline (NS) during transport (refer to eye irrigation protocol in Section Three).
- Do not use emetics. For ingestion, rinse mouth and administer 5 ml/kg up to 200 ml of water for dilution if the patient can swallow, has a strong gag reflex, and does not drool. Administer Fullers' Earth, 7% bentonite USP or activated charcoal (refer to ingestion protocol in Section Three and activated charcoal protocol in Section Four). Do not delay GI decontamination.
- Cover skin burns with dry, sterile dressings after decontamination (refer to chemical burn protocol in Section Three).

ADVANCED TREATMENT

- Consider orotracheal or nasotracheal intubation for airway control in the patient who is unconscious, has severe pulmonary edema, or is in severe respiratory distress.
- Positive-pressure ventilation techniques with a bag-valve-mask device, (without supplemental oxygen in cases of paraquat or diquat exposure) may be beneficial.
- Consider drug therapy for pulmonary edema (refer to pulmonary edema protocol in Section Three).
- Monitor cardiac rhythm and treat arrhythmias if necessary (refer to cardiac protocol in Section Three).
- Start IV administration of D_5W TKO. Use 0.9% saline (NS) or lactated Ringer's (LR) if signs of hypovolemia are present. For hypotension with signs of hypovolemia, administer fluid cautiously, Consider vasopressors if patient is hypotensive with a normal fluid volume. Watch for signs of pulmonary edema (refer to shock protocol in Section Three).
- Use proparacaine hydrochloride to assist eye irrigation (refer to proparacaine hydrochloride protocol in Section Four).

INITIAL EMERGENCY DEPARTMENT CONSIDERATIONS

- Useful initial laboratory studies include complete blood count, serum electrolytes, blood urea nitrogen (BUN), creatinine, glucose, urinalysis, and baseline biochemical profile, including serum aminotransferases (AST and ALT), lactic dehydrogenase (LDH), calcium, phosphorus, magnesium, and plasma paraquat/diquat concentrations. Determination of anion and osmolar gaps may be helpful. Arterial blood gases (ABGs), chest radiograph, and electrocardiogram may be required. Plasma paraquat concentrations are useful in predicting prognosis.
- Rapid Dithionite Test: to detect urinary paraquat/diquat:
  - Add 5 ml 1% sodium dithionite (sodium hydrosulfate) in sodium hydroxide (1N) to 10 ml urine. Wait 60 seconds.
  - Use positive and negative controls: dark blue color = paraquat or diquat; green color = diquat.

- The vividness of the color approximates the paraquat/diquat concentration. This is a semiquantitative test.

- Positive end-expiratory pressure (PEEP)–assisted ventilation may be necessary in patients with acute parenchymal injury who develop pulmonary edema or acute respiratory distress syndrome.
- Administer Fuller's Earth or 7% bentonite USP: Adult dosage: 100 to 150 g via lavage tube; Pediatric dosage: 1 to 2 g/kg.
- If above are not available, use activated charcoal (refer to activated charcoal protocol in Section Four).
- Do not delay GI decontamination.
- Charcoal hemoperfusion within the first 2 hours of ingestion may be useful.
- Obtain toxicological consultation as necessary.

SPECIAL CONSIDERATIONS

- Oxygen enhances paraquat pulmonary toxicity. Although diquat does not cause pulmonary fibrosis, oxygen promotes the formation of superoxide (O_2^-) radicals that may cause multiorgan damage. Avoid supplemental oxygen administration with either paraquat or diquat poisoning unless the patient shows signs of severe cyanosis, respiratory compromise, or respiratory or cardiac arrest.
- Paraquat is actively transported into the lungs even after oral ingestion, causing pulmonary edema and irreversible fibrosis.
- Two phases of paraquat pulmonary toxicity:

  Phase I: Types I and II pulmonary epithelial cells destroyed, causing alveolitis

  Phase II: Intraalveolar and interalveolar fibrosis

Pentachlorophenol and Related Compounds

SUBSTANCE IDENTIFICATION

Found as a dark gray or light brown solid with a phenolic odor. Used as an emulsifiable concentrate, pellets, pills, and in solution forms. Used in making pesticides, fungicides, and herbicides and as a wood preservative. Compounds may be contaminated with polychlorinated dibenzodioxins and dibenzofurans.

ROUTES OF EXPOSURE

Skin and eye contact
Inhalation
Ingestion
Skin absorption

TARGET ORGANS

Primary
Skin
Eyes
Central nervous system
Cardiovascular system
Respiratory system
Hepatic system
Metabolism
Secondary
Gastrointestinal system
Renal system

LIFE THREAT

Respiratory and circulatory collapse. Severe increase in body temperature (hyperthermia).

SIGNS AND SYMPTOMS BY SYSTEM

Cardiovascular: Initially, blood pressure increase followed by hypotension. Ventricular arrhythmias and tachycardia.

Respiratory: Sneezing, respiratory tract irritation, deep breathing followed by dyspnea, decreased rate, and arrest. Bronchitis is a common symptom. Pulmonary edema may occur secondary to massive inhalation exposures.

CNS: CNS excitation followed by depression, coma, and seizures. Extreme fatigue, headache, dizziness, incoordination, and weakness. Cerebral edema.

Gastrointestinal: Nausea, vomiting, diarrhea, and abdominal pains.

Eye: Chemical conjunctivitis, dilated pupils, and opacification of the cornea.

Skin: Dermatitis, chloracne, diaphoresis, and chemical burns.

Renal: Kidney damage. Renal output increased, then decreased.

Hepatic: Liver damage.

Metabolism: Metabolic acidosis. Uncouplers of oxidative phosphorylation.

Other: Exposure may alter metabolism and cause severe hyperthermia. Response personnel should be warned against overheating, since the toxicity of these products may be exaggerated by high-temperature environments. NOTE: Some of these products may be mixed with a hydrocarbon solvent as a vehicle. Toxicity may result from the solvent.

SYMPTOM ONSET FOR ACUTE EXPOSURE

Immediate

Some symptoms possibly delayed

CO-EXPOSURE CONCERNS

Polychlorinated dibenzodioxins

Polychlorinated dibenzofurans

High-temperature environments

THERMAL DECOMPOSITION PRODUCTS INCLUDE

Carbon dioxide

Carbon monoxide

Chlorine

Chlorinated hydrocarbons

Chlorinated phenols

Hydrogen chloride

Phosgene

MEDICAL CONDITIONS POSSIBLY AGGRAVATED BY EXPOSURE

Kidney disorders

Liver disorders

DECONTAMINATION

- Wear positive-pressure SCBA and protective equipment specified by references such as the *North American Emergency Response Guidebook*. If special chemical protective clothing is required, consult the chemical manufacturer or specific protective clothing compatibility charts. A qualified, experienced person should make decisions regarding the type of personal protective equipment necessary.
- Delay entry until trained personnel and proper protective equipment are available.
- Remove patient from contaminated area.
- Quickly remove and isolate patient's clothing, jewelry, and shoes.
- Gently brush away dry particles and blot excess liquids with absorbent material.
- Rinse patient with warm water, 32° C to 35° C (90° F to 95° F), if possible.
- Wash patient with a mild liquid soap and large quantities of water.
- Refer to decontamination protocol in Section Three.

IMMEDIATE FIRST AID

- Ensure that adequate decontamination has been carried out.
- If patient is not breathing, start artificial respiration, preferably with a demand-valve resuscitator, bag-valve-mask device, or pocket mask, as trained. Perform CPR if necessary.
- Immediately flush contaminated eyes with gently flowing water.
- Do not induce vomiting. If vomiting occurs, lean patient forward or place on left side (head-down position, if possible) to maintain an open airway and prevent aspiration.
- Keep patient quiet and maintain normal body temperature.
- Obtain medical attention.

BASIC TREATMENT

- Establish a patent airway (oropharyngeal or nasopharyngeal airway, if needed). Suction if necessary.
- Watch for signs of respiratory insufficiency and assist ventilations if necessary.
- Administer oxygen by nonrebreather mask at 10 to 15 L/min.
- Monitor for shock and treat if necessary (refer to shock protocol in Section Three).
- Monitor for pulmonary edema and treat if necessary (refer to pulmonary edema protocol in Section Three).
- Anticipate seizures and treat if necessary (refer to seizure protocol in Section Three).
- For eye contamination, flush eyes immediately with water. Irrigate each eye continuously with 0.9% saline (NS) during transport (refer to eye irrigation protocol in Section Three).
- Do not use emetics. For ingestion, rinse mouth and administer 5 ml/kg up to 200 ml of water for dilution if the patient can swallow, has a strong gag reflex, and does not drool. Administer activated charcoal (refer to ingestion protocol in Section Three and activated charcoal protocol in Section Four).
- Cover skin burns with dry sterile dressings after decontamination (refer to chemical burn protocol in Section Three).
- Rapid body cooling may be necessary in case of hyperthermia. Use of salicylates is contraindicated.

ADVANCED TREATMENT

- Consider orotracheal or nasotracheal intubation for airway control in the patient who is unconscious, has severe pulmonary edema, or is in severe respiratory distress.
- Positive-pressure ventilation techniques with a bag-valve-mask device may be beneficial.
- Consider drug therapy for pulmonary edema (refer to pulmonary edema protocol in Section Three).
- Monitor cardiac rhythm and treat arrhythmias if necessary (refer to cardiac protocol in Section Three).
- Start IV administration of 0.9% saline (NS) or lactated Ringer's (LR) TKO. For dehydration and hypotension with signs of hypovolemia, administer fluid cautiously. Consider vasopressors if patient is hypotensive with a normal fluid volume. Watch for signs of fluid overload, cerebral edema, and pulmonary edema (refer to shock protocol in Section Three).
- Treat seizures with diazepam (Valium) or lorazepam (Ativan) (refer to diazepam and lorazepam protocols in Section Four and seizure protocol in Section Three).
- Use proparacaine hydrochloride to assist eye irrigation (refer to proparacaine hydrochloride protocol in Section Four).

INITIAL EMERGENCY DEPARTMENT CONSIDERATIONS

- Useful initial laboratory studies include complete blood count, serum electrolytes, blood urea nitrogen (BUN), creatinine, glucose, urinalysis, and baseline biochemical profile, including serum aminotransferases (AST and ALT), serum alkaline phosphatase, lactic dehydrogenase (LDH), calcium, phosphorus, and magnesium. Determination of anion and osmolar gaps may be helpful.

Arterial blood gases (ABGs), chest radiograph, and electrocardiogram may be required.

- Positive end-expiratory pressure (PEEP)–assisted ventilation may be necessary in patients with acute parenchymal injury who develop pulmonary edema or acute respiratory distress syndrome.
- Products may cause acidosis; hyperventilation and sodium bicarbonate may be beneficial. Bicarbonate therapy should be guided by patient presentation, ABG determination, and serum electrolytes considerations.
- Obtain toxicological consultation as necessary.

SPECIAL CONSIDERATIONS

- Identify the solvent involved and consult the appropriate guideline.
- Atropine is contraindicated.

Glyphosate (Roundup) and Related Compounds

SUBSTANCE IDENTIFICATION

Colorless or white, odorless crystals. Also found in water-based solution form with a 15% surfactant (polyoxyethyleneamine) to aid in emulsification of the herbicide. This surfactant adds to the toxicity of the mixture. Used as an organic herbicide in the form of the mono (isopropylammonium) salt. Used in forestry, agriculture, and general weed-killing.

ROUTES OF EXPOSURE

Skin and eye contact
Inhalation
Ingestion

TARGET ORGANS

Primary
Skin
Eyes
Cardiovascular system
Respiratory system
Gastrointestinal tract
Blood
Secondary
Central nervous system
Hepatic system
Renal system
Metabolism

LIFE THREAT

Hypotension, cardiac arrhythmias, and pulmonary edema.

SIGNS AND SYMPTOMS BY SYSTEM

Cardiovascular: Cardiovascular collapse with hypotension. Ventricular arrhythmias and bradycardia.
Respiratory: Irritation of the upper airway. Pulmonary edema.
CNS: Ataxia, vertigo, incoordination, stupor, and coma.
Gastrointestinal: Nausea, vomiting, diarrhea, abdominal pain, pharyngitis, and erosions of GI tract mucosa.
Eye: Chemical conjunctivitis.
Skin: Dermatitis and chemical burns.
Renal: Kidney damage.
Hepatic: Liver damage.
Metabolism: Metabolic acidosis.
Blood: May cause red blood cell hemolysis.
Other: May cause hypothermia or hyperthermia.

SYMPTOM ONSET FOR ACUTE EXPOSURES

Immediate

Some symptoms possibly delayed

CO-EXPOSURE CONCERNS

Polyoxyethyleneamine

THERMAL DECOMPOSITION PRODUCTS INCLUDE

Carbon dioxide

Carbon monoxide

Nitrogen oxides

Phosphorus oxides

MEDICAL CONDITIONS POSSIBLY AGGRAVATED BY EXPOSURE

Anemia

Respiratory disorders (COPD)

Cardiovascular disorders

DECONTAMINATION

- Wear positive-pressure SCBA and protective equipment specified by references such as the *North American Emergency Response Guidebook*. If special chemical protective clothing is required, consult the chemical manufacturer or specific protective clothing compatibility charts. A qualified, experienced person should make decisions regarding the type of personal protective equipment necessary.
- Delay entry until trained personnel and proper protective equipment are available.
- Remove patient from contaminated area.
- Quickly remove and isolate patient's clothing, jewelry, and shoes.
- Gently brush away dry particles and blot excess liquids with absorbent material.
- Rinse patient with warm water, 32° C to 35° C (90° F to 95° F), if possible.
- Wash patient with a mild liquid soap and large quantities of water.
- Refer to decontamination protocol in Section Three.

IMMEDIATE FIRST AID

- Ensure that adequate decontamination has been carried out.
- If patient is not breathing, start artificial respiration, preferably with a demand-valve resuscitator, bag-valve-mask device, or pocket mask, as trained. Perform CPR if necessary.
- Immediately flush contaminated eyes with gently flowing water.
- Do not induce vomiting. If vomiting occurs, lean patient forward or place on left side (head-down position, if possible) to maintain an open airway and prevent aspiration.
- Keep patient quiet and maintain normal body temperature.
- Obtain medical attention.

BASIC TREATMENT

- Establish a patent airway (oropharyngeal or nasopharyngeal airway, if needed). Suction if necessary.
- Watch for signs of respiratory insufficiency and assist ventilations if necessary.
- Administer oxygen by nonrebreather mask at 10 to 15 L/min.
- Monitor for pulmonary edema and treat if necessary (refer to pulmonary edema protocol in Section Three).
- Monitor for shock and treat if necessary (refer to shock protocol in Section Three).

- For eye contamination, flush eyes immediately with water. Irrigate each eye continuously with 0.9% saline (NS) during transport (refer to eye irrigation protocol in Section Three).
- Do not use emetics. For ingestion, rinse mouth and administer 5 ml/kg up to 200 ml of water for dilution if the patient can swallow, has a strong gag reflex, and does not drool. Administer activated charcoal (refer to ingestion protocol in Section Three and activated charcoal protocol in Section Four).
- Monitor body temperature and treat if necessary.
- Cover skin burns with dry sterile dressings after decontamination (refer to chemical burn protocol in Section Three).

ADVANCED TREATMENT

- Consider orotracheal or nasotracheal intubation for airway control in the patient who is unconscious, has severe pulmonary edema, or is in severe respiratory distress.
- Positive-pressure ventilation techniques with a bag-valve-mask-device may be beneficial.
- Consider drug therapy for pulmonary edema (refer to pulmonary edema protocol in Section Three).
- Monitor and treat cardiac arrhythmias if necessary (refer to cardiac protocol in Section Three).
- Start IV administration of 0.9% saline (NS) or lactated Ringer's (LR) TKO. Titrate to maintain adequate urine flow. For hypotension with signs of hypovolemia, administer fluid cautiously. Consider vasopressors if patient is hypotensive with a normal fluid volume. Watch for signs of fluid overload (refer to shock protocol in Section Three).
- Use proparacaine hydrochloride to assist eye irrigation (refer to proparacaine hydrochloride protocol in Section Four).

INITIAL EMERGENCY DEPARTMENT CONSIDERATIONS

- Useful initial laboratory studies include complete blood count, serum electrolytes, blood urea nitrogen (BUN), creatinine, glucose, urinalysis, and baseline biochemical profile, including serum aminotransferases (AST and ALT), calcium, phosphorus, and magnesium. Determination of anion and osmolar gaps may be helpful. Arterial blood gases (ABGs), chest radiograph, and electrocardiogram may be required.
- Positive end-expiratory pressure (PEEP)–assisted ventilation may be necessary in patients with acute parenchymal injury who develop pulmonary edema or acute respiratory distress syndrome.
- Products may cause acidosis; hyperventilation and sodium bicarbonate may be beneficial. Bicarbonate therapy should be guided by patient presentation, ABG determination, and serum electrolyte considerations.
- Monitor for myoglobinuria. If present, maintain adequate hydration state and urine output. Diuretics and urinary alkalinization may be required in severe cases.
- Obtain toxicological consultation as necessary.

Strychnine and Related Compounds

SUBSTANCE IDENTIFICATION

Colorless, odorless solid. Found as grains, crystals, or powders. Used as a rodenticide and in veterinary products. Also found as a common adulterant of many street drugs.

ROUTES OF EXPOSURE

Skin and eye contact
Inhalation
Ingestion

TARGET ORGANS

Primary
Eyes
Central nervous system
Respiratory system
Secondary
Skin
Cardiovascular system
Gastrointestinal system
Hepatic system
Renal system
Metabolism

LIFE THREAT

Convulsions leading to acidosis and diaphragmatic spasm causing respiratory arrest.

SIGNS AND SYMPTOMS BY SYSTEM

Cardiovascular: Tachycardia and hypertension followed by cardiovascular collapse.

Respiratory: Hypoxemia and respiratory arrest secondary to convulsions.

CNS: Stiffness of face and neck. Restlessness, hyperexcitability, hyperreflexia, and muscle cramps. Mild sensory stimulus may produce violent paroxysmal convulsions. Body typically arches in hyperextension (opisthotonos): legs are adducted and extended, arms are rigidly extended, fists are tightly clenched, and the jaw is rigidly clamped. Patients are usually conscious and oriented during the convulsive episode.

Gastrointestinal: Occasional vomiting.

Eye: Chemical conjunctivitis.

Skin: Cyanosis and diaphoresis.

Renal: Kidney damage secondary to acidosis, rhabdomyolysis, and myoglobinuria.

Hepatic: Liver damage secondary to acidosis.

Metabolism: Lactic acidosis.

Other: Hyperthermia.

SYMPTOM ONSET FOR ACUTE EXPOSURE

Immediate

Symptoms possibly delayed 15 to 30 minutes

THERMAL DECOMPOSITION PRODUCTS INCLUDE

Carbon dioxide

Carbon monoxide

Nitrogen oxides

Sulfur dioxide

DECONTAMINATION

- Wear positive-pressure SCBA and protective equipment specified by references such as the *North American Emergency Response Guidebook*. If special chemical protective clothing is required, consult the chemical manufacturer or specific protective clothing compatibility charts. A qualified, experienced person should make decisions regarding the type of personal protective equipment necessary.
- Delay entry until trained personnel and proper protective equipment are available.
- Remove patient from contaminated area.
- Quickly remove and isolate patient's clothing, jewelry, and shoes.
- Gently brush away dry particles and blot excess liquids with absorbent material.
- Rinse patient with warm water, 32° C to 35° C (90° F to 95° F), if possible.
- Wash patient with a mild liquid soap and large quantities of water.
- Refer to decontamination protocol in Section Three.

IMMEDIATE FIRST AID

- Ensure that adequate decontamination has been carried out.
- If patient is not breathing, start artificial respiration, preferably with a demand-valve resuscitator, bag-valve-mask device, or pocket mask, as trained. Perform CPR if necessary.
- Immediately flush contaminated eyes with gently flowing water until medical treatment is obtained.
- Do not induce vomiting. If vomiting occurs, lean patient forward or place on left side (head-down position, if possible) to maintain an open airway and prevent aspiration.
- Keep patient quiet and maintain normal body temperature.
- Obtain medical attention.

BASIC TREATMENT

- Establish a patent airway (oropharyngeal or nasopharyngeal airway, if needed). Suction if necessary.
- Watch for signs of respiratory insufficiency and assist ventilations if necessary.
- Administer oxygen by nonrebreather mask at 10 to 15 L/min.
- Anticipate convulsions and treat if necessary (refer to seizure protocol in Section Three).
- For eye contamination, flush eyes immediately with water. Irrigate each eye continuously with 0.9% saline (NS) during transport (refer to eye irrigation protocol in Section Three).
- Do not use emetics. Administer activated charcoal (refer to ingestion protocol in Section Three and activated charcoal protocol in Section Four).
- Use rapid cooling measures to treat hyperthermia.

ADVANCED TREATMENT

- Consider orotracheal or nasotracheal intubation for airway control in the patient who is unconscious or is in severe respiratory distress.
- Monitor cardiac rhythm and treat arrhythmias if necessary (refer to cardiac protocol in Section Three).
- Start IV administration of D_5W TKO. Use 0.9% saline (NS) or lactated Ringer's (LR) if signs of hypovolemia are present. For hypotension with signs of hypovolemia, administer fluid cautiously. Consider vasopressors if patient is hypotensive with a normal fluid volume. Watch for signs of fluid overload (refer to shock protocol in Section Three).
- Treat convulsions with diazepam (Valium) or lorazepam (Ativan) (refer to diazepam and lorazepam protocols in Section Four and seizure protocol in Section Three).
- Use proparacaine hydrochloride to assist eye irrigation (refer to proparacaine hydrochloride protocol in Section Four).

INITIAL EMERGENCY DEPARTMENT CONSIDERATIONS

- Useful initial laboratory studies include complete blood count, serum electrolytes, blood urea nitrogen (BUN), creatinine, glucose, urinalysis, and baseline biochemical profile, including serum aminotransferases (AST and ALT), calcium, phosphorus, and magnesium. Determination of anion and osmolar gaps may be helpful. Arterial blood gases (ABGs), chest radiograph, and electrocardiogram may be required.
- Monitor for myoglobinuria. If present, maintain adequate hydration state and urinary output. Diuretic therapy may be necessary. Avoid alkalinization therapies, since this will delay excretion of strychnine.
- If convulsions are not controlled by diazepam or lorazepam, paralyzing agents (succinylcholine) may be needed.
- Acid diuresis is of questionable benefit and not indicated if myoglobinuria is present.
- Obtain toxicological consultation as necessary.

SPECIAL CONSIDERATIONS

- Very slight stimuli may cause convulsions; try to keep all external stimuli to a minimum.

Thiabendazoles and Related Compounds

SUBSTANCE IDENTIFICATION

A white, odorless solid. Formed as wettable powders, flowable suspension, thermal fumigation tablets, dusts, and 40% solutions. Used as systemic fungicides and in paint manufacturing. Thiabendazole (Mintezol) is used as a prescription anthelmintic.

ROUTES OF EXPOSURE

Skin and eye contact
Inhalation
Ingestion
Skin absorption

TARGET ORGANS

Primary
Skin
Eyes
Cardiovascular system
Respiratory system
Secondary
Central nervous system
Gastrointestinal system
Hepatic system
Renal system
Metabolism
Blood

LIFE THREAT

Cardiovascular collapse and respiratory tract irritation.

SIGNS AND SYMPTOMS BY SYSTEM

Cardiovascular: Bradycardia, hypotension, and cardiovascular collapse.
Respiratory: Respiratory tract irritation, wheezing, and hypersensitivity reaction possible.
CNS: Headache, drowsiness, giddiness, tinnitus, numbness, muscle incoordination, vertigo, hyperexcitability, seizures, and CNS depression.
Gastrointestinal: Epigastric distress, excessive salivation, anorexia, nausea, vomiting, and diarrhea.
Eye: Conjunctivitis.
Skin: Allergic dermatitis, erythema multiforme, and Stevens-Johnson syndrome (severe toxic cutaneous reaction with mucosal erosions).
Renal: Involuntary urination.
Hepatic: Liver damage.
Metabolism: Hyperglycemia.

Blood: Low white blood cell count (leukopenia).

Other: Some products have a carbamate structure but do not cause cholinesterase inhibitory effects. NOTE: Some of these products may be mixed with a hydrocarbon solvent as a vehicle. Toxicity may result from the solvent.

SYMPTOM ONSET FOR ACUTE EXPOSURE

Immediate

Some symptoms possibly delayed

THERMAL DECOMPOSITION PRODUCTS INCLUDE

n-Butylisocyanate

Hydrogen sulfide

Sulfides

Sulfur oxides

MEDICAL CONDITIONS POSSIBLY AGGRAVATED BY EXPOSURE

Allergic reactions

Asthma

Dermatitis

DECONTAMINATION

- Wear positive-pressure SCBA and protective equipment specified by references such as the *North American Emergency Response Guidebook*. If special chemical protective clothing is required, consult the chemical manufacturer or specific protective clothing compatibility charts. A qualified, experienced person should make decisions regarding the type of personal protective equipment necessary.
- Delay entry until trained personnel and proper protective equipment are available.
- Remove patient from contaminated area.
- Quickly remove and isolate patient's clothing, jewelry, and shoes.
- Gently brush away dry particles and blot excess liquids with absorbent material.
- Rinse patient with warm water, 32° C to 35° C (90° F to 95° F), if possible.
- Wash patient with a mild liquid soap and large quantities of water.
- Refer to decontamination protocol in Section Three.

IMMEDIATE FIRST AID

- Ensure that adequate decontamination has been carried out.
- If patient is not breathing, start artificial respiration, preferably with a demand-valve resuscitator, bag-valve-mask device, or pocket mask, as trained. Perform CPR if necessary.
- Immediately flush contaminated eyes with gently flowing water.
- Do not induce vomiting. If vomiting occurs, lean patient forward or place on left side (head-down position, if possible) to maintain an open airway and prevent aspiration.
- Keep patient quiet and maintain normal body temperature.
- Obtain medical attention.

BASIC TREATMENT

- Establish a patent airway (oropharyngeal or nasopharyngeal airway, if needed). Suction if necessary.
- Watch for signs of respiratory insufficiency and assist ventilations if necessary.
- Administer oxygen by nonrebreather mask at 10 to 15 L/min.
- Monitor for shock and treat if necessary (refer to shock protocol in Section Three).

- Anticipate seizures and treat if necessary (refer to seizure protocol in Section Three).
- For eye contamination, flush eyes immediately with water. Irrigate each eye continuously with 0.9% saline (NS) during transport (refer to eye irrigation protocol in Section Three).
- Do not use emetics. For ingestion, rinse mouth and administer 5 ml/kg up to 200 ml of water for dilution if the patient can swallow, has a strong gag reflex, and does not drool. Administer activated charcoal (refer to ingestion protocol in Section Three and activated charcoal protocol in Section Four).

ADVANCED TREATMENT

- Consider orotracheal or nasotracheal intubation for airway control in the patient who is unconscious or in severe respiratory distress.
- Consider administering a beta agonist such as albuterol for severe bronchospasm (refer to albuterol protocol in Section Four).
- Monitor cardiac rhythm and treat arrhythmias if necessary (refer to cardiac protocol in Section Three).
- Start IV administration of D_5W TKO. Use 0.9% saline (NS) or lactated Ringer's (LR) if signs of hypovolemia are present. For hypotension with signs of hypovolemia, administer fluid cautiously. Consider vasopressors if patient is hypotensive with a normal fluid volume. Watch for signs of fluid overload (refer to shock protocol in Section Three).
- Treat seizures with diazepam (Valium) or lorazepam (Ativan) (refer to diazepam and lorazepam protocols in Section Four and seizure protocol in Section Three).
- Use proparacaine hydrochloride to assist eye irrigation (refer to proparacaine hydrochloride protocol in Section Four).

INITIAL EMERGENCY DEPARTMENT CONSIDERATIONS

- Useful initial laboratory studies include complete blood count, serum electrolytes, blood urea nitrogen (BUN), creatinine, glucose, urinalysis, and baseline biochemical profile, including serum aminotransferases (AST and ALT), calcium, phosphorus, and magnesium. Determination of anion and osmolar gaps may be helpful. Arterial blood gases (ABGs), chest radiograph, and electrocardiogram may be required.
- Bronchospastic symptoms should be treated with an inhalation medication regimen similar to that used for reactive airways disease. Inhaled corticosteroids may be of value in severe bronchospasm.
- Obtain toxicological consultation as necessary.

SPECIAL CONSIDERATIONS

- Identify the solvent involved and consult the appropriate guideline.
- Acute toxicity problems are usually related to allergic dermatitis and hypersensitivity reactions.
- Thiabendazole has been reported to inhibit theophylline metabolism.

71

Warfarin, Hydroxycoumarin, Indandione, and Related Compounds

SUBSTANCE IDENTIFICATION

Colorless, odorless solids. Used as solids, pellets, dusts, and solutions. Used as rodenticides. A variety of products are on the market. Warfarin is marketed as the anticoagulant drug, brand name Coumadin.

ROUTES OF EXPOSURE

Skin and eye contact
Inhalation
Ingestion
Skin absorption

TARGET ORGANS

Primary
Eyes
Cardiovascular system
Hepatic system
Secondary
Skin
Central nervous system
Respiratory system
Gastrointestinal system
Renal system

LIFE THREAT

Impairs the clotting ability of the blood and causes internal hemorrhage.

SIGNS AND SYMPTOMS BY SYSTEM

Cardiovascular: Tachycardia and hypotension.
Respiratory: Mild tachypnea.
CNS: Possibly paralysis or other signs of cerebral vascular accident caused by cerebral hemorrhage.
Gastrointestinal: Hematemesis, epistaxis, and bleeding gums. Bloody or tar-like stools.
Eye: Chemical conjunctivitis.
Skin: Ecchymosis at knees, elbows, and buttocks.
Renal: Kidney damage.
Hepatic: Liver damage.
Other: Some products may present a human teratogenic risk. Symptoms usually result from repeated exposures. Newer products, the so-called "superwarfarins" (indandiones), may cause symptoms after a single exposure.

SYMPTOM ONSET FOR ACUTE EXPOSURE

Delayed maximum anticoagulation effect usually reached in 36 to 72 hours.

THERMAL DECOMPOSITION PRODUCTS INCLUDE

Acrid smoke and fumes
Carbon dioxide
Carbon monoxide

MEDICAL CONDITIONS POSSIBLY AGGRAVATED BY EXPOSURE

Blood disorders/bleeding tendencies

DECONTAMINATION

- Wear positive-pressure SCBA and protective equipment specified by references such as the *North American Emergency Response Guidebook*. If special chemical protective clothing is required, consult the chemical manufacturer or specific protective clothing compatibility charts. A qualified, experienced person should make decisions regarding the type of personal protective equipment necessary.
- Delay entry until trained personnel and proper protective equipment are available.
- Remove patient from contaminated area.
- Quickly remove and isolate patient's clothing, jewelry, and shoes.
- Gently brush away dry particles and blot excess liquids with absorbent material.
- Rinse patient with warm water, 32° C to 35° C (90° F to 95° F), if possible.
- Wash patient with a mild liquid soap and large quantities of water.
- Refer to decontamination protocol in Section Three.

IMMEDIATE FIRST AID

- Ensure that adequate decontamination has been carried out.
- If patient is not breathing, start artificial respiration, preferably with a demand-valve resuscitator, bag-valve-mask device, or pocket mask, as trained. Perform CPR if necessary.
- Immediately flush contaminated eyes with gently flowing water.
- Do not induce vomiting. If vomiting occurs, lean patient forward or place on left side (head-down position, if possible) to maintain an open airway and prevent aspiration.
- Keep patient quiet and maintain normal body temperature.
- Obtain medical attention.

BASIC TREATMENT

- Establish a patent airway (oropharyngeal or nasopharyngeal airway, if needed). Suction if necessary.
- Watch for signs of respiratory insufficiency and assist ventilations if necessary.
- Administer oxygen by nonrebreather mask at 10 to 15 L/min.
- Monitor for shock and treat if necessary (refer to shock protocol in Section Three).
- For eye contamination, flush eyes immediately with water. Irrigate each eye continuously with 0.9% saline (NS) during transport (refer to eye irrigation protocol in Section Three).
- Do not use emetics. For ingestion, rinse mouth and administer 5 ml/kg up to 200 ml of water for dilution if the patient can swallow, has a strong gag reflex, and does not drool. Administer activated charcoal (refer to ingestion protocol in Section Three and activated charcoal protocol in Section Four).

ADVANCED TREATMENT

- Consider orotracheal or nasotracheal intubation for airway control in the patient who is unconscious or is in severe respiratory distress.

- Start IV administration of 0.9% saline (NS) or lactated Ringer's (LR) TKO. For hypotension with signs of hypovolemia, administer fluid cautiously. Watch for signs of fluid overload (refer to shock protocol in Section Three).
- Use proparacaine hydrochloride to assist eye irrigation (refer to proparacaine hydrochloride protocol in Section Four).

INITIAL EMERGENCY DEPARTMENT CONSIDERATIONS

- Monitor clotting parameters, including prothrombin and partial thromboplastin times.
- Useful initial laboratory studies include complete blood count, serum electrolytes, blood urea nitrogen (BUN), creatinine, glucose, urinalysis, and baseline biochemical profile, including serum aminotransferases (AST and ALT), lactic dehydrogenase (LDH), calcium, phosphorus, and magnesium. Determination of anion and osmolar gaps may be helpful. Arterial blood gases (ABGs), chest radiograph, and electrocardiogram may be required.
- IM administration of vitamin K_1 (Aquamyphyton) may be beneficial (adult dosage: 5 to 10 mg; pediatric dosage: 1 to 5 mg).
- In severe poisoning cases with hemorrhage, vitamin K_1 may be given intravenously (adult dosage: 10 mg; pediatric dosage: 5 mg). Do not use vitamin K_3 (Synkavite). NOTE: IV use has increased risk of anaphylaxis.
- Fresh frozen plasma may be necessary.
- Obtain toxicological consultation as necessary.

SPECIAL CONSIDERATIONS

- Use caution with invasive therapeutic measures. Intubation may cause upper airway hemorrhage.
- Persons taking sulfa drugs (Bactrim), aspirin, NSAIDs, anti-platelet medications (e.g., Ticlid), amiodarone, metronidazole, erythromycin, and tetracycline may have an augmented response.

Arsenic and Related Compounds

SUBSTANCE IDENTIFICATION

A silver-gray, crystalline, solid or black and yellow amorphous form. Used in the manufacture of glass, metallurgy, alloys, and electrical and semiconductor devices. Also used in the manufacture of many commercial products, including insecticides, herbicides, desiccants, and wood preservatives.

ROUTES OF EXPOSURE

Skin and eye contact
Inhalation
Ingestion
Skin absorption

TARGET ORGANS

Primary
Skin
Eyes
Respiratory system
Hepatic system
Renal system
Blood
Secondary
Central nervous system
Cardiovascular system
Gastrointestinal system

LIFE THREAT

Heavy metal toxicity. Vomiting with GI bleeding. CNS depression, pulmonary edema, and cardiac arrest.

SIGNS AND SYMPTOMS BY SYSTEM

Cardiovascular: Hypovolemic shock and circulatory collapse. Tachycardia and ventricular arrhythmias. QT interval prolongation and T wave changes.

Respiratory: Respiratory tract irritation, depression, and pulmonary edema.

CNS: Headache, vertigo, delirium, syncope, CNS depression, muscle cramps, coma, and seizures. Peripheral neuropathy with chronic exposure.

Gastrointestinal: Burning pain, nausea, vomiting, and bloody diarrhea. GI bleeding with hematemesis and hematochezia. Intense thirst, garlic-type breath odor.

Eye: Chemical conjunctivitis, corneal damage.

Skin: Dermatitis and burns. Cyanosis and cold extremities.

Renal: Kidney damage and hemoglobinuria.

Hepatic: Liver damage.

Blood: Anemia, low white blood cell count (leukopenia), decreased platelet count (thrombocytopenia), bone marrow suppression (pancytopenia), and increased bone marrow vascularity.

Other: Some products may present a human carcinogenic or teratogenic risk. Arsenic in contact with acid or acid mist may produce arsine gas.

SYMPTOM ONSET FOR ACUTE EXPOSURE

Immediate

Some symptoms (blood, hepatic, renal) possibly delayed

THERMAL DECOMPOSITION PRODUCTS INCLUDE

Metal oxide fumes

Arsenic trioxide

MEDICAL CONDITIONS POSSIBLY AGGRAVATED BY EXPOSURE

Respiratory system disorders

Nervous system disorders

Liver disorders

Kidney disorders

DECONTAMINATION

- Wear positive-pressure SCBA and protective equipment specified by references such as the North American Emergency Response Guidebook. If special chemical protective clothing is required, consult the chemical manufacturer or specific protective clothing compatibility charts. A qualified, experienced person should make decisions regarding the type of personal protective equipment necessary.
- Delay entry until trained personnel and proper protective equipment are available.
- Remove patient from contaminated area.
- Quickly remove and isolate patient's clothing, jewelry, and shoes.
- Gently brush away dry particles and blot excess liquids with absorbent material.
- Rinse patient with warm water, 32° C to 35° C (90° F to 95° F), if possible.
- Wash patient with a mild liquid soap and large quantities of water.
- Refer to decontamination protocol in Section Three.

IMMEDIATE FIRST AID

- Remove patient from contact with the material.
- Ensure that adequate decontamination has been carried out.
- If patient is not breathing, start artificial respiration, preferably with a demand-valve resuscitator, bag-valve-mask device, or pocket mask, as trained. Perform CPR if necessary.
- Immediately flush contaminated eyes with gently flowing water.
- Do not induce vomiting. If vomiting occurs, lean patient forward or place on left side (head-down position, if possible) to maintain an open airway and prevent aspiration.
- Keep patient quiet and maintain normal body temperature.
- Obtain medical attention.

BASIC TREATMENT

- Establish a patent airway (oropharyngeal or nasopharyngeal airway, if needed). Suction if necessary.
- Watch for signs of respiratory insufficiency and assist ventilations if necessary.
- Administer oxygen by nonrebreather mask at 10 to 15 L/min.
- Monitor for shock and treat if necessary (refer to shock protocol in Section Three).

- Monitor for pulmonary edema and treat if necessary (refer to pulmonary edema protocol in Section Three).
- Treat seizures if necessary (refer to seizure protocol in Section Three).
- For eye contamination, flush eyes immediately with water. Irrigate each eye continuously with 0.9% saline (NS) during transport (refer to eye irrigation protocol in Section Three).
- Do not use emetics. For ingestion, rinse mouth and administer 5 ml/kg up to 200 ml of water for dilution if the patient can swallow, has a strong gag reflex, and does not drool. Administer activated charcoal (refer to ingestion protocol in Section Three and activated charcoal protocol in Section Four).

ADVANCED TREATMENT

- Consider orotracheal or nasotracheal intubation for airway control in the patient who is unconscious, has severe pulmonary edema, or is in severe respiratory distress.
- Positive-pressure ventilation techniques with a bag-valve-mask device may be beneficial.
- Consider drug therapy for pulmonary edema (refer to pulmonary edema protocol in Section Three).
- Monitor cardiac rhythm and treat arrhythmias if necessary (refer to cardiac protocol in Section Three).
- Start IV administration of D_5W TKO. Use 0.9% saline (NS) or lactated Ringer's (LR) if signs of hypovolemia are present. For hypotension with signs of hypovolemia, administer fluid cautiously. Consider vasopressors if patient is hypotensive with a normal fluid volume. Watch for signs of fluid overload and pulmonary edema (refer to shock protocol in Section Three).
- Treat seizures with diazepam (Valium) or lorazepam (Ativan) (refer to diazepam and lorazepam protocols in Section Four and seizure protocol in Section Three).
- Use proparacaine hydrochloride to assist eye irrigation (refer to proparacaine hydrochloride protocol in Section Four).

INITIAL EMERGENCY DEPARTMENT CONSIDERATIONS

- Useful initial laboratory studies include complete blood count, serum electrolytes, blood urea nitrogen (BUN), creatinine, glucose, urinalysis, coagulation profile, and baseline biochemical profile, including serum aminotransferases (AST and ALT), calcium, phosphorus, and magnesium. Determination of anion and osmolar gaps may be helpful. Arterial blood gases (ABGs), chest radiograph, and electrocardiogram may be required.
- Blood and urine arsenic determinations should be done. Treatment should not be delayed in the symptomatic patient, since results may take several days to obtain.
- Positive end-expiratory pressure (PEEP)–assisted ventilation may be necessary in patients with acute parenchymal injury who develop pulmonary edema or acute respiratory distress syndrome.
- Closely monitor hydration state and urinary output and maintain if necessary.
- Urine alkalinization and chelation therapy with BAL or D-penicillamine may be beneficial in symptomatic patients. Therapy should be guided by patient presentation and renal test values.
- Hemodialysis may be required in cases of acute renal failure.
- Obtain toxicological consultation as necessary.

73

Arsine and Related Compounds

SUBSTANCE IDENTIFICATION

Found as a colorless gas that may have a garlic-type odor. Arsine may be found wherever hydrogen is generated in the presence of arsenic. Arsine is formed by the action of a weak acid on arsenic-containing iron or other nonferrous metals. Used in the electronics industry in doping gas mixtures for semiconductors and in organic synthesis. Most common type of exposure is during cleaning of tanks and tank cars.

ROUTES OF EXPOSURE

Skin and eye contact
Inhalation

TARGET ORGANS

Primary
Cardiovascular system
Hepatic system
Renal system
Blood
Secondary
Skin
Eyes
Central nervous system
Respiratory system
Gastrointestinal system

LIFE THREAT

Intravascular hemolysis, pulmonary edema, and acute renal failure. Latent period of 2 to 24 hours may precede jaundice and renal failure. Exposure may cause cardiac and respiratory arrest.

SIGNS AND SYMPTOMS BY SYSTEM

Cardiovascular: Tachycardia, ventricular arrhythmias, and hypotension.
Respiratory: Dyspnea and pulmonary edema. Respiratory tract irritation.
CNS: Headache, dizziness, paresthesia, delirium, and coma.
Gastrointestinal: Nausea, vomiting, and abdominal pain.
Eye: Chemical conjunctivitis, corneal damage. Red staining of the conjunctiva.
Skin: Dermatitis and burns. Bronzing of the skin and jaundice.
Renal: Red or bronze-colored urine. Painless hematuria leading to renal damage or acute renal failure.
Hepatic: Liver damage with jaundice.
Blood: Intravascular hemolysis, anemia, bone marrow depression. Decreased erythrocyte glutathione (GSH) reported.
Other: Some products may present a human carcinogen or teratogenic risk. Can be fatal or cause severe injuries at concentrations below the odor threshold (0.5 ppm).

SYMPTOM ONSET FOR ACUTE EXPOSURE

Immediate
Some symptoms possibly delayed for minutes to hours

CO-EXPOSURE CONCERNS

Chlorine
Fluorine
Nitric acid
Nitrogen trifluoride

THERMAL DECOMPOSITION PRODUCTS INCLUDE

Arsenic trioxide
Arsine generation from gallium arsenide

MEDICAL CONDITIONS COMMONLY AGGRAVATED BY EXPOSURE

Kidney disease
Congenital deficiency of reduced erythrocyte glutathione (GSH)
Anemia

DECONTAMINATION

- Wear positive-pressure SCBA and protective equipment specified by references such as the *North American Emergency Response Guidebook.* If special chemical protective clothing is required, consult the chemical manufacturer or specific protective clothing compatibility charts. A qualified, experienced person should make decisions regarding the type of personal protective equipment necessary.
- Delay entry until trained personnel and proper protective equipment are available.
- Remove patient from contaminated area.
- Quickly remove and isolate patient's clothing, jewelry, and shoes.
- If any concurrent liquid or solid contamination exists:
  Gently brush away dry particles and blot excess liquids with absorbent material.
  Rinse patient with warm water, 32° C to 35° C (90° F to 95° F), if possible.
  Wash patient with a mild liquid soap and large quantities of water.
- Refer to decontamination protocol in Section Three.

IMMEDIATE FIRST AID

- Ensure that adequate decontamination has been carried out.
- If patient is not breathing, start artificial respiration, preferably with a demand-valve resuscitator, bag-valve-mask device, or pocket mask, as trained. Perform CPR if necessary.
- Immediately flush contaminated eyes with gently flowing water.
- Do not induce vomiting. If vomiting occurs, lean patient forward or place on left side (head-down position, if possible) to maintain an open airway and prevent aspiration.
- Keep patient quiet and maintain normal body temperature.
- Obtain medical attention.

BASIC TREATMENT

- Establish a patent airway (oropharyngeal or nasopharyngeal airway, if needed). Suction if necessary.
- Watch for signs of respiratory insufficiency and assist ventilations if necessary.
- Administer oxygen by nonrebreather mask at 10 to 15 L/min.
- Monitor for shock and treat if necessary (refer to shock protocol in Section Three).

- Monitor for pulmonary edema and treat if necessary (refer to pulmonary edema protocol in Section Three).
- For eye contamination, flush eyes immediately with water. Irrigate each eye continuously with 0.9% saline (NS) during transport (refer to eye irrigation protocol in Section Three).

ADVANCED TREATMENT

- Consider orotracheal or nasotracheal intubation for airway control in the patient who is unconscious, has severe pulmonary edema, or is in severe respiratory distress.
- Positive-pressure ventilation techniques with a bag-valve-mask device may be beneficial.
- Consider drug therapy for pulmonary edema (refer to pulmonary edema protocol in Section Three).
- Administer furosemide (Lasix) (refer to furosemide protocol in Section Four).
- Monitor cardiac rhythm and treat arrhythmias if necessary (refer to cardiac protocol in Section Three).
- Start IV administration of 0.9% saline (NS) or lactated Ringer's (LR). Titrate flow to maintain urine output. Treat hypotension with cautious fluid administration. Vasopressors should be used only if fluid administration cannot maintain an adequate blood pressure. Watch for signs of fluid overload (refer to shock protocol in Section Three).
- Administer sodium bicarbonate IV push, by DIRECT PHYSICIAN ORDER ONLY. This will alkalinize the urine and prevent hemoglobin precipitation and acute renal failure (refer to sodium bicarbonate protocol in Section Four).
- Cover skin burns with dry sterile dressings after decontamination (refer to chemical burn protocol in Section Three).
- Use proparacaine hydrochloride to assist eye irrigation (refer to proparacaine hydrochloride protocol in Section Four).

INITIAL EMERGENCY DEPARTMENT CONSIDERATIONS

- Useful initial laboratory studies include complete blood count, serum electrolytes, blood urea nitrogen (BUN), creatinine, glucose, urinalysis, coagulation profile, blood and urine arsenic concentrations, and baseline biochemical profile, including serum aminotransferases (AST and ALT), calcium, phosphorus, and magnesium. Determination of anion and osmolar gaps may be helpful. Arterial blood gases (ABGs), chest radiograph, and electrocardiogram may be required.
- Positive end-expiratory pressure (PEEP)–assisted ventilation may be necessary in patients with acute parenchymal injury who develop pulmonary edema or acute respiratory distress syndrome.
- Hemodialysis may be beneficial in the severely poisoned patient.
- Obtain toxicological consultation as necessary.

Barium and Related Compounds

SUBSTANCE IDENTIFICATION

Found in a white or yellowish metal powder that will evolve gas. Contained in rodenticides, alloys, paints, soap, paper, rubber, ceramics, glass, depilatories of animal hair, and fireworks. Also found in x-ray contrast (barium sulfate) media and in the textile industry and steel-hardening procedures. Also used in spark plugs and engine rod bearings and in gas removal from vacuum tubes during manufacturing.

ROUTES OF EXPOSURE

Skin and eye exposure
Inhalation
Ingestion

TARGET ORGANS

Primary
Skin
Eyes
Central nervous system
Cardiovascular system
Respiratory system
Secondary
Gastrointestinal system
Renal system
Metabolism

LIFE THREAT

Cardiac arrhythmias leading to cardiac arrest and respiratory arrest caused by hypokalemia and muscle paralysis.

SIGNS AND SYMPTOMS BY SYSTEM

Cardiovascular: Ventricular arrhythmias with premature ventricular contractions (PVCs) leading to bradycardia, episodes of ventricular tachycardia, ventricular fibrillation, and asystole. Vasoconstriction and transient hypertension. Hypotension caused by fluid loss from vomiting and diarrhea.

Respiratory: Failure due to respiratory muscle paralysis. A corrosive action that may cause irritation and bronchial pneumonia.

CNS: Dizziness, tinnitus, muscle spasms, and seizures followed by coma and paralysis.

Gastrointestinal: Severe gastroenteritis causing cramp-type pain, nausea, vomiting, and bloody diarrhea. Excessive salivation.

Eye: Chemical conjunctivitis and severe burns with corneal damage possible. Dilated pupils may be present.

Skin: May be alkaline in solution and cause severe skin burns.

Renal: Kidney damage.
Metabolism: Hypokalemia.

SYMPTOM ONSET FOR ACUTE EXPOSURE

Immediate
Some symptoms possibly delayed

CO-EXPOSURE CONCERNS

Other metals

THERMAL DECOMPOSITION PRODUCTS INCLUDE

Oxides
Barium hydride

MEDICAL CONDITIONS POSSIBLY AGGRAVATED BY EXPOSURE

Respiratory disorders
Cardiac dysrhythmias
Low serum potassium

DECONTAMINATION

- Wear positive-pressure SCBA and protective equipment specified by references such as the *North American Emergency Response Guidebook.* If special chemical protective clothing is required, consult the chemical manufacturer or specific protective clothing compatibility charts. A qualified, experienced person should make decisions regarding the type of personal protective equipment necessary.
- Delay entry until trained personnel and proper protective equipment are available.
- Remove patient from contaminated area.
- Quickly remove and isolate patient's clothing, jewelry, and shoes.
- Gently brush away dry particles and blot excess liquids with absorbent material.
- Rinse patient with warm water, 32° C to 35° C (90° F to 95° F), if possible.
- Wash patient with a mild liquid soap and large quantities of water.
- Refer to decontamination protocol in Section Three.

IMMEDIATE FIRST AID

- Ensure that adequate decontamination has been carried out.
- If patient is not breathing, start artificial respiration, preferably with a demand-valve resuscitator, bag-valve-mask device, or pocket mask, as trained. Perform CPR if necessary.
- Immediately flush contaminated eyes with gently flowing water.
- Do not induce vomiting. If vomiting occurs, lean patient forward or place on left side (head-down position, if possible) to maintain an open airway and prevent aspiration.
- Keep patient quiet and maintain normal body temperature.
- Obtain medical attention.

BASIC TREATMENT

- Establish a patent airway (oropharyngeal or nasopharyngeal airway, if needed). Suction if necessary.
- Watch for signs of respiratory insufficiency and assist ventilations if necessary.
- Administer oxygen by nonrebreather mask at 10 to 15 L/min.
- Monitor for shock and treat if necessary (refer to shock protocol in Section Three).
- Anticipate seizures and treat if necessary (refer to seizure protocol in Section Three).

- For eye contamination, flush eyes immediately with water. Irrigate each eye continuously with 0.9% saline (NS) during transport (refer to eye irrigation protocol in Section Three).
- Do not use emetics. For ingestion, rinse mouth and administer 5 ml/kg up to 200 ml of water for dilution if the patient can swallow, has a strong gag reflex, and does not drool (refer to ingestion protocol in Section Three).
- Do not attempt to neutralize, because of exothermic reaction.
- Cover skin burns with dry sterile dressings after decontamination (refer to chemical burn protocol in Section Three).

ADVANCED TREATMENT

- Consider orotracheal or nasotracheal intubation for airway control in the patient who is unconscious or is in severe respiratory distress.
- Monitor cardiac rhythm and treat arrhythmias if necessary (refer to cardiac protocol in Section Three).
- Start IV administration of 0.9% saline (NS) or lactated Ringer's (LR) TKO. For hypotension with signs of hypovolemia, administer fluid cautiously. Watch for signs of fluid overload (refer to shock protocol in Section Three).
- Treat seizures with diazepam (Valium) or lorazepam (Ativan) (refer to diazepam and lorazepam protocols in Section Four and seizure protocol in Section Three).
- Use proparacaine hydrochloride to assist eye irrigation (refer to proparacaine hydrochloride protocol in Section Four).

INITIAL EMERGENCY DEPARTMENT CONSIDERATIONS

- Useful initial laboratory studies include complete blood count, serum electrolytes, blood urea nitrogen (BUN), creatinine, glucose, urinalysis, and baseline biochemical profile, including serum aminotransferases (AST and ALT), calcium, phosphorus, and magnesium. Determination of anion and osmolar gaps may be helpful. Arterial blood gases (ABGs), chest radiograph, and electrocardiogram may be required.
- Serum potassium should be monitored and hypokalemia treated if necessary.
- Forced diuresis and hemodialysis may be beneficial in the severely poisoned patient.
- Obtain toxicological consultation as necessary.

Beryllium and Related Compounds

SUBSTANCE IDENTIFICATION

A hard, light, grayish-white metal. May exist as fume (beryllium oxide), respirable dust, metal, or alloy. Used in the manufacture of electrical components, chemicals, ceramics, and x-ray tubes. Beryllium is also added to many alloys to increase strength and corrosion resistance.

ROUTES OF EXPOSURE

Skin and eye contact
Inhalation
Ingestion

TARGET ORGANS

Primary
Skin
Eyes
Respiratory system
Secondary
Central nervous system
Cardiovascular system
Gastrointestinal system
Hepatic system
Renal system

LIFE THREAT

Acute beryllium pneumonitis and pulmonary edema.

SIGNS AND SYMPTOMS BY SYSTEM

Cardiovascular: Tachycardia.

Respiratory: Irritation of respiratory tract. Epistaxis, feeling of facial fullness with pain, nonproductive cough, dyspnea, and pulmonary edema. Chest pain or tightness of the chest may be present. Berylliosis (chronic beryllium disease).

CNS: Weakness, dizziness, and fatigue. Seizures.

Gastrointestinal: Irritation of the mucous membranes.

Eye: Chemical conjunctivitis, corneal damage, and severe burns.

Skin: Dermatitis. If solid beryllium is implanted under broken or abraded skin, lesions with central nonhealing areas may result. Cyanosis may be present.

Renal: Kidney dysfunction.

Hepatic: Liver damage.

Other: Some products may present a human carcinogen risk.

SYMPTOM ONSET FOR ACUTE EXPOSURE

Immediate
Some symptoms possibly delayed

THERMAL DECOMPOSITION PRODUCTS INCLUDE

Beryllium oxide fumes
Hydrogen chloride
Hydrogen
Nitrogen oxides
Sulfur dioxide

MEDICAL CONDITIONS GENERALLY AGGRAVATED BY EXPOSURE

Pulmonary disorders
Cardiac disorders
Skin disorders
Liver disorders
Kidney disorders

DECONTAMINATION

- Wear positive-pressure SCBA and protective equipment specified by references such as the *North American Emergency Response Guidebook*. If special chemical protective clothing is required, consult the chemical manufacturer or specific protective clothing compatibility charts. A qualified, experienced person should make decisions regarding the type of personal protective equipment necessary.
- Delay entry until trained personnel and proper protective equipment are available.
- Remove patient from contaminated area.
- Quickly remove and isolate patient's clothing, jewelry, and shoes.
- Gently brush away dry particles and blot excess liquids with absorbent material.
- Rinse patient with warm water, 32° C to 35° C (90° F to 95° F), if possible.
- Wash patient with a mild liquid soap and large quantities of water.
- Refer to decontamination protocol in Section Three.

IMMEDIATE FIRST AID

- Ensure that adequate decontamination has been carried out.
- If patient is not breathing, start artificial respiration, preferably with a demand-valve resuscitator, bag-valve-mask device, or pocket mask, as trained. Perform CPR if necessary.
- Immediately flush contaminated eyes with gently flowing water.
- Do not induce vomiting. If vomiting occurs, lean patient forward or place on left side (head-down position, if possible) to maintain an open airway and prevent aspiration.
- Keep patient quiet and maintain normal body temperature.
- Obtain medical attention.

BASIC TREATMENT

- Establish a patent airway (oropharyngeal or nasopharyngeal airway, if needed). Suction if necessary.
- Watch for signs of respiratory insufficiency and assist ventilations if necessary.
- Administer oxygen by nonrebreather mask at 10 to 15 L/min.
- Monitor for pulmonary edema and treat if necessary (refer to pulmonary edema protocol in Section Three).
- Anticipate seizures and treat if necessary (refer to seizure protocol in Section Three).
- For eye contamination, flush eyes immediately with water. Irrigate each eye continuously with 0.9% saline (NS) during transport (refer to eye irrigation protocol in Section Three).

- Do not use emetics. For ingestion, rinse mouth and administer 5 ml/kg up to 200 ml of water for dilution if the patient can swallow, has a strong gag reflex, and does not drool. Administer activated charcoal (refer to ingestion protocol in Section Three and activated charcoal protocol in Section Four).

ADVANCED TREATMENT

- Consider orotracheal or nasotracheal intubation for airway control in the patient who is unconscious, has severe pulmonary edema, or is in severe respiratory distress.
- Positive-pressure ventilation techniques with a bag-valve-mask device may be beneficial.
- Consider drug therapy for pulmonary edema (refer to pulmonary edema protocol in Section Three).
- Monitor cardiac rhythm and treat arrhythmias if necessary (refer to cardiac protocol in Section Three).
- Start IV administration of D_5W TKO. Use 0.9% saline (NS) or lactated Ringer's (LR) if signs of hypovolemia are present. For hypotension with signs of hypovolemia, administer fluid cautiously. Watch for signs of fluid overload (refer to shock protocol in Section Three).
- Treat seizures with diazepam (Valium) or lorazepam (Ativan) (refer to diazepam and lorazepam protocols in Section Four and seizure protocol in Section Three).
- Use proparacaine hydrochloride to assist eye irrigation (refer to proparacaine hydrochloride protocol in Section Four).

INITIAL EMERGENCY DEPARTMENT CONSIDERATIONS

- Useful initial laboratory studies include complete blood count, serum electrolytes, blood urea nitrogen (BUN), creatinine, glucose, urinalysis, and baseline biochemical profile, including serum aminotransferases (AST and ALT), calcium, phosphorus, and magnesium. Determination of anion and osmolar gaps may be helpful. Arterial blood gases (ABGs), chest radiograph, and electrocardiogram may be required. Beryllium blood concentrations not helpful in management.
- Positive end-expiratory pressure (PEEP)–assisted ventilation may be necessary in patients with acute parenchymal injury who develop pulmonary edema or acute respiratory distress syndrome.
- Obtain toxicological consultation as necessary.

SPECIAL CONSIDERATIONS

- Beryllium lymphocyte transformation test useful in assessing risk of developing lung fibrosis (berylliosis) from beryllium exposure.

Cadmium and Related Compounds

SUBSTANCE IDENTIFICATION

Odorless, white, metallic solid. Found as a powder, pure sticks, ingots, slabs, or crystals. Used in various silver and copper alloys; in rustproofing; in the production of phosphors, paints, pigments, and batteries; and in various metallurgical processes, including metal electroplating. Also a by-product of zinc-smelting operations. May be released from welding cadmium-containing objects or soldering (copper, lead, tin, zinc, and silver solder) and brazing with rods or wire containing cadmium.

ROUTES OF EXPOSURE

Skin and eye contact
Inhalation
Ingestion

TARGET ORGANS

Primary
Skin
Eyes
Cardiovascular system
Respiratory system
Renal system
Secondary
Central nervous system
Gastrointestinal system
Hepatic system
Metabolism

LIFE THREAT

Respiratory irritant that can cause pulmonary edema.

SIGNS AND SYMPTOMS BY SYSTEM

Cardiovascular: Tachycardia and arrhythmias.

Respiratory: Respiratory tract irritation. Productive cough, stridor, dyspnea, tachypnea, and noncardiac chest pain. Cadmium fume pneumonitis, acute pulmonary edema (sometimes hemorrhagic), and pulmonary fibrosis.

CNS: Headache, weakness, vertigo, and metallic taste in the mouth. CNS depression to coma. Seizures are rare. Muscle cramps may be present.

Gastrointestinal: Nausea, vomiting, hemorrhagic gastritis, and diarrhea. Abdominal cramps and excessive salivation.

Eye: Chemical conjunctivitis.

Skin: Dermatitis.

Renal: Kidney damage.

Hepatic: Liver damage.

Metabolism: Metabolic acidosis. Altered calcium metabolism.
Other: Fever. Some products may present a human carcinogenic risk.

SYMPTOM ONSET FOR ACUTE EXPOSURE

Immediate
Some symptoms possibly delayed for days

CO-EXPOSURE CONCERNS

Metals capable of causing a metal fume fever-type syndrome.
Cigarette smoking (cigarette smoking increases normal cadmium intake)

THERMAL DECOMPOSITION PRODUCTS INCLUDE

Cadmium oxides
Sulfur dioxide

MEDICAL CONDITIONS POSSIBLY AGGRAVATED BY EXPOSURE

Respiratory disorders
Kidney disorders

DECONTAMINATION

- Wear positive-pressure SCBA and protective equipment specified by references such as the *North American Emergency Response Guidebook*. If special chemical protective clothing is required, consult the chemical manufacturer or specific protective clothing compatibility charts. A qualified, experienced person should make decisions regarding the type of personal protective equipment necessary.
- Delay entry until trained personnel and proper protective equipment are available.
- Remove patient from contaminated area.
- Quickly remove and isolate patient's clothing, jewelry, and shoes.
- Gently brush away dry particles and blot excess liquids with absorbent material.
- Rinse patient with warm water, 32° C to 35° C (90° F to 95° F), if possible.
- Wash patient with a mild liquid soap and large quantities of water.
- Refer to decontamination protocol in Section Three.

IMMEDIATE FIRST AID

- Ensure that adequate decontamination has been carried out.
- If patient is not breathing, start artificial respiration, preferably with a demand-valve resuscitator, bag-valve-mask device, or pocket mask, as trained. Perform CPR if necessary.
- Immediately flush contaminated eyes with gently flowing water.
- Do not induce vomiting. If vomiting occurs, lean patient forward or place on left side (head-down position, if possible) to maintain an open airway and prevent aspiration.
- Keep patient quiet and maintain normal body temperature.
- Obtain medical attention.

BASIC TREATMENT

- Establish a patent airway (oropharyngeal or nasopharyngeal airway, if needed). Suction if necessary.
- Watch for signs of respiratory insufficiency and assist ventilations if necessary.
- Administer oxygen by nonrebreather mask at 10 to 15 L/min.
- Monitor for pulmonary edema and treat if necessary (refer to pulmonary edema protocol in Section Three).
- Anticipate seizures and treat if necessary (refer to seizure protocol in Section Three).

- For eye contamination, flush eyes immediately with water. Irrigate each eye continuously with 0.9% saline (NS) during transport (refer to eye irrigation protocol in Section Three).
- Do not use emetics. For ingestion, rinse mouth and administer 5 ml/kg up to 200 ml of water for dilution if the patient can swallow, has a strong gag reflex, and does not drool. Administer activated charcoal (refer to ingestion protocol in Section Three and activated charcoal protocol in Section Four).

ADVANCED TREATMENT

- Consider orotracheal or nasotracheal intubation for airway control in the patient who is unconscious, has severe pulmonary edema, or is in severe respiratory distress.
- Positive-pressure ventilation techniques with a bag-valve-mask device may be beneficial.
- Consider drug therapy for pulmonary edema (refer to pulmonary edema protocol in Section Three).
- Monitor cardiac rhythm and treat arrhythmias if necessary (refer to cardiac protocol in Section Three).
- Start IV administration of D_5W TKO. Use 0.9% saline (NS) or lactated Ringer's (LR) if signs of hypovolemia are present. For hypotension with signs of hypovolemia, administer fluid cautiously. Watch for signs of fluid overload (refer to shock protocol in Section Three).
- Treat seizures with diazepam (Valium) or lorazepam (Ativan) (refer to diazepam and lorazepam protocols in Section Four and seizure protocol in Section Three).
- Use proparacaine hydrochloride to assist eye irrigation (refer to proparacaine hydrochloride protocol in Section Four).

INITIAL EMERGENCY DEPARTMENT CONSIDERATIONS

- Useful initial laboratory studies include complete blood count, serum electrolytes, blood urea nitrogen (BUN), creatinine, glucose, urinalysis, and baseline biochemical profile, including serum aminotransferases (ALT and AST), calcium, phosphorus, and magnesium. Blood and urine cadmium concentrations may be obtained. Determination of anion and osmolar gaps may be helpful. Arterial blood gases (ABGs), chest radiograph, and electrocardiogram may be required.
- Urinary cadmium concentrations provide an indication of recent cadmium exposure and body burden. Beta$_2$-microglobulin determination in urine may be increased in acute cadmium induced nephropathy.
- Serum cadmium concentrations range from 0.0005 to 0.002 mg/L, with blood cadmium averaging 0.004 mg/L in nonexposed workers to 0.009 mg/L in asymptomatic individuals exposed to cadmium fumes. Urine cadmium concentrations over 0.005 mg/L may indicate excessive exposure.
- Positive end-expiratory pressure (PEEP)–assisted ventilation may be necessary in patients with acute parenchymal injury who develop pulmonary edema or acute respiratory distress syndrome.
- There are no effective chelating agents. Calcium and vitamin D therapy have proven useful in cases of severe bone loss.
- Obtain toxicological consultation as necessary.

SPECIAL CONSIDERATIONS

- Cadmium has a half-life in humans of 25 to 30 years.

77

Cobalt and Related Compounds

SUBSTANCE IDENTIFICATION

Silvery gray to silvery, bluish white odorless solid or found in solution form. Used in the manufacture of cobalt-bearing alloys, permanent magnets, lacquers, paint driers, cutting materials, and wear-resistant materials; in the production of inks, enamels, glazes, glass/ceramic pigments, and catalysts; and in the synthesis of heating fuels and as a catalyst in hydrocarbon production. Pyrophoric cobalt is a black powder that burns in contact with air.

ROUTES OF EXPOSURE

Skin and eye contact
Inhalation
Ingestion
Skin absorption

TARGET ORGANS

Primary
Skin
Eyes
Cardiovascular system
Respiratory system
Blood
Secondary
Central nervous system
Gastrointestinal system
Renal system
Metabolism

LIFE THREAT

Respiratory irritant that may cause pulmonary edema and fibrosis.

SIGNS AND SYMPTOMS BY SYSTEM

Cardiovascular: Tachycardia, arrhythmias, and hypotension.

Respiratory: Respiratory tract irritation. Cough, wheezing, stridor, dyspnea, tachypnea, and noncardiac chest pain. Interstitial fibrosis and pulmonary edema. Reactive airways disease.

CNS: CNS depression.

Gastrointestinal: Nausea, vomiting, diarrhea, abdominal cramps, and pancreatitis.

Eye: Chemical conjunctivitis and corneal damage.

Skin: Irritant or allergic dermatitis.

Renal: Hematuria and kidney damage.

Metabolism: Metabolic acidosis. Hypothyroidism.

Blood: Coagulation abnormalities.

SYMPTOM ONSET FOR ACUTE EXPOSURE

Immediate
Some symptoms possibly delayed for days

CO-EXPOSURE CONCERNS

Nickel
Chromium

MEDICAL CONDITIONS POSSIBLY AGGRAVATED BY EXPOSURE

Cardiovascular disorders
Respiratory disorders
Skin disorders

DECONTAMINATION

- Wear positive-pressure SCBA and protective equipment specified by references such as the *North American Emergency Response Guidebook*. If special chemical protective clothing is required, consult the chemical manufacturer or specific protective clothing compatibility charts. A qualified, experienced person should make decisions regarding the type of personal protective equipment necessary.
- Delay entry until trained personnel and proper protective equipment are available.
- Remove patient from contaminated area.
- Quickly remove and isolate patient's clothing, jewelry, and shoes.
- Gently brush away dry particles and blot excess liquids with absorbent material.
- Rinse patient with warm water, 32° C to 35° C (90° F to 95° F), if possible.
- Wash patient with a mild liquid soap and large quantities of water.
- Refer to decontamination protocol in Section Three.

IMMEDIATE FIRST AID

- Ensure that adequate decontamination has been carried out.
- If patient is not breathing, start artificial respiration, preferably with a demand-valve resuscitator, bag-valve-mask device, or pocket mask, as trained. Perform CPR if necessary.
- Immediately flush contaminated eyes with gently flowing water.
- Do not induce vomiting. If vomiting occurs, lean patient forward or place on left side (head-down position, if possible) to maintain an open airway and prevent aspiration.
- Keep patient quiet and maintain normal body temperature.
- Obtain medical attention.

BASIC TREATMENT

- Establish a patent airway (oropharyngeal or nasopharyngeal airway, if needed). Suction if necessary.
- Watch for signs of respiratory insufficiency and assist ventilations if necessary.
- Administer oxygen by nonrebreather mask at 10 to 15 L/min.
- Monitor for pulmonary edema and treat if necessary (refer to pulmonary edema protocol in Section Three).
- Monitor for shock and treat if necessary (refer to shock protocol in Section Three).
- For eye contamination, flush eyes immediately with water. Irrigate each eye continuously with 0.9% saline (NS) during transport (refer to eye irrigation protocol in Section Three).

- Do not use emetics. For ingestion, rinse mouth and administer 5 ml/kg up to 200 ml of water for dilution if the patient can swallow, has a strong gag reflex, and does not drool. Administer activated charcoal (refer to ingestion protocol in Section Three and activated charcoal protocol in Section Four).

ADVANCED TREATMENT

- Consider orotracheal or nasotracheal intubation for airway control in the patient who is unconscious, has severe pulmonary edema, or is in severe respiratory distress.
- Positive-pressure ventilation techniques with a bag-valve-mask device may be beneficial.
- Consider drug therapy for pulmonary edema (refer to pulmonary edema protocol in Section Three).
- Consider administering a beta agonist such as albuterol for severe bronchospasm (refer to albuterol protocol in Section Four).
- Monitor cardiac rhythm and treat arrhythmias if necessary (refer to cardiac protocol in Section Three).
- Start IV administration of D_5W TKO. Use 0.9% saline (NS) or lactated Ringer's (LR) if signs of hypovolemia are present. For hypotension with signs of hypovolemia, administer fluids cautiously. Consider vasopressors if patient is hypotensive with a normal fluid volume. Watch for signs of fluid overload (refer to shock protocol in Section Three).
- Use proparacaine hydrochloride to assist eye irrigation (refer to proparacaine hydrochloride protocol in Section Four).

INITIAL EMERGENCY DEPARTMENT CONSIDERATIONS

- Useful initial laboratory studies include complete blood count, coagulation profile, serum electrolytes, blood urea nitrogen (BUN), creatinine, glucose, urinalysis, and baseline biochemical profile, including serum aminotransferases (ALT and AST), amylase, calcium, phosphorus, and magnesium and thyroid profile. Determination of anion and osmolar gaps may be helpful. Arterial blood gases (ABGs), chest radiograph, and electrocardiogram may be required.
- Positive end-expiratory pressure (PEEP)–assisted ventilation may be necessary in patients with acute parenchymal injury who develop pulmonary edema or acute respiratory distress syndrome.
- Bronchospastic symptoms should be treated with an inhalation medication regimen similar to that used for reactive airways disease. Inhaled corticosteroids may be of value in severe bronchospasm.
- Products may cause acidosis; hyperventilation and sodium bicarbonate may be beneficial. Bicarbonate therapy should be guided by patient presentation, ABG determination, and serum electrolyte considerations.
- Obtain toxicological consultation if necessary.

Copper and Related Compounds

SUBSTANCE IDENTIFICATION

Reddish, lustrous, odorless metal. Found as solids, dusts, or mists. May be found in paint pigments, coloring agents, electroplating baths, wood preservation, and textile treatments. Also used in the manufacture of copper wire, rod, piping, and tubing. Product can be liberated from production and application of insecticides, germicides, and fungicides. Also produced during mining and refining of copper ore. Elemental copper is an essential enzyme co-factor.

ROUTES OF EXPOSURE

Skin and eye contact
Inhalation
Ingestion

TARGET ORGANS

Primary
Skin
Eyes
Respiratory system
Renal system
Hepatic system
Blood
Secondary
Central nervous system
Cardiovascular system
Gastrointestinal system

LIFE THREAT

Respiratory tract irritation. Respiratory arrest. Hemorrhagic gastritis.

SIGNS AND SYMPTOMS BY SYSTEM

Cardiovascular: Tachycardia, weak pulse, and hypotension.

Respiratory: Irritation of respiratory tract mucous membranes, ulcerations of nasal septum. May aggravate other respiratory problems. Chest pain, dyspnea, and apnea leading to respiratory arrest.

CNS: Headache, fatigue, and coma.

Gastrointestinal: Nausea, vomiting (blue-green emesis), abdominal pain, hemorrhagic gastritis, and diarrhea. Metallic taste in the mouth.

Eye: Chemical conjunctivitis, corneal ulceration, and palpebral edema.

Skin: Irritant dermatitis. Skin may be pale, cool, and clammy. Greenish discoloration of the skin and hair possible.

Renal: Kidney damage, hematuria, oliguria, increased BUN, and acute tubular necrosis.

Hepatic: Liver damage.

Blood: Hemolytic anemia.

Other: Exposure may cause metal fume fever: a self-limited, flu-type illness with symptoms of metallic taste, fever, chills, aches, chest tightness, and cough.

SYMPTOM ONSET FOR ACUTE EXPOSURE

Immediate

Symptoms possibly delayed 48 hours

CO-EXPOSURE CONCERNS

Other metals

THERMAL DECOMPOSITION PRODUCTS INCLUDE

Copper fumes

Metal oxides

Carbon monoxide

Carbon dioxide

MEDICAL CONDITIONS POSSIBLY AGGRAVATED BY EXPOSURE

Wilson's disease (an autosomal recessive genetic condition resulting in excess copper storage in the body).

DECONTAMINATION

- Wear positive-pressure SCBA and protective equipment specified by references such as the *North American Emergency Response Guidebook*. If special chemical protective clothing is required, consult the chemical manufacturer or specific protective clothing compatibility charts. A qualified, experienced person should make decisions regarding the type of personal protective equipment necessary.
- Delay entry until trained personnel and proper protective equipment are available.
- Remove patient from contaminated area.
- Quickly remove and isolate patient's clothing, jewelry, and shoes.
- Gently brush away dry particles and blot excess liquids with absorbent material.
- Rinse patient with warm water, 32° C to 35° C (90° F to 95° F), if possible.
- Wash patient with a mild liquid soap and large quantities of water.
- Refer to decontamination protocol in Section Three.

IMMEDIATE FIRST AID

- Ensure that adequate decontamination has been carried out.
- If patient is not breathing, start artificial respiration, preferably with a demand-valve resuscitator, bag-valve-mask device, or pocket mask, as trained. Perform CPR if necessary.
- Immediately flush contaminated eyes with gently flowing water.
- Do not induce vomiting. If vomiting occurs, lean patient forward or place on left side (head-down position, if possible) to maintain an open airway and prevent aspiration.
- Keep patient quiet and maintain normal body temperature.
- Obtain medical attention.

BASIC TREATMENT

- Establish a patent airway (oropharyngeal or nasopharyngeal airway, if needed). Suction if necessary.
- Watch for signs of respiratory insufficiency and assist ventilations if necessary.
- Administer oxygen by nonrebreather mask at 10 to 15 L/min.
- Monitor for shock and treat if necessary (refer to shock protocol in Section Three).

- For eye contamination, flush eyes immediately with water. Irrigate each eye continuously with 0.9% saline (NS) during transport (refer to eye irrigation protocol in Section Three).
- Do not use emetics. For ingestion, rinse mouth and administer 5 ml/kg up to 200 ml of water for dilution if the patient can swallow, has a strong gag reflex, and does not drool. Administer activated charcoal (refer to ingestion protocol in Section Three and activated charcoal protocol in Section Four).

ADVANCED TREATMENT

- Consider orotracheal or nasotracheal intubation for airway control in the patient who is unconscious or is in severe respiratory distress.
- Start IV administration of 0.9% saline (NS) or lactated Ringer's (LR) TKO. For hypotension with signs of hypovolemia, administer fluid cautiously. Consider vasopressors if patient is hypotensive with a normal fluid volume. Watch for signs of fluid overload (refer to shock protocol in Section Three).
- Use proparacaine hydrochloride to assist eye irrigation (refer to proparacaine hydrochloride protocol in Section Four).

INITIAL EMERGENCY DEPARTMENT CONSIDERATIONS

- Useful initial laboratory studies include complete blood count, coagulation profile, serum electrolytes, blood urea nitrogen (BUN), creatinine, glucose, urinalysis, and baseline biochemical profile, including bilirubin, serum aminotransferases (ALT and AST), calcium, phosphorus, magnesium, and serum or blood copper. Determination of anion and osmolar gaps may be helpful. Arterial blood gases (ABGs), chest radiograph, and electrocardiogram may be required.
- Normal serum copper concentrations vary widely and range up to 1.09 mg/L in men and 1.2 mg/L in women. Copper concentrations may double in pregnancy. Blood copper concentrations average 0.89 mg/L in both men and women. Blood copper levels correlate more closely than serum copper levels with acute poisoning. Blood concentrations greater than 3 mg/L may be indicative of toxicity.
- Chelating agents (BAL, D-penicillamine) may be beneficial in symptomatic patients. Therapy should be guided by patient presentation and laboratory values.
- Obtain toxicological consultation as necessary.

SPECIAL CONSIDERATIONS

- Copper sulfate is a strong emetic. This emetic action may limit toxicity in case of mild to moderate ingestion.
- Metal fume fever, also called "Monday morning fever," may develop from exposure to copper fumes. Symptoms include metallic taste, dry cough, shortness of breath, diaphoresis, fever, chills, fatigue, and myalgia. Symptoms usually begin 4 to 12 hours after exposure, are self-limited, and remit during the work week and reappear with exposure after the weekend. This is most likely an immune-mediated problem related to occupational exposures.

79

Iron and Related Compounds

SUBSTANCE IDENTIFICATION

Greenish or yellowish solid in fine or lumpy crystals. Can be found in solution form. Used as fertilizers; herbicides; water treatment processes; reducing agent in chemical processes; and in process engraving. Elemental iron is an essential metal for hemoglobin synthesis.

ROUTES OF EXPOSURE

Skin and eye contact
Inhalation
Ingestion

TARGET ORGANS

Primary
Respiratory system
Gastrointestinal system
Hepatic system
Metabolism
Blood

Secondary
Skin
Eyes
Central nervous system
Cardiovascular system

LIFE THREAT

Hypovolemic shock from fluid loss.

SIGNS AND SYMPTOMS BY SYSTEM

Cardiovascular: Cardiovascular collapse, hypovolemic shock, increased venous pooling, hypotension, and tachycardia.

Respiratory: Rapid, shallow respirations. Occasionally acidosis may cause a rapid and deep breathing pattern, similar to Kussmaul respirations. Chronic occupational inhalation of iron oxides may produce pulmonary fibrosis (pulmonary siderosis).

CNS: Drowsiness and hyporeflexia. CNS depression, cerebral edema, and coma.

Gastrointestinal: Nausea, prolonged vomiting (hematemesis), bloody diarrhea, and abdominal pain.

Eye: Dilated pupils.

Skin: Cool skin with pallor and cyanosis.

Hepatic: Liver damage ranging from hepatocyte iron accumulation (hemochromatosis) to fulminant hepatic failure.

Metabolism: Metabolic acidosis and hyperglycemia.

Blood: Coagulation defects.

Other: Acute iron ingestion has been classically categorized into four stages: Stage I—nausea, hematemesis, abdominal pain (0.5 to 2 hours); Stage II—

apparent symptom remission or latent period (6 to 24 hours); Stage III—multisystem toxicity, including shock, coma, acidosis, hepatic necrosis, and coagulopathy (2 to 96 hours); Stage IV—late complications of GI system and obstruction (2 to 4 weeks). Agreement does not exist on the exact number of phases or time frame of each phase. Patients may not exhibit all phases.

Toxicity levels:

- < 20 mg/kg: minimal to no toxicity
- 20-60 mg/kg: mild to moderate toxicity
- > 60 mg/kg: potentially serious toxicity

SYMPTOM ONSET FOR ACUTE EXPOSURE

Immediate

Some symptoms may be delayed.

There may be a period of apparent recovery followed by severe symptoms.

THERMAL DECOMPOSITION PRODUCTS INCLUDE

Ferrous sulfate: Sulfur oxides

Ferrous chloride: Hydrogen chloride

Ferrous ammonium sulfate: Sulfur oxides, ammonia, nitrogen oxides

MEDICAL CONDITIONS POSSIBLY AGGRAVATED BY EXPOSURE

Eye disorders

Skin disorders

Respiratory disorders

Liver disorders

Kidney disorders

Hemosiderosis, hemochromatosis

DECONTAMINATION

- Wear positive-pressure SCBA and protective equipment specified by references such as the *North American Emergency Response Guidebook*. If special chemical protective clothing is required, consult the chemical manufacturer or specific protective clothing compatibility charts. A qualified, experienced person should make decisions regarding the type of personal protective equipment necessary.
- Delay entry until trained personnel and proper protective equipment are available.
- Remove patient from contaminated area.
- Quickly remove and isolate patient's clothing, jewelry, and shoes.
- Gently brush away dry particles and blot excess liquids with absorbent material.
- Rinse patient with warm water, 32° C to 35° C (90° F to 95° F), if possible.
- Wash patient with a mild liquid soap and large quantities of water.
- Refer to decontamination protocol in Section Three.

IMMEDIATE FIRST AID

- Ensure that adequate decontamination has been carried out.
- If patient is not breathing, start artificial respiration, preferably with a demand-valve resuscitator, bag-valve-mask device, or pocket mask, as trained. Perform CPR if necessary.
- Immediately flush contaminated eyes with gently flowing water.
- Do not induce vomiting. If vomiting occurs, lean patient forward or place on left side (head-down position, if possible) to maintain an open airway and prevent aspiration.

- Keep patient quiet and maintain normal body temperature.
- Obtain medical attention.

BASIC TREATMENT

- Establish a patent airway (oropharyngeal or nasopharyngeal airway, if needed). Suction if necessary.
- Watch for signs of respiratory insufficiency and assist ventilations if necessary.
- Administer oxygen by nonrebreather mask at 10 to 15 L/min.
- Monitor for shock and treat if necessary (refer to shock protocol in Section Three).
- For eye contamination, flush eyes immediately with water. Irrigate each eye continuously with 0.9% saline (NS) during transport (refer to eye irrigation protocol in Section Three).
- Do not use emetics. For ingestion, rinse mouth and administer 5 ml/kg up to 200 ml of water for dilution if the patient can swallow, has a strong gag reflex, and does not drool (refer to ingestion protocol in Section Three).

ADVANCED TREATMENT

- Consider orotracheal or nasotracheal intubation for airway control in the patient who is unconscious or is in severe respiratory distress.
- Monitor cardiac rhythm and treat arrhythmias if necessary (refer to cardiac protocol in Section Three).
- Start IV administration of 0.9% saline (NS) or lactated Ringer's (LR) TKO. For hypotension with signs of hypovolemia, administer fluid cautiously. Watch for signs of fluid overload (refer to shock protocol in Section Three).
- Use proparacaine hydrochloride to assist eye irrigation (refer to proparacaine hydrochloride protocol in Section Four).

INITIAL EMERGENCY DEPARTMENT

- Useful initial laboratory studies include complete blood count, platelet count and coagulation profile (prothrombin and partial thromboplastin times), serum electrolytes, blood urea nitrogen (BUN), creatinine, glucose, urinalysis, and baseline biochemical profile, including serum aminotransferases (AST and ALT), calcium, phosphorus, and magnesium. Determination of anion and osmolar gaps may be helpful. Arterial blood gases (ABGs), chest radiograph, and electrocardiogram may be required.
- Monitor serum iron and total iron-binding capacity (TIBC) initially and 4 to 6 hours after ingestion. Serum iron concentration greater than 450 to 500 μg/dl and/or higher than the TIBC usually means that acute poisoning is possible. CAUTION: In acute iron ingestion, the TIBC may be falsely elevated, thus negating its diagnostic usefulness. Serum iron concentrations may need to be repeated at 8 to 12 hours after exposure if delayed toxicity expected.
- Increased white blood cell count greater than 15,000 and/or glucose greater than 150 mg/dl may indicate acute iron toxicity.
- Products may cause acidosis; hyperventilation and sodium bicarbonate may be beneficial. Bicarbonate therapy should be guided by patient presentation, ABG determination, and serum electrolyte considerations.
- Deferoxamine (Desferal) chelation may be beneficial in symptomatic patients (refer to deferoxamine protocol in Section Four).

- Abdominal radiograph may be helpful in oral ingestions, as iron tablets are radiopaque.
- Consider lavage and/or whole bowel irrigation with polyethylene glycol electrolyte solution (Go-LYTELY).
- Obtain toxicological consultation as necessary.

80 Lead and Related Compounds

SUBSTANCE IDENTIFICATION

A heavy, soft, gray metal. Usually found as a solid but can also be a component of liquid compounds. Used in storage batteries, printers' type, solder, pipes, shot, paints, rustproofers, primers, pottery, alloys (antimony, tin, arsenic), and insecticide sprays.

ROUTES OF EXPOSURE

Skin and eye contact
Inhalation
Ingestion
Skin absorption

TARGET ORGANS

Primary
Skin
Eyes
Central nervous system
Gastrointestinal system
Renal system
Blood

Secondary
Cardiovascular system
Respiratory system
Hepatic system

LIFE THREAT

Circulatory collapse, coma, and rare seizures. Toxicity from multiple exposures (i.e., chronic) is more common than from a single exposure.

SIGNS AND SYMPTOMS BY SYSTEM

Cardiovascular: Cardiovascular collapse and shock.

Respiratory: Tachypnea.

CNS: Muscle weakness with muscle and joint pain, paresthesias, depression, and headache. Mild anxiety, delirium, hallucinations, memory loss, insomnia, delusions, and decreased level of consciousness to coma (lead encephalopathy) may be present with severe acute or chronic exposure. Increased intracranial pressure and seizures.

Gastrointestinal: Anorexia, nausea, vomiting, diarrhea, constipation, and abdominal pain of a burning nature. Pain may become colicky and severe in nature. Metallic taste in the mouth.

Eye: Chemical conjunctivitis.

Skin: Irritation from some liquid compounds.

Renal: Kidney damage.

Hepatic: Liver damage.

Blood: Anemia (microcytic or normocytic), basophilic stipling.

SYMPTOM ONSET FOR ACUTE EXPOSURE

Usually delayed

CO-EXPOSURE CONCERNS

Other heavy metals

THERMAL DECOMPOSITION PRODUCTS INCLUDE

Lead oxide fumes

Hydrogen chloride

MEDICAL CONDITIONS POSSIBLY AGGRAVATED BY EXPOSURE

Diseases of the blood and bone marrow

Diseases of kidneys, nervous system

Diseases of reproductive system

DECONTAMINATION

- Wear positive-pressure SCBA and protective equipment specified by references such as the *North American Emergency Response Guidebook*. If special chemical protective clothing is required, consult the chemical manufacturer or specific protective clothing compatibility charts. A qualified, experienced person should make decisions regarding the type of personal protective equipment necessary.
- Delay entry until trained personnel and proper protective equipment are available.
- Remove patient from contaminated area.
- Quickly remove and isolate patient's clothing, jewelry, and shoes.
- Gently brush away dry particles and blot excess liquids with absorbent material.
- Rinse patient with warm water, 32° C to 35° C (90° F to 95° F), if possible.
- Wash patient with a mild liquid soap and large quantities of water.
- Refer to decontamination protocol in Section Three.

IMMEDIATE FIRST AID

- Ensure that adequate decontamination has been carried out.
- If patient is not breathing, start artificial respiration, preferably with a demand-valve resuscitator, bag-valve-mask device, or pocket mask, as trained. Perform CPR if necessary.
- Immediately flush contaminated eyes with gently flowing water.
- Do not induce vomiting. If vomiting occurs, lean patient forward or place on left side (head-down position, if possible) to maintain an open airway and prevent aspiration.
- Keep patient quiet and maintain normal body temperature.
- Obtain medical attention.

BASIC TREATMENT

- Establish a patent airway (oropharyngeal or nasopharyngeal airway, if needed). Suction if necessary.
- Watch for signs of respiratory insufficiency and assist ventilations if necessary.
- Administer oxygen by nonrebreather mask at 10 to 15 L/min.
- Monitor for shock and treat if necessary (refer to shock protocol in Section Three).
- Anticipate seizures and treat if necessary (refer to seizure protocol in Section Three).
- For eye contamination, flush eyes immediately with water. Irrigate each eye continuously with 0.9% saline (NS) during transport (refer to eye irrigation protocol in Section Three).

- Do not use emetics. For ingestion, rinse mouth and administer 5 ml/kg up to 200 ml of water for dilution if the patient can swallow, has a strong gag reflex, and does not drool. Administer activated charcoal (refer to ingestion protocol in Section Three and activated charcoal protocol in Section Four).

ADVANCED TREATMENT

- Consider orotracheal or nasotracheal intubation for airway control in the patient who is unconscious or is in severe respiratory distress.
- Moderate hyperventilation (20 respirations per minute) may be beneficial for increased intracranial pressure.
- Start IV administration of 0.9% saline (NS) or lactated Ringer's (LR) TKO. For hypotension with signs of hypovolemia, administer fluid cautiously. Watch for signs of fluid overload (refer to shock protocol in Section Three).
- Treat seizures with diazepam (Valium) or lorazepam (Ativan) (refer to diazepam and lorazepam protocols in Section Four and seizure protocol in Section Three).
- Use proparacaine hydrochloride to assist eye irrigation (refer to proparacaine hydrochloride protocol in Section Four).

INITIAL EMERGENCY DEPARTMENT CONSIDERATIONS

- Useful initial laboratory studies include complete blood count, serum electrolytes, blood urea nitrogen (BUN), creatinine, glucose, urinalysis, and baseline biochemical profile, including serum aminotransferases (AST and ALT), calcium, phosphorus, and magnesium. Determination of anion and osmolar gaps may be helpful. Arterial blood gases (ABGs), chest radiograph, and electrocardiogram may be required.
- Specific laboratory measurements include blood or 24-hour urine lead, free erythrocyte protoporphyrin (FEP) or zinc protoporphyrin (ZPP), ALA-D (δ-aminolevulinic dehydratase). There is some question as to whether FEP or ZPP determinations should be used to give the most accurate picture of body lead burden. This is not as critical as consistently using the same method to follow an individual.
- Hyperventilation and diuretics (mannitol and furosemide) may be beneficial in treating increased intracranial pressure.
- Chelation therapy (calcium EDTA, BAL, D-penicillamine, succimer [DMSA]) may be beneficial in treating symptomatic patients. Therapy should be guided by patient presentation and laboratory values.
- Obtain toxicological consultation as necessary.

SPECIAL CONSIDERATIONS

- Children are especially sensitive to CNS lead effects. This has prompted the removal of lead from house paints and organic lead compounds (tetraethyl lead) from gasoline.
- Lead exposure effects are cumulative. These include fatigue, mood changes, stomach pains, arthralgias, myalgias, difficulty sleeping, hypertension, gout, and bone marrow damage. Peripheral nerve disorders: motor nerve axonal neuropathy, ulnar nerve neuropathy, and nerve entrapment syndrome such as carpal tunnel/tarsal tunnel. Kidney and reproductive system damage (reduced fertility, decreased sperm count, and abnormal spermatogenesis). Some products may present a human teratogenic and carcinogenic risk.

Lithium and Related Compounds

SUBSTANCE IDENTIFICATION

Silvery white, odorless metal that becomes yellowish or gray on exposure to moist air. Also found in a soluble form that is clear to yellow liquid. Used in metallurgy, in the production of grease and ceramics, in alkaline storage batteries and the nuclear power industry, in photographic products, as corrosion inhibitors, and as a catalyst for chemical reactions. Lithium carbonate is used to treat manic-depressive and other psychiatric illnesses.

ROUTES OF EXPOSURE

Skin and eye contact
Inhalation
Ingestion

TARGET ORGANS

Primary
Skin
Eyes
Respiratory system
Gastrointestinal system
Secondary
Central nervous system
Cardiovascular system
Renal system
Metabolism

LIFE THREAT

Products can be extremely corrosive and cause damage to the respiratory tract leading to pulmonary edema.

SIGNS AND SYMPTOMS BY SYSTEM

Cardiovascular: Cardiovascular collapse, arrhythmias, and hypotension.

Respiratory: Irritation of respiratory tract, sore throat, cough, dyspnea, pneumonitis, pulmonary edema, and respiratory arrest.

CNS: Coarse tremors, confusion, ataxia, hyperreflexia, dysarthria, CNS depression, and coma. Seizures. Neurobehavioral changes.

Gastrointestinal: Mucosal burns, abdominal pain, nausea, vomiting, and diarrhea.

Eye: Conjunctivitis and burns.

Skin: Irritant dermatitis and chemical burns.

Renal: Albuminuria and kidney damage.

Metabolism: Thyroid enlargement, hypothyroidism (rare), hyponatremia, and elevated serum calcium (hypercalcemia).

SYMPTOM ONSET FOR ACUTE EXPOSURE

Immediate

Some symptoms (respiratory) possibly delayed

THERMAL DECOMPOSITION PRODUCTS INCLUDE

Hydrogen gas

Lithium hydroxide

Lithium oxide

MEDICAL CONDITIONS POSSIBLY AGGRAVATED BY EXPOSURE

Current therapy with lithium medication

Hyponatremia

DECONTAMINATION

- Wear positive-pressure SCBA and protective equipment specified by references such as the *North American Emergency Response Guidebook*. If special chemical protective clothing is required, consult the chemical manufacturer or specific protective clothing compatibility charts. A qualified, experienced person should make decisions regarding the type of personal protective equipment necessary.
- Delay entry until trained personnel and proper protective equipment are available.
- Remove patient from contaminated area.
- Quickly remove and isolate patient's clothing, jewelry, and shoes.
- Gently brush away dry particles and blot excess liquids with absorbent material.
- If water-reactive products are embedded in the skin, no water should be applied. The embedded products should be covered with a light oil (mineral or cooking oil), and the patient transported for surgical debridement. If products are not embedded, gently brush away as much as possible and flush with copious amounts of water to rapidly remove any residual product.
- Rinse patient with warm water, 32° C to 35° C (90° F to 95° F), if possible.
- Wash patient with a mild liquid soap and large quantities of water.
- Refer to decontamination protocol in Section Three.

IMMEDIATE FIRST AID

- Ensure that adequate decontamination has been carried out.
- If patient is not breathing, start artificial respiration, preferably with a demand-valve resuscitator, bag-valve-mask device, or pocket mask, as trained. Perform CPR if necessary.
- Immediately flush contaminated eyes with gently flowing water.
- Do not induce vomiting. If vomiting occurs, lean patient forward or place on left side (head-down position, if possible) to maintain an open airway and prevent aspiration.
- Keep patient quiet and maintain normal body temperature.
- Obtain medical attention.

BASIC TREATMENT

- Establish a patent airway (oropharyngeal or nasopharyngeal airway, if needed). Suction if necessary.
- Watch for signs of respiratory insufficiency and assist ventilations if necessary.
- Administer oxygen by nonrebreather mask at 10 to 15 L/min.
- Monitor for pulmonary edema and treat if necessary (refer to pulmonary edema protocol in Section Three).

- Monitor for shock and treat if necessary (refer to shock protocol in Section Three).
- Anticipate seizures and treat if necessary (refer to seizure protocol in Section Three).
- For eye contamination, flush eyes immediately with water. Irrigate each eye continuously with 0.9% saline (NS) during treatment (refer to eye irrigation protocol in Section Three).
- Do not use emetics. For ingestion, rinse mouth and administer 5 ml/kg up to 200 ml of water for dilution if the patient can swallow, has a strong gag reflex, and does not drool (refer to ingestion protocol in Section Three).
- Cover skin burns with dry sterile dressings after decontamination (refer to chemical burn protocol in Section Three).

ADVANCED TREATMENT

- Consider orotracheal or nasotracheal intubation for airway control in the patient who is unconscious, has severe pulmonary edema, or is in severe respiratory distress.
- Positive-pressure ventilation techniques with a bag-valve-mask device may be beneficial.
- Consider drug therapy for pulmonary edema (refer to pulmonary edema protocol in Section Three).
- Monitor cardiac rhythm and treat arrhythmias if necessary (refer to cardiac protocol in Section Three).
- Start IV administration of D_5W TKO. Use 0.9% saline (NS) or lactated Ringer's (LR) if signs of hypovolemia are present. For hypotension with signs of hypovolemia, administer fluid cautiously. Consider vasopressors if patient is hypotensive with a normal fluid volume. Watch for signs of fluid overload (refer to shock protocol in Section Three).
- Treat seizures with diazepam (Valium) or lorazepam (Ativan) (refer to diazepam and lorazepam protocols in Section Four and seizure protocol in Section Three).
- Use proparacaine hydrochloride to assist eye irrigation (refer to proparacaine hydrochloride protocol in Section Four).

INITIAL EMERGENCY DEPARTMENT CONSIDERATIONS

- Useful initial laboratory studies include complete blood count, serum electrolytes, blood urea nitrogen (BUN), creatinine, glucose, urinalysis, and baseline biochemical profile, including serum aminotransferases (ALT and AST), thyroid profile, calcium, phosphorus, and magnesium. Arterial blood gases (ABGs), chest radiograph, and electrocardiogram may be required.
- Monitor serum lithium concentrations. Lithium has a very low therapeutic index. Patients on lithium therapy have concentrations ranging from 0.5 to 1.3 mmol/L. Acute toxicity is usually seen with concentrations greater than 2 mmol/L. Chronic poisoning patients may have lithium concentrations near the therapeutic range.
- Positive end-expiratory pressure (PEEP)–assisted ventilation may be necessary in patients with acute parenchymal injury who develop pulmonary edema or acute respiratory distress syndrome.
- Maintain adequate fluid and electrolyte balance (especially sodium concentration).

- Hemodialysis may be beneficial in the symptomatic patient. Therapy should be guided by clinical presentation and laboratory results.
- Obtain toxicological consultation as necessary.

SPECIAL CONSIDERATIONS

- Persistent neurobehavioral changes are possible, even after acute symptoms have resolved.

Magnesium and Related Compounds

SUBSTANCE IDENTIFICATION

Bright, silvery or colorless metal. Found in powder, crystal, or in solution form. Used as drying agents and in making refractory materials, magnesia cements, petroleum additives, and fertilizers. Also used in optical instruments and semiconductors, in the paper industry, and in the manufacture of structural parts. Magnesium has a variety of medical uses, including in oral cathartics and antacids, magnesium sulfate (Epsom salts), magnesium hydroxide (Milk of Magnesia), and magnesium citrate.

ROUTES OF EXPOSURE

Skin and eye contact
Inhalation
Ingestion

TARGET ORGANS

Primary
Skin
Eyes
Respiratory system
Secondary
Central nervous system
Cardiovascular system
Gastrointestinal system
Renal system

LIFE THREAT

Cardiovascular collapse, cardiac arrhythmias, and respiratory depression

SIGNS AND SYMPTOMS BY SYSTEM

Cardiovascular: Cardiovascular collapse, hypotension. Prolongation of PR, QRS, and QT intervals may be observed. Asystole.

Respiratory: Irritation of respiratory tract with dyspnea and pulmonary edema. Hypoventilation and respiratory paralysis secondary to muscle paralysis.

CNS: Headache, dizziness, CNS depression, seizures, neuromuscular paralysis, and hyporeflexia.

Gastrointestinal: Nausea, vomiting, diarrhea. Irritation and hypomotility of the gastrointestinal tract.

Eye: Conjunctivitis.

Skin: Drying of the skin, cyanosis, and dermatitis. Particles may become embedded in skin.

Renal: Kidney damage.

Other: Metal fume fever (flu-type symptoms).

SYMPTOM ONSET FOR ACUTE EXPOSURE

Immediate

Most symptoms can be delayed

CO-EXPOSURE CONCERNS

Calcium and ammonium compounds

THERMAL DECOMPOSITION PRODUCTS INCLUDE

Carbon dioxide

Carbon monoxide

Hydrogen

Hydrogen chloride

Magnesium oxide fumes

Nitrogen oxides

MEDICAL CONDITIONS POSSIBLY AGGRAVATED BY EXPOSURE

Respiratory conditions

Dermatitis

Central nervous system dysfunction

Impaired kidney function

DECONTAMINATION

- Wear positive-pressure SCBA and protective equipment specified by references such as the *North American Emergency Response Guidebook*. If special chemical protective clothing is required, consult the chemical manufacturer or specific protective clothing compatibility charts. A qualified, experienced person should make decisions regarding the type of personal protective equipment necessary.
- Delay entry until trained personnel and proper protective equipment are available.
- Remove patient from contaminated area.
- Quickly remove and isolate patient's clothing, jewelry, and shoes.
- Gently brush away dry particles and blot excess liquids with absorbent material.
- If water-reactive products are embedded in the skin, no water should be applied. The embedded products should be covered with a light oil (mineral or cooking oil) and the patient transported for surgical debridement. If products are not embedded, gently brush away as much as possible and flush with copious amounts of water to rapidly remove any residual product.
- Rinse patient with warm water, 32° C to 35° C (90° F to 95° F), if possible.
- Wash patient with a mild liquid soap and large quantities of water.
- Refer to decontamination protocol in Section Three.

IMMEDIATE FIRST AID

- Ensure that adequate decontamination has been carried out.
- If patient is not breathing, start artificial respiration, preferably with a demand-valve resuscitator, bag-valve-mask device, or pocket mask, as trained. Perform CPR if necessary.
- Immediately flush contaminated eyes with gently flowing water.
- Do not induce vomiting. If vomiting occurs, lean patient forward or place on left side (head-down position, if possible) to maintain an open airway and prevent aspiration.
- Keep patient quiet and maintain normal body temperature.
- Obtain medical attention.

BASIC TREATMENT

- Establish a patent airway (oropharyngeal or nasopharyngeal airway, if needed). Suction if necessary.
- Watch for signs of respiratory insufficiency and assist ventilations if necessary.
- Administer oxygen by nonrebreather mask at 10 to 15 L/min.
- Monitor for pulmonary edema and treat if necessary (refer to pulmonary edema protocol in Section Three).
- Monitor for shock and treat if necessary (refer to shock protocol in Section Three).
- For eye contamination, flush eyes immediately with water. Irrigate each eye continuously with 0.9% saline (NS) during transport (refer to eye irrigation protocol in Section Three).
- Do not use emetics. For ingestion, rinse mouth and administer 5 ml/kg up to 200 ml of water for dilution if the patient can swallow, has a strong gag reflex, and does not drool (refer to ingestion protocol in Section Three).

ADVANCED TREATMENT

- Consider orotracheal or nasotracheal intubation for airway control in the patient who is unconscious, has severe pulmonary edema, or is in severe respiratory distress.
- Positive-pressure ventilation techniques with a bag-valve-mask device may be beneficial.
- Consider drug therapy for pulmonary edema (refer to pulmonary edema protocol in Section Three).
- Monitor cardiac rhythm and treat arrhythmias if necessary (refer to cardiac protocol in Section Three).
- Start IV administration of D_5W TKO. Use 0.9% saline (NS) or lactated Ringer's (LR) if signs of hypovolemia are present. For hypotension with signs of hypovolemia, administer fluid cautiously. Consider vasopressors if patient is hypotensive with a normal fluid volume. Watch for signs of fluid overload (refer to shock protocol in Section Three).
- Use proparacaine hydrochloride to assist eye irrigation (refer to proparacaine hydrochloride protocol in Section Four).

INITIAL EMERGENCY DEPARTMENT CONSIDERATIONS

- Useful initial laboratory studies include complete blood count, serum electrolytes, blood urea nitrogen (BUN), creatinine, glucose, urinalysis, and baseline biochemical profile, including serum aminotransferases (ALT and AST), calcium, phosphorus, and magnesium. Arterial blood gases (ABGs), chest radiograph, and electrocardiogram may be required.
- Normal plasma magnesium concentrations range from 1.5 to 2.2 mEq/L. Symptoms of toxicity usually become evident at 3.0 mEq/L or above.
- Products may cause acidosis; hyperventilation and sodium bicarbonate may be beneficial. Bicarbonate therapy should be guided by patient presentation and ABG determination.
- Hemodialysis or forced diuresis may be beneficial in the symptomatic patient. Treatment should be guided by clinical presentation and laboratory results.
- Obtain toxicological consultation as necessary.

SPECIAL CONSIDERATIONS

- Metal fume fever, also termed "Monday morning fever," may develop from exposure to magnesium fumes. Symptoms include metallic taste, dry cough, shortness of breath, diaphoresis, fever, chills, fatigue, and myalgia. Symptoms usually begin 4 to 12 hours after exposure, are self-limited, remit during the work week, and reappear with exposure after the weekend. This is most likely an immune-mediated problem related to occupational exposures.

Manganese and Related Compounds

SUBSTANCE IDENTIFICATION

Reddish-gray or silvery metallic element. Found in solid, dust, and solution forms. Used in the manufacture of steel, ceramics, matches, glass, dyes, welding rods; and in dry cell batteries.

ROUTES OF EXPOSURE

Skin and eye contact
Inhalation
Ingestion

TARGET ORGANS

Primary
Skin
Eyes
Central nervous system
Respiratory system
Secondary
Cardiovascular system
Gastrointestinal system
Hepatic system

LIFE THREAT

Respiratory tract irritation and pulmonary edema

SIGNS AND SYMPTOMS BY SYSTEM

Cardiovascular: Cardiovascular collapse, hypotension.

Respiratory: Metal fume fever (flu-type symptoms), manganese pneumonitis (fever, chills, coughing, and congestion). Irritation of respiratory tract, dyspnea, and possibly pulmonary edema.

CNS: No acute symptoms reported. Chronic symptoms include intoxication-type symptoms, speech impairment, loss of balance, incoordination, and muscle cramps.

Gastrointestinal: Nausea, irritation, and burns to GI tract.

Eye: Conjunctivitis and corneal damage.

Skin: Irritation and dermatitis.

Hepatic: Liver damage.

Other: Some products may present a human carcinogenic risk.

SYMPTOM ONSET FOR ACUTE EXPOSURE

Metal fume fever symptoms immediate
Other symptoms delayed

THERMAL DECOMPOSITION PRODUCTS INCLUDE

Manganese chloride
Manganese oxide

MEDICAL CONDITIONS POSSIBLY AGGRAVATED BY EXPOSURE

Respiratory system disorders
Neurological disorders
Anemia
COPD

DECONTAMINATION

- Wear positive-pressure SCBA and protective equipment specified by references such as the *North American Emergency Response Guidebook.* If special chemical protective clothing is required, consult the chemical manufacturer or specific protective clothing compatibility charts. A qualified, experienced person should make decisions regarding the type of personal protective equipment necessary.
- Delay entry until trained personnel and proper protective equipment are available.
- Remove patient from contaminated area.
- Quickly remove and isolate patient's clothing, jewelry, and shoes.
- Gently brush away dry particles and blot excess liquids with absorbent material.
- If water-reactive products are embedded in the skin, no water should be applied. The embedded products should be covered with a light oil (mineral or cooking oil), and the patient transported for surgical debridement. If products are not embedded, gently brush away as much as possible and flush with copious amounts of water to rapidly remove any residual product.
- Rinse patient with warm water, 32° C to 35° C (90° F to 95° F), if possible.
- Wash patient with a mild liquid soap and large quantities of water.
- Refer to decontamination protocol in Section Three.

IMMEDIATE FIRST AID

- Ensure that adequate decontamination has been carried out.
- If patient is not breathing, start artificial respiration, preferably with a demand-valve resuscitator, bag-valve-mask device, or pocket mask, as trained. Perform CPR if necessary.
- Immediately flush contaminated eyes with gently flowing water.
- Do not induce vomiting. If vomiting occurs, lean patient forward or place on left side (head-down position, if possible) to maintain an open airway and prevent aspiration.
- Keep patient quiet and maintain normal body temperature.
- Obtain medical attention.

BASIC TREATMENT

- Establish a patent airway (oropharyngeal or nasopharyngeal airway, if needed). Suction if necessary.
- Watch for signs of respiratory insufficiency and assist ventilations if necessary.
- Administer oxygen by nonrebreather mask at 10 to 15 L/min.
- Monitor for pulmonary edema and treat if necessary (refer to pulmonary edema protocol in Section Three).
- Monitor for shock and treat if necessary (refer to shock protocol in Section Three).
- For eye contamination, flush eyes immediately with water. Irrigate each eye continuously with 0.9% saline (NS) during transport (refer to eye irrigation protocol in Section Three).

- Do not use emetics. For ingestion, rinse mouth and administer 5 ml/kg up to 200 ml of water for dilution if the patient can swallow, has a strong gag reflex, and does not drool (refer to ingestion protocol in Section Three).

ADVANCED TREATMENT

- Consider orotracheal or nasotracheal intubation for airway control in the patient who is unconscious, has severe pulmonary edema, or is in severe respiratory distress.
- Positive-pressure ventilation techniques with a bag-valve-mask device may be beneficial.
- Consider drug therapy for pulmonary edema (refer to pulmonary edema protocol in Section Three).
- Consider administering a beta agonist such as albuterol for severe bronchospasm (refer to albuterol protocol in Section Four).
- Monitor cardiac rhythm and treat arrhythmias if necessary (refer to cardiac protocol in Section Three).
- Start IV administration of D_5W TKO. Use 0.9% saline (NS) or lactated Ringer's (LR) if signs of hypovolemia are present. For hypotension with signs of hypovolemia, administer fluid cautiously. Consider vasopressors if patient is hypotensive with a normal fluid volume. Watch for signs of fluid overload (refer to shock protocol in Section Three).
- Use proparacaine hydrochloride to assist eye irrigation (refer to proparacaine hydrochloride protocol in Section Four).

INITIAL EMERGENCY DEPARTMENT CONSIDERATIONS

- Useful initial laboratory studies include complete blood count, serum electrolytes, blood urea nitrogen (BUN), creatinine, glucose, urinalysis, and baseline biochemical profile, including serum aminotransferases (AST and ALT), calcium, phosphorus, and magnesium. Arterial blood gases (ABGs), chest radiograph, and electrocardiogram may be required.
- Positive end-expiratory pressure (PEEP)–assisted ventilation may be necessary in patients with acute parenchymal injury who develop pulmonary edema or acute respiratory distress syndrome.
- Manganese pneumonitis may require bronchodilator and antibiotic therapy.

SPECIAL CONSIDERATIONS

- Metal fume fever, also termed "Monday morning fever," may develop from exposure to manganese fumes. Symptoms include metallic taste, dry cough, shortness of breath, diaphoresis, fever, chills, fatigue, and myalgia. Symptoms usually begin 4 to 12 hours after exposure, are self-limited, remit during the work week, and reappear with exposure after the weekend. This is most likely an immune-mediated problem related to occupational exposures.
- Chronic occupational exposure produces the following clinical picture:
  - *Prodromal phase*: Cognitive dysfunction, emotional disturbances, muscular pain.
  - *Intermediate phase*: Inappropriate emotional outbursts, clumsiness of movement, hyperreflexia in lower extremities, manganese facies (mask-type expression),visual hallucinations, excessive salivation, confusion.
  - *Established phase*: General muscle weakness, difficulty in walking, impaired speech, tremors.

84 Mercury and Related Compounds

SUBSTANCE IDENTIFICATION

Found as a silvery, odorless liquid. In many inorganic and organic forms such as dusts, wettable powders, solutions, and vapors. Used in dental amalgams, thermometers, and barometers; in the manufacture of industrial and medical equipment; and in gold extraction. Also found in the manufacture of pesticides, antiseptics, paints, explosives, and germicides.

ROUTES OF EXPOSURE

Skin and eye contact
Inhalation
Ingestion
Skin absorption

TARGET ORGANS

Primary
Skin
Eyes
Central nervous system
Respiratory system
Hepatic system
Renal system
Secondary
Cardiovascular system
Gastrointestinal system
Blood

LIFE THREAT

Circulatory collapse, arrhythmias, respiratory failure, pulmonary edema, and neurotoxic effects.

SIGNS AND SYMPTOMS BY SYSTEM

Cardiovascular: Cardiovascular collapse with a rapid, weak pulse. Ventricular arrhythmias.

Respiratory: Severe respiratory tract irritant. Manifested by acute bronchitis and interstitial pneumonitis. Dyspnea, cough, chest pain, and tightness of the chest may be present. Large vapor exposures may induce pulmonary edema.

CNS: Headache, irritability, indecision, malaise, neurobehavioral changes, excessive fatigue, muscle weakness, and tremors. Seizures and cerebral edema may occur.

Gastrointestinal: Corrosive ulceration and hemorrhage of mucous membranes. Burning pain and cramps in mouth and stomach. Nausea, profuse vomiting, and bloody diarrhea. Excessive salivation, thirst, and metallic taste in the mouth.

Eye: Chemical conjunctivitis.

Skin: Irritation, pallor, and pruritus.

Renal: Acute renal failure, nephrotic syndrome, and glomerulonephritis.
Blood: Thrombocytopenia, neutropenia, and agranulocytosis.
Other: Some products may present a human teratogenic risk.

SYMPTOM ONSET FOR ACUTE EXPOSURE

Immediate

Many symptoms possibly delayed

CO-EXPOSURE CONCERNS

Copper

THERMAL DECOMPOSITION PRODUCTS INCLUDE

Mercury vapor

MEDICAL CONDITIONS POSSIBLY AGGRAVATED BY EXPOSURE

CNS disorders

Alcoholism

Kidney disorders

DECONTAMINATION

- Wear positive-pressure SCBA and protective equipment specified by references such as the *North American Emergency Response Guidebook*. If special chemical protective clothing is required, consult the chemical manufacturer or specific protective clothing compatibility charts. A qualified, experienced person should make decisions regarding the type of personal protective equipment necessary.
- Delay entry until trained personnel and proper protective equipment are available.
- Remove patient from contaminated area.
- Quickly remove and isolate patient's clothing, jewelry, and shoes.
- Gently brush away dry particles and blot excess liquids with absorbent material.
- Rinse patient with warm water, 32° C to 35° C (90° F to 95° F), if possible.
- Wash patient with a mild liquid soap and large quantities of water.
- Refer to decontamination protocol in Section Three.

IMMEDIATE FIRST AID

- Ensure that adequate decontamination has been carried out.
- If patient is not breathing, start artificial respiration, preferably with a demand-valve resuscitator, bag-valve-mask device, or pocket mask, as trained. Perform CPR if necessary.
- Immediately flush contaminated eyes with gently flowing water.
- Do not induce vomiting. If vomiting occurs, lean patient forward or place on left side (head-down position, if possible) to maintain an open airway and prevent aspiration.
- Keep patient quiet and maintain normal body temperature.
- Obtain medical attention.

BASIC TREATMENT

- Establish a patent airway (oropharyngeal or nasopharyngeal airway, if needed). Suction if necessary.
- Watch for signs of respiratory insufficiency and assist ventilations if necessary.
- Administer oxygen by nonrebreather mask at 10 to 15 L/min.
- Monitor for pulmonary edema and treat if necessary (refer to pulmonary edema protocol in Section Three).
- Monitor for shock and treat if necessary (refer to shock protocol in Section Three).

- Anticipate seizures and treat if necessary (refer to seizure protocol in Section Three).
- For eye contamination, flush eyes immediately. Irrigate each eye continuously with 0.9% saline (NS) during transport (refer to eye irrigation protocol in Section Three).
- Do not use emetics. For ingestion, rinse mouth and administer 5 ml/kg up to 200 ml of water for dilution if the patient can swallow, has a strong gag reflex, and does not drool. Administer activated charcoal (refer to ingestion protocol in Section Three and activated charcoal protocol in Section Four).

ADVANCED TREATMENT

- Consider orotracheal or nasotracheal intubation for airway control in the patient who is unconscious, has severe pulmonary edema, or is in severe respiratory distress.
- Positive-pressure ventilation techniques with a bag-valve-mask device may be beneficial.
- Consider drug therapy for pulmonary edema (refer to pulmonary edema protocol in Section Three).
- Monitor cardiac rhythm and treat arrhythmias if necessary (refer to cardiac protocol in Section Three).
- Start IV administration of D_5W. Use 0.9% saline (NS) or lactated Ringer's (LR) if signs of hypovolemia are present. For hypotension with signs of hypovolemia, administer fluid cautiously. Consider vasopressors if patient is hypotensive with a normal fluid volume. Watch for signs of fluid overload (refer to shock protocol in Section Three).
- Treat seizures with diazepam (Valium) or lorazepam (Ativan) (refer to diazepam and lorazepam protocols in Section Four and seizure protocol in Section Three).
- Use proparacaine hydrochloride to assist eye irrigation (refer to proparacaine hydrochloride protocol in Section Four).

INITIAL EMERGENCY DEPARTMENT CONSIDERATIONS

- Useful initial laboratory studies include complete blood count, serum electrolytes, blood urea nitrogen (BUN), creatinine, glucose, urinalysis, and baseline biochemical profile, including serum aminotransferases (ALT and AST), calcium, phosphorus, and magnesium. Arterial blood gases (ABGs), chest radiograph, and electrocardiogram may be required.
- Blood and 24-hour urine mercury concentrations may be done. Urine mercury is helpful in assessing body burden. Background mercury levels will vary with occupational exposure and fish consumption. Normal range usually less than 5 μg/dl. Toxicity is usually seen with concentrations over 20 μg/dl in blood or 50 μg/L in urine.
- Positive end-expiratory pressure (PEEP)–assisted ventilation may be necessary in patients with acute parenchymal injury who develop pulmonary edema or acute respiratory distress syndrome.
- Chelation therapy (D-penicillamine, BAL, *N*-acetyl-penicillamine [NAP], 2,3-dimercaptosuccinic acid [DMSA]) may be beneficial in the symptomatic patient. Therapy should be guided by clinical presentation and laboratory results.
- Hemodialysis may be required for renal failure.
- Obtain toxicological consultation as necessary.

SPECIAL CONSIDERATIONS

- Chronic poisoning with either elemental, inorganic, or organic mercury compounds produces cumulative effects: neurobehavioral changes, personality and mood disorders, paresthesia, weakness, muscle tremors, gait disturbances, thyroid enlargement, gingivitis, loss of teeth and excessive salivation, digestive disorders, dermatitis, dermographism, nephrotic syndrome, glomerulonephritis, renal failure, liver damage, and anemia.

85

Nickel and Related Compounds

SUBSTANCE IDENTIFICATION

Found as a silvery, white metal. Nickel salts are blue or green, clear or opaque crystals. Most products are odorless. Used in nickel-plating, electroplating, coinage, blackening zinc and brass, storage batteries, and dying and printing fabric. Also used in the production of catalysts, spark plugs, enamels, ceramics, and glass and in the manufacture of corrosion-resistant copper, manganese, zinc and steel alloys. Reaction of unrefined nickel and carbon monoxide during the nickel refining process produces nickel carbonyl ($Ni[CO_4]$), which is an extremely toxic gas. Dermal or oral exposure toxicity effects from nickel and nickel compounds are primarily allergic in nature, causing either allergic dermatitis or acute allergic reactions. Inhalational exposure of nickel carbonyl, other gas compounds, or dusts may produce pneumonitis or pulmonary edema.

ROUTES OF EXPOSURE

Skin and eye contact
Inhalation
Ingestion
Skin absorption

TARGET ORGANS

Primary
Respiratory system
Skin
Eyes
Secondary
Central nervous system
Cardiovascular system
Gastrointestinal system
Hepatic system
Renal system

LIFE THREAT

Respiratory failure, cerebral edema, allergic reactions.

SIGNS AND SYMPTOMS BY SYSTEM

Cardiovascular: Arrhythmias, electrocardiogram changes, hypotension, cardiovascular collapse.

Respiratory: Dyspnea, hyperpnea, rhinitis, sinusitis, chest pain, and pneumonitis with a nonproductive cough. Wheezing, asthma, bronchitis, or anaphylactoid reaction. Pulmonary edema. Pulmonary fibrosis may occur as a late complication.

CNS: Headache, giddiness, blurred vision, and dizziness. Cerebral edema.

Gastrointestinal: Irritation of the GI tract, epigastric pain, nausea, vomiting, and diarrhea.

Eye: Chemical conjunctivitis, ocular burns, and corneal damage.

Skin: Allergic dermatitis. Irritant dermatitis. Dermatitis symptoms include burning sensations, itching, and inflammation. Some compounds may produce severe dermal burns. Cyanosis with respiratory failure.

Hepatic: Liver damage.

Renal: Kidney dysfunction.

Other: Nickel is an occupational respiratory tract (nasal and lung) carcinogen.

SYMPTOM ONSET FOR ACUTE EXPOSURE

Immediate

Some symptoms such as pulmonary edema, may be delayed

CO-EXPOSURE CONCERNS

Benz(a)pyrene

Alkaline materials

THERMAL DECOMPOSITION PRODUCTS INCLUDE

Nickel carbonyl

Nitrogen oxides

Nickel sulfates: Sulfur oxides, carbon monoxide, and carbon dioxide

Nickel acetates: Carbon monoxide and carbon dioxide

MEDICAL CONDITIONS POSSIBLY AGGRAVATED BY EXPOSURE

Respiratory disorders

Kidney disorders

Liver disorders

Nervous system disorders

DECONTAMINATION

- Wear positive-pressure SCBA and protective equipment specified by references such as the *North American Emergency Response Guidebook.* If special chemical protective clothing is required, consult the chemical manufacturer or specific protective clothing compatibility charts. A qualified, experienced person should make decisions regarding the type of personal protective equipment necessary.
- Delay entry until trained personnel and proper protective equipment are available.
- Remove patient from contaminated area.
- Quickly remove and isolate patient's clothing, jewelry, and shoes.
- Gently brush away dry particles and blot excess liquids with absorbent material.
- Rinse patient with warm water, 32° C to 35° C (90° F to 95° F), if possible.
- Wash patient with a mild liquid soap and large quantities of water.
- Refer to decontamination protocol in Section Three.

IMMEDIATE FIRST AID

- Ensure that adequate decontamination has been carried out.
- If patient is not breathing, start artificial respiration, preferably with a demand-valve resuscitator, bag-valve-mask device, or pocket mask, as trained. Perform CPR if necessary.
- Immediately flush contaminated eyes with gently flowing water.
- Do not induce vomiting. If vomiting occurs, lean patient forward or place on left side (head-down position, if possible) to maintain an open airway and prevent aspiration.
- Keep patient quiet and maintain normal body temperature.
- Obtain medical attention.

BASIC TREATMENT

- Establish a patent airway (oropharyngeal or nasopharyngeal airway, if needed). Suction if necessary.
- Watch for signs of respiratory insufficiency and assist ventilations if necessary.
- Administer oxygen by nonrebreather mask at 10 to 15 L/min.
- Monitor for shock and treat if necessary (refer to shock protocol in Section Three).
- Monitor for pulmonary edema and treat if necessary (refer to pulmonary edema protocol in Section Three).
- For eye contamination, flush eyes immediately with water. Irrigate each eye continuously with 0.9% saline (NS) during transport (refer to eye irrigation protocol in Section Three).
- Do not use emetics. For ingestion, rinse mouth and administer 5 ml/kg up to 200 ml of water for dilution if the patient can swallow, has a strong gag reflex, and does not drool (refer to ingestion protocol in Section Three).

ADVANCED TREATMENT

- Consider orotracheal or nasotracheal intubation for airway control in the patient who is unconscious, has severe pulmonary edema, or is in severe respiratory distress.
- Positive-pressure ventilation techniques with a bag-valve-mask device may be beneficial.
- Consider drug therapy for pulmonary edema (refer to pulmonary edema protocol in Section Three).
- Monitor cardiac rhythm and treat arrhythmias if necessary (refer to cardiac protocol in Section Three).
- Start IV administration of D_5W TKO. Use 0.9% saline (NS) or lactated Ringer's (LR) if signs of hypovolemia are present. For hypotension with signs of hypovolemia, administer fluid cautiously. Consider vasopressors if patient is hypotensive with a normal fluid volume. Watch for signs of fluid overload (refer to shock protocol in Section Three).
- Use proparacaine hydrochloride to assist eye irrigation (refer to proparacaine hydrochloride protocol in Section Four).

INITIAL EMERGENCY DEPARTMENT CONSIDERATIONS

- Useful initial laboratory studies include complete blood count, serum electrolytes, blood urea nitrogen (BUN), creatinine, glucose, urinalysis, and baseline biochemical profile, including serum aminotransferases (ALT and AST), calcium, phosphorus, and magnesium. Arterial blood gases (ABGs), chest radiograph, and electrocardiogram may be required.
- Monitor urine, plasma, or blood nickel levels. Decision to institute chelation therapy should be based on clinical presentation and urinary nickel concentrations.
- Chelation may be required in cases of acute poisoning with nickel carbonyl. D-penicillamine is possibly effective. Diethyldithiocarbamate (DDC) is an investigational drug showing the most therapeutic promise for nickel carbonyl poisoning. Disulfiram (tetraethylthiuram disulfide) has also been proposed as a chelating agent because it converts to two molecules of DDC.

- Severe divalent nickel (Ni^{2+}): poisoning with renal failure, cardiac toxicity or neurotoxicity may require hemodialysis. DDC is not indicated for nickel poisoning.
- Obtain toxicological consultation as necessary.

Selenium and Related Compounds

SUBSTANCE IDENTIFICATION

Found as a red crystalline solid or amorphous powder. May be found as a gas (hydrogen selenide) or in solution. Used in the manufacture of glass, ceramics, pigments, paints and glazes, pharmaceuticals, inks, photographic processes, and insecticides. Also used in the manufacture of many commercial products, including rubber (vulcanizing agent), steel, various alloys, and electronic and semiconductor devices (selenium photocells). Selenious acid is found in gun-blueing solution. Environmental exposure is seen in copper smelting and lead and uranium mining. Selenium is used in antidandruff shampoos. Selenium is an essential dietary trace element. Selenium may be found as elemental selenium (Se^0), selenite (Se^{+4}), selanate (Se^{+6}), and selenide (Se^{-2}). Selenium deficiency has been associated with cardiomyopathy.

ROUTES OF EXPOSURE

Skin and eye contact
Inhalation
Ingestion
Skin absorption

TARGET ORGANS

Primary
Skin
Eyes
Central nervous system
Cardiovascular system
Respiratory system
Gastrointestinal system
Hepatic system
Renal system
Secondary
Blood
Metabolism

LIFE THREAT

Arrhythmias, pulmonary edema, bronchospasm, and seizures. Vomiting with GI bleeding.

SIGNS AND SYMPTOMS BY SYSTEM

Cardiovascular: Hypovolemic shock and circulatory collapse. Tachycardia and ventricular arrhythmias. Electrocardiogram changes: QT interval prolongation, ST elevation, and T wave changes.

Respiratory: Rhinitis, respiratory tract irritation, depression, or arrest, wheezes (reactive airways disease), and pulmonary edema.

CNS: Headache, fatigue, vertigo, anxiety, delirium, syncope, CNS depression, muscle cramps, paresthesias, coma, and seizures.

Gastrointestinal: Burning pain, nausea, vomiting, excess salivation, and bloody diarrhea. GI burns and bleeding with hematemesis and hematochezia. Intense thirst. Metallic taste and garlic odor of breath.

Eye: Chemical conjunctivitis and corneal injury.

Skin: Irritant dermatitis and burns. Loss of hair and nails or discoloration of nails. Pallor, cyanosis, and cold extremities.

Renal: Kidney damage.

Hepatic: Liver damage.

Metabolism: Metabolic acidosis and hyperglycemia

Blood: Increased white blood count (leukocytosis).

SYMPTOM ONSET FOR ACUTE EXPOSURE

Immediate

Some symptoms possibly delayed

CO-EXPOSURE CONCERNS

Mercury

Thallium

THERMAL DECOMPOSITION PRODUCTS INCLUDE

Hydrogen selenide gas

Metal oxide fumes

Nitrogen oxides

Selenious acid

MEDICAL CONDITIONS POSSIBLY AGGRAVATED BY EXPOSURE

Respiratory system disorders

Nervous system disorders

Liver disorders

Kidney disorders

Skin disorders

Eye disorders

DECONTAMINATION

- Wear positive-pressure SCBA and protective equipment specified by references such as the *North American Emergency Response Guidebook*. If special chemical protective clothing is required, consult the chemical manufacturer or specific protective clothing compatibility charts. A qualified, experienced person should make decisions regarding the type of personal protective equipment necessary.
- Delay entry until trained personnel and proper protective equipment are available.
- Remove patient from contaminated area.
- Quickly remove and isolate patient's clothing, jewelry, and shoes.
- Gently brush away dry particles and blot excess liquids with absorbent material.
- Rinse patient with warm water, 32° C to 35° C (90° F to 95° F), if possible.
- Wash patient with a mild liquid soap and large quantities of water.
- Refer to decontamination protocol in Section Three.

IMMEDIATE FIRST AID

- Ensure that adequate decontamination has been carried out.

- If patient is not breathing, start artificial respiration, preferably with a demand-valve resuscitator, bag-valve-mask device, or pocket mask, as trained. Perform CPR if necessary.
- Immediately flush contaminated eyes with gently flowing water.
- Do not induce vomiting. If vomiting occurs, lean patient forward or place on left side (head-down position, if possible) to maintain an open airway and prevent aspiration.
- Keep patient quiet and maintain normal body temperature.
- Obtain medical attention.

BASIC TREATMENT

- Establish a patent airway (oropharyngeal or nasopharyngeal airway, if needed). Suction if necessary.
- Watch for signs of respiratory insufficiency and assist ventilations if necessary.
- Administer oxygen by nonrebreather mask at 10 to 15 L/min.
- Monitor for shock and treat if necessary (refer to shock protocol in Section Three).
- Monitor for pulmonary edema and treat if necessary (refer to pulmonary edema protocol in Section Three).
- Treat seizures if necessary (refer to seizure protocol in Section Three).
- For eye contamination, flush eyes immediately with water. Irrigate each eye continuously with 0.9% saline (NS) during transport (refer to eye irrigation protocol in Section Three).
- Do not use emetics. For ingestion, rinse mouth and administer 5 ml/kg up to 200 ml of water for dilution if the patient can swallow, has a strong gag reflex, and does not drool. Administer activated charcoal (refer to ingestion protocol in Section Three and activated charcoal protocol in Section Four).

ADVANCED TREATMENT

- Consider orotracheal or nasotracheal intubation for airway control in the patient who is unconscious, has severe pulmonary edema, or is in severe respiratory distress.
- Positive-pressure ventilation techniques with a bag-valve-mask device may be beneficial.
- Consider drug therapy for pulmonary edema (refer to pulmonary edema protocol in Section Three).
- Consider administering a beta agonist such as albuterol for severe bronchospasm (refer to albuterol protocol in Section Four).
- Monitor cardiac rhythm and treat arrhythmias if necessary (refer to cardiac protocol in Section Three).
- Start IV administration of D_5W TKO. Use 0.9% saline (NS) or lactated Ringer's (LR) if signs of hypovolemia are present. For hypotension with signs of hypovolemia, administer fluid cautiously. Consider vasopressors if patient is hypotensive with a normal fluid volume. Watch for signs of fluid overload (refer to shock protocol in Section Three).
- Treat seizures with diazepam (Valium) or lorazepam (Ativan) (refer to diazepam and lorazepam protocols in Section Four and seizure protocol in Section Three).
- Use proparacaine hydrochloride to assist eye irrigation (refer to proparacaine hydrochloride protocol in Section Four).

INITIAL EMERGENCY DEPARTMENT CONSIDERATIONS

- Useful initial laboratory studies include complete blood count, serum electrolytes, blood urea nitrogen (BUN), creatinine, glucose, urinalysis, and baseline biochemical profile, including serum aminotransferases (ALT and AST), alkaline phosphatase, calcium, phosphorus, and magnesium. Determination of the anion gap may be helpful. Arterial blood gases (ABGs), chest radiograph, and electrocardiogram may be required.
- Positive end-expiratory pressure (PEEP)–assisted ventilation may be necessary in patients with acute parenchymal injury developing pulmonary edema or acute respiratory distress syndrome.
- Products may cause acidosis; hyperventilation and sodium bicarbonate may be beneficial. Bicarbonate therapy should be guided by patient presentation, ABG determination, and serum electrolyte considerations.
- Bronchospastic symptoms should be treated with an inhalation medication regimen similar to that used for reactive airways disease. Inhaled corticosteroids may be of value in severe bronchospasm.
- Closely monitor hydration state and urinary output and maintain if necessary.
- Obtain toxicological consultation if necessary.

87 Thallium and Related Compounds

SUBSTANCE IDENTIFICATION

Found as a colorless to bluish white, odorless solid. Used as fungicides, pesticides, and insecticides. Also used in the manufacture of many products, including semiconductors, dyes, pigments, optical lenses, cement factories, and fireworks. Thallium metal is acid-soluble and very reactive. Home use of thallium was stopped by the U.S. Department of Agriculture in 1965. It is used in medical diagnostic imaging procedures for myocardial scans.

ROUTES OF EXPOSURE

Skin and eye contact
Inhalation
Ingestion
Skin absorption

TARGET ORGANS

Primary
Skin
Eyes
Central nervous system
Respiratory system
Gastrointestinal system
Hepatic system
Renal system
Secondary
Cardiovascular system

LIFE THREAT

Pulmonary edema, respiratory failure, circulatory collapse, and seizures.

SIGNS AND SYMPTOMS BY SYSTEM

Cardiovascular: Tachycardia, arrhythmias, and hypertension, followed by circulatory collapse and shock.

Respiratory: Pulmonary edema, dyspnea, and respiratory depression. Nasal discharge and tightness of the chest.

CNS: Ptosis, crossed eyes, weakness, ataxia, paralysis, cranial nerve neuropathy, tremor, paresthesia of arms and legs, peripheral neuropathy, lethargy, and jumbled speech. Psychosis, delirium, coma, and seizures.

Gastrointestinal: Nausea, vomiting, and diarrhea. Abdominal pain and GI hemorrhage. Vomitus and stools often contain blood.

Eye: Chemical conjunctivitis.

Skin: Irritation and cyanosis.

Renal: Proteinuria and kidney damage.

Hepatic: Liver damage.

Other: Hair loss and muscular atrophy may occur. Some products may present a human teratogenic risk.

SYMPTOM ONSET FOR ACUTE EXPOSURE

Immediate

Some symptoms possibly delayed

CO-EXPOSURE CONCERNS

Other metals

Potassium metal

THERMAL DECOMPOSITION PRODUCTS INCLUDE

Metal oxide fumes

Nitrogen oxide fumes

MEDICAL CONDITIONS POSSIBLY AGGRAVATED BY EXPOSURE

Liver disorders

Kidney disorders

Nervous system disorders

DECONTAMINATION

- Wear positive-pressure SCBA and protective equipment specified by references such as the *North American Emergency Response Guidebook.* If special chemical protective clothing is required, consult the chemical manufacturer or specific protective clothing compatibility charts. A qualified, experienced person should make decisions regarding the type of personal protective equipment necessary.
- Delay entry until trained personnel and proper protective equipment are available.
- Remove patient from contaminated area.
- Quickly remove and isolate patient's clothing, jewelry, and shoes.
- Gently brush away dry particles and blot excess liquids with absorbent material.
- Rinse patient with warm water, 32° C to 35° C (90° F to 95° F), if possible.
- Wash patient with a mild liquid soap and large quantities of water.
- Refer to decontamination protocol in Section Three.

IMMEDIATE FIRST AID

- Ensure that adequate decontamination has been carried out.
- If patient is not breathing, start artificial respiration, preferably with a demand-valve resuscitator, bag-valve-mask device, or pocket mask, as trained. Perform CPR if necessary.
- Immediately flush contaminated eyes with gently flowing water.
- Do not induce vomiting. If vomiting occurs, lean patient forward or place on left side (head-down position, if possible) to maintain an open airway and prevent aspiration.
- Keep patient quiet and maintain normal body temperature.
- Obtain medical attention.

BASIC TREATMENT

- Establish a patent airway (oropharyngeal or nasopharyngeal airway, if needed). Suction if necessary.
- Watch for signs of respiratory insufficiency and assist ventilations if necessary.
- Administer oxygen by nonrebreather mask at 10 to 15 L/min.
- Monitor for pulmonary edema and treat if necessary (refer to pulmonary edema protocol in Section Three).
- Monitor for shock and treat if necessary (refer to shock protocol in Section Three).

- Anticipate seizures and treat if necessary (refer to seizure protocol in Section Three).
- For eye contamination, flush eyes immediately with water. Irrigate each eye continuously with 0.9% saline (NS) during transport (refer to eye irrigation protocol in Section Three).
- Do not use emetics. For ingestion, rinse mouth and administer 5 ml/kg up to 200 ml of water for dilution if the patient can swallow, has a strong gag reflex, and does not drool. Administer activated charcoal (refer to ingestion protocol in Section Three and activated charcoal protocol in Section Four).

ADVANCED TREATMENT

- Consider orotracheal or nasotracheal intubation for airway control in the patient who is unconscious, has severe pulmonary edema, or is in severe respiratory distress.
- Positive-pressure ventilation techniques with a bag-valve-mask device may be beneficial.
- Consider drug therapy for pulmonary edema (refer to pulmonary edema protocol in Section Three).
- Monitor cardiac rhythm and treat arrhythmias if necessary (refer to cardiac protocol in Section Three).
- Start IV administration of D_5W TKO. Use 0.9% saline (NS) or lactated Ringer's (LR) if signs of hypovolemia are present. For hypotension with signs of hypovolemia, administer fluid cautiously. Watch for signs of fluid overload (refer to shock protocol in Section Three).
- Treat seizures with diazepam (Valium) or lorazepam (Ativan) (refer to diazepam and lorazepam protocols in Section Four and seizure protocol in Section Three).
- Use proparacaine hydrochloride to assist eye irrigation (refer to proparacaine hydrochloride protocol in Section Four).

INITIAL EMERGENCY DEPARTMENT CONSIDERATIONS

- Useful initial laboratory studies include complete blood count, serum electrolytes, blood urea nitrogen (BUN), creatinine, glucose, urinalysis, and baseline biochemical profile, including serum aminotransferases (AST and ALT), calcium, phosphorus, and magnesium. Arterial blood gases (ABGs), chest radiograph, and electrocardiogram may be required.
- Blood or urine thallium determinations may be done. Urine thallium concentration is probably the most useful. Blood thallium in normal individuals may average 3 μg/L with most individuals less than 5 μg/L. Urine concentration should be less than 2 μg/L.
- Positive end-expiratory pressure (PEEP)–assisted ventilation may be necessary in patients with acute parenchymal injury who develop pulmonary edema or acute respiratory distress syndrome.
- Hemoperfusion and hemodialysis may be beneficial in the symptomatic patient. This therapy is controversial and should be guided by clinical presentation and laboratory findings.
- There is no effective chelator for thallium poisoning.
- Combination oral therapy with potassium chloride and activated charcoal has been successful: ADULT DOSAGE: Oral KCL 20 mEq with 20 to 30 g of activated charcoal and cathartic QID.
- Obtain toxicological consultation as necessary.

Zinc and Related Compounds

SUBSTANCE IDENTIFICATION

Odorless gray dust, lustrous powder, or ingot. May be found in solution form. Used in alloys, galvanizing and electroplating other metals, dry cell batteries, and manufactured metal goods. Compounds are used as paint pigments, coatings, and inks; as an ingredient of cosmetics, driers, quick-setting cements, dental cements; in the manufacture of opaque and transparent glass, enamels, automobile tires, white glue, matches, porcelains, and zinc chromates; as a reagent in analytical chemistry; in electrostatic copying paper; as a flame retardant; in electronics as a semiconductor; and in medicine as an antiseptic, astringent, and topical protectant. Zinc is an essential dietary trace metal.

ROUTES OF EXPOSURE

Skin and eye contact
Inhalation
Ingestion

TARGET ORGANS

Primary
Skin
Eyes
Cardiovascular system
Respiratory system
Secondary
Gastrointestinal system
Renal system
Blood

LIFE THREAT

Respiratory irritant that may cause metal fume fever or pulmonary edema.

SIGNS AND SYMPTOMS BY SYSTEM

Cardiovascular: Tachycardia and cardiovascular collapse.

Respiratory: Respiratory tract irritation, metal fume fever (flu-type symptoms), bronchospasm, or pulmonary edema.

CNS: Lethargy, CNS depression, and seizures.

Gastrointestinal: Burning pain in the mouth, throat, and abdomen. Nausea, vomiting, abdominal pain, and bloody diarrhea.

Eye: Metal particles can irritate the eyes. Irritation and severe burns with some compounds. Corneal damage.

Skin: Dryness, irritation, dermatitis, and dermal burns.

Renal: Kidney damage.

Blood: Anemia, low white blood cell count (leukopenia), copper deficiency.

SYMPTOM ONSET FOR ACUTE EXPOSURE

Immediate
Some symptoms possibly delayed for days

CO-EXPOSURE CONCERNS

Other metals

THERMAL DECOMPOSITION PRODUCTS INCLUDE

Zinc oxide
Hydrogen gas when wet
Hydrochloric acid–zinc chloride
Sulfur oxides–zinc sulfate

MEDICAL CONDITIONS POSSIBLY AGGRAVATED BY EXPOSURE

Respiratory system disorders
Anemia

DECONTAMINATION

- Wear positive-pressure SCBA and protective equipment specified by references such as the *North American Emergency Response Guidebook*. If special chemical protective clothing is required, consult the chemical manufacturer or specific protective clothing compatibility charts. A qualified, experienced person should make decisions regarding the type of personal protective equipment necessary.
- Delay entry until trained personnel and proper protective equipment are available.
- Remove patient from contaminated area.
- Quickly remove and isolate patient's clothing, jewelry, and shoes.
- Gently brush away dry particles and blot excess liquids with absorbent material.
- Rinse patient with warm water, 32° C to 35° C (90° F to 95° F), if possible.
- Wash patient with a mild liquid soap and large quantities of water.
- Refer to decontamination protocol in Section Three.

IMMEDIATE FIRST AID

- Ensure that adequate decontamination has been carried out.
- If patient is not breathing, start artificial respiration, preferably with a demand-valve resuscitator, bag-valve-mask device, or pocket mask, as trained. Perform CPR if necessary.
- Immediately flush contaminated eyes with gently flowing water.
- Do not induce vomiting. If vomiting occurs, lean patient forward or place on left side (head-down position, if possible) to maintain an open airway and prevent aspiration.
- Keep patient quiet and maintain normal body temperature.
- Obtain medical attention.

BASIC TREATMENT

- Establish a patent airway (oropharyngeal or nasopharyngeal airway, if needed). Suction if necessary.
- Watch for signs of respiratory insufficiency and assist ventilations if necessary.
- Administer oxygen by nonrebreather mask at 10 to 15 L/min.
- Monitor for pulmonary edema and treat if necessary (refer to pulmonary edema protocol in Section Three).
- Anticipate seizures and treat if necessary (refer to seizure protocol in Section Three).
- Monitor for shock and treat if necessary (refer to shock protocol in Section Three).
- For eye contamination, flush eyes immediately with water. Irrigate each eye continuously with 0.9% saline (NS) during transport (refer to eye irrigation protocol in Section Three).

- Do not use emetics. For ingestion, rinse mouth and administer 5 ml/kg up to 200 ml of water for dilution if the patient can swallow, has a strong gag reflex, and does not drool. Administer activated charcoal (refer to ingestion protocol in Section Three and activated charcoal protocol in Section Four).

ADVANCED TREATMENT

- Consider orotracheal or nasotracheal intubation for airway control in the patient who is unconscious, has severe pulmonary edema, or is in severe respiratory distress.
- Positive-pressure ventilation techniques with a bag-valve-mask device may be beneficial.
- Consider drug therapy for pulmonary edema (refer to pulmonary edema protocol in Section Three).
- Consider administering a beta agonist such as albuterol for severe bronchospasm (refer to albuterol protocol in Section Four).
- Monitor cardiac rhythm and treat arrhythmias if necessary (refer to cardiac protocol in Section Three).
- Start IV administration of D_5W TKO. Use 0.9% saline (NS) or lactated Ringer's (LR) if signs of hypovolemia are present. For hypotension with signs of hypovolemia, administer fluids cautiously. Consider vasopressors if patient is hypotensive with a normal fluid volume. Watch for signs of fluid overload (refer to shock protocol in Section Three).
- Treat seizures with diazepam (Valium) or lorazepam (Ativan) (refer to diazepam and lorazepam protocols in Section Four and seizure protocol in Section Three).
- Use proparacaine hydrochloride to assist eye irrigation (refer to proparacaine hydrochloride protocol in Section Four).

INITIAL EMERGENCY DEPARTMENT CONSIDERATIONS

- Useful initial laboratory studies include complete blood count, serum electrolytes, blood urea nitrogen (BUN), creatinine, glucose, urinalysis, and baseline biochemical profile, including serum aminotransferases (ALT and AST), calcium, phosphorus, and magnesium. Arterial blood gases (ABGs), chest radiograph, and electrocardiogram may be required.
- Zinc may be measured in blood and urine. Concentrations are not necessarily related to toxicity.
- Positive end-expiratory pressure (PEEP)–assisted ventilation may be necessary in patients with acute parenchymal injury who develop pulmonary edema or acute respiratory distress syndrome.
- Bronchospastic symptoms should be treated with an inhalation medication regimen similar to that used for reactive airway disease. Inhaled corticosteroids may be of value in severe bronchospasm.
- Obtain toxicological consultation as necessary.

SPECIAL CONSIDERATIONS

- Metal fume fever, also termed "Monday morning fever," may develop from exposure to zinc oxide. Symptoms include metallic taste, dry cough, shortness of breath, diaphoresis, fever, chills, fatigue, and myalgia. Symptoms usually begin 4 to 12 hours after exposure, are self-limited, remit during the work week, and reappear with exposure after the weekend. This is most likely an immune-mediated problem related to occupational exposures.

89

Carbon Monoxide and Related Compounds

SUBSTANCE IDENTIFICATION

Colorless, tasteless, and odorless gas that is formed when organic material undergoes incomplete combustion. Found in exhaust fumes of internal combustion engines and furnace flues. Also used in metallurgy, organic synthesis, and the manufacture of metal carbonyls. Rarely found in liquid form. Metabolite of methylene chloride (example of lethal synthesis).

ROUTES OF EXPOSURE

Skin and eye contact
Inhalation

TARGET ORGANS

Primary
Central nervous system
Cardiovascular system
Respiratory system
Blood
Secondary
Skin
Eyes
Gastrointestinal system
Hepatic system
Renal system
Metabolism

LIFE THREAT

Hemoglobin has a 200 to 300 times greater affinity for carbon monoxide (CO) than oxygen. The oxygen transport function of hemoglobin in the blood is reduced when it binds with carbon monoxide, forming carboxyhemoglobin. Carboxyhemoglobin cannot bind with oxygen. This cellular poison causes death via hypoxia.

SIGNS AND SYMPTOMS BY SYSTEM

Cardiovascular: Cardiovascular collapse, arrhythmias, and angina. Exposure may precipitate an acute myocardial infarction.

Respiratory: Tachypnea, followed by slow irregular respirations and respiratory arrest. Signs of pulmonary edema.

CNS: CNS depression and coma. Dizziness, headache, tinnitus, weakness, hallucinations, and seizures. Confusion, visual disturbances, irritability, impaired judgment, loss of memory, and fatigue. Increased intracranial pressure from cerebral edema.

Gastrointestinal: Nausea and vomiting.

Eye: Chemical conjunctivitis.

Skin: Cyanosis, pallor, and rare cherry red color.

Renal: Kidney damage and myoglobinuria.
Hepatic: Liver damage.
Metabolism: Lactic acidosis.
Blood: Carboxyhemoglobin formation.
Other: The period between exposure and toxic signs and symptoms is shortened by any factor that speeds circulation or respiration, such as exercise, exertion, or trauma.

SYMPTOM ONSET FOR ACUTE EXPOSURES

Immediate
Neurological and neurobehavioral effects possibly delayed

CO-EXPOSURE CONCERNS

Simple asphyxiants
Other chemical asphyxiants
Trauma

THERMAL DECOMPOSITION PRODUCTS INCLUDE

Carbon
Carbon dioxide

MEDICAL CONDITIONS POSSIBLY AGGRAVATED BY EXPOSURE

Respiratory disorders
Cardiovascular disorders

DECONTAMINATION

- Wear positive-pressure SCBA and protective equipment specified by references such as the *North American Emergency Response Guidebook*. If special chemical protective clothing is required, consult the chemical manufacturer or specific protective clothing compatibility charts. A qualified, experienced person should make decisions regarding the type of personal protective equipment necessary.
- Delay entry until trained personnel and proper protective equipment are available.
- Remove patient from contaminated area.
- Quickly remove and isolate patient's clothing, jewelry, and shoes.
- If any concurrent liquid or solid contamination exists:
  - Gently brush away dry particles and blot excess liquids with absorbent material.
  - Rinse patient with warm water, 32° C to 35° C (90° F to 95° F), if possible.
  - Wash patient with a mild liquid soap and large quantities of water.

  Refer to decontamination protocol in Section Three.

IMMEDIATE FIRST AID

- Ensure that adequate decontamination has been carried out.
- If patient is not breathing, start artificial respiration, preferably with a demand-valve resuscitator, bag-valve-mask device, or pocket mask, as trained. Perform CPR if necessary.
- Immediately flush contaminated eyes with gently flowing water.
- Do not induce vomiting. If vomiting occurs, lean patient forward or place on left side (head-down position, if possible) to maintain an open airway and prevent aspiration.
- Keep patient quiet and maintain normal body temperature.
- Obtain medical attention.

BASIC TREATMENT

- Establish a patent airway (oropharyngeal or nasopharyngeal airway, if needed). Suction if necessary.
- Watch for signs of respiratory insufficiency and assist ventilations if necessary.
- Administer 100% oxygen by nonrebreather mask at 10 to 15 L/min.
- Monitor for shock and treat if necessary (refer to shock protocol in Section Three).
- Monitor for signs of an acute myocardial infarction and treat if necessary.
- Monitor for pulmonary edema and treat if necessary (refer to pulmonary edema protocol in Section Three).
- Anticipate seizures and treat if necessary (refer to seizure protocol in Section Three).
- For eye contamination, flush eyes immediately with water. Irrigate each eye continuously with 0.9% saline (NS) during transport (refer to eye irrigation protocol in Section Three).

ADVANCED TREATMENT

- Consider orotracheal or nasotracheal intubation for airway control in the patient who is unconscious, has severe pulmonary edema, or is in severe respiratory distress.
- Positive-pressure ventilation techniques with a bag-valve-mask device may be beneficial.
- Consider drug therapy for pulmonary edema (refer to pulmonary edema protocol in Section Three).
- Moderate hyperventilation (20 respirations per minute) may be beneficial for increased intracranial pressure.
- Monitor cardiac rhythm and treat arrhythmias if necessary (refer to cardiac protocol in Section Three).
- Start IV administration of D_5W TKO. Use 0.9% saline (NS) or lactated Ringer's (LR) if signs of hypovolemia are present. For hypotension with signs of hypovolemia, administer fluid cautiously. Consider vasopressors if patient is hypotensive with a normal fluid volume. Watch for signs of fluid overload (refer to shock protocol in Section Three).
- Treat seizures with diazepam (Valium) or lorazepam (Ativan) (refer to diazepam and lorazepam protocols in Section Four and seizure protocol in Section Three).
- Proparacaine hydrochloride should be used to assist eye irrigation (refer to proparacaine hydrochloride protocol in Section Four).

INITIAL EMERGENCY DEPARTMENT CONSIDERATIONS

- Useful initial laboratory studies include carboxyhemoglobin, complete blood count, serum electrolytes, blood urea nitrogen (BUN), creatinine, glucose, urinalysis, and baseline biochemical profile, including serum aminotransferases (AST and ALT), calcium, phosphorus, and magnesium. Determination of anion and osmolar gaps may be helpful. Arterial blood gases (ABGs) with measured (not calculated) oxygen saturation, chest radiograph, and electrocardiogram may be required.
- Use caution with interpretation of pulse oximetry because readings may be inaccurate.

- Hyperbaric oxygen (HBO) may be required for optimal treatment. Absolute indications for HBO therapy are neurological dysfunction such as seizures, decreased level of consciousness, and/or cardiac arrhythmias. Also, because of delayed neurotoxic effects of CO, carboxyhemoglobin blood concentrations of 25% to 30% may require HBO therapy.
- Fetal hemoglobin binds CO more tightly (half-life 15 hours) than adult hemoglobin. Pregnant women therefore require longer administration of 100% oxygen and, in cases of severe poisoning, probably should be considered for HBO therapy. Severe maternal exposures have caused fetal morbidity and mortality.
- Hyperventilation and osmotic therapy may be beneficial in treating increased intracranial pressure.
- Positive end-expiratory pressure (PEEP)–assisted ventilation may be necessary in patients with acute parenchymal injury who develop pulmonary edema or acute respiratory distress syndrome.
- Obtain toxicological consultation as necessary.

SPECIAL CONSIDERATIONS

Pulse oximetry readings may not be accurate in these exposures.

Cyanide and Related Compounds

SUBSTANCE IDENTIFICATION

May be found in liquid, solid, or gaseous form. In solid form it is white, with a faint almond odor (an estimated 20% of the population is genetically unable to detect this odor). Used as a fumigant, in metal treatment, and in the welding/cutting of heat-resistant metals. Also used in paper manufacturing, photography, electroplating, blueprinting, and engraving. By-product liberated during ore extraction and metal purification. Thermal decomposition product of many plastics and other combustible products. Present in most smoke inhalation cases.

ROUTES OF EXPOSURE

Skin and eye contact
Inhalation
Ingestion
Skin absorption

TARGET ORGANS

Primary
Skin
Eyes
Central nervous system
Cardiovascular system
Secondary
Respiratory system
Gastrointestinal system
Hepatic system
Renal system
Metabolism

LIFE THREAT

Death caused by an inhibitory action on the cytochrome oxidase system, preventing mitochondrial use of oxygen to make adenosine triphosphate (ATP). Cyanide brings cellular respiration to a halt.

SIGNS AND SYMPTOMS BY SYSTEM

Cardiovascular: At first, pulse rate decreases and blood pressure rises. As poisoning continues, bradycardia, heart blocks, ventricular arrhythmias, hypotension, and cardiovascular collapse may occur. Palpitations and tightness of the chest.

Respiratory: May cause immediate respiratory arrest. Initially, respiratory rate and depth are increased; as poisoning progresses, respirations become slow, gasping, and finally apneic. Respiratory tract irritation and pulmonary edema.

CNS: Immediate coma. Early symptoms include anxiety, agitation, vertigo, weakness, paralysis, headache, confusion, and lethargy. Seizures.

Gastrointestinal: Nausea, vomiting, excessive salivation, and hemorrhage.
Eye: Chemical conjunctivitis. Dilated pupils.
Skin: Dermatitis and, in some cases, ulcers. Pale or reddish skin color with diaphoresis. Cyanosis is not always present.
Renal: Kidney damage.
Hepatic: Hepatic damage.
Metabolism: Anion gap metabolic acidosis and rhabdomyolysis.
Other: May be rapidly fatal without early symptoms.

SYMPTOM ONSET FOR ACUTE EXPOSURE

Immediate
Symptoms possibly delayed

CO-EXPOSURE CONCERNS

Other oxygen excluders
Simple asphyxiants

THERMAL DECOMPOSITION PRODUCTS INCLUDE

Ammonia gases
Carbon monoxide
Hydrogen cyanide
Nitrogen oxides

MEDICAL CONDITIONS POSSIBLY AGGRAVATED BY EXPOSURE

Central nervous system disorders
Liver disorders
Kidney disorders
Lung disorders
Thyroid gland dysfunction

DECONTAMINATION

- Wear positive-pressure SCBA and protective equipment specified by references such as the *North American Emergency Response Guidebook*. If special chemical protective clothing is required, consult the chemical manufacturer or specific protective clothing compatibility charts. A qualified, experienced person should make decisions regarding the type of personal protective equipment necessary.
- Delay entry until trained personnel and proper protective equipment are available.
- Remove patient from contaminated area.
- Quickly remove and isolate patient's clothing, jewelry, and shoes.
- Gently brush away dry particles and blot excess liquids with absorbent material.
- Rinse patient with warm water, 32° C to 35° C (90° F to 95° F), if possible.
- Wash patient with a mild liquid soap and large quantities of water.
- Refer to decontamination protocol in Section Three.

IMMEDIATE FIRST AID

- Ensure that adequate decontamination has been carried out.
- If patient is not breathing, start artificial respiration, preferably with a demand-valve resuscitator, bag-valve-mask device, or pocket mask, as trained. Perform CPR if necessary.
- Immediately flush contaminated eyes with gently flowing water.
- Do not induce vomiting. If vomiting occurs, lean patient forward or place on left side (head-down position, if possible) to maintain an open airway and prevent aspiration.

- Keep patient quiet and maintain normal body temperature.
- Obtain medical attention.

BASIC TREATMENT

- Establish a patent airway (oropharyngeal or nasopharyngeal airway, if needed). Suction if necessary.
- Watch for signs of respiratory insufficiency and assist ventilations if necessary.
- Administer oxygen by nonrebreather mask at 10 to 15 L/min.
- Administer amyl nitrite ampules as per protocol and physician order (refer to cyanide kit protocol in Section Four).
- Monitor for shock and treat if necessary (refer to shock protocol in Section Three).
- Monitor for pulmonary edema and treat if necessary (refer to pulmonary edema protocol in Section Three).
- Anticipate seizures and treat if necessary (refer to seizure protocol in Section Three).
- For eye contamination, flush eyes immediately with water. Irrigate each eye continuously with 0.9% saline (NS) during transport (refer to eye irrigation protocol in Section Three).
- Do not use emetics. For ingestion, rinse mouth and administer 5 ml/kg up to 200 ml of water for dilution if the patient can swallow, has a strong gag reflex, and does not drool (refer to ingestion protocol in Section Three).

ADVANCED TREATMENT

- Consider orotracheal or nasotracheal intubation for airway control in the patient who is unconscious, has severe pulmonary edema, or is in severe respiratory distress.
- Positive-pressure ventilation techniques with a bag-valve-mask device may be beneficial.
- Consider drug therapy for pulmonary edema (refer to pulmonary edema protocol in Section Three).
- Monitor and treat cardiac arrhythmias if necessary (refer to cardiac protocol in Section Three).
- Start IV administration of D_5W TKO. Use 0.9% saline (NS) or lactated Ringer's (LR) if signs of hypovolemia are present. For hypotension with signs of hypovolemia, administer fluid cautiously. Consider vasopressors if patient is hypotensive with a normal fluid volume. Watch for signs of fluid overload (refer to shock protocol in Section Three).
- Administer cyanide antidote kit as per protocol and physician order (refer to cyanide antidote kit protocol in Section Four).
- Treat seizures with diazepam (Valium) or lorazepam (Ativan) (refer to diazepam and lorazepam protocols in Section Four and seizure protocol in Section Three).
- Use proparacaine hydrochloride to assist eye irrigation (refer to proparacaine hydrochloride protocol in Section Four).

INITIAL EMERGENCY DEPARTMENT CONSIDERATIONS

- Useful initial laboratory studies include complete blood count, serum electrolytes, blood urea nitrogen (BUN), creatinine, glucose, urinalysis, and baseline biochemical profile, including serum aminotransferases (ALT and AST), calcium, phosphorus, and magnesium. Determination of anion and osmolar gaps may be helpful. Arterial blood gases (ABGs), chest radiograph, and electrocardiogram may be required.

- Whole blood cyanide concentrations may be drawn. Background and postexposure values are extremely variable. Smokers demonstrate higher background concentrations than non-smokers.
- Treatment should not be withheld pending laboratory cyanide determinations. Treatment must be based on exposure history and clinical presentation.
- Positive end-expiratory pressure (PEEP)–assisted ventilation may be necessary in patients with acute parenchymal injury who develop pulmonary edema or acute respiratory distress syndrome.
- Obtain toxicological consultation as necessary.

SPECIAL CONSIDERATIONS

- Administration of sodium nitrite may cause hypotension.
- Pulse oximetry readings may not be accurate in these exposures.
- Asymptomatic individuals who may have transiently inhaled cyanide vapors are not at risk for delayed systemic symptoms once removed from the contaminated environment, unless they have ingested the product or continue to have skin exposure to liquids or solids.

Hydrogen Sulfide and Related Compounds

SUBSTANCE IDENTIFICATION

Colorless gases with strong offensive odor. Colorless liquid at low temperature or under high pressure. Used as an agricultural disinfectant and fumigant, a laboratory reagent, an additive in cutting oils and lubricants, and in the preparation of heavy water for nuclear reactions. By-products of numerous manufacturing processes and petroleum refining. Naturally occurs when organic matter decays; may be found in sewers, sewage treatment facilities, natural gas/crude oil operations, and manure tanks. Products may have an odor of "rotten eggs," but may prove to have an inadequate warning property. Olfactory nerve fatigue develops after a relatively brief exposure time.

ROUTES OF EXPOSURE

Skin and eye contact
Inhalation
Skin absorption with some compounds

TARGET ORGANS

Primary
Eyes
Respiratory system
Secondary
Skin
Central nervous system
Cardiovascular system
Gastrointestinal system
Metabolism

LIFE THREAT

Severe respiratory irritant that can cause pulmonary edema and respiratory paralysis (especially hydrogen sulfide). Products may inhibit the cytochrome oxidase system and interfere with cellular respiration.

SIGNS AND SYMPTOMS BY SYSTEM

Cardiovascular: Cardiovascular collapse, tachycardia or bradycardia, and arrhythmias.

Respiratory: Respiratory tract irritant, cough, dyspnea, tachypnea, laryngitis, pneumonitis or bronchitis. Pulmonary edema and respiratory arrest may occur with severe exposures.

CNS: Headache, confusion, vertigo, dizziness, excitement, tiredness, olfactory fatigue, and a garlic taste in mouth. Decreased level of consciousness, delirium, coma, and seizures.

Gastrointestinal: Nausea, vomiting, diarrhea, and profuse salivation.

Eye: Chemical conjunctivitis (sometimes termed "gas eye"), lacrimation, and photophobia. Permanent damage, including corneal ulceration.

Skin: Dermatitis, sweating, and local pain. Cyanosis. Contact with liquid may cause frostbite.
Metabolism: Lactic acidosis.

SYMPTOM ONSET FOR ACUTE EXPOSURE

High concentrations have an immediate effect
Pulmonary edema possibly delayed

CO-EXPOSURE CONCERNS

Alcohol
Other chemical asphyxiants
Simple asphyxiants

THERMAL DECOMPOSITION PRODUCTS INCLUDE

Hydrogen
Sulfur
Sulfur oxides

MEDICAL CONDITIONS POSSIBLY AGGRAVATED BY EXPOSURE

Eye conditions
Asthma and fibrotic pulmonary diseases
Reactive airways disease

DECONTAMINATION

- Wear positive-pressure SCBA and protective equipment specified by references such as the *North American Emergency Response Guidebook*. If special chemical protective clothing is required, consult the chemical manufacturer or specific protective clothing compatibility charts. A qualified, experienced person should make decisions regarding the type of personal protective equipment necessary.
- Delay entry until trained personnel and proper protective equipment are available.
- Remove patient from contaminated area.
- Quickly remove and isolate patient's clothing, jewelry, and shoes.
- If any concurrent liquid or solid contamination exists:
  Gently brush away dry particles and blot excess liquids with absorbent material.
  Rinse patient with warm water, 32° C to 35° C (90° F to 95° F), if possible.
  Wash patient with a mild liquid soap and large quantities of water.
  Refer to decontamination protocol in Section Three.

IMMEDIATE FIRST AID

- Ensure that adequate decontamination has been carried out.
- If patient is not breathing, start artificial respiration, preferably with a demand-valve resuscitator, bag-valve-mask device, or pocket mask, as trained. Perform CPR if necessary.
- Immediately flush contaminated eyes with gently flowing water.
- Do not induce vomiting. If vomiting occurs, lean patient forward or place on left side (head-down position, if possible) to maintain an open airway and prevent aspiration.
- Keep patient quiet and maintain normal body temperature.
- Obtain medical attention.

BASIC TREATMENT

- Establish a patent airway (oropharyngeal or nasopharyngeal airway, if needed). Suction if necessary.

- Watch for signs of respiratory insufficiency and assist ventilations if necessary.
- Administer oxygen by nonrebreather mask at 10 to 15 L/min.
- Monitor for pulmonary edema and treat if necessary (refer to pulmonary edema protocol in Section Three).
- Monitor for shock and treat if necessary (refer to shock protocol in Section Three).
- Anticipate seizures and treat if necessary (refer to seizure protocol in Section Three).
- For eye contamination, flush eyes immediately with water. Irrigate each eye continuously with 0.9% saline (NS) during transport (refer to eye irrigation protocol in Section Three).
- Treat with rapid rewarming techniques if frostbite occurs (refer to frostbite protocol in Section Three).

ADVANCED TREATMENT

- Consider orotracheal or nasotracheal intubation for airway control in the patient who is unconscious, has severe pulmonary edema, or is in severe respiratory distress.
- Positive-pressure ventilation techniques with a bag-valve-mask device may be beneficial.
- Consider drug therapy for pulmonary edema (refer to pulmonary edema protocol in Section Three).
- Monitor cardiac rhythm and treat arrhythmias if necessary (refer to cardiac protocol in Section Three).
- Start IV administration of D_5W TKO. Use 0.9% saline (NS) or lactated Ringer's (LR) if signs of hypovolemia are present. For hypotension with signs of hypovolemia, administer fluid cautiously. Consider vasopressors if patient is hypotensive with a normal fluid volume. Watch for signs of fluid overload (refer to shock protocol in Section Three).
- Treat seizures with diazepam (Valium) or lorazepam (Ativan) (refer to diazepam and lorazepam protocols in Section Four and seizure protocol in Section Three).
- In severe cases use amyl nitrite and sodium nitrite (from the cyanide antidote kit) as described for cyanide poisoning; omit the sodium thiosulfate injection. Early administration will be the most effective. DIRECT PHYSICIAN ORDER ONLY (refer to cyanide kit protocol in Section Four).
- Use proparacaine hydrochloride to assist eye irrigation (refer to proparacaine hydrochloride protocol in Section Four).

INITIAL EMERGENCY DEPARTMENT CONSIDERATIONS

- Useful initial laboratory studies include complete blood count, serum electrolytes, blood urea nitrogen (BUN), creatinine, glucose, urinalysis, and baseline biochemical profile, including serum aminotransferases (ALT and AST), calcium, phosphorus, and magnesium. Determination of anion and osmolar gaps may be helpful. Arterial blood gases (ABGs), chest radiograph, and electrocardiogram may be required.
- Positive end-expiratory pressure (PEEP)–assisted ventilation may be necessary in patients with acute parenchymal injury who develop pulmonary edema or acute respiratory distress syndrome.

- Products may cause acidosis; hyperventilation and sodium bicarbonate may be beneficial. Bicarbonate therapy should be guided by patient presentation, ABG determination, and serum electrolyte considerations.
- Obtain toxicological consultation as necessary.

SPECIAL CONSIDERATIONS

- Hydrogen sulfide inhibits the cytochrome oxidase P_{450} system.
- Pulse oximetry readings may not be accurate in these exposures.

92

Simple Asphyxiants and Related Compounds

SUBSTANCE IDENTIFICATION

Found as colorless and usually odorless gases. Some compounds may have odorants added. These gases are used in a variety of manufacturing processes. Simple asphyxiants usually have no or very little inherent toxicity. Their primary hazard is the displacement of atmospheric oxygen below normal. The hazard is increased in confined areas. Use caution in scene operations, since many of these products have inadequate warning properties. They are shipped as a compressed or liquefied gas or in a cryogenic state. Liquefied gases present a frostbite hazard when released. Cryogenics are gases compressed into liquids with a temperature below –150° F. Cryogenic and liquefied gases have a large expansion ratio; a small amount of liquid vaporizes to a large amount of gas.

ROUTES OF EXPOSURE

Inhalation
Skin contact

TARGET ORGANS

Primary
Respiratory system
Central nervous system
Skin
Secondary
Cardiovascular system
Gastrointestinal system

LIFE THREAT

Asphyxia caused by atmospheric oxygen deficiency.

SIGNS AND SYMPTOMS BY SYSTEM

Cardiovascular: Tachycardia, arrhythmias, hypotension, and cardiovascular collapse caused by hypoxia.
Respiratory: Increased respiratory rate and dyspnea followed by apnea and death.
CNS: Headache, dizziness, and confusion. Decreased level of consciousness, coma, and seizures.
Gastrointestinal: Nausea and vomiting.
Eye: Vision deficits.
Skin: Frostbite or frozen tissue from product at low temperatures. Cyanosis.
Other: At low atmospheric oxygen concentrations, coordination and judgment may be lost without warning, making self-rescue impossible.

SYMPTOM ONSET FOR ACUTE EXPOSURE

Immediate

CO-EXPOSURE CONCERNS

Carbon monoxide

Hydrogen sulfide
Methemoglobin formers
Trauma

THERMAL DECOMPOSITION PRODUCTS INCLUDE

Numerous; varies with compound

MEDICAL CONDITIONS POSSIBLY AGGRAVATED BY EXPOSURE

Respiratory disorders
Cardiovascular disorders

DECONTAMINATION

- Wear positive-pressure SCBA and protective equipment specified by references such as the *North American Emergency Response Guidebook*. If special chemical protective clothing is required, consult the chemical manufacturer or specific protective clothing compatibility charts. A qualified, experienced person should make decisions regarding the type of personal protective equipment necessary.
- Delay entry until trained personnel and proper protective equipment are available.
- Remove patient from contaminated area.
- If any concurrent liquid or solid contamination exists:
  Quickly remove and isolate patient's clothing, jewelry, and shoes.
  Gently brush away dry particles and blot excess liquids with absorbent material.
  Rinse patient with warm water, 32° C to 35° C (90° F to 95° F), if possible.
  Wash patient with a mild liquid soap and large quantities of water.
  Refer to decontamination protocol in Section Three.

IMMEDIATE FIRST AID

- Ensure that adequate decontamination has been carried out.
- If patient is not breathing, start artificial respiration, preferably with a demand-valve resuscitator, bag-valve-mask device, or pocket mask, as trained. Perform CPR if necessary.
- Immediately flush contaminated eyes with gently flowing water.
- Do not induce vomiting. If vomiting occurs, lean patient forward or place on left side (head-down position, if possible) to maintain an open airway and prevent aspiration.
- Keep patient quiet and maintain normal body temperature.
- Obtain medical attention.

BASIC TREATMENT

- Establish a patent airway (oropharyngeal or nasopharyngeal airway, if needed). Suction if necessary.
- Watch for signs of respiratory insufficiency and assist ventilations if necessary.
- Administer oxygen by nonrebreather mask at 10 to 15 L/min.
- Anticipate seizures and treat if necessary (refer to seizure protocol in Section Three).
- Use rapid rewarming techniques if frostbite occurs (refer to frostbite protocol in Section Three).

ADVANCED TREATMENT

- Consider orotracheal or nasotracheal intubation for airway control in the patient who is unconscious or is in severe respiratory distress.
- Monitor cardiac rhythm and treat arrhythmias if necessary (refer to cardiac protocol in Section Three).

- Start IV administration of D_5W TKO.
- Treat seizures with diazepam (Valium) or lorazepam (Ativan) (refer to diazepam and lorazepam protocols in Section Four and seizure protocol in Section Three).

INITIAL EMERGENCY DEPARTMENT CONSIDERATIONS

- Useful initial laboratory studies include complete blood count, serum electrolytes, blood urea nitrogen (BUN), creatinine, glucose, urinalysis, and baseline biochemical profile, including serum aminotransferases (ALT and AST), calcium, phosphorus, and magnesium. Determination of anion and osmolar gaps may be helpful. Arterial blood gases (ABGs), chest radiograph, and electrocardiogram may be required.
- Obtain toxicological consultation if necessary.

SPECIAL CONSIDERATIONS

- Assess the scene and exposure history carefully to rule out other toxic or physical mechanisms of injury.

Carbon Disulfide and Related Compounds

SUBSTANCE IDENTIFICATION

Clear, colorless to faintly yellow liquids with a strong, sweet odor; in commercial grades, an offensive odor like decaying cabbage. Used in the manufacture of viscose rayon, carbon tetrachloride, cellophane, dyes, and rubber. Also found in solvents, waxes, and cleaners. Used in vapor form as a disinfectant, insecticide, and fumigant. Products may be extremely flammable.

ROUTES OF EXPOSURE

Skin and eye contact
Inhalation
Ingestion
Skin absorption

TARGET ORGANS

Primary
Skin
Eyes
Central nervous system
Cardiovascular system
Renal system
Hepatic system
Secondary
Respiratory system
Gastrointestinal system

LIFE THREAT

Respiratory paralysis and arrest caused by CNS depression.

SIGNS AND SYMPTOMS BY SYSTEM

- **Cardiovascular:** Arrhythmias, cardiovascular collapse, and hypotension.
- **Respiratory:** Irritation to the respiratory tract and respiratory arrest. Garlicky odor on breath.
- **CNS:** Mood and personality disturbances. Dizziness, unsteady gait, fatigue, muscle weakness, headache, and hallucinations. CNS depression, seizures, and coma. Neurobehavioral changes.
- **Gastrointestinal:** Irritation of mucous membranes, nausea, vomiting, diarrhea, and abdominal cramps.
- **Eye:** Chemical conjunctivitis, corneal burns, and optic nerve damage.
- **Skin:** Irritant dermatitis and burns.
- **Renal:** Kidney damage.
- **Hepatic:** Liver damage.

SYMPTOM ONSET FOR ACUTE EXPOSURE

Immediate

CO-EXPOSURE

Alcohol
Disulfiram (Antabuse)
Hydrogen sulfide

THERMAL DECOMPOSITION PRODUCTS INCLUDE

Carbon dioxide
Carbon monoxide
Sulfur dioxide

MEDICAL CONDITIONS POSSIBLY AGGRAVATED BY EXPOSURE

Central nervous system disorders
Cardiovascular disorders
Gastrointestinal disorders
Liver or kidney disorders

DECONTAMINATION

- Wear positive-pressure SCBA and protective equipment specified by references such as the *North American Emergency Response Guidebook.* If special chemical protective clothing is required, consult the chemical manufacturer or specific protective clothing compatibility charts. A qualified, experienced person should make decisions regarding the type of personal protective equipment necessary.
- Delay entry until trained personnel and proper protective equipment are available.
- Remove patient from contaminated area.
- Quickly remove and isolate patient's clothing, jewelry, and shoes.
- Gently blot excess liquids with absorbent material.
- Rinse patient with warm water, 32° C to 35° C (90° F to 95° F), if possible.
- Wash patient with a mild liquid soap and large quantities of water.
- Refer to decontamination protocol in Section Three.

IMMEDIATE FIRST AID

- Ensure that adequate decontamination has been carried out.
- If patient is not breathing, start artificial respiration, preferably with a demand-valve resuscitator, bag-valve-mask device, or pocket mask, as trained. Perform CPR if necessary.
- Immediately flush contaminated eyes with gently flowing water.
- Do not induce vomiting. If vomiting occurs, lean patient forward or place on left side (head-down position, if possible) to maintain an open airway and prevent aspiration.
- Keep patient quiet and maintain normal body temperature.
- Obtain medical attention.

BASIC TREATMENT

- Establish a patent airway (oropharyngeal or nasopharyngeal airway, if needed). Suction if necessary.
- Watch for signs of respiratory insufficiency and assist ventilations if necessary.
- Administer oxygen by nonrebreather mask at 10 to 15 L/min.
- Anticipate seizures and treat if necessary (refer to seizure protocol in Section Three).
- Monitor for shock and treat if necessary (refer to shock protocol in Section Three).

- For eye contamination, flush eyes immediately with water. Irrigate each eye continuously with 0.9% saline (NS) during transport (refer to eye irrigation protocol in Section Three).
- Do not use emetics. For ingestion, rinse mouth and administer 5 ml/kg up to 200 ml of water for dilution if the patient can swallow, has a strong gag reflex, and does not drool. Administer activated charcoal (refer to ingestion protocol in Section Three and activated charcoal protocol in Section Four).
- Cover skin burns with sterile dressings after decontamination (refer to chemical burn protocol in Section Three).

ADVANCED TREATMENT

- Consider orotracheal or nasotracheal intubation for airway control in the patient who is unconscious or is in severe respiratory distress.
- Monitor cardiac rhythm and treat arrhythmias if necessary (refer to cardiac protocol in Section Three).
- Start IV administration of 0.9% saline (NS) or lactated Ringer's (LR) TKO. For hypotension with signs of hypovolemia, administer fluid cautiously. Watch for signs of fluid overload (refer to shock protocol in Section Three)
- Treat seizures with diazepam (Valium) or lorazepam (Ativan) (refer to diazepam and lorazepam protocols in Section Four and seizure protocol in Section Three).
- Use proparacaine hydrochloride to assist eye irrigation (refer to proparacaine hydrochloride protocol in Section Four).

INITIAL EMERGENCY DEPARTMENT CONSIDERATIONS

- Useful initial laboratory studies include complete blood count, serum electrolytes, blood urea nitrogen (BUN), creatinine, glucose, urinalysis, and baseline biochemical profile, including serum aminotransferases (ALT and AST), calcium, phosphorus, and magnesium. Determination of anion and osmolar gaps may be helpful. Arterial blood gases (ABGs), chest radiograph, and electrocardiogram may be required.
- Obtain toxicological consultation as necessary.

SPECIAL CONSIDERATIONS

- Avoid epinephrine and related beta agonists (unless patient is in cardiac arrest or has reactive airways disease refractory to other treatment) because of the possible irritable condition of the myocardium. Use of these medications may lead to ventricular fibrillation.

Isocyanates, Aliphatic Thiocyanates, and Related Compounds

SUBSTANCE IDENTIFICATION

Found in oil bases, powder, liquids, and gases in diluted and concentrated forms. Used as contact insecticides; as two-part automobile, boat, and bus paints; in the manufacture of rigid polyurethane foams, adhesives, varnishes, wire enamels, protective coatings, and foundry core binders; and as mediators in chemical reactions. Certain products may have a synergistic effect when combined with organophosphates or other insecticides. Toxicity may result from the hydrocarbon vehicle, which is often kerosene (consult the appropriate guideline).

ROUTES OF EXPOSURE

Skin and eye contact
Inhalation
Ingestion
Skin absorption

TARGET ORGANS

Primary
Skin
Eyes
Respiratory system
Secondary
Central nervous system
Cardiovascular system
Gastrointestinal system
Hepatic system
Renal system

LIFE THREAT

Respiratory arrest caused by CNS depression, paralysis of the respiratory center, and pulmonary edema. Certain thiocyanates (see "Other" below) may cause cyanide toxicity.

SIGNS AND SYMPTOMS BY SYSTEM

Cardiovascular: Arrhythmias, cardiovascular collapse.

Respiratory: Respiratory tract irritation, rhinitis, sinusitis, pharyngitis, cough, chest pain, dyspnea, increased secretions, wheezing, hyperpnea, and respiratory arrest. Pulmonary edema, bronchitis, hypersensitivity pneumonitis, or asthma/reactive airways disease.

CNS: Restlessness, irritability, ataxia, seizures, decreased level of consciousness or coma.

Gastrointestinal: Mucous membrane irritation, nausea, vomiting, and abdominal pain.

Eye: Lacrimation, chemical conjunctivitis, severe ocular burns, and corneal damage.
Skin: Irritation, irritant or allergic dermatitis with erythema, edema, or blistering.
Renal: Kidney damage.
Hepatic: Liver damage.
Other:
Thiocyanates (cyanide-producing): Certain aliphatic thiocyantes such as methyl, ethyl, and isopropyl thiocyanates, Lethane 60, Lethane 384, and Thanite. These thiocyanate compounds may release cyanide ions when metabolized and therefore produce acute cyanide poisoning.
Thiocyanates (noncyanide-producing): Ammonium thiocyanate, laurel thiocyanate, methyl isothiocyanate, potassium thiocyanate, and sodium thiocyanate. The thiocyanate ion is slowly excreted in the urine intact and does not generally produce cyanide toxicity.
Isocyanates: Methyl isocyanate, ethyl isocyanate, and toluene diisocyanate (TDI). These chemicals act as primary pulmonary irritants and do not release cyanide on exposure. Acute, life-threatening pulmonary edema can develop. Acute exposure may precipitate asthma/reactive airways disease, bronchitis, chest tightness, and dyspnea. These conditions may persist from months to years and may be permanent after a single exposure.

SYMPTOM ONSET FOR ACUTE EXPOSURE

Symptoms possibly immediate or delayed
Reactive airway symptoms may appear after acute exposure

CO-EXPOSURE CONCERNS

Other isocyanates
Organophosphates
Other insecticides

THERMAL DECOMPOSITION PRODUCTS INCLUDE

Carbon dioxide
Carbon monoxide
Hydrocarbons
Hydrogen cyanide
Nitrogen oxides

MEDICAL CONDITIONS POSSIBLY AGGRAVATED BY EXPOSURE

Respiratory system disorders
Asthma/reactive airways disease

DECONTAMINATION

- Wear positive-pressure SCBA and protective equipment specified by references such as the *North American Emergency Response Guidebook*. If special chemical protective clothing is required, consult the chemical manufacturer or specific protective clothing compatibility charts. A qualified, experienced person should make decisions regarding the type of personal protective equipment necessary.
- Delay entry until trained personnel and proper protective equipment are available.
- Remove patient from contaminated area.
- Quickly remove and isolate patient's clothing, jewelry, and shoes.
- Gently brush away dry particles and blot excess liquids with absorbent material.
- Rinse patient with warm water, 32° C to 35° C (90° F to 95° F), if possible.

- Wash patient with a mild liquid soap and large quantities of water.
- Refer to decontamination protocol in Section Three.

IMMEDIATE FIRST AID

- Ensure that adequate decontamination has been carried out.
- If patient is not breathing, start artificial respiration, preferably with a demand-valve resuscitator, bag-valve-mask device, or pocket mask, as trained. Perform CPR if necessary.
- Immediately flush contaminated eyes with gently flowing water.
- Do not induce vomiting. If vomiting occurs, lean patient forward or place on left side (head-down position, if possible) to maintain an open airway and prevent aspiration.
- Keep patient quiet and maintain normal body temperature.
- Obtain medical attention.

BASIC TREATMENT

- Establish a patent airway (oropharyngeal or nasopharyngeal airway, if needed). Suction if necessary.
- Watch for signs of respiratory insufficiency and assist ventilations if necessary.
- Administer oxygen by nonrebreather mask at 10 to 15 L/min.
- Monitor for pulmonary edema and treat if necessary (refer to pulmonary edema protocol in Section Three).
- Monitor for shock and treat if necessary (refer to shock protocol in Section Three).
- Monitor for seizures and treat if necessary (refer to seizure protocol in Section Three).
- For eye contamination, flush eyes immediately with water. Irrigate each eye continuously with 0.9% saline (NS) during transport (refer to eye irrigation protocol in Section Three).
- Do not use emetics. For ingestion, rinse mouth and administer 5 ml/kg up to 200 ml of water for dilution if the patent can swallow, has a strong gag reflex, and does not drool. Administer activated charcoal (refer to ingestion protocol in Section Three and activated charcoal protocol in Section Four).

ADVANCED TREATMENT

- Consider orotracheal or nasotracheal intubation for airway control in the patient who is unconscious, has severe pulmonary edema, or is in severe respiratory distress.
- Positive-pressure ventilation techniques with a bag-valve-mask device may be beneficial.
- Consider drug therapy for pulmonary edema (refer to pulmonary edema protocol in Section Three).
- Consider administering a beta agonist such as albuterol for severe bronchospasm (refer to albuterol protocol in Section four).
- Monitor cardiac rhythm and treat arrhythmias if necessary (refer to cardiac protocol in Section Three).
- Start IV administration of D_5W TKO. Use 0.9% saline (NS) or lactated Ringer's (LR) if signs of hypovolemia are present. For hypotension with signs of hypovolemia, administer fluid cautiously. Consider vasopressors if patient is hypotensive with a normal fluid volume. Watch for signs of fluid overload (refer to shock protocol in Section Three).

- Treat seizures with diazepam (Valium) or lorazepam (Ativan) (refer to diazepam and lorazepam protocols in Section Four and seizure protocol in Section Three).
- Treat exposure to Lethane 60, Lethane 384, Thanite, methyl, ethyl, or isopropyl thiocyanates with the cyanide antidote kit. (DIRECT PHYSICIAN ORDER ONLY; refer to cyanide guideline and cyanide protocol in Section Four.)
- Use proparacaine hydrochloride to assist eye irrigation (refer to proparacaine hydrochloride protocol in Section Four).

INITIAL EMERGENCY DEPARTMENT CONSIDERATIONS

- Useful initial laboratory studies include complete blood count, serum electrolytes, blood urea nitrogen (BUN), creatinine, glucose, urinalysis, anion gap calculation, and baseline biochemical profile, including serum aminotransferases (ALT and AST), calcium, phosphorus, and magnesium. Arterial blood gases (ABGs), chest radiograph, and electrocardiogram may be required.
- IgE antibodies to certain isocyanates have been detected in individuals sensitive to isocyanates.
- Positive end-expiratory pressure (PEEP)–assisted ventilation may be necessary in patients with acute parenchymal injury who develop pulmonary edema or acute respiratory distress syndrome.
- Bronchospastic symptoms should be treated with an inhalation medication regimen similar to that used for reactive airways disease. Inhaled corticosteroids may be of value in severe bronchospasm.
- Products may cause acidosis; hyperventilation and sodium bicarbonate may be beneficial. Bicarbonate therapy should be guided by patient presentation, ABG determination, and serum electrolyte considerations.
- With products that release cyanide, hyperbaric oxygen therapy may be beneficial as an adjunct to the cyanide antidote kit (nitrite therapy) (refer to cyanide antidote kit protocol in Section Four).
- Obtain toxicological consultation as necessary.

SPECIAL CONSIDERATIONS

- Isocyanates produce reversible airflow obstruction by direct irritation of the airways or by sensitizing the airway to isocyanates. Isocyanate-induced asthma may persist for years after the exposure.
- Emergency medical transportation should be rapid.
- Toxicity may result from the hydrocarbon vehicle (often kerosene). Identify the vehicle and consult the appropriate guideline.
- Some products may present a human carcinogenic risk.

Bromine, Methyl Bromide, and Related Compounds

SUBSTANCE IDENTIFICATION

Colorless liquid or gas with no odor at low concentrations and a chloroform-like odor at high concentrations. Used as insecticides and as a fumigant for grain elevators, mills, ships, greenhouses, and food-processing facilities; as a soil fumigant; in fire extinguishers, refrigerants, and solvents; and as a methylating agent in chemical manufacturing processes.

ROUTES OF EXPOSURE

Skin and eye contact
Inhalation
Ingestion
Skin absorption

TARGET ORGANS

Primary
Skin
Eyes
Central nervous system
Respiratory system
Secondary
Cardiovascular system
Gastrointestinal system
Hepatic system
Renal system
Blood
Metabolism

LIFE THREAT

Severe respiratory irritation progressing to pulmonary edema and respiratory failure. Neurotoxin that may cause coma, convulsions, and death.

SIGNS AND SYMPTOMS BY SYSTEM

Cardiovascular: Arrhythmias and cardiovascular collapse.

Respiratory: Irritation of respiratory tract mucosa, rhinitis, sinusitis, pneumonitis, and pneumonia. Acute pulmonary edema, dyspnea, tachypnea, and bronchospasm. Noncardiac chest pain.

CNS: Headache, weakness, confusion, dizziness, slurred speech, tremors, diplopia, and jacksonian seizures. Temporary blindness, hearing loss, and a staggering gait. Decreased level of consciousness, paraesthesias, paralysis, coma, and seizures. Neurobehavioral changes.

Gastrointestinal: Nausea, vomiting, and abdominal pain.

Eye: Chemical conjunctivitis to severe eye injury. Blurred vision.

Skin: Cyanosis, chemical burns, and irritant dermatitis (low-level exposures). Allergic dermatitis.
Renal: Kidney damage.
Hepatic: Liver damage.
Blood: Hemolysis and/or decreased white blood cell count (leukocytosis).
Metabolism: Metabolic acidosis.
Other: Human carcinogenic risk of methyl bromide is under review.

SYMPTOM ONSET FOR ACUTE EXPOSURE

Immediate
Pulmonary edema possibly delayed

CO-EXPOSURE CONCERNS

Other halogens
Other neurotoxins
Other respiratory irritants

THERMAL DECOMPOSITION PRODUCTS INCLUDE

Bromide fumes
Carbon dioxide
Carbon monoxide

MEDICAL CONDITIONS POSSIBLY AGGRAVATED BY EXPOSURE

Nervous system disorders
Respiratory system disorders
Skin disorders

DECONTAMINATION

- Wear positive-pressure SCBA and protective equipment specified by references such as the *North American Emergency Response Guidebook*. If special chemical protective clothing is required, consult the chemical manufacturer or specific protective clothing compatibility charts. A qualified, experienced person should make decisions regarding the type of personal protective equipment necessary.
- Delay entry until trained personnel and proper protective equipment are available.
- Remove patient from contaminated area.
- Quickly remove and isolate patient's clothing, jewelry, and shoes.
- Gently blot excess liquids with absorbent material.
- Rinse patient with warm water, 32° C to 35° C (90° F to 95° F), if possible.
- Wash patient with a mild liquid soap and large quantities of water.
- Refer to decontamination protocol in Section Three.

IMMEDIATE FIRST AID

- Ensure that adequate decontamination has been carried out.
- If patient is not breathing, start artificial respiration, preferably with a demand-valve resuscitator, bag-valve-mask device, or pocket mask, as trained. Perform CPR if necessary.
- Immediately flush contaminated eyes with gently flowing water.
- Do not induce vomiting. If vomiting occurs, lean patient forward or place on left side (head-down position, if possible) to maintain an open airway and prevent aspiration.
- Keep patient quiet and maintain normal body temperature.
- Obtain medical attention.

BASIC TREATMENT

- Establish a patent airway (oropharyngeal or nasopharyngeal airway, if needed). Suction if necessary.
- Watch for signs of respiratory insufficiency and assist ventilations if necessary.
- Administer oxygen by nonrebreather mask at 10 to 15 L/min.
- Monitor for pulmonary edema and treat if necessary (refer to pulmonary edema protocol in Section Three).
- Monitor for shock and treat if necessary (refer to shock protocol in Section Three).
- Anticipate seizures and treat if necessary (refer to seizure protocol in Section Three).
- For eye contamination, flush eyes immediately with water. Irrigate each eye continuously with 0.9% saline (NS) during transport (refer to eye irrigation protocol in Section Three).
- Do not use emetics. For ingestion, rinse mouth and administer 5 ml/kg up to 200 ml of water for dilution if the patient can swallow, has a strong gag reflex, and does not drool. Administer activated charcoal (refer to ingestion protocol in Section Three and activated charcoal protocol in Section Four).
- Cover skin burns with dry sterile dressings after decontamination (refer to chemical burn protocol in Section Three).

ADVANCED TREATMENT

- Consider orotracheal or nasotracheal intubation for airway control in the patient who is unconscious, has severe pulmonary edema, or is in severe respiratory distress.
- Positive-pressure ventilation techniques with a bag-valve-mask device may be beneficial.
- Consider drug therapy for pulmonary edema (refer to pulmonary edema protocol in Section Three).
- Consider administering a beta agonist such as albuterol for severe bronchospasm (refer to albuterol protocol in Section four).
- Monitor cardiac rhythm and treat arrhythmias if necessary (refer to cardiac protocol in Section Three).
- Start IV administration of D_5W TKO. Use 0.9% saline (NS) or lactated Ringer's (LR) if signs of hypovolemia are present. For hypotension with signs of hypovolemia, administer fluid cautiously. Consider vasopressors if patient is hypotensive with a normal fluid volume. Watch for signs of fluid overload (refer to shock protocol in Section Three).
- Treat seizures with diazepam (Valium) or lorazepam (Ativan) (refer to diazepam and lorazepam protocols in Section Four and seizure protocol in Section Three).
- Use proparacaine hydrochloride to assist eye irrigation (refer to proparacaine hydrochloride protocol in Section Four).

INITIAL EMERGENCY DEPARTMENT CONSIDERATIONS

- Useful initial laboratory studies include complete blood count, serum electrolytes, blood urea nitrogen (BUN), creatinine, glucose, urinalysis, and baseline biochemical profile, including serum aminotransferases (ALT and AST), calcium, phosphorus, and magnesium. Determination of anion and osmolar gaps may be helpful. Arterial blood gases (ABGs), chest radiograph, and electrocardiogram may be required.

- Positive end-expiratory pressure (PEEP)–assisted ventilation may be necessary in patients with acute parenchymal injury who develop pulmonary edema or acute respiratory distress syndrome.
- Bronchospastic symptoms should be treated with an inhalation medication regimen similar to that used for reactive airways disease. Inhaled corticosteroids may be of value in severe bronchospasm.
- Products may cause acidosis; hyperventilation and sodium bicarbonate may be beneficial. Bicarbonate therapy should be guided by patient presentation, ABG determination, and serum electrolyte considerations.
- Obtain toxicological consultation as necessary.

SPECIAL CONSIDERATIONS

- Acute occupational exposure and resultant symptoms may be superimposed over chronic toxicity effects.

Bromates and Related Compounds

SUBSTANCE IDENTIFICATION

White, crystalline powders in solid form; may also be found in solutions. Products are used as laboratory reagents and oxidizing agents and in the manufacture of fireworks, matches, weed killers, and dyes.

ROUTES OF EXPOSURE

Skin and eye contact
Inhalation
Ingestion
Skin absorption

TARGET ORGANS

Primary
Eyes
Central nervous system
Respiratory system
Renal system
Secondary
Skin
Cardiovascular system
Gastrointestinal system
Metabolism
Blood

LIFE THREAT

CNS and respiratory system depression. Renal failure, usually days to weeks after exposure.

SIGNS AND SYMPTOMS BY SYSTEM

Cardiovascular: Tachycardia and hypotension.

Respiratory: Tachypnea and dyspnea. Irritation of the respiratory tract. Respiratory system depression. Pulmonary edema.

CNS: Headaches and restlessness followed by apathy. Seizures are rare, usually occurring in the later stages of renal failure. Coma. Hearing loss.

Gastrointestinal: Mucous membrane irritation. Nausea, vomiting, diarrhea, and abdominal pain.

Eye: Chemical conjunctivitis. Visual disturbances.

Skin: Cyanosis followed by pallor. Irritation and burns.

Renal: Kidney damage and renal failure.

Metabolism: Metabolic acidosis.

Blood: Methemoglobinemia may be present but not apparent until hours after exposure. Decreased platelet count (thrombocytopenia) and hemolysis.

Other: The patient may present with lumbar pain.

SYMPTOM ONSET FOR ACUTE EXPOSURE

Immediate

Renal symptoms possibly delayed

CO-EXPOSURE CONCERNS

Chlorates

THERMAL DECOMPOSITION PRODUCTS INCLUDE

Bromine

MEDICAL CONDITIONS POSSIBLY AGGRAVATED BY EXPOSURE

Respiratory system disorders

Kidney disorders

DECONTAMINATION

- Wear positive-pressure SCBA and protective equipment specified by references such as the *North American Emergency Response Guidebook.* If special chemical protective clothing is required, consult the chemical manufacturer or specific protective clothing compatibility charts. A qualified, experienced person should make decisions regarding the type of personal protective equipment necessary.
- Delay entry until trained personnel and proper protective equipment are available.
- Remove patient from contaminated area.
- Quickly remove and isolate patient's clothing, jewelry, and shoes.
- Gently brush away dry particles and blot excess liquids with absorbent material.
- Rinse patient with warm water, 32° C to 35° C (90° F to 95° F), if possible.
- Wash patient with a mild liquid soap and large quantities of water.
- Refer to decontamination protocol in Section Three.

IMMEDIATE FIRST AID

- Ensure that adequate decontamination has been carried out.
- If patient is not breathing, start artificial respiration, preferably with a demand-valve resuscitator, bag-valve-mask device, or pocket mask, as trained. Perform CPR if necessary.
- Immediately flush contaminated eyes with gently flowing water.
- Do not induce vomiting. If vomiting occurs, lean patient forward or place on left side (head-down position, if possible) to maintain an open airway and prevent aspiration.
- Keep patient quiet and maintain normal body temperature.
- Obtain medical attention.

BASIC TREATMENT

- Establish a patent airway (oropharyngeal or nasopharyngeal airway, if needed). Suction if necessary.
- Watch for signs of respiratory insufficiency and assist ventilations if necessary.
- Administer oxygen by nonrebreather mask at 10 to 15 L/min.
- Anticipate seizures and treat if necessary (refer to seizure protocol in Section Three).
- Monitor for pulmonary edema and treat if necessary (refer to pulmonary edema protocol in Section Three).
- Monitor for shock and treat if necessary (refer to shock protocol in Section Three).
- For eye contamination, flush eyes immediately with water. Irrigate each eye continuously with 0.9% saline (NS) during transport (refer to eye irrigation protocol in Section Three).

- Do not use emetics. For ingestion, rinse mouth and administer 5 ml/kg up to 200 ml of water for dilution if the patient can swallow, has a strong gag reflex, and does not drool (refer to ingestion protocol in Section Three).

ADVANCED TREATMENT

- Consider orotracheal or nasotracheal intubation for airway control in the patient who is unconscious or is in severe respiratory distress.
- Positive-pressure ventilation techniques with a bag-valve-mask device may be beneficial.
- Start IV administration of D_5W TKO. Use 0.9% saline (NS) or lactated Ringer's (LR) if signs of hypovolemia are present. For hypotension with signs of hypovolemia, administer fluid cautiously. Watch for signs of fluid overload (refer to shock protocol in Section Three).
- Treat seizures with diazepam (Valium) or lorazepam (Ativan) (refer to diazepam and lorazepam protocols in Section Four and seizure protocol in Section Three).
- Use proparacaine hydrochloride to assist eye irrigation (refer to proparacaine hydrochloride protocol in Section Four).

INITIAL EMERGENCY DEPARTMENT CONSIDERATIONS

- Useful initial laboratory studies include complete blood count, platelet count, coagulation profile, methemoglobin, serum electrolytes, blood urea nitrogen (BUN), creatinine, glucose, urinalysis, and baseline biochemical profile, including serum aminotransferases (ALT and AST), calcium, phosphorus, and magnesium. Determination of anion and osmolar gaps may be helpful. Arterial blood gases (ABGs), chest radiograph, and electrocardiogram may be required.
- Positive end-expiratory pressure (PEEP)–assisted ventilation may be necessary in patients with acute parenchymal injury who develop pulmonary edema or acute respiratory distress syndrome.
- Products may cause acidosis; hyperventilation and sodium bicarbonate may be beneficial. Bicarbonate therapy should be guided by patient presentation, ABG determination, and serum electrolyte considerations.
- Sodium thiosulfate may reduce bromate to bromide ion, which may be less toxic. ADULT DOSAGE: 10 to 50 ml (0.2 to 1 ml/kg; maximum 50 ml) of 10% sodium thiosulfate solution, slow IV over 30 minutes. Rapid administration may cause hypotension.
- Hemodialysis may be required for renal failure. Therapy should be guided by patient presentation and laboratory values.
- Titrate hydration status to maintain adequate urine output.
- Obtain toxicological consultation as necessary.

SPECIAL CONSIDERATIONS

- Methylene blue has little or no effect on this form of methemoglobinemia and may intensify the bromate-catalyzed oxidative hemolysis; therefore it should not be used.
- Exchange transfusion has been advocated for severe poisoning.
- Pulse oximetry readings may not be accurate in these exposures.

Chlorates and Related Compounds

SUBSTANCE IDENTIFICATION

White or colorless crystals. Also found in solutions. Products are used in the production of chlorine dioxide; as analytical agents, herbicides, and oxidizing agents; and in the manufacture of fireworks, matches, throat gargles, and dyes.

ROUTES OF EXPOSURE

Skin and eye contact
Inhalation
Ingestion

TARGET ORGANS

Primary
Skin
Eyes
Renal system
Blood
Secondary
Central nervous system
Cardiovascular system
Respiratory system
Gastrointestinal system
Hepatic system
Metabolism

LIFE THREAT

Hemolysis and methemoglobinemia causing chlorate catalyzed hypoperfusion and CNS depression. Renal failure, usually 2 to 14 days after exposure.

SIGNS AND SYMPTOMS BY SYSTEM

Cardiovascular: Tachycardia. Myocardial injury.
Respiratory: Irritation of the respiratory tract, tachypnea, and dyspnea.
CNS: Restlessness followed by apathy. Seizures are rare, usually in the later stages of renal failure or from hypoxia. Coma.
Gastrointestinal: Nausea, vomiting, irritation of the GI tract, hemorrhage, diarrhea, and abdominal pain.
Eye: Chemical conjunctivitis.
Skin: Cyanosis, pallor, and dermatitis.
Renal: Hemoglobinuria, proteinuria, kidney damage, and renal failure.
Hepatic: Liver damage.
Metabolism: Hyperkalemia.
Blood: Hemolysis. Methemoglobinemia and decreased platelet count (thrombocytopenia) are prominent features but may not be apparent until several hours after exposure.

Other: Lumbar pain.

SYMPTOM ONSET FOR ACUTE EXPOSURE

Immediate
Some symptoms possibly delayed

CO-EXPOSURE CONCERNS

Bromates
Arsine

THERMAL DECOMPOSITION PRODUCTS INCLUDE

Chlorine dioxide
Hydrogen chloride
Oxygen
Sodium perchlorate

MEDICAL CONDITIONS POSSIBLY AGGRAVATED BY EXPOSURE

Respiratory system disorders
Kidney disorders

DECONTAMINATION

- Wear positive-pressure SCBA and protective equipment specified by references such as the *North American Emergency Response Guidebook*. If special chemical protective clothing is required, consult the chemical manufacturer or specific protective clothing compatibility charts. A qualified, experienced person should make decisions regarding the type of personal protective equipment necessary.
- Delay entry until trained personnel and proper protective equipment are available.
- Remove patient from contaminated area.
- Quickly remove and isolate patient's clothing, jewelry, and shoes.
- Gently brush away dry particles and blot excess liquids with absorbent material.
- Rinse patient with warm water, 32° C to 35° C (90° F to 95° F), if possible.
- Wash patient with a mild liquid soap and large quantities of water.
- Refer to decontamination protocol in Section Three.

IMMEDIATE FIRST AID

- Ensure that adequate decontamination has been carried out.
- If patient is not breathing, start artificial respiration, preferably with a demand-valve resuscitator, bag-valve-mask device, or pocket mask, as trained. Perform CPR if necessary.
- Immediately flush contaminated eyes with gently flowing water.
- Do not induce vomiting. If vomiting occurs, lean patient forward or place on left side (head-down position, if possible) to maintain an open airway and prevent aspiration.
- Keep patient quiet and maintain normal body temperature.
- Obtain medical attention.

BASIC TREATMENT

- Establish a patent airway (oropharyngeal or nasopharyngeal airway, if needed). Suction if necessary.
- Watch for signs of respiratory insufficiency and assist ventilations if necessary.
- Administer oxygen by nonrebreather mask at 10 to 15 L/min.
- Anticipate seizures and treat if necessary (refer to seizure protocol in Section Three).

- For eye contamination, flush eyes immediately with water. Irrigate each eye continuously with 0.9% saline (NS) during transport (refer to eye irrigation protocol in Section Three).
- Do not use emetics. For ingestion, rinse mouth and administer 5 ml/kg up to 200 ml of water for dilution if the patient can swallow, has a strong gag reflex, and does not drool (refer to ingestion protocol in Section Three).

ADVANCED TREATMENT

- Consider orotracheal or nasotracheal intubation for airway control in the patient who is unconscious or is in severe respiratory distress.
- Start IV administration of D_5W TKO. Use 0.9% saline (NS) or lactated Ringer's (LR) if signs of hypovolemia are present. For hypotension with signs of hypovolemia, administer fluids cautiously. Watch for signs of fluid overload. (refer to shock protocol in Section Three).
- Treat seizures with diazepam (Valium) or lorazepam (Ativan) (refer to diazepam and lorazepam protocols in Section Four and seizure protocol in Section Three).
- Use proparacaine hydrochloride to assist eye irrigation (refer to proparacaine hydrochloride protocol in Section Four).

INITIAL EMERGENCY DEPARTMENT CONSIDERATIONS

- Useful initial laboratory studies include complete blood count, platelet count, coagulation profile, methemoglobin, serum electrolytes, blood urea nitrogen (BUN), creatinine, glucose, urinalysis, and baseline biochemical profile, including serum aminotransferases (ALT and AST), calcium, phosphorus, and magnesium. Determination of anion and osmolar gaps may be helpful. Arterial blood gases (ABGs), chest radiograph, and electrocardiogram may be required.
- Positive end-expiratory pressure (PEEP)–assisted ventilation may be necessary in patients with acute parenchymal injury who develop pulmonary edema or acute respiratory distress syndrome.
- Products may cause acidosis; hyperventilation and sodium bicarbonate may be beneficial. Bicarbonate therapy should be guided by patient presentation, ABG determination, and serum electrolyte considerations.
- Sodium thiosulfate may reduce chlorate to chloride ion, which may be less toxic. ADULT DOSAGE: 10 to 50 ml (0.2 to 1 ml/kg; maximum 50 ml) of 10% sodium thiosulfate solution, slow IV over 30 minutes. Rapid administration may cause hypotension.
- Hemodialysis may be required for renal failure. Therapy should be guided by patient presentation and laboratory values.
- Titrate hydration status to maintain adequate urine output.
- Obtain toxicological consultation as necessary.

SPECIAL CONSIDERATIONS

- Methylene blue has little or no effect on this form of methemoglobinemia and may intensify the chlorate catalyzed oxidative hemolysis; therefore it should not be used.
- Exchange transfusion has been advocated for severe poisoning.
- Pulse oximetry readings may not be accurate in these exposures.

98

Chlorine and Related Compounds

SUBSTANCE IDENTIFICATION

Found in liquid and gaseous forms. Colorless to amber-colored liquid and greenish-yellow gas with a characteristic odor. Some solid compounds may generate chlorine when in contact with water. Used in the production of chlorinated inorganic and organic chemicals and in the manufacture of solvents, automotive compounds, and plastics. Also used in metallurgy and disinfectants and as a bacteriostat in water treatment and a bleaching/cleaning agent. Some are used as fumigants, rodenticides, and insecticides.

ROUTES OF EXPOSURE

Skin and eye contact
Inhalation
Ingestion

TARGET ORGANS

Primary
Skin
Eyes
Respiratory system
Secondary
Central nervous system
Cardiovascular system
Gastrointestinal system
Renal system
Hepatic system
Metabolism

LIFE THREAT

Severe respiratory tract irritant that may cause pulmonary edema. Skin, eye, and mucous membrane irritant.

SIGNS AND SYMPTOMS BY SYSTEM

Cardiovascular: Cardiovascular collapse and possible ventricular arrhythmias.

Respiratory: Acute or delayed noncardiogenic pulmonary edema, dyspnea, and tachypnea. Upper airway irritation and burns to the mucous membranes and lungs. Cough, choking sensation, rhinitis, sinusitis, rhinorrhea, pneumonitis, and pneumonia.

CNS: Decreased level of consciousness to coma. Headache and dizziness.

Gastrointestinal: Nausea and vomiting.

Eye: Chemical conjunctivitis with lacrimation. Severe and painful irritation and burns.

Skin: Irritation and chemical burns. Cyanosis. Possible frostbite secondary to exposure to expanding gas.

Renal: Kidney damage.
Hepatic: Liver damage.
Other: Metabolic acidosis.

SYMPTOM ONSET FOR ACUTE EXPOSURE

Immediate
Respiratory symptoms may be delayed for hours

CO-EXPOSURE CONCERNS

Caustics/corrosives
Phosgene
Other respiratory irritants

THERMAL DECOMPOSITION PRODUCTS INCLUDE

Reacts with water to form hydrochloric and hypochlorous acid
Reacts with carbon monoxide to form phosgene
Toxic substances are formed when combustibles burn in chlorine

MEDICAL CONDITIONS POSSIBLY AGGRAVATED BY EXPOSURE

Respiratory disorders
Chronic skin disorders

DECONTAMINATION

- Wear positive-pressure SCBA and protective equipment specified by references such as the *North American Emergency Response Guidebook*. If special chemical protective clothing is required, consult the chemical manufacturer or specific protective clothing compatibility charts. A qualified, experienced person should make decisions regarding the type of personal protective equipment necessary.
- Delay entry until trained personnel and proper protective equipment are available.
- Remove patient from contaminated area.
- Quickly remove and isolate patient's clothing, jewelry, and shoes.
- Gently brush away dry particles and blot excess liquids with absorbent material.
- Rinse patient with warm water, 32° C to 35° C (90° F to 95° F), if possible.
- Wash patient with a mild liquid soap and large quantities of water.
- Refer to decontamination protocol in Section Three.

IMMEDIATE FIRST AID

- Ensure that adequate decontamination has been carried out.
- If patient is not breathing, start artificial respiration, preferably with a demand-valve resuscitator, bag-valve-mask device, or pocket mask, as trained. Perform CPR if necessary.
- Immediately flush contaminated eyes with gently flowing water.
- Do not induce vomiting. If vomiting occurs, lean patient forward or place on left side (head-down position, if possible) to maintain an open airway and prevent aspiration.
- Keep patient quiet and maintain normal body temperature.
- Obtain medical attention.

BASIC TREATMENT

- Establish a patent airway (oropharyngeal or nasopharyngeal airway, if needed). Suction if necessary.
- Watch for signs of respiratory insufficiency and assist ventilations if necessary.
- Administer oxygen by nonrebreather mask at 10 to 15 L/min.

- Monitor for pulmonary edema and treat if necessary (refer to pulmonary edema protocol in Section Three).
- Monitor for shock and treat if necessary (refer to shock protocol in Section Three).
- For eye contamination, flush eyes immediately with water. Irrigate each eye continuously with 0.9% saline (NS) during transport (refer to eye irrigation protocol in Section Three).
- Do not use emetics. For ingestion, rinse mouth and administer 5 ml/kg up to 200 ml of water for dilution if the patient can swallow, has a strong gag reflex, and does not drool (refer to ingestion protocol in Section Three).
- Cover skin burns with dry sterile dressings after decontamination (refer to chemical burn protocol in Section Three).

ADVANCED TREATMENT

- Consider orotracheal or nasotracheal intubation for airway control in the patient who is unconscious, has severe pulmonary edema, or is in severe respiratory distress.
- Positive-pressure ventilation techniques with a bag-valve-mask device may be beneficial.
- Consider drug therapy for pulmonary edema (refer to pulmonary edema protocol in Section Three).
- Monitor cardiac rhythm and treat arrhythmias if necessary (refer to cardiac protocol in Section Three).
- Start IV administration of D_5W TKO. Use 0.9% saline (NS) or lactated Ringer's (LR) if signs of hypovolemia are present. For hypotension with signs of hypovolemia, administer fluid cautiously. Consider vasopressors if patient is hypotensive with normal fluid volume. Watch for signs of fluid overload (refer to shock protocol in Section Three).
- Use proparacaine hydrochloride to assist eye irrigation (refer to proparacaine hydrochloride protocol in Section Four).

INITIAL EMERGENCY DEPARTMENT CONSIDERATIONS

- Useful initial laboratory studies include complete blood count, serum electrolytes, blood urea nitrogen (BUN), creatinine, glucose, urinalysis, and baseline biochemical profile, including serum aminotransferases (AST and ALT), calcium, phosphorus, and magnesium. Determination of anion and osmolar gaps may be helpful. Arterial blood gases (ABGs), chest radiograph, and electrocardiogram may be required.
- Positive end-expiratory pressure (PEEP)–assisted ventilation may be necessary in patients with acute parenchymal injury who develop pulmonary edema or acute respiratory distress syndrome.
- Products may cause acidosis; hyperventilation and sodium bicarbonate may be beneficial. Bicarbonate therapy should be guided by patient presentation, ABG determination, and serum electrolyte considerations.
- Obtain toxicological consultation as necessary.

SPECIAL CONSIDERATIONS

- Chlorine's relatively high water solubility accounts for the early upper airway symptoms.
- Mixing chlorine and ammonia cleaners may result in the release of hydrochloric acid, nitrogen oxides, and chlorine active compounds.

Fluorine and Related Compounds

SUBSTANCE IDENTIFICATION

Found in liquid, yellowish gas and in solid forms with various colors. Most have an irritating odor. Used in the manufacture of fluorinated organic and inorganic chemicals, pesticides, refrigerants, fertilizer, microelectronic circuits, and rocket fuel. Also used for etching, electroplating, and water treatment.

ROUTES OF EXPOSURE

Skin and eye contact
Inhalation
Ingestion
Skin absorption

TARGET ORGANS

Primary
Skin
Eyes
Respiratory system
Renal system
Metabolism
Secondary
Central nervous system
Cardiovascular system
Gastrointestinal system

LIFE THREAT

CNS depression and respiratory arrest. Cardiovascular collapse, shock, and arrhythmias may be found.

SIGNS AND SYMPTOMS BY SYSTEM

Cardiovascular: Cardiovascular collapse with a weak, rapid pulse and arrhythmias.

Respiratory: Shallow respirations and respiratory arrest caused by laryngospasm and CNS depression. Respiratory tract irritation, rhinitis, sinusitis, pneumonitis, pneumonia, and pulmonary edema.

CNS: CNS depression, coma, and seizures. Headache, dizziness, muscle weakness, and tremors. Hyperactive reflexes, painful muscle spasms, and carpopedal spasm.

Gastrointestinal: Nausea, vomiting, diarrhea, and abdominal pain.

Eye: Chemical conjunctivitis and corneal damage.

Skin: Local or generalized rash; deep, painful skin burns. Cyanotic, cold, and wet skin.

Renal: Kidney damage.

Metabolism: Systemic exposure may result in life-threatening reduction in serum calcium (hypocalcemia) and serum magnesium (hypomagnesemia) and increased serum potassium (hyperkalemia).

SYMPTOM ONSET FOR ACUTE EXPOSURE

Immediate

Some symptoms such as pulmonary edema may be delayed for hours

CO-EXPOSURE CONCERNS

Chlorine

Other halogens

THERMAL DECOMPOSITION PRODUCTS INCLUDE

Hydrogen fluoride

Nitrogen oxides

MEDICAL CONDITIONS POSSIBLY AGGRAVATED BY EXPOSURE

Cardiovascular disorders

Respiratory disorders

DECONTAMINATION

- Wear positive-pressure SCBA and protective equipment specified by references such as the *North American Emergency Response Guidebook.* If special chemical protective clothing is required, consult the chemical manufacturer or specific protective clothing compatibility charts. A qualified, experienced person should make decisions regarding the type of personal protective equipment necessary.
- Delay entry until trained personnel and proper protective equipment are available.
- Remove patient from contaminated area.
- Quickly remove and isolate patient's clothing, jewelry, and shoes.
- Gently brush away dry particles and blot excess liquids with absorbent material.
- Rinse patient with warm water, 32° C to 35° C (90° F to 95° F), if possible.
- Wash patient with a mild liquid soap and large quantities of water.
- Refer to decontamination protocol in Section Three.

IMMEDIATE FIRST AID

- Ensure that adequate decontamination has been carried out.
- If patient is not breathing, start artificial respiration, preferably with a demand-valve resuscitator, bag-valve-mask device, or pocket mask, as trained. Perform CPR if necessary.
- Immediately flush contaminated eyes with gently flowing water.
- Do not induce vomiting. If vomiting occurs, lean patient forward or place on left side (head-down position, if possible) to maintain an open airway and prevent aspiration.
- Keep patient quiet and maintain normal body temperature.
- Obtain medical attention.

BASIC TREATMENT

- Establish a patent airway (oropharyngeal or nasopharyngeal airway, if needed). Suction if necessary.
- Watch for signs of respiratory insufficiency and assist ventilations if necessary.
- Administer oxygen by nonrebreather mask at 10 to 15 L/min.
- Monitor for pulmonary edema and treat if necessary (refer to pulmonary edema protocol in Section Three).
- Monitor for shock and treat if necessary (refer to shock protocol in Section Three).
- Anticipate seizures and treat if necessary (refer to seizure protocol in Section Three).

- For eye contamination, flush eyes immediately with water. Irrigate each eye continuously with 0.9% saline (NS) during transport (refer to eye irrigation protocol in Section Three).
- Do not use emetics. For ingestion, rinse mouth and administer 5 ml/kg up to 200 ml of water for dilution if the patent can swallow, has a strong gag reflex, and does not drool (refer to ingestion protocol in Section Three).
- Cover skin burns with dry sterile dressings after decontamination (refer to chemical burn protocol in Section Three).

ADVANCED TREATMENT

- Consider orotracheal or nasotracheal intubation for airway control in the patient who is unconscious, has severe pulmonary edema, or is in severe respiratory distress.
- Positive-pressure ventilation techniques with a bag-valve-mask device may be beneficial.
- Consider drug therapy for pulmonary edema (refer to pulmonary edema protocol in Section Three).
- Monitor cardiac rhythm and treat arrhythmias if necessary (refer to cardiac protocol in Section Three).
- Start IV administration of D_5W. Use 0.9% saline (NS) or lactated Ringer's (LR) if signs of hypovolemia are present. For hypotension with signs of hypovolemia, administer fluid cautiously. Consider vasopressors if patient is hypotensive with a normal fluid volume. Watch for signs of fluid overload (refer to shock protocol in Section Three).
- Treat seizures with diazepam (Valium) or lorazepam (Ativan) (refer to diazepam and lorazepam protocols in Section Four and seizure protocol in Section Three).
- Use proparacaine hydrochloride to assist eye irrigation (refer to proparacaine hydrochloride protocol in Section Four).

INITIAL EMERGENCY DEPARTMENT CONSIDERATIONS

- Useful initial laboratory studies include complete blood count, serum electrolytes, blood urea nitrogen (BUN), creatinine, glucose, urinalysis, and baseline biochemical profile, including serum aminotransferases (ALT and AST), calcium, phosphorus, and magnesium. Determination of anion and osmolar gaps may be helpful. Arterial blood gases (ABGs), chest radiograph, and electrocardiogram may be required.
- Positive end-expiratory pressure (PEEP)–assisted ventilation may be necessary in patients with acute parenchymal injury who develop pulmonary edema or acute respiratory distress syndrome.
- IV calcium gluconate may be needed for severe systemic hypocalcemia. Therapy should be guided by patient presentation and laboratory values. See calcium gluconate protocol in Section Four.
- Massive hypocalcemia/hypomagnesemia from concentrated HF exposure demonstrates high morbidity/mortality. Rapid, aggressive treatment is required, with close monitoring of electrocardiogram, serum electrolytes, calcium, and magnesium.
- Monitor and treat if necessary for hyperkalemia.
- Obtain toxicological consultation as necessary.

SPECIAL CONSIDERATIONS

- See hydrogen fluoride (Guideline 16).

100

Iodine and Related Compounds

SUBSTANCE IDENTIFICATION

Powders, purple crystalline solids, or colorless liquids that may darken on exposure to light. Used in the separation of mixtures of minerals; in the manufacture of germicides, antiseptics, pharmaceuticals, and medical imaging contrast media; and in water treatment, laboratory tests, and the photographic industry.

ROUTES OF EXPOSURE

Skin and eye contact
Inhalation
Ingestion
Skin absorption

TARGET ORGANS

Primary
Skin
Eyes
Respiratory system
Gastrointestinal system
Secondary
Central nervous system
Cardiovascular system
Hepatic system
Renal system
Metabolism

LIFE THREAT

Hypotension, circulatory collapse, and pulmonary edema.

SIGNS AND SYMPTOMS BY SYSTEM

Cardiovascular: Cardiovascular collapse. Weak, rapid pulse and arrhythmias.
Respiratory: Respiratory tract irritation, rhinitis, bronchitis, pneumonitis, pneumonia, and pulmonary edema.
CNS: Headache, delirium, dizziness, decreased consciousness, and coma.
Gastrointestinal: Severe corrosive gastroenteritis and parotid gland inflammation (parotitis). Nausea, vomiting, diarrhea, and abdominal pain. A metallic taste in the mouth.
Eye: Pain, chemical conjunctivitis, blepharitis, burns, and corneal damage.
Skin: Erythema, irritant dermatitis, burns, and/or hypersensitivity reaction.
Renal: Kidney damage.
Hepatic: Liver damage.
Metabolism: Metabolism acidosis.
Other: Severe allergic reactions have been reported.

SYMPTOM ONSET FOR ACUTE EXPOSURE
Immediate
Some symptoms may be delayed for hours
CO-EXPOSURE CONCERNS
Other halogens and halogenated compounds
THERMAL DECOMPOSITION PRODUCTS INCLUDE
Carbon dioxide
Carbon monoxide
Iodine
Iodine compounds
MEDICAL CONDITIONS POSSIBLY AGGRAVATED BY EXPOSURE
Thyroid disorders
Respiratory disorders
Kidney disorders
Skin disorders
DECONTAMINATION
- Wear positive-pressure SCBA and protective equipment specified by references such as the *North American Emergency Response Guidebook.* If special chemical protective clothing is required, consult the chemical manufacturer or specific protective clothing compatibility charts. A qualified, experienced person should make decisions regarding the type of personal protective equipment necessary.
- Delay entry until trained personnel and proper protective equipment are available.
- Remove patient from contaminated area.
- Quickly remove and isolate patient's clothing, jewelry, and shoes.
- Gently brush away dry particles and blot excess liquids with absorbent material.
- Rinse patient with warm water, 32° C to 35° C (90° F to 95° F), if possible.
- Wash patient with a mild liquid soap and large quantities of water.
- Refer to decontamination protocol in Section Three.
IMMEDIATE FIRST AID
- Ensure that adequate decontamination has been carried out.
- If patient is not breathing, start artificial respiration, preferably with a demand-valve resuscitator, bag-valve-mask device, or pocket mask, as trained. Perform CPR if necessary.
- Immediately flush contaminated eyes with gently flowing water.
- Do not induce vomiting. If vomiting occurs, lean patient forward or place on left side (head-down position, if possible) to maintain an open airway and prevent aspiration.
- Keep patient quiet and maintain normal body temperature.
- Obtain medical attention.
- **BASIC TREATMENT**
- Establish a patent airway (oropharyngeal or nasopharyngeal airway, if needed). Suction if necessary.
- Watch for signs of respiratory insufficiency and assist ventilations if necessary.
- Administer oxygen by nonrebreather mask at 10 to 15 L/min.
- Monitor for pulmonary edema and treat if necessary (refer to pulmonary edema protocol in Section Three).
- Monitor for shock and treat if necessary (refer to shock protocol in Section Three).

- For eye contamination, flush eyes immediately with water. Irrigate each eye continuously with 0.9% saline (NS) during transport (refer to eye irrigation protocol in Section Three).
- Do not use emetics. For ingestion, rinse mouth and administer 5 ml/kg up to 200 ml of water for dilution if the patent can swallow, has a strong gag reflex, and does not drool. Administer activated charcoal (refer to ingestion protocol in Section Three and activated charcoal protocol in Section Four).
- Cover skin burns with dry sterile dressings after decontamination (refer to chemical burn protocol in Section Three).

ADVANCED TREATMENT

- Consider orotracheal or nasotracheal intubation for airway control in the patient who is unconscious, has severe pulmonary edema, or is in severe respiratory distress.
- Positive-pressure ventilation techniques with a bag-valve-mask device may be beneficial.
- Consider drug therapy for pulmonary edema (refer to pulmonary edema protocol in Section Three).
- Monitor cardiac rhythm and treat arrhythmias if necessary (refer to cardiac protocol in Section Three).
- Start IV administration of D_5W. Use 0.9% saline (NS) or lactated Ringer's (LR) if signs of hypovolemia are present. For hypotension with signs of hypovolemia, administer fluids cautiously. Consider vasopressors if patient is hypotensive with a normal fluid volume. Watch for signs of fluid overload (refer to shock protocol in Section Three)
- Use proparacaine hydrochloride to assist eye irrigation (refer to proparacaine hydrochloride protocol in Section Four).

INITIAL EMERGENCY DEPARTMENT CONSIDERATIONS

- Useful initial laboratory studies include complete blood count, serum electrolytes, blood urea nitrogen (BUN), creatinine, glucose, urinalysis, and baseline biochemical profile, including serum aminotransferases (ALT and AST), calcium, phosphorus, and magnesium. Determination of anion and osmolar gaps may be helpful. Arterial blood gases (ABGs), chest radiograph, and electrocardiogram may be required.
- Positive end-expiratory pressure (PEEP)–assisted ventilation may be necessary in patients with acute parenchymal injury who develop pulmonary edema or acute respiratory distress syndrome.
- Products may cause acidosis; hyperventilation and sodium bicarbonate may be beneficial. Bicarbonate therapy should be guided by patient presentation, ABG determination, and serum electrolyte considerations.
- Obtain toxicological consultation if necessary.

Phosgene and Related Compounds

SUBSTANCE IDENTIFICATION

Found as a colorless liquid or gas with a low water solubility. At low air concentrations, compounds have a sweet odor, like hay. A sharp, pungent odor is present at higher concentrations. Can be liberated from the combustion of chlorinated hydrocarbons. Used in the manufacture of insecticides, plastics, dyes, and pharmaceuticals and in metallurgy. Prepared for military use as a choking agent known as CG.

ROUTES OF EXPOSURE

Skin and eye contact
Inhalation
Ingestion
Skin absorption

TARGET ORGANS

Primary
Skin
Eyes
Respiratory system
Secondary
Central nervous system
Cardiovascular system
Gastrointestinal system

LIFE THREAT

Severe respiratory irritant that can cause damage to the alveoli and resultant pulmonary edema. Phosgene has been used as a chemical warfare agent gas and is extremely toxic.

SIGNS AND SYMPTOMS BY SYSTEM

Cardiovascular: Cardiovascular collapse, hypovolemia, shock, and arrhythmias.

Respiratory: Throat dryness, pharyngitis, with primarily lower respiratory tract mucous membrane irritation, including pneumonitis and pneumonia. Acute or delayed pulmonary edema, dyspnea, and tachypnea. Cough with thick, bloody, foamy sputum. Noncardiac chest pain. Pulmonary damage (bronchitis, emphysema, fibrosis) may be late sequela.

CNS: Headache, CNS depression to coma and seizures.

Gastrointestinal: Nausea, vomiting, and abdominal pain.

Eye: Chemical conjunctivitis, corneal damage, and burns. Lacrimation and spasm of the eyelids (blepharospasm).

Skin: Irritant dermatitis and chemical burns. Cyanosis.

Other: Ability to detect product by smell may be lost after a relatively brief exposure time (olfactory nerve fatigue).

SYMPTOM ONSET FOR ACUTE EXPOSURE

Immediate

Some symptoms, especially pulmonary edema, may be delayed 2 to 24 hours

CO-EXPOSURE CONCERNS

Chlorine active compounds

Corrosive vapors

THERMAL DECOMPOSITION PRODUCTS INCLUDE

Carbon monoxide

Chloride

Hydrochloric acid if moisture or steam is present

MEDICAL CONDITIONS POSSIBLY AGGRAVATED BY EXPOSURE

Respiratory system disorders

DECONTAMINATION

- Wear positive-pressure SCBA and protective equipment specified by references such as the *North American Emergency Response Guidebook*. If special chemical protective clothing is required, consult the chemical manufacturer or specific protective clothing compatibility charts. A qualified, experienced person should make decisions regarding the type of personal protective equipment necessary.
- Delay entry until trained personnel and proper protective equipment are available.
- Remove patient from contaminated area.
- Quickly remove and isolate patient's clothing, jewelry, and shoes.
- Gently blot excess liquids with absorbent material.
- Rinse patient with warm water, 32° C to 35° C (90° F to 95° F), if possible.
- Wash patient with a mild liquid soap and large quantities of water.
- Refer to decontamination protocol in Section Three.

IMMEDIATE FIRST AID

- Ensure that adequate decontamination has been carried out.
- If patient is not breathing, start artificial respiration, preferably with a demand-valve resuscitator, bag-valve-mask device, or pocket mask, as trained. Perform CPR if necessary.
- Immediately flush contaminated eyes with gently flowing water.
- Do not induce vomiting. If vomiting occurs, lean patient forward or place on left side (head-down position, if possible) to maintain an open airway and prevent aspiration.
- Keep patient quiet and maintain normal body temperature.
- Obtain medical attention.

BASIC TREATMENT

- Establish a patent airway (oropharyngeal or nasopharyngeal airway, if needed). Suction if necessary.
- Watch for signs of respiratory insufficiency and assist ventilations if necessary.
- Administer oxygen by nonrebreather mask at 10 to 15 L/min.
- Monitor for pulmonary edema and treat if necessary (refer to pulmonary edema protocol in Section Three).
- Anticipate seizures and treat if necessary (refer to seizure protocol in Section Three).

- For eye contamination, flush eyes immediately with water. Irrigate each eye continuously with 0.9% saline (NS) during transport (refer to eye irrigation protocol in Section Three).
- Do not use emetics. For ingestion, rinse mouth and administer 5 ml/kg up to 200 ml of water for dilution if the patient can swallow, has a strong gag reflex, and does not drool (refer to ingestion protocol in Section Three).
- Cover skin burns with dry sterile dressings after decontamination (refer to chemical burn protocol in Section Three).

ADVANCED TREATMENT

- Consider orotracheal or nasotracheal intubation for airway control in the patient who is unconscious, has severe pulmonary edema, or is in severe respiratory distress.
- Positive-pressure ventilation techniques with a bag-valve-mask device may be beneficial.
- Consider drug therapy for pulmonary edema (refer to pulmonary edema protocol in Section Three).
- Monitor cardiac rhythm and treat arrhythmias if necessary (refer to cardiac protocol in Section Three).
- Start IV administration of D_5W TKO. Use 0.9% saline (NS) or lactated Ringer's (LR) if signs of hypovolemia are present. For hypotension with signs of hypovolemia, administer fluid cautiously. Watch for signs of fluid overload (refer to shock protocol in Section Three).
- Treat seizures with diazepam (Valium) or lorazepam (Ativan) (refer to diazepam and lorazepam protocols in Section Four and seizure protocol in Section Three).
- Use proparacaine hydrochloride to assist eye irrigation (refer to proparacaine hydrochloride protocol in Section Four).

INITIAL EMERGENCY DEPARTMENT CONSIDERATIONS

- Useful initial laboratory studies include complete blood count, serum electrolytes, blood urea nitrogen (BUN), creatinine, glucose, urinalysis, and baseline biochemical profile, including serum aminotransferases (ALT and AST), calcium, phosphorus, and magnesium. Determination of anion and osmolar gaps may be helpful. Arterial blood gases (ABGs) and electrocardiogram may be required.
- Obtain serial chest radiographs and monitor ABGs and respiratory function.
- Positive end-expiratory pressure (PEEP)–assisted ventilation may be necessary in patients with acute parenchymal injury who develop pulmonary edema or acute respiratory distress syndrome.
- Obtain toxicological consultation as necessary.

SPECIAL CONSIDERATIONS

- Phosgene's poor water solubility limits its effects on the upper airway, allowing most of the product to penetrate into the lower airways. Phosgene reacts with moisture in the lower airways to form hydrochloric acid and carbon dioxide with resulting pulmonary edema. This is the mechanism for the delayed onset pulmonary edema.

Asbestos

SUBSTANCE IDENTIFICATION

Found as odorless, grayish-white, flexible fibers with a soft texture. Asbestos is a generic term used for a number of naturally occurring amphibole and serpentine hydrated magnesium silicates that are incombustible and can be separated into fibers. Types of fibers include actinolite, amosite (brown asbestos), anthophyllite, chrysotile (white asbestos), crocidolite (blue asbestos), and tremolite. All fibers belong to the amphibole group—long, straight fibers packed in parallel rows—with the exception of chrysolite, which is the only member of the serpentine group, with wavy fibers packed as intertwined bundles. The most widely used asbestos fiber in the United States was chrysolite [$Mg_6Si_4O_{10}(OH)_8$]. Asbestos has been used in noise and thermal insulation materials, cement products, floor-covering materials, friction products (brake linings), gaskets, and fireproof textiles. Asbestos fibers may be firmly bonded in the product or easily broken apart. The latter are considered to be friable and will generate more airborne fibers.

ROUTES OF EXPOSURE

Inhalation
Ingestion

TARGET ORGANS

Primary
Respiratory system
Gastrointestinal system

LIFE THREAT

Asbestosis/lung cancer/malignant mesothelioma

SIGNS AND SYMPTOMS BY SYSTEM

Cardiovascular: None.
Respiratory: Irritation of the nose and throat.
Gastrointestinal: No acute effects from ingestion.

SYMPTOM ONSET FOR ACUTE EXPOSURE

Delayed. Usual latency period 10 to 20 years for asbestosis. Malignancies may have longer latent periods.

CHRONIC EXPOSURE/CARCINOGENIC EFFECTS

Asbestosis
Pleural plaques
Pleural thickening
Benign pleural effusion
Lung cancer
Malignant mesothelioma
Possibly increased cancer risk of the larynx, GI tract, pancreas, and colon

CO-EXPOSURE CONCERNS

Smoking

Other agents capable of causing pneumoconiosis (e.g., barium, beryllium, coal dust, nitrogen oxides, talc)

MEDICAL CONDITIONS POSSIBLY AGGRAVATED BY EXPOSURE

Pulmonary disease
Coalworker's pneumoconiosis
Silo filler's disease (nitrogen oxides)

DECONTAMINATION

- Wear positive-pressure SCBA and protective equipment specified by references such as the *North American Emergency Response Guidebook.* If special chemical protective clothing is required, consult the chemical manufacturer or specific protective clothing compatibility charts. A qualified, experienced person should make decisions regarding the type of personal protective equipment necessary.
- Delay entry until trained personnel and proper protective equipment are available.
- Remove patient from contaminated area.
- Quickly remove and isolate patient's clothing, jewelry, and shoes.
- Gently brush away dry particles and blot excess liquids with absorbent material.
- Rinse patient with warm water, 32° C to 35° C (90° F to 95° F), if possible.
- Wash patient with a mild liquid soap and large quantities of water.
- Refer to decontamination protocol in Section Three.

IMMEDIATE FIRST AID

- Ensure that adequate decontamination has been carried out.
- Obtain medical attention.

BASIC TREATMENT

- Establish a patent airway (oropharyngeal or nasopharyngeal airway, if needed). Suction if necessary.
- Assist ventilations if necessary.
- Administer oxygen by nonrebreather mask at 10 to 15 L/min.
- Treat any associated injury and/or illness if necessary.

ADVANCED TREATMENT

- Treat any associated injury and/or illness if necessary.

INITIAL EMERGENCY DEPARTMENT CONSIDERATIONS

- Initial examination should include a chest radiograph and pulmonary function testing.
- Obtain toxicological consultation as necessary.

SPECIAL CONSIDERATIONS

- Risk of asbestos exposure should be considered in cases of building fires or explosions where encapsulated or previously unknown/undisturbed sources of asbestos insulation may be released. The risk of asbestos exposure is also increased at asbestos abatement projects where large quantities of removed product may be stored.
- Asbestos-related diseases have developed in family members of workers who inadvertently brought fibers home on contaminated clothing.
- Hazardous material personnel exposed to asbestos or at risk for asbestos exposure require ongoing medical monitoring programs.

103

Boron and Related Compounds

SUBSTANCE IDENTIFICATION

Boron compounds may be found as solids, liquids, or gases. For example, decaborane ($B_{10}H_{14}$) is a colorless, crystalline powder with a strong pungent odor; pentaborane (B_5H_9) is a colorless, volatile liquid; and boron hydride (B_2H_6, diborane) is a flammable, colorless gas that fumes in moist air with a sharp, irritating odor. Can be found as liquids at low temperatures or when stored under pressure. Used as solvents, in cleaning operations, in metal treatment, and in various manufacturing processes.

ROUTES OF EXPOSURE

Skin and eye contact
Inhalation
Ingestion
Skin absorption

TARGET ORGANS

Primary
Skin
Eyes
Central nervous system
Respiratory system
Renal system
Secondary
Cardiovascular system
Gastrointestinal system
Hepatic system

LIFE THREAT

Respiratory tract irritant that may cause laryngeal spasm, laryngeal edema, and pulmonary edema. May cause severe chemical burns.

SIGNS AND SYMPTOMS BY SYSTEM

Cardiovascular: Tachycardia and cardiovascular collapse.

Respiratory: Severe irritation of the respiratory system, coughing, and choking; causes pulmonary edema, laryngeal spasm. Upper airway obstruction.

CNS: CNS depression, coma, dizziness, muscle tremors, ataxia, seizures. Neurobehavioral changes.

Gastrointestinal: Nausea, vomiting, and abdominal pain.

Eye: Chemical conjunctivitis and severe burns, possibly causing permanent loss of vision.

Skin: Irritant dermatitis and severe chemical burns.

Renal: Kidney damage.

Hepatic: Liver damage.

SYMPTOM ONSET FOR ACUTE EXPOSURE

Immediate

Some symptoms may be delayed

CO-EXPOSURE CONCERNS

Corrosives

Other boron compounds

THERMAL DECOMPOSITION PRODUCTS INCLUDE

Ammonia

Hydrochloric acid

Nitrogen oxides

Oxides

MEDICAL CONDITIONS POSSIBLY AGGRAVATED BY EXPOSURE

Respiratory system disorders

Skin disorders

DECONTAMINATION

- Wear positive-pressure SCBA and protective equipment specified by references such as the *North American Emergency Response Guidebook*. If special chemical protective clothing is required, consult the chemical manufacturer or specific protective clothing compatibility charts. A qualified, experienced person should make decisions regarding the type of personal protective equipment necessary.
- Delay entry until trained personnel and proper protective equipment are available.
- Remove patient from contaminated area.
- Quickly remove and isolate patient's clothing, jewelry, and shoes.
- Gently brush away dry particles and blot excess liquids with absorbent material.
- Rinse patient with warm water, 32° C to 35° C (90° F to 95° F), if possible.
- Wash patient with a mild liquid soap and large quantities of water.
- Refer to decontamination protocol in Section Three.

IMMEDIATE FIRST AID

- Ensure that adequate decontamination has been carried out.
- If patient is not breathing, start artificial respiration, preferably with a demand-valve resuscitator, bag-valve-mask device, or pocket mask, as trained. Perform CPR if necessary.
- Immediately flush contaminated eyes with gently flowing water.
- Do not induce vomiting. If vomiting occurs, lean patient forward or place on left side (head-down position, if possible) to maintain an open airway and prevent aspiration.
- Keep patient quiet and maintain normal body temperature.
- Obtain medical attention.

BASIC TREATMENT

- Establish a patent airway (oropharyngeal or nasopharyngeal airway, if needed). Suction if necessary.
- Aggressive airway management may be necessary.
- Watch for signs of respiratory insufficiency and assist ventilations if necessary.
- Administer oxygen by nonrebreather mask at 10 to 15 L/min.
- Monitor for pulmonary edema and treat if necessary (refer to pulmonary edema protocol in Section Three).
- Monitor for shock and treat if necessary (refer to shock protocol in Section Three).

- For eye contamination, flush eyes immediately with water. Irrigate each eye continuously with 0.9% saline (NS) during transport (refer to eye irrigation protocol in Section Three).
- Do not use emetics. For ingestion, rinse mouth and administer 5 ml/kg up to 200 ml of water for dilution if the patient can swallow, has a strong gag reflex, and does not drool. Administer activated charcoal (refer to ingestion protocol in Section Three and activated charcoal protocol in Section Four).
- Cover skin burns with dry sterile dressings after decontamination (refer to chemical burn protocol in Section Three).

ADVANCED TREATMENT

- Consider orotracheal or nasotracheal intubation for airway control in the patient who is unconscious, has severe pulmonary edema, or is in severe respiratory distress. Early intubation at the first sign of upper airway obstruction may be necessary.
- Positive-pressure ventilation techniques with a bag-valve-mask device may be beneficial.
- Consider drug therapy for pulmonary edema (refer to pulmonary edema protocol in Section Three).
- Monitor cardiac rhythm and treat arrhythmias if necessary (refer to cardiac protocol in Section Three).
- Start IV administration of D_5W TKO. Use 0.9% saline (NS) or lactated Ringer's (LR) if signs of hypovolemia are present. For hypotension with signs of hypovolemia, administer fluid cautiously. Consider vasopressors if patient is hypotensive with a normal fluid volume. Watch for signs of fluid overload (refer to shock protocol in Section Three).
- Use proparacaine hydrochloride to assist eye irrigation (refer to proparacaine hydrochloride protocol in Section Four).

INITIAL EMERGENCY DEPARTMENT CONSIDERATIONS

- Useful initial laboratory studies include complete blood count, serum electrolytes, blood urea nitrogen (BUN), creatinine, glucose, urinalysis, and baseline biochemical profile, including serum aminotransferases (ALT and AST), calcium, phosphorus, and magnesium. Determination of anion and osmolar gaps may be helpful. Arterial blood gases (ABGs), chest radiograph, and electrocardiogram may be required.
- Positive end-expiratory pressure (PEEP)–assisted ventilation may be necessary in patients with acute parenchymal injury who develop pulmonary edema or acute respiratory distress syndrome.
- Obtain toxicological consultation as necessary.

SPECIAL CONSIDERATIONS

- Some products may cause olfactory fatigue and therefore have poor warning properties.

Ozone (O_3) and Related Compounds

SUBSTANCE IDENTIFICATION

A colorless gas with a sharp odor. At very low temperatures, ozone is found as a dark blue liquid. Used for purifying air and water; as an oxidizing agent, disinfectant, and bleaching agent; and in the treatment of industrial wastes.

ROUTES OF EXPOSURE

Skin and eye contact
Inhalation

TARGET ORGANS

Primary
Skin
Eyes
Respiratory system
Secondary
Central nervous system
Cardiovascular system
Gastrointestinal system

LIFE THREAT

Pulmonary edema and airway obstruction

SIGNS AND SYMPTOMS BY SYSTEM

Cardiovascular: Cardiovascular collapse and hypotension.

Respiratory: Irritation of respiratory tract, coughing, choking, dyspnea, and in severe exposures, pulmonary edema. Chest pain or tightness of the chest may be present.

CNS: Headache, fatigue, dizziness, insomnia, inability to concentrate, and drowsiness.

Gastrointestinal: Gastroenteritis symptoms including nausea and vomiting.

Eye: Chemical conjunctivitis.

Skin: Dermatitis, burns with liquid product exposure. Expanding gases may cause frostbite.

Other: The ability to detect the product by smell may be lost shortly after exposure.

SYMPTOM ONSET FOR ACUTE EXPOSURE

Immediate

CO-EXPOSURE CONCERNS

Other airway irritants

MEDICAL CONDITIONS POSSIBLY AGGRAVATED BY EXPOSURE

Respiratory system disorders
Asthma/reactive airways disease disorders

DECONTAMINATION

- Wear positive-pressure SCBA and protective equipment specified by references such as the *North American Emergency Response Guidebook*. If special chemical protective clothing is required, consult the chemical manufacturer or specific protective clothing compatibility charts. A qualified, experienced person should make decisions regarding the type of personal protective equipment necessary.

- Delay entry until trained personnel and proper protective equipment are available.
- Remove patient from contaminated area.
- If concurrent liquid or solid exposure exists:
  Quickly remove and isolate patient's clothing, jewelry, and shoes.
  Gently brush away dry particles and blot excess liquids with absorbent material.
  Rinse patient with warm water, 32° C to 35° C (90° F to 95° F), if possible.
  Wash patient with a mild liquid soap and large quantities of water.
  Refer to decontamination protocol in Section Three.

IMMEDIATE FIRST AID

- Ensure that adequate decontamination has been carried out.
- If patient is not breathing, start artificial respiration, preferably with a demand-valve resuscitator, bag-valve-mask device, or pocket mask, as trained. Perform CPR if necessary.
- Immediately flush contaminated eyes with gently flowing water.
- Do not induce vomiting. If vomiting occurs, lean patient forward or place on left side (head-down position, if possible) to maintain an open airway and prevent aspiration.
- Keep patient quiet and maintain normal body temperature.
- Obtain medical attention.

BASIC TREATMENT

- Establish a patent airway (oropharyngeal or nasopharyngeal airway, if needed). Suction if necessary.
- Watch for signs of respiratory insufficiency and assist ventilations if necessary.
- Administer oxygen by nonrebreather mask at 10 to 15 L/min.
- Monitor for pulmonary edema and treat if necessary (refer to pulmonary edema protocol in Section Three).
- Monitor for shock and treat if necessary (refer to shock protocol in Section Three).
- For eye contamination, flush eyes immediately with water. Irrigate each eye continuously with 0.9% saline (NS) during transport (refer to eye irrigation protocol in Section Three).
- Use rapid rewarming techniques for frostbite (refer to frostbite protocol in Section Three).

ADVANCED TREATMENT

- Consider orotracheal or nasotracheal intubation for airway control in the patient who is unconscious, has severe pulmonary edema, or is in severe respiratory distress.
- Positive-pressure ventilation techniques with a bag-valve-mask device may be beneficial.
- Consider drug therapy for pulmonary edema (refer to pulmonary edema protocol in Section Three).
- Consider administering a beta agonist such as albuterol for severe bronchospasm (refer to albuterol protocol in Section Four).
- Monitor cardiac rhythm and treat arrhythmias if necessary (refer to cardiac protocol in Section Three).

- Start IV administration of D_5W TKO. Use 0.9% saline (NS) or lactated Ringer's (LR) if signs of hypovolemia are present. For hypotension with signs of hypovolemia, administer fluid cautiously. Consider vasopressors if patient is hypotensive with a normal fluid volume. Watch for signs of fluid overload (refer to shock protocol in Section Three).
- Use proparacaine hydrochloride to assist eye irrigation (refer to proparacaine hydrochloride protocol in Section Four).

INITIAL EMERGENCY DEPARTMENT CONSIDERATIONS

- Useful initial laboratory studies include complete blood count, serum electrolytes, blood urea nitrogen (BUN), creatinine, glucose, urinalysis, and baseline biochemical profile, including serum aminotransferases (ALT and AST), calcium, phosphorus, and magnesium. Determination of anion and osmolar gaps may be helpful. Arterial blood gases (ABGs), chest radiograph, and electrocardiogram may be required.
- Positive end-expiratory pressure (PEEP)–assisted ventilation may be necessary in patients with acute parenchymal injury who develop pulmonary edema or acute respiratory distress syndrome.
- Asthma/reactive airways disease symptoms may require inhaled bronchodilator therapy. Pulmonary function testing is recommended.
- Obtain toxicological consultation as necessary.

105

Sulfur and Related Compounds

SUBSTANCE IDENTIFICATION

Sulfur compounds are commonly found as odorless, brown to yellow solids or as a yellow dispersion. Used in the manufacture of insecticides, chemicals, gunpowder, plastics, dyes, rubber, matches, pharmaceuticals, sulfuric acid, enamels, and metal-glass cement and in wood pulp processes. Organic sulfur compounds such as methyl mercaptan are added as odorants to natural gas. Sulfur dioxide (SO_2) is a colorless gas with a sharp, irritating odor. It is commonly used as a disinfectant; for bleaching textile fibers; in wood pulp treatment; in ore and metal refining; and in the manufacture of preservatives, bleaches, and glues. A by-product of coal-burning power plants, sulfur dioxide contributes to air pollution. Sulfites are used as food preservatives and parenteral medication additives.

ROUTES OF EXPOSURE

Skin and eye contact
Inhalation
Ingestion

TARGET ORGANS

Primary
Skin
Eyes
Respiratory system
Secondary
Central nervous system
Cardiovascular system
Gastrointestinal system
Renal system
Metabolism

LIFE THREAT

Respiratory tract irritation leading to pulmonary edema. Anaphylaxis.

SIGNS AND SYMPTOMS BY SYSTEM

Cardiovascular: Tachycardia, hypotension, and cardiovascular collapse.

Respiratory: Respiratory tract irritation, rhinitis, sinusitis, pharyngitis, upper airway edema, coughing, bronchoconstriction, chest discomfort, and failure. Pulmonary edema. Exposure may cause asthma/reactive airways disease.

CNS: Headaches, vertigo, memory loss, decreased level of consciousness, seizures, and coma.

Gastrointestinal: Nausea, vomiting, and abdominal pain.

Eye: Irritation, lacrimation, and chemical burns.

Skin: Irritation and chemical burns. Frostbite may occur from exposure to liquefied product or expanding gas. Urticaria and allergic reactions with sulfites.

Renal: Kidney damage.
Metabolism: Acidosis and hyperkalemia.

SYMPTOM ONSET FOR ACUTE EXPOSURE

Immediate
Some symptoms (renal) may be delayed

CO-EXPOSURE CONCERNS

Other respiratory irritants

THERMAL DECOMPOSITION PRODUCTS INCLUDE

Carbon disulfide
Hydrogen sulfide
Sulfur dioxide

MEDICAL CONDITIONS POSSIBLY AGGRAVATED BY EXPOSURE

Respiratory system disorders
Cardiovascular disorders

DECONTAMINATION

- Wear positive-pressure SCBA and protective equipment specified by references such as the *North American Emergency Response Guidebook*. If special chemical protective clothing is required, consult the chemical manufacturer or specific protective clothing compatibility charts. A qualified, experienced person should make decisions regarding the type of personal protective equipment necessary.
- Delay entry until trained personnel and proper protective equipment are available.
- Remove patient from contaminated area.
- Quickly remove and isolate patient's clothing, jewelry, and shoes.
- Gently brush away dry particles and blot excess liquids with absorbent material.
- Rinse patient with warm water, 32° C to 35° C (90° F to 95° F), if possible.
- Wash patient with a mild liquid soap and large quantities of water.
- Refer to decontamination protocol in Section Three.

IMMEDIATE FIRST AID

- Ensure that adequate decontamination has been carried out.
- If patient is not breathing, start artificial respiration, preferably with a demand-valve resuscitator, bag-valve-mask device, or pocket mask, as trained. Perform CPR if necessary.
- Immediately flush contaminated eyes with gently flowing water.
- Do not induce vomiting. If vomiting occurs, lean patient forward or place on left side (head-down position, if possible) to maintain an open airway and prevent aspiration.
- Keep patient quiet and maintain normal body temperature.
- Obtain medical attention.

BASIC TREATMENT

- Establish a patent airway (oropharyngeal or nasopharyngeal airway, if needed). Suction if necessary.
- Watch for signs of respiratory insufficiency and assist ventilations if necessary.
- Administer oxygen by nonrebreather mask at 10 to 15 L/min.
- Monitor for pulmonary edema and treat if necessary (refer to pulmonary edema protocol in Section Three).
- Anticipate seizures and treat if necessary (refer to seizure protocol in Section Three).

- Monitor for shock and treat if necessary (refer to shock protocol in Section Three).
- For eye contamination, flush eyes immediately with water. Irrigate each eye continuously with 0.9% saline (NS) during transport (refer to eye irrigation protocol in Section Three).
- Do not use emetics. For ingestion, rinse mouth and administer 5 ml/kg up to 200 ml of water for dilution if the patient can swallow, has a strong gag reflex, and does not drool. Administer activated charcoal (refer to ingestion protocol in Section Three and activated charcoal protocol in Section Four).
- Cover skin burns with sterile dressings after decontamination (refer to chemical burn protocol in Section Three).

ADVANCED TREATMENT

- Consider orotracheal or nasotracheal intubation for airway control in the patient who is unconscious, has severe pulmonary edema, or is in severe respiratory distress. Early intubation at the first sign of upper airway obstruction may be necessary.
- Positive-pressure ventilation techniques with a bag-valve-mask device may be beneficial.
- Consider drug therapy for pulmonary edema (refer to pulmonary edema protocol in Section Three).
- Consider administering a beta agonist such as albuterol for severe bronchospasm (refer to albuterol protocol in Section Four).
- Monitor cardiac rhythm and treat arrhythmias if necessary (refer to cardiac protocol in Section Three).
- Start IV administration of D_5W TKO. Use 0.9% saline (NS) or lactated Ringer's (LR) if signs of hypovolemia are present. For hypotension with signs of hypovolemia, administer fluid cautiously. Consider vasopressors if patient is hypotensive with a normal fluid volume. Watch for signs of fluid overload (refer to shock protocol in Section Three)
- Treat seizures with diazepam (Valium) or lorazepam (Ativan) (refer to diazepam and lorazepam protocols in Section Four and seizure protocol in Section Three).
- Use proparacaine hydrochloride to assist eye irrigation (refer to proparacaine hydrochloride protocol in Section Four).

INITIAL EMERGENCY DEPARTMENT CONSIDERATIONS

- Useful initial laboratory studies include complete blood count, serum electrolytes, blood urea nitrogen (BUN), creatinine, glucose, urinalysis, and baseline biochemical profile, including serum aminotransferases (ALT and AST), calcium, phosphorus, and magnesium. Determination of anion and osmolar gaps may be helpful. Arterial blood gases (ABGs), chest radiograph, and electrocardiogram may be required.
- Positive end-expiratory pressure (PEEP)–assisted ventilation may be necessary in patients with acute parenchymal injury who develop pulmonary edema or acute respiratory distress syndrome.
- Bronchodilator therapy may be indicated in cases of severe bronchospasm. Observe for signs of anaphylaxis.

- Products may cause acidosis; hyperventilation and sodium bicarbonate may be beneficial. Bicarbonate therapy should be guided by patient presentation, ABG determination, and serum electrolyte considerations.
- Obtain toxicological consultation as necessary.

SPECIAL CONSIDERATIONS

- Sulfite compounds may cause bronchospasm and/or allergic reactions in asthmatics. Individuals not known to be asthmatic or allergic to sulfites may develop anaphylaxis or anaphylactoid reactions as well.

106

Tri-Ortho-Cresyl Phosphate (TOCP) and Related Compounds

SUBSTANCE IDENTIFICATION

Found as a colorless, odorless liquid. Used as a flame retardant, a plasticizer in lacquers and varnishes, and a gasoline/hydraulic fluid additive. Tri-ortho-cresyl phosphate (TOCP) is an organophosphate compound that may cause a peripheral axonopathy without the acute symptoms of cholinergic poisoning (SLUDGE syndrome) that are commonly seen in cases of other organophosphate insecticide poisonings.

ROUTES OF EXPOSURE

Skin and eye contact
Inhalation
Ingestion
Skin absorption

TARGET ORGANS

Primary
Central nervous system

Secondary
Skin
Eyes
Gastrointestinal system

LIFE THREAT

A delayed neurotoxin that causes an ascending paralysis of the extremities

SIGNS AND SYMPTOMS BY SYSTEM

Cardiovascular: Acute symptoms unlikely.

Respiratory: Acute symptoms unlikely.

CNS: Delayed 3 to 30 days; sharp, cramping pain in the calves and sensory disturbances, including paresthesias of the lower extremities. There is an abrupt onset of flaccid paralysis of the extremities 10 to 14 days later. The paralysis can spread to the upper extremities. Upper extremity recovery may occur with a resultant, permanent lower-extremity paralysis with spasticity, hyperreflexia, hypertonicity, clonus, and slapping gait.

Gastrointestinal: Sudden onset of nausea, vomiting, diarrhea, and abdominal pain starting shortly after exposure. This lasts for approximately 48 hours and is followed by an asymptomatic, latent period of 8 to 35 days.

Eye: Conjunctivitis after latent period.

Skin: Excessive sweating with cold, cyanotic, and moist hands and feet.

Other: Symptoms are generally nonfatal, but may take years to recover from and may leave permanent damage.

SYMPTOM ONSET FOR ACUTE EXPOSURE

Delayed

CO-EXPOSURE CONCERNS

Carbamates

Organophosphates

THERMAL DECOMPOSITION PRODUCTS INCLUDE

Phosphorus fumes

MEDICAL CONDITIONS POSSIBLY AGGRAVATED BY EXPOSURE

Neurological disorders

DECONTAMINATION

- Wear positive-pressure SCBA and protective equipment specified by references such as the *North American Emergency Response Guidebook*. If special chemical protective clothing is required, consult the chemical manufacturer or specific protective clothing compatibility charts. A qualified, experienced person should make decisions regarding the type of personal protective equipment necessary.
- Delay entry until trained personnel and proper protective equipment are available.
- Remove patient from contaminated area.
- Quickly remove and isolate patient's clothing, jewelry, and shoes.
- Gently blot excess liquids with absorbent material.
- Rinse patient with warm water, 32° C to 35° C (90° F to 95° F), if possible.
- Wash patient with a mild liquid soap and large quantities of water.
- Refer to decontamination protocol in Section Three.

IMMEDIATE FIRST AID

- Ensure that adequate decontamination has been carried out.
- If patient is not breathing, start artificial respiration, preferably with a demand-valve resuscitator, bag-valve-mask device, or pocket mask, as trained. Perform CPR if necessary.
- Immediately flush contaminated eyes with gently flowing water
- Do not induce vomiting. If vomiting occurs, lean patient forward or place on left side (head-down position, if possible) to maintain an open airway and prevent aspiration.
- Keep patient quiet and maintain normal body temperature.
- Obtain medical attention.

BASIC TREATMENT

- Establish a patent airway (oropharyngeal or nasopharyngeal airway, if needed). Suction if necessary.
- Watch for signs of respiratory insufficiency and assist ventilations if necessary.
- Administer oxygen by nonrebreather mask at 10 to 15 L/min.
- For eye contamination, flush eyes immediately with water. Irrigate each eye continuously with 0.9% saline (NS) during transport (refer to eye irrigation protocol in Section Three).
- Do not use emetics. For ingestion, rinse mouth and administer 5 ml/kg up to 200 ml of water for dilution if the patient can swallow, has a strong gag reflex, and does not drool. Administer activated charcoal (refer to ingestion protocol in Section Three and activated charcoal protocol in Section Four).

ADVANCED TREATMENT

- Use proparacaine hydrochloride to assist eye irrigation (refer to proparacaine hydrochloride protocol in Section Four).

INITIAL EMERGENCY DEPARTMENT CONSIDERATIONS

- Careful history and baseline neurological examination should be done.
- Useful initial laboratory studies include complete blood count, serum electrolytes, blood urea nitrogen (BUN), creatinine, glucose, urinalysis, and baseline biochemical profile, including serum aminotransferases (ALT and AST), calcium, phosphorus, and magnesium. Obtain baseline plasma and red blood cell cholinesterase levels. Baseline chest radiograph and electrocardiogram may be required.
- Treatment is supportive.
- For additional information on organophosphate poisoning, see Guideline 49.
- Obtain toxicological consultation as necessary.

SPECIAL CONSIDERATIONS

- Since the only symptoms in the acute phase are GI in nature, treatment should be supportive and to ensure follow-up medical treatment.
- In 1930, during Prohibition, an epidemic known as "ginger jake paralysis" occurred in 15,000 to 20,000 individuals consuming Jamaica ginger extract contaminated with TOCP. Similar outbreaks have occurred with ingestion of similarly adulterated products.
- Tri-tolyl phosphate is made up of three isomers. Only the ortho isomer (TOCP) is responsible for the delayed neurotoxicity.

Silane, Chlorosilane, and Related Compounds

SUBSTANCE IDENTIFICATION

Silane (SiH_4) is found as a gas with an unpleasant odor. Silane is used in semiconductor manufacture for the deposition of thin dielectric films. It is spontaneously combustible (pyrophoric) in air or may accumulate and detonate. The toxicity of silane is limited to its irritant properties. Chlorosilanes (e.g., trichlorosilane [$SiCl_3H$]) and organochlorosilanes (e.g., methylchlorosilane [CH_3SiCl_3]) are found as clear to white fuming liquids with a sharp odor. They are used in chemical synthesis; in the production of silicon fluids, silicon resins, and amorphous silicon; and in semiconductor manufacture. Trichlorosilane is used to clean silicon wafer surfaces. Chlorosilanes or organochlorosilanes on contact with water form hydrochloric acid. There are limited human toxicity data on these compounds.

ROUTES OF EXPOSURE

Skin and eye contact
Inhalation
Ingestion
Skin absorption

TARGET ORGANS

Primary
Skin
Eyes
Respiratory system
Gastrointestinal system
Blood

Secondary
Central nervous system
Cardiovascular system
Renal system

LIFE THREAT

Respiratory tract irritation; pulmonary edema.

SIGNS AND SYMPTOMS BY SYSTEM

Cardiovascular: Tachycardia, hypotension, arrhythmias, and cardiovascular collapse.

Respiratory: Respiratory tract irritation, rhinitis, sinusitis, pharyngitis, coughing, dyspnea, and hypoxia. Pulmonary edema.

CNS: Headaches, dizziness, incoordination, decreased level of consciousness, seizures, and coma.

Gastrointestinal: Salivation, nausea, vomiting, diarrhea, and abdominal pain. GI tract irritation and mucosal burns.

Eye: Irritation, lacrimation, corneal damage, and chemical burns.
Skin: Irritant dermatitis and severe chemical burns.
Renal: Kidney damage.
Blood: Red blood cell destruction (hemolysis) may occur with exposure to tetrachlorosilane.

SYMPTOM ONSET FOR ACUTE EXPOSURE

Immediate
Some symptoms such as pulmonary edema may be delayed

CO-EXPOSURE CONCERNS

Other respiratory irritants

THERMAL DECOMPOSITION PRODUCTS INCLUDE

Carbon dioxide
Carbon monoxide
Hydrogen chloride
Silicon dioxide
Silicates
Silane exhibits almost complete combustion above 450° C

MEDICAL CONDITIONS POSSIBLY AGGRAVATED BY EXPOSURE

Respiratory system disorders

DECONTAMINATION

- Wear positive-pressure SCBA and protective equipment specified by references such as the *North American Emergency Response Guidebook*. If special chemical protective clothing is required, consult the chemical manufacturer or specific protective clothing compatibility charts. A qualified, experienced person should make decisions regarding the type of personal protective equipment necessary.
- Delay entry until trained personnel and proper protective equipment are available.
- Remove patient from contaminated area.
- Quickly remove and isolate patient's clothing, jewelry, and shoes.
- Gently brush away dry particles and blot excess liquids with absorbent material.
- Rinse patient with warm water, 32° C to 35° C (90° F to 95° F), if possible.
- Wash patient with a mild liquid soap and large quantities of water.
- Refer to decontamination protocol in Section Three.

IMMEDIATE FIRST AID

- Ensure that adequate decontamination has been carried out.
- If patient is not breathing, start artificial respiration, preferably with a demand-valve resuscitator, bag-valve-mask device, or pocket mask, as trained. Perform CPR if necessary.
- Immediately flush contaminated eyes with gently flowing water.
- Do not induce vomiting. If vomiting occurs, lean patient forward or place on left side (head-down position, if possible) to maintain an open airway and prevent aspiration.
- Keep patient quiet and maintain normal body temperature.
- Obtain medical attention.

BASIC TREATMENT

- Establish a patent airway (oropharyngeal or nasopharyngeal airway, if needed). Suction if necessary.
- Watch for signs of respiratory insufficiency and assist ventilations if necessary.

- Administer oxygen by nonrebreather mask at 10 to 15 L/min.
- Monitor for pulmonary edema and treat if necessary (refer to pulmonary edema protocol in Section Three).
- Anticipate seizures and treat if necessary (refer to seizure protocol in Section Three).
- Monitor for shock and treat if necessary (refer to shock protocol in Section Three).
- For eye contamination, flush eyes immediately with water. Irrigate each eye continuously with 0.9% saline (NS) during transport (refer to eye irrigation protocol in Section Three).
- Do not use emetics. For ingestion, rinse mouth and administer 5 ml/kg up to 200 ml of water for dilution if the patient can swallow, has a strong gag reflex, and does not drool. Administer activated charcoal (refer to ingestion protocol in Section Three and activated charcoal protocol in Section Four).
- Cover skin burns with sterile dressings after decontamination (refer to chemical burn protocol in Section Three).

ADVANCED TREATMENT

- Consider orotracheal or nasotracheal intubation for airway control in the patient who is unconscious, has severe pulmonary edema, or is in severe respiratory distress. Early intubation at the first sign of upper airway obstruction may be necessary.
- Positive-pressure ventilation techniques with a bag-valve-mask device may be beneficial.
- Consider drug therapy for pulmonary edema (refer to pulmonary edema protocol in Section Three).
- Monitor cardiac rhythm and treat arrhythmias if necessary (refer to cardiac protocol in Section Three).
- Start IV administration of D_5W TKO. Use 0.9% saline (NS) or lactated Ringer's (LR) if signs of hypovolemia are present. For hypotension with signs of hypovolemia, administer fluid cautiously. Consider vasopressors if patient is hypotensive with a normal fluid volume. Watch for signs of fluid overload (refer to shock protocol in Section Three)
- Treat seizures with diazepam (Valium) or lorazepam (Ativan) (refer to diazepam and lorazepam protocols in Section Four and seizure protocol in Section Three).
- Use proparacaine hydrochloride to assist eye irrigation (refer to proparacaine hydrochloride protocol in Section Four).

INITIAL EMERGENCY DEPARTMENT CONSIDERATIONS

- Useful initial laboratory studies include complete blood count, serum electrolytes, blood urea nitrogen (BUN), creatinine, glucose, urinalysis, and baseline biochemical profile, including serum aminotransferases (ALT and AST), calcium, phosphorus, and magnesium. Arterial blood gases (ABGs), chest radiograph, and electrocardiogram may be required.
- Positive end-expiratory pressure (PEEP)–assisted ventilation may be necessary in patients with acute parenchymal injury who develop pulmonary edema or acute respiratory distress syndrome.
- Endoscopy may be needed to assess extent of gastrointestinal damage.
- Obtain toxicological consultation if necessary.

SPECIAL CONSIDERATIONS

- Products may be mixed in a variety of hydrocarbon solvents (e.g., methanol or toluene). The solvent may contribute to the overall toxicity. Identify solvent vehicle and consult the appropriate guideline.

Phosphine and Related Compounds

SUBSTANCE IDENTIFICATION

A colorless gas with an odor of decaying fish. The reaction of hydrogen and various metal phosphides (e.g., aluminum, zinc, or gallium phosphide) forms phosphine gas (PH_3). Phosphides may also release phosphine gas on contact with water. Used in fumigation and as a doping agent in semiconductor manufacture, a polymerization inhibitor, and a chemical intermediate. Products may be toxic at air concentrations below the odor threshold of 1 to 2 ppm.

ROUTES OF EXPOSURE

Inhalation

TARGET ORGANS

Primary
Cardiovascular system
Respiratory system
Secondary
Central nervous system
Gastrointestinal system
Renal system
Hepatic system

LIFE THREAT

Severe pulmonary irritation leading to pulmonary edema.

SIGNS AND SYMPTOMS BY SYSTEM

Cardiovascular: Cardiac arrhythmias, hypotension, and cardiovascular collapse. Direct myocardial muscle damage with elevated MB-CPK (MB–creatine phosphokinase) myocardial enzyme release.

Respiratory: Acute pulmonary edema, respiratory tract irritation, chest tightness, cough, dyspnea and tachypnea.

CNS: Headache, dizziness, tremors, fatigue, ataxia, paresthesia, seizures, and coma.

Gastrointestinal: Nausea, vomiting, diarrhea, and abdominal pain. Intense thirst.

Skin: Diaphoresis.

Renal: Kidney damage.

Hepatic: Liver damage, jaundice with associated elevations in serum aminotransferases.

Metabolism: Metabolic acidosis.

Other: Products may spontaneously ignite.

SYMPTOM ONSET FOR ACUTE EXPOSURE

Immediate
Some respiratory symptoms (pulmonary edema) may be delayed

THERMAL DECOMPOSITION PRODUCTS INCLUDE

Hydrogen
Phosphorus

MEDICAL CONDITIONS POSSIBLY AGGRAVATED BY EXPOSURE

Respiratory disorders
Cardiovascular disorders

DECONTAMINATION

- Wear positive-pressure SCBA and protective equipment specified by references such as the *North American Emergency Response Guidebook.* If special chemical protective clothing is required, consult the chemical manufacturer or specific protective clothing compatibility charts. A qualified, experienced person should make decisions regarding the type of personal protective equipment necessary.
- Delay entry until trained personnel and proper protective equipment are available.
- Remove patient from contaminated area.
- Quickly remove and isolate patient's clothing, jewelry, and shoes.
- If any concurrent liquid or solid contamination exists:
  Gently brush away dry particles and blot excess liquids with absorbent material.
  Rinse patient with warm water, 32° C to 35° C (90° F to 95° F), if possible.
  Wash patient with a mild liquid soap and large quantities of water.
- Refer to decontamination protocol in Section Three.

IMMEDIATE FIRST AID

- Ensure that adequate decontamination has been carried out.
- If patient is not breathing, start artificial respiration, preferably with a demand-valve resuscitator, bag-valve-mask device, or pocket mask, as trained. Perform CPR if necessary.
- Immediately flush contaminated eyes with gently flowing water.
- Do not induce vomiting. If vomiting occurs, lean patient forward or place on left side (head-down position, if possible) to maintain an open airway and prevent aspiration.
- Keep patient quiet and maintain normal body temperature.
- Obtain medical attention.

BASIC TREATMENT

- Establish a patent airway (oropharyngeal or nasopharyngeal airway, if needed). Suction if necessary.
- Watch for signs of respiratory insufficiency and assist ventilations if necessary.
- Administer oxygen by nonrebreather mask at 10 to 15 L/min.
- Monitor for pulmonary edema and treat if necessary (refer to pulmonary edema protocol in Section Three).
- Monitor for shock and treat if necessary (refer to shock protocol in Section Three).
- Anticipate seizures and treat if necessary (refer to seizure protocol in Section Three).
- For eye contamination, flush eyes immediately with water. Irrigate each eye continuously with 0.9% saline (NS) during transport (refer to eye irrigation protocol in Section Three).

ADVANCED TREATMENT

- Consider orotracheal or nasotracheal intubation for airway control in the patient who is unconscious, has severe pulmonary edema, or is in severe respiratory distress.
- Positive-pressure ventilation techniques with a bag-valve-mask device may be beneficial.
- Consider drug therapy for pulmonary edema (refer to pulmonary edema protocol in Section Three).
- Monitor cardiac rhythm and treat arrhythmias if necessary (refer to cardiac protocol in Section Three).
- Start IV administration of D_5W TKO. Use 0.9% saline (NS) or lactated Ringer's (LR) if signs of hypovolemia are present. For hypotension with signs of hypovolemia, administer fluid cautiously. Consider vasopressors if patient is hypotensive with a normal fluid volume. Watch for signs of fluid overload (refer to shock protocol in Section Three).
- Treat seizures with diazepam (Valium) or lorazepam (Ativan) (refer to diazepam and lorazepam protocols in Section Four and seizure protocol in Section Three).
- Use proparacaine hydrochloride to assist eye irrigation (refer to proparacaine hydrochloride protocol in Section Four).

INITIAL EMERGENCY DEPARTMENT CONSIDERATIONS

- Useful initial laboratory studies include complete blood count, prothrombin time, serum electrolytes, blood urea nitrogen (BUN), creatinine, glucose, urinalysis, and baseline biochemical profile, including bilirubin, serum aminotransferases (ALT and AST), calcium, phosphorus, and magnesium. Determination of anion and osmolar gaps may be helpful. Arterial blood gases (ABGs), chest radiograph, and electrocardiogram may be required.
- Positive end-expiratory pressure (PEEP)–assisted ventilation may be necessary in patients with acute parenchymal injury who develop pulmonary edema or acute respiratory distress syndrome.
- Products may cause acidosis; hyperventilation and sodium bicarbonate may be beneficial. Bicarbonate therapy should be guided by patient presentation, ABG determination, and serum electrolyte considerations.
- Obtain toxicological consultation as necessary.

109

Phosphorus and Related Compounds

SUBSTANCE IDENTIFICATION

Found as solids and liquids. In solid form, phosphorus exists as a white to yellow, soft, waxy substance that spontaneously burns in air. It can be found as a yellow fuming liquid. Also found in a red granular form. Red phosphorus is relatively nontoxic, since it has low volatility and is not well absorbed. Used in the manufacture of many products, including fertilizers, water treatment products, food products, and explosives. Also used in rat poisons and roach powders. Many of these products can spontaneously burn in air.

ROUTES OF EXPOSURE

Skin and eye contact
Inhalation
Ingestion
Skin absorption

TARGET ORGANS

Primary
Skin
Eyes
Respiratory system
Gastrointestinal system
Hepatic system
Renal system
Secondary
Central nervous system
Cardiovascular system
Metabolism

LIFE THREAT

Hypovolemic shock and severe tissue burns. Severe respiratory irritant that can cause pulmonary edema and respiratory arrest. Cardiac rhythm and electrocardiogram changes leading to sudden death have also been reported.

SIGNS AND SYMPTOMS BY SYSTEM

Cardiovascular: Cardiac arrhythmias and hypovolemic shock.

Respiratory: Acute pulmonary edema, which may be delayed. Dyspnea, tachypnea, and irritation of the respiratory tract.

CNS: Headache, dizziness, fatigue, and photophobia. May cause seizures and coma.

Gastrointestinal: Mucosal burns. Nausea, vomiting, and abdominal pain. Excessive salivation with tooth and jaw pain. Vomitus and feces may be phosphorescent, and the breath may exhibit a garlic odor (all are rare findings).

Eye: Lacrimation, eyelid spasm (blepharospasm), conjunctivitis, corneal damage, and photophobia.

Skin: Severe chemical and thermal burns. Irritant dermatitis.
Renal: Kidney damage, including renal failure.
Hepatic: Fatty degeneration of the liver and jaundice.
Metabolism: Hypoglycemia and hypocalcemia.
Other: After initial symptoms, a symptom-free period of several days may occur, followed by signs of severe systemic poisoning. Red phosphorus is less toxic than white or yellow. Although red phosphorus is poorly absorbed and nontoxic in a single dose, repeated doses may demonstrate enhanced absorption, causing toxicity. The ability to detect the product by smell may be lost after a short exposure time (olfactory nerve fatigue).

SYMPTOM ONSET FOR ACUTE EXPOSURE

Immediate
Some symptoms, especially respiratory and hepatic, may be delayed

THERMAL DECOMPOSITION PRODUCTS INCLUDE

Hydrogen
Hydrogen chloride
Phosphine
Phosphoric acid fumes
Phosphorus oxides

MEDICAL CONDITIONS POSSIBLY AGGRAVATED BY EXPOSURE

Respiratory disorders (COPD)
Liver disorders

DECONTAMINATION

- Wear positive-pressure SCBA and protective equipment specified by references such as the *North American Emergency Response Guidebook*. If special chemical protective clothing is required, consult the chemical manufacturer or specific protective clothing compatibility charts. A qualified, experienced person should make decisions regarding the type of personal protective equipment necessary.
- Delay entry until trained personnel and proper protective equipment are available.
- Remove patient from contaminated area.
- Quickly remove and isolate patient's clothing, jewelry, and shoes.
- Gently brush away dry particles and blot excess liquids with absorbent material.
- If phosphorus particles are embedded in the skin, continuous water irrigation, water immersion, or sterile water-soaked dressings should be applied during transport to hospital for surgical debridement. Do not use oil for phosphorus exposure because this may promote dermal absorption.
- Rinse patient with cool water.
- Wash patient with a mild liquid soap and large quantities of water.
- Refer to decontamination protocol in Section Three.

IMMEDIATE FIRST AID

- Ensure that adequate decontamination has been carried out.
- If patient is not breathing, start artificial respiration, preferably with a demand-valve resuscitator, bag-valve-mask device, or pocket mask, as trained. Perform CPR if necessary.
- Immediately flush contaminated eyes with gently flowing water.

- Do not induce vomiting. If vomiting occurs, lean patient forward or place on left side (head-down position, if possible) to maintain an open airway and prevent aspiration.
- Keep patient quiet and maintain normal body temperature.
- Obtain medical attention.

BASIC TREATMENT

- Establish a patent airway (oropharyngeal or nasopharyngeal airway, if needed). Suction if necessary.
- Watch for signs of respiratory insufficiency and assist ventilations if necessary.
- Administer oxygen by nonrebreather mask at 10 to 15 L/min.
- Monitor for pulmonary edema and treat if necessary (refer to pulmonary edema protocol in Section Three).
- Monitor for shock and treat if necessary (refer to shock protocol in Section Three).
- Anticipate seizures and treat if necessary (refer to seizure protocol in Section Three).
- For eye contamination, flush eyes immediately with water. Irrigate each eye continuously with 0.9% saline (NS) during transport (refer to eye irrigation protocol in Section Three).
- Do not use emetics. For ingestion, rinse mouth and administer 5 ml/kg up to 200 ml of water for dilution if the patent can swallow, has a strong gag reflex, and does not drool. Administer activated charcoal (refer to ingestion protocol in Section Three and activated charcoal protocol in Section Four).
- If product was ingested, protect yourself from contact with vomitus, as it may cause burns.

ADVANCED TREATMENT

- Consider orotracheal or nasotracheal intubation for airway control in the patient who is unconscious, has severe pulmonary edema, or is in severe respiratory distress.
- Positive-pressure ventilation techniques with a bag-valve-mask device may be beneficial.
- Consider drug therapy for pulmonary edema (refer to pulmonary edema protocol in Section Three).
- Monitor cardiac rhythm and treat arrhythmias if necessary (refer to cardiac protocol in Section Three).
- Start IV administration of D_5W TKO. Use 0.9% saline (NS) or lactated Ringer's (LR) if signs of hypovolemia are present. For hypotension with signs of hypovolemia, administer fluid cautiously. Watch for signs of fluid overload (refer to shock protocol in Section Three).
- Treat seizures with diazepam (Valium) or lorazepam (Ativan) (refer to diazepam and lorazepam protocols in Section Four and seizure protocol in Section Three).
- Monitor for signs of hypoglycemia (decreased LOC, tachycardia, pallor, dilated pupils, diaphoresis, and/or dextrose stick or glucometer readings below 50 mg/dl) and administer 50% dextrose if necessary. Draw blood sample before administration (refer to 50% dextrose protocol in Section Four).
- Use proparacaine hydrochloride to assist eye irrigation (refer to proparacaine hydrochloride protocol in Section Four).

INITIAL EMERGENCY DEPARTMENT CONSIDERATIONS

- Useful initial laboratory studies include complete blood count, prothrombin time, serum electrolytes, blood urea nitrogen (BUN), creatinine, glucose, urinalysis, and baseline biochemical profile, including bilirubin, serum aminotransferases (ALT and AST), calcium, phosphorus, and magnesium. Determination of anion and osmolar gaps may be helpful. Arterial blood gases (ABGs), chest radiograph, and electrocardiogram may be required.
- Positive end-expiratory pressure (PEEP)–assisted ventilation may be necessary in patients with acute parenchymal injury who develop pulmonary edema or acute respiratory distress syndrome.
- Calcium supplementation (IV calcium gluconate) may be required to correct hypocalcemia. Therapy should be guided by clinical presentation and laboratory findings.
- Obtain toxicological consultation as necessary.

SPECIAL CONSIDERATIONS

- Products are extremely toxic; rapid transport is essential. If solids are embedded in the skin, keep area submerged in water during transport to hospital for surgical debridement.
- Three stages of acute phosphorus poisoning:
  - Stage I: GI symptoms and shock (0 to 24 hours).
  - Stage II: Quiescent period of 1 to 3 days.
  - Stage III: Hepatic damage/failure, renal failure, arrhythmias, seizures, and coma.

110

Radiological Threats: Simple Radiological Device

SUBSTANCE IDENTIFICATION

A simple radiological device could be a hidden radioactive source (usually a gamma source) that is placed in a heavily populated/congested area. It can consist of any material or combination of materials that spontaneously emit ionizing radiation. Potential sources include hospital radiation therapy (cobalt-60, cesium-137), nuclear power fuel rods (uranium-235, plutonium), and sources from universities, laboratories, radiography (cobalt-60, cesium-137, iridium-192, radium-226). Patients exposed to electromagnetic radiation sources emitting gamma rays will be irradiated. These patients are not contaminated and do not pose a secondary contamination risk. Conversely, exposure to particle radiation sources (alpha and beta particles, neutrons, protons, and positrons) in the form of dusts, liquids, or gases contaminates the patient and presents a secondary contamination risk unless properly handled.

ROUTES OF EXPOSURE

Skin and eye contact
Inhalation
Ingestion
Skin absorption
Proximity exposure risk with certain products

LIFE THREAT

Radiation ionizes atoms, resulting in intracellular formation of free radicals that damage DNA and RNA. Cells with high metabolic turnover rates such as those in the GI tract and hematopoietic system are affected the most. Massive radiation exposures may result in extensive neurological and GI damage. Loss of bone marrow function may also occur with resulting immunocompromise and systemic infection. Soluble radioactive compounds may cause local symptoms as well. Products may act as carcinogens.

SIGNS AND SYMPTOMS BY SYSTEM

Cardiovascular: Tachycardia and cardiovascular collapse.

Respiratory: Dyspnea, cough with irritation and edema to the upper airway, and pneumonitis.

CNS: Decreased level of consciousness and coma, ataxia, headache, lethargy, weakness, tremors, and convulsions.

Gastrointestinal: Nausea, vomiting, and diarrhea.

Eye: Lacrimation, conjunctivitis, and corneal damage.

Skin: Symptoms range from mild irritation to burns. Hair loss.

Blood: Bone marrow suppression.

Other: In most cases symptoms are delayed for hours to days.

DECONTAMINATION

- In most cases patients will present away from the source of exposure and will not require any decontamination.
- If a particulate source was used in the form of a dust or liquid, decontamination will be required. Wear positive-pressure SCBA and protective equipment specified by references such as the *North American Emergency Response Guidebook*. If special chemical protective clothing is required, consult the chemical manufacturer or specific protective clothing compatibility charts. A qualified, experienced person should make decisions regarding the type of personal protective equipment necessary.
- Responders should delay entry until properly trained and equipped personnel are on scene.
- For small numbers of patients with life-threatening injuries and particle or liquid exposure:

  Quickly remove and isolate patient's clothing, jewelry, and shoes.

  Package the patient, using reverse isolation procedures such as transportation bags, plastic, or blankets. This helps prevent the spread of contamination during transport.

  Provide adequate ambulance ventilation (intake and exhaust fans of proper size).

  Use adequate personal protective equipment. See Useful EMS/HAZMAT Equipment Procedure in Section Five.

  Notify the emergency department that a potentially contaminated patient is en route and supply them with all available information concerning the identity and nature of the contaminant.
- In mass casualty cases the number of contaminated patients will quickly overwhelm the available resources if field decontamination is not carried out.
- With large numbers or patients or if high levels of radioactive contamination are present or other chemical contaminants are suspected:

  Gently brush away dry particles and blot excess liquids with absorbent material.

  Rinse patient with warm water, 32° C to 35° C (90° F to 95° F), if possible. Use caution not to rinse contamination to areas of tissue damage or body cavity openings.

  Wash patient with a mild liquid soap and large quantities of water.

  Refer to decontamination protocol in Section Three.

IMMEDIATE FIRST AID

- Ensure that adequate decontamination has been carried out as needed.
- If patient is not breathing, start artificial respiration, preferably with a demand-valve resuscitator, bag-valve-mask device, or pocket mask, as trained. Perform CPR if necessary.
- Immediately flush contaminated eyes with gently flowing water.
- Do not induce vomiting. If vomiting occurs, lean patient forward or place on left side (head-down position, if possible) to maintain an open airway and prevent aspiration.
- Keep patient quiet and maintain normal body temperature.
- Obtain medical attention.

BASIC TREATMENT

- Establish a patent airway (oropharyngeal or nasopharyngeal airway, if needed). Suction if necessary.
- Watch for signs of respiratory insufficiency and assist ventilations if necessary.
- Administer oxygen by nonrebreather mask at 10 to 15 L/min.
- Monitor for shock and treat if necessary (refer to shock protocol in Section Three).
- Anticipate seizures and treat if necessary (refer to seizure protocol in Section Three).
- Perform routine emergency care for associated injuries.
- For eye contamination, flush eyes immediately with water. Irrigate each eye continuously during transport (refer to eye irrigation protocol in Section Three).
- Do not use emetics. For ingestion, rinse mouth and administer 5 ml/kg up to 200 ml of water for dilution if the patent can swallow, has a good gag reflex, and does not drool (refer to ingestion protocol in Section Three).
- Perform routine BLS care as necessary.

ADVANCED TREATMENT

- Consider orotracheal or nasotracheal intubation for airway control in the patient who is unconscious or is in severe respiratory distress.
- Monitor cardiac rhythm and treat arrhythmias as necessary (refer to cardiac protocol in Section Three).
- Start IV administration of 0.9% saline (NS) or lactated Ringer's (LR) TKO. For hypotension with signs of hypovolemia, administer fluid cautiously. Watch for signs of fluid overload (refer to shock protocol in Section Three).
- Treat seizures with diazepam (Valium) or lorazepam (Ativan) (refer to diazepam and lorazepam protocols in Section Four).
- Perform routine advanced life support care as needed
- Use proparacaine hydrochloride to assist eye irrigation (refer to proparacaine hydrochloride protocol in Section Four).

INITIAL EMERGENCY DEPARTMENT CONSIDERATIONS

- Chelating agents or pharmacologic blocking drugs (potassium iodine, diethylenetriamine pentaacetic acid [DTPA], dimercaprol [British antilewisite, BAL], sodium bicarbonate, Prussian blue, calcium gluconate, ammonium chloride, barium sulfate, sodium alginate, D-penicillamine) may be useful if given before or immediately after exposure. The Oak Ridge number listed at the end of this guideline can be contacted for specific treatment advice.

SPECIAL CONSIDERATIONS

- Most symptoms from radioactive product exposure are delayed; treat other medical or trauma problems according to normal protocols.
- An accurate history of the exposure is essential to determine risk and proper treatment modalities.
- The dose of radiation determines the type and clinical course of exposure:
  100 rads: GI symptoms (nausea, vomiting, abdominal cramps, diarrhea). Symptom onset within a few hours.
  600 rads: Severe GI symptoms (necrotic gastroenteritis) may result in dehydration and death within a few days.

Several thousand rads: neurological/cardiovascular symptoms (confusion, lethargy, ataxia, seizures, coma, cardiovascular collapse) within minutes to hours. Bone marrow depression, leukopenia, and infections usually follow severe exposures.

- Assistance and advice on patient care concerns may be obtained from the Oak Ridge Radiation Emergency Assistance Center and Training Site 24 hours a day by calling (615) 576-3131 or (615) 481-1000, ext. 1502 or beeper 241.

Radiological Threats: Radiological Dispersal Devices or Weapons

SUBSTANCE IDENTIFICATION

A radiological dispersal device (RDD), sometimes called a "dirty bomb," is designed to spread radioactive material contaminating patients, structures, and terrain. Unlike a nuclear weapon it does not release radioactivity in a massive burst of energy. Radioactive contaminants can be delivered by a variety of means. A common device consists of a radioactive source and a conventional explosive. Potential sources for the radioactive component of these devices include hospital radiation therapy (cobalt-60, cesium-137), nuclear power fuel rods (uranium-235, plutonium), and sources from universities, laboratories, and radiography (cobalt-60, cesium-137, iridium-192, radium-226). The advantage of these devices is that nuclear technology is not required. While an RDD may cause traumatic injuries secondary to the conventional explosion, their primary value is the psychological effect on patients and the need to carry out extensive structural decontamination procedures. Patients may be contaminated by the radiological material and require decontamination.

ROUTES OF EXPOSURE

Skin and eye contact
Inhalation
Ingestion
Skin absorption
Proximity exposure risk with certain products

LIFE THREAT

Initial injuries will be from the blast effect of the conventional explosive. If patients accumulate a large enough dose through ingestion, inhalation, or exposure, radiation sickness may occur. Radiation ionizes atoms, resulting in intracellular formation of free radicals that damage DNA and RNA. Cells with high metabolic turnover rates such as those in the GI tract and hematopoietic system are affected the most. Massive radiation exposures may result in extensive neurological and GI damage. Loss of bone marrow function may also occur with resulting immunocompromise and systemic infection. Soluble radioactive compounds may cause local symptoms as well. Products may act as carcinogens.

SIGNS AND SYMPTOMS BY SYSTEM

Cardiovascular: Tachycardia and cardiovascular collapse.

Respiratory: Dyspnea, cough, with irritation and edema to the upper airway, and pneumonitis.

CNS: Decreased level of consciousness and coma, ataxia, headache, lethargy, weakness, tremors, and convulsions.

Gastrointestinal: Nausea, vomiting, and diarrhea.
Eye: Lacrimation, conjunctivitis, and corneal damage.
Skin: Symptoms range from mild irritation to burns. Hair loss.
Blood: Bone marrow suppression.
Other: In most cases symptoms are delayed for hours to days.

The explosive device that is used will cause physical injuries. There are four different injury classes that are commonly seen from blast scenarios.

Primary Blast Injury

Explosive devices when detonated turn from a solid into a superheated gas in 1/10,000 of a second. These gases expand at a rate of 13,000 mph (Mach 17.6). After the device explodes, waves of pressure, called "blast waves" are sent out from the seat of the blast. These are the first to cause injury to patients by smashing and shattering anything in the way. Four main target organs are affected by this wave:

- Ears
- Lungs
- Gastrointestinal system
- Central nervous system

Secondary Injury

Secondary injuries are injuries caused by shrapnel from the fragments of the device and from things that have been attached to the explosive device. This trauma is just like any other penetrating trauma. The patient may also have bruising, bleeding, broken bones, and shock.

Tertiary Injuries

Tertiary injuries are caused by the patient being thrown like a projectile. The injuries are similar to injuries seen from falls or motor vehicle accidents. The treatment will also be the same as for these injuries. These patients may also have primary and secondary blast injuries.

Type IV injuries (Miscellaneous)

These are all the other injuries caused by the incident. These can include burns, chemical/radiation exposure, and psychological injuries.

DECONTAMINATION

- Wear positive-pressure SCBA and protective equipment specified by references such as the *North American Emergency Response Guidebook.* If special chemical protective clothing is required, consult the chemical manufacturer or specific protective clothing compatibility charts. A qualified, experienced person should make decisions regarding the type of personal protective equipment necessary.
- Immediate rescue and lifesaving care is of primary importance, taking all reasonable precautions to avoid contact with the radioactive materials or their containers. The time responders spend in any potentially contaminated area should be guided by experts and contamination assessment findings.
- Remove patient from contaminated area.
- Patients with electromagnetic radiation (gamma) exposure require no further decontamination.
- Experts and contamination assessment techniques should guide the need for individual patient decontamination.
- In mass casualty cases the number of contaminated patients will quickly overwhelm the available resources if field decontamination is not carried out.

With large numbers or patients or if high levels of radioactive contamination are present or other chemical contaminants are suspected:

Gently brush away dry particles and blot excess liquids with absorbent material.

Rinse patient with warm water, 32°C to 35°C (90° F to 95° F), if possible. Use caution not to rinse contamination to areas of tissue damage or body cavity openings.

Wash patient with a mild liquid soap and large quantities of water.

Refer to decontamination protocol in Section Three.

- If transportation is required before decontamination can be accomplished:

Quickly remove and isolate patient's clothing, jewelry, and shoes.

Package the patient, using reverse isolation procedures such as transportation bags, plastic, or blankets. This helps prevent the spread of contamination during transport.

Provide adequate ambulance ventilation (intake and exhaust fans of proper size).

Use adequate personal protective equipment. See Useful EMS/HAZMAT Equipment Procedure in Section Five.

Notify the emergency department that a potentially contaminated patient is en route and supply them with all available information concerning the identity and nature of the contaminant.

IMMEDIATE FIRST AID

- Ensure that adequate decontamination has been carried out as needed
- If patient is not breathing, start artificial respiration, preferably with a demand-valve resuscitator, bag-valve-mask device, or pocket mask, as trained. Perform CPR if necessary.
- Immediately flush contaminated eyes with gently flowing water.
- Do not induce vomiting. If vomiting occurs, lean patient forward or place on left side (head-down position, if possible) to maintain an open airway and prevent aspiration.
- Keep patient quiet and maintain normal body temperature.
- Obtain medical attention.

BASIC TREATMENT

- Establish a patent airway (oropharyngeal or nasopharyngeal airway, if needed). Suction if necessary.
- Watch for signs of respiratory insufficiency and assist ventilations if necessary.
- Administer oxygen by nonrebreather mask at 10 to 15 L/min.
- Monitor for shock and treat if necessary (refer to shock protocol in Section Three).
- Anticipate seizures and treat if necessary (refer to seizure protocol in Section Three).
- Perform routine emergency care for associated injuries.
- For eye contamination, flush eyes immediately with water. Irrigate each eye continuously during transport (refer to eye irrigation protocol in Section Three).
- Do not use emetics. For ingestion, rinse mouth and administer 5 ml/kg up to 200 ml of water for dilution if the patent can swallow, has a good gag reflex, and does not drool (refer to ingestion protocol in Section Three).
- Perform routine BLS care as necessary.

ADVANCED TREATMENT

- Consider orotracheal or nasotracheal intubation for airway control in the patient who is unconscious or is in severe respiratory distress.
- Monitor cardiac rhythm and treat arrhythmias as necessary (refer to cardiac protocol in Section Three).
- Start IV administration of 0.9% saline (NS) or lactated Ringer's (LR). For hypotension with signs of hypovolemia, administer fluid cautiously. Watch for signs of fluid overload (refer to shock protocol in Section Three).
- Treat seizures with diazepam (Valium) or lorazepam (Ativan) (refer to Seizure protocol in Section Three and diazepam and lorazepam protocols in Section Four).
- Perform routine advanced life support care as needed.
- Use proparacaine hydrochloride to assist eye irrigation (refer to proparacaine hydrochloride protocol in Section Four).

INITIAL EMERGENCY DEPARTMENT CONSIDERATIONS

- Chelating agents or pharmacologic blocking drugs (potassium iodine, diethylenetriamine pentaacetic acid [DTPA], dimercaprol [British antilewisite, BAL], sodium bicarbonate, Prussian blue, calcium gluconate, ammonium chloride, barium sulfate, sodium alginate, D-penicillamine) may be useful if given before or immediately after exposure. The Oak Ridge number listed at the end of this guideline can be contacted for specific treatment advice.

SPECIAL CONSIDERATIONS

- Radiation monitors should be available to evaluate the radiation dose rates and compute/verify safe times to remain in contaminated areas. Experts are needed to review the data and provide specific recommendations to the Incident Commander as to the hazards present in the affected areas. Medical radiation experts should be available to guide patient treatment.
- Most symptoms from radioactive product exposure are delayed; treat other medical or trauma problems according to normal protocols.
- An accurate history of the exposure is essential to determine risk and proper treatment modalities.
- The dose of radiation determines the type and clinical course of exposure:
  100 rads: GI symptoms (nausea, vomiting, abdominal cramps, diarrhea). Symptom onset within a few hours.
  600 rads: Severe GI symptoms (necrotic gastroenteritis) may result in dehydration and death within a few days.
  Several thousand rads: neurological/cardiovascular symptoms (confusion, lethargy, ataxia, seizures, coma, cardiovascular collapse) within minutes to hours. Bone marrow depression, leukopenia, and infections usually follow severe exposures.
- Assistance and advice on patient care concerns may be obtained from the Oak Ridge Radiation Emergency Assistance Center and Training Site 24 hours a day by calling (615) 576-3131 or (615) 481-1000, ext. 1502 or beeper 241.

Radiological Threats: Nuclear Detonation

SUBSTANCE IDENTIFICATION

The physical effects of a nuclear weapon detonation are blast, thermal radiation, and nuclear radiation. The effects depend on the size (yield) of the weapon, its physical design, and how the weapon is employed (air, surface, or subsurface burst). An enhanced radiation weapon (ERW) is designed to concentrate a much greater portion of the total energy release into neutrons and x-rays than a comparably sized standard nuclear weapon. Thus, an ERW will produce less thermal radiation but much greater nuclear radiation. Significant prompt radiation occurs only within the area of severe blast damage for ground bursts. Radiation from a large enhanced radiation weapon exploded above the surface would cause radiation injuries beyond the blast-damaged area. Fallout and residual radiation is a hazard for survivors, rescuers, and medical response personnel.

The altitude at which a nuclear weapon is detonated will determine the relative damage of blast, heat, and nuclear radiation.

Airburst

An airburst is an explosion from the weapon detonated in the air at an altitude below 30 km but high enough that the fireball does not contact the earth. An airburst causes significant structural damage, skin burns, and eye injuries. There may be a significant, initial radiation hazard and some neutron-induced activity in the vicinity of ground zero. Fallout hazard is minimal with an airburst.

Surface Burst

Detonated on or slightly above the earth surface, the fireball actually touches the land or water surface. The area that is affected by the blast, thermal radiation, and initial nuclear radiation will be less extensive than for an airburst of similar yield. There will be extensive damage and cratering at ground zero. Radioactive fallout will be a hazard over a much larger downwind area than that which is affected by the blast and thermal radiation.

Subsurface Burst

Detonated beneath the surface of the land or water. Cratering will result. If the burst does not penetrate the surface, the only other hazard will be from ground and water shock. If the surface is penetrated, there will be blast, thermal, and initial radiation effects. Local fallout will also be heavy.

High-Altitude Burst

A high-altitude burst above 30 km is designed to create significant ionization of the upper atmosphere, causing severe disruption of communications. These bursts also result in an intense electromagnetic pulse.

A nuclear detonation will result in the generation of four types of ionizing radiation: neutron, gamma, beta, and alpha. Neutrons and gamma rays characterize the initial burst while the residual radiation is primarily alpha, beta, and gamma rays. There may also be neutron-induced radioactive material in a small area around ground zero. In most cases, blast and thermal effects will far outnumber radiation injuries.

Nuclear detonation is accompanied by an electromagnetic pulse (EMP) that will greatly impact operations by interfering with electronic medical equipment. This happens immediately after the blast and should not affect units arriving later.

Patients exposed to electromagnetic radiation sources emitting gamma rays will be irradiated. These patients are not contaminated and do not pose a secondary contamination risk. Conversely, exposure to particle radiation sources (alpha and beta particles, neutrons, protons, and positrons) in the form of dusts, dirt, and fallout contaminates the patient and presents a secondary contamination risk unless properly handled.

ROUTES OF EXPOSURE

Skin and eye contact
Inhalation
Ingestion
Skin absorption
Proximity exposure risk with certain products

LIFE THREAT

Most injuries will be from the thermal and blast effects of the weapon. Radiation ionizes atoms, resulting in intracellular formation of free radicals that damage DNA and RNA. Cells with high metabolic turnover rates such as those in the GI tract and hematopoietic system are affected the most. Massive radiation exposures may result in extensive neurological and GI damage. Loss of bone marrow function may also occur, with resulting immunocompromise and systemic infection. Soluble radioactive compounds may cause local symptoms as well. Products may act as carcinogens.

SIGNS AND SYMPTOMS BY SYSTEM

Cardiovascular: Tachycardia and cardiovascular collapse.

Respiratory: Dyspnea, cough, with irritation and edema to the upper airway, and pneumonitis.

CNS: Decreased level of consciousness and coma, ataxia, headache, lethargy, weakness, tremors, and convulsions.

Gastrointestinal: Nausea, vomiting, and diarrhea.

Eye: Lacrimation, conjunctivitis, and corneal damage.

Skin: Symptoms range from mild irritation to burns. Hair loss.

Blood: Bone marrow suppression.

Other: In most cases symptoms are delayed for hours to days.

The explosive device that is used will cause physical injuries. There are four different injury classes that are commonly seen from blast scenarios.

Primary Blast Injury

Explosive devices when detonated turn from a solid into a superheated gas in 1/10,000 of a second. These gases expand at a rate of 13,000 mph (Mach 17.6). After the device explodes, waves of pressure, called "blast waves" are sent out from the seat of the blast. These are the first to cause injury to patients by smashing and shattering anything in the way. Four main target organs are affected by this wave:

- Ears
- Lungs

- Gastrointestinal system
- Central nervous system

Secondary Injury

Secondary injuries are injuries caused by shrapnel from the fragments of the device and from things that have been attached to the explosive device. This trauma is just like any other penetrating trauma. The patient may also have bruising, bleeding, broken bones, and shock.

Tertiary Injuries

Tertiary injuries are caused by the patient being thrown like a projectile. The injuries are similar to injuries seen from falls or motor vehicle accidents. The treatment will also be the same as for these injuries. These patients may also have primary and secondary blast injuries.

Type IV injuries (Miscellaneous)

These are all the other injuries caused by the incident. These can include burns, chemical/radiation exposure, and psychological injuries.

DECONTAMINATION

- Wear positive-pressure SCBA and protective equipment specified by references such as the *North American Emergency Response Guidebook.* If special chemical protective clothing is required, consult the chemical manufacturer or specific protective clothing compatibility charts. A qualified, experienced person should make decisions regarding the type of personal protective equipment necessary.
- Immediate rescue and lifesaving care is of primary importance, taking all reasonable precautions to avoid contact with the radioactive materials or their containers. The time responders spend in any potentially contaminated area should be guided by experts and contamination assessment findings.
- Remove patient from contaminated area.
- Patients with electromagnetic radiation (gamma) exposure require no further decontamination.
- Experts and contamination assessment techniques should guide the need for individual patient decontamination.
- In mass casualty cases the number of contaminated patients will quickly overwhelm the available resources if field decontamination is not carried out. With large numbers or patients or if high levels of radioactive contamination are present or other chemical contaminants are suspected:

  Gently brush away dry particles and blot excess liquids with absorbent material.

  Rinse patient with warm water, 32° C to 35° C (90° F to 95° F), if possible. Use caution not to rinse contamination to areas of tissue damage or body cavity openings.

  Wash patient with a mild liquid soap and large quantities of water.

  Refer to decontamination protocol in Section Three.
- If transportation is required before decontamination can be accomplished:

  Quickly remove and isolate patient's clothing, jewelry, and shoes.

  Package the patient, using reverse isolation procedures such as transportation bags, plastic, or blankets. This helps prevent the spread of contamination during transport.

  Provide adequate ambulance ventilation (intake and exhaust fans of proper size).

Use adequate personal protective equipment. See Useful EMS/HAZMAT Equipment Procedure in Section Five.

Notify the emergency department that a potentially contaminated patient is en route and supply them with all available information concerning the identity and nature of the contaminant.

IMMEDIATE FIRST AID

- Ensure that adequate decontamination has been carried out as needed.
- If patient is not breathing, start artificial respiration, preferably with a demand-valve resuscitator, bag-valve-mask device, or pocket mask, as trained. Perform CPR if necessary.
- Immediately flush contaminated eyes with gently flowing water.
- Do not induce vomiting. If vomiting occurs, lean patient forward or place on left side (head-down position, if possible) to maintain an open airway and prevent aspiration.
- Keep patient quiet and maintain normal body temperature.
- Obtain medical attention.

BASIC TREATMENT

- Establish a patent airway (oropharyngeal or nasopharyngeal airway, if needed). Suction if necessary.
- Watch for signs of respiratory insufficiency and assist ventilations if necessary.
- Administer oxygen by nonrebreather mask at 10 to 15 L/min.
- Monitor for shock and treat if necessary (refer to shock protocol in Section Three).
- Anticipate seizures and treat if necessary (refer to seizure protocol in Section Three).
- Perform routine emergency care for associated injuries.
- For eye contamination, flush eyes immediately with water. Irrigate each eye continuously during transport (refer to eye irrigation protocol in Section Three).
- Do not use emetics. For ingestion, rinse mouth and administer 5 ml/kg up to 200 ml of water for dilution if the patent can swallow, has a good gag reflex, and does not drool (refer to ingestion protocol in Section Three).
- Perform routine BLS care as necessary.

ADVANCED TREATMENT

- Consider orotracheal or nasotracheal intubation for airway control in the patient who is unconscious or is in severe respiratory distress.
- Monitor cardiac rhythm and treat arrhythmias as necessary (refer to cardiac protocol in Section Three).
- Start IV administration of 0.9% saline (NS) or lactated Ringer's (LR) TKO. For hypotension with signs of hypovolemia, administer fluid cautiously. Watch for signs of fluid overload (refer to shock protocol in Section Three).
- Treat seizures with diazepam (Valium) or lorazepam (Ativan) (refer to seizure protocol in Section Three and diazepam and lorazepam protocols in Section Four).
- Perform routine advanced life support care as needed
- Use proparacaine hydrochloride to assist eye irrigation (refer to proparacaine hydrochloride protocol in Section Four).

INITIAL EMERGENCY DEPARTMENT CONSIDERATIONS

- Chelating agents or pharmacologic blocking drugs (potassium iodine, diethylenetriamine pentaacetic acid [DTPA], dimercaprol [British antilewisite, BAL], sodium bicarbonate, Prussian blue, calcium gluconate, ammonium chloride, barium sulfate, sodium alginate, D-penicillamine) may be useful if given before or immediately after exposure. The Oak Ridge number listed at the end of this guideline can be contacted for specific treatment advice.

SPECIAL CONSIDERATIONS

- Radiation monitors should be available to evaluate the radiation dose rates and compute/verify safe times to remain in contaminated areas. Experts are needed to review the data and provide specific recommendations to the Incident Commander as to the hazards present in the affected areas. Medical radiation experts should be available to guide patient treatment.
- Most symptoms from radioactive product exposure are delayed; treat other medical or trauma problems according to normal protocols.
- An accurate history of the exposure is essential to determine risk and proper treatment modalities.
- The dose of radiation determines the type and clinical course of exposure:
  - 100 rads: GI symptoms (nausea, vomiting, abdominal cramps, diarrhea). Symptom onset within a few hours.
  - 600 rads: Severe GI symptoms (necrotic gastroenteritis) may result in dehydration and death within a few days.
  - Several thousand rads: neurological/cardiovascular symptoms (confusion, lethargy, ataxia, seizures, coma, cardiovascular collapse) within minutes to hours. Bone marrow depression, leukopenia, and infections usually follow severe exposures.
- Assistance and advice on patient care concerns may be obtained from the Oak Ridge Radiation Emergency Assistance Center and Training Site 24 hours a day by calling (615) 576-3131 or (615) 481-1000, ext. 1502 or beeper 241.

Anthrax *(Bacillus anthracis)*

SUBSTANCE IDENTIFICATION

Anthrax is disease caused by the gram-positive, spore-forming bacterium *Bacillus anthracis*. It occurs naturally as a zoonotic disease most commonly in hoofed mammals such as cattle, sheep, goats, camels, antelopes, and other herbivores. However, it can also occur in humans when they are exposed to infected animals, animal tissue, or anthrax spores used as a bioterrorism weapon. Human cases of anthrax sometimes occur because of occupational exposures among leather and wool industry workers.

Three forms of anthrax disease may occur, depending on the route of exposure. *Inhalational anthrax disease* is the most lethal form of disease, with a historical mortality rate greater than 80% throughout the twentieth century. However, advances in critical care are lessening the mortality of the disease. It occurs after the inhalation of spores and is the most likely form of disease to be seen following an act of bioterrorism. *Cutaneous anthrax disease* is the most common form, with a mortality of 10% to 20% if not treated. It occurs following the exposure of compromised skin to anthrax spores. *Gastrointestinal anthrax disease* is highly lethal but very rare. It occurs after the ingestion of live *B. anthracis* in contaminated meat. The bacterium is an extremely small organism composed of a single cell. It is considered by many experts in biological warfare to be a perfect bioweapon due to its ability to survive and remain virulent as a spore under conditions that destroy most pathogens. As a spore, it can remain dormant for years and begin replicating and generating toxins again under the right conditions, such as introduction into the human body. It has also proven to be a very effective agent for bioterrorism, causing 22 cases of anthrax disease and 5 deaths in the fall of 2001 when circulated through the U.S. Postal System in contaminated letters.

ROUTES OF EXPOSURE

Inhalation
Cutaneous (via cut or abrasion on the skin)
Ingestion

TARGET ORGANS

Primary
Respiratory system
Skin
Gastrointestinal system
Secondary
Lymphatic system
Hematologic system
Neurological system

LIFE THREAT

Toxemia, sepsis, septic shock, and hemorrhagic meningitis. Without treatment during the prodromal phase of inhalational anthrax, the fulminant stage may progress to include the development of high-grade bacteremia characterized by fever, respiratory distress, profuse sweating, cyanosis, and shock. Patients displaying these symptoms usually progress to death within several days. Other forms of anthrax disease untreated may also progress to bacteremia.

SIGNS AND SYMPTOMS BY SYSTEM

Cardiovascular: Tachycardia, dysrhythmias (commonly bradycardia, pulseless electrical activity [PEA], ventricular tachycardia, or ventricular fibrillation), hypotension, and cardiovascular collapse. Septic shock may occur.

Respiratory (inhalational anthrax disease): Initial symptoms of chest tightness and pleuritic pain that progress to nonproductive cough, dyspnea, and eventually to severe respiratory distress. CXR may show widened mediastinum, mediastinal adenopathy, pleural effusion, and infiltrates.

CNS: Headache, malaise, mental status changes, decreased level of consciousness, and coma. Meningitis and seizures may occur.

Gastrointestinal (gastrointestinal anthrax disease): Nausea, vomiting, hematemesis, hematochezia, abdominal pain, tenderness, guarding, and rebound.

Skin (cutaneous anthrax disease): Small, pruritic papule evolving to a vesicle and progressing to a small ulcer by the second day. Over the following 3 to 5 days, progressing to a depressed black eschar. Without antimicrobial therapy, may lead to systemic infection and death.

Metabolic: Fever

Blood: Elevated white blood cell count. Gram stain and culture of blood may show gram-positive bacilli once severe disease has developed.

INCUBATION PERIOD/SYMPTOM PROGRESSION

Inhalational anthrax typically has an incubation period of 1 to 10 days but may be as long as several weeks. The incubation period for this form of disease is usually followed by two-stage illness. The *prodromal phase* consists of nonspecific flulike symptoms lasting for a few hours to a few days. This is followed by a *fulminant stage* of a high-grade bacteremia that normally progresses to death within 2 days.

Cutaneous anthrax has an incubation period of 1 to 12 days. A small, pruritic papule usually appears on the arms, hands, neck, or head. It evolves to a vesicle and progresses to a small ulcer within two days. Over the next 3 to 5 days, it progresses to a depressed black eschar. Without antimicrobial therapy, it may lead to systemic infection and death. The lesion usually resolves within 2 weeks.

Gastrointestinal anthrax has an incubation period of 3 to 5 days. Initial presentation includes 1 to 2 days of fever, nausea, vomiting, and anorexia. These symptoms quickly become more severe to include hematemesis, hematochezia, abdominal pain, tenderness, guarding, and rebound. Without treatment, mortality is high.

MEDICAL CONDITIONS THAT MAY INCREASE RISK FOLLOWING EXPOSURE

Preexisting acute or chronic respiratory disease (inhalational disease)

Compromised skin conditions (cutaneous disease)

DECONTAMINATION

- If a covert release is successfully accomplished, patients seen days or weeks later will not pose a risk to providers and do not require decontamination. Patient decontamination is warranted only in the immediate aftermath of a known release. Surfaces, bedding, and dressings in contact with body fluids, as well as instruments used for invasive procedures on patients with known or suspected disease, should be sterilized with a sporicidal agent such as hypochlorite (bleach).

- If a suspected overt release has occurred:

  Wear respiratory protection such as an air-purifying respirator with appropriate cartridges/filters or positive-pressure SCBA. Protective equipment such as gloves, suits, boot covers, and eye protection should be used. A qualified, experienced person should make decisions regarding the type of personal protective equipment necessary.

  Delay entry into the suspected release area until trained personnel and proper protective equipment are available.

  Remove patient from contaminated area.

  Quickly remove and isolate patient's clothing, jewelry, and shoes.

  Gently brush away dry particles and blot excess liquids with absorbent material.

  Rinse patient with warm water, 32° C to 35° C (90° F to 95° F), if possible.

  Wash patient with a mild liquid soap and large quantities of water.

  Refer to decontamination protocol in Section Three.

IMMEDIATE FIRST AID

- For overt releases:

  Ensure that adequate decontamination has been carried out as needed.

  If patient is not breathing, start artificial respiration, preferably with a demand-valve resuscitator, bag-valve-mask device, or pocket mask, as trained. Perform CPR as necessary.

  Immediately flush contaminated eyes with gently flowing water.

  Do not induce vomiting. If vomiting occurs, lean patient forward or place on left side (head-down position, if possible) to maintain an open airway and prevent aspiration.

  Keep patient quiet and maintain normal body temperature.

  Obtain medical attention.

BASIC TREATMENT

- Establish a patent airway (oropharyngeal or nasopharyngeal airway, if needed). Suction if necessary.
- Watch for signs of respiratory insufficiency and assist ventilations if necessary.
- Administer oxygen by nonrebreather mask at 10 to 15 L/min.
- Monitor for shock and treat if necessary (refer to shock protocol in Section Three).
- Anticipate seizures and treat if necessary (refer to seizure protocol in Section Three).
- For eye contamination, flush eyes immediately with water. Irrigate each eye continuously with 0.9% saline (NS) during transport (refer to eye irrigation protocol in Section Three).

ADVANCED TREATMENT

- Consider orotracheal or nasotracheal intubation for airway control in the patient who is unconscious or is in severe respiratory distress.
- Positive-pressure ventilation techniques with a bag-valve-mask device may be beneficial.

- Monitor cardiac rhythm and treat arrhythmias as necessary (refer to cardiac protocol in Section Three).
- Start IV administration of D_5W TKO. Use 0.9% saline (NS) or lactated Ringer's (LR) if signs of hypovolemia are present. For hypotension with signs of hypovolemia, administer fluid cautiously. Consider vasopressors if patient is hypotensive with a normal fluid volume. Watch for signs of fluid overload (refer to shock protocol in Section Three).
- Treat seizures with diazepam (Valium) or lorazepam (Ativan) (refer to diazepam and lorazepam protocols in Section Four and seizure protocol in Section Three).
- Consider antimicrobial therapy as soon as exposure or diagnosis is suspected. If antibiotics are administered during the incubation period, morbidity and mortality can be greatly reduced. Treatment of 60 days may be required. The course of antibiotic therapy for prophylactic therapy is the same duration but may be reduced if acellular vaccine is also used (available only from the Centers for Disease Prevention and Control [CDC]).
- The primary drugs of choice for postexposure prophylaxis are ciprofloxacin, doxycycline, and amoxicillin. The primary drugs of choice for treating anthrax disease are ciprofloxacin or doxycycline, plus one or two additional antibiotics, including penicillin, rifampin, clindamycin, vancomycin, imipenem, and chloramphenicol (refer to antibiotic protocols in Section Four).
- Use proparacaine hydrochloride to assist eye irrigation (refer to proparacaine hydrochloride protocol in Section Four).

INITIAL EMERGENCY DEPARTMENT CONSIDERATIONS

- Initial presentation of inhalational anthrax disease includes mild and nonspecific flulike symptoms. Without treatment during the prodromal phase of the inhalational form of illness, the fulminant stage may progress to include the development of high-grade bacteremia characterized by fever, respiratory distress, profuse sweating, cyanosis, and shock. Patients displaying these symptoms usually progress to death within several days. Other forms of anthrax disease untreated may also progress to bacteremia. Presumptive diagnosis should be made on signs and symptoms alone in the setting of a known or suspected outbreak. Treatment should be initiated any time anthrax is suspected. Do not delay treatment while waiting on confirmatory testing results.
- Useful initial studies include chest radiograph, gram stain and culture of blood, ABGs, pulse oximetry, CBC, electrolytes, and renal and liver function tests. Peripheral blood smears may show gram-positive rods. Cultures are often positive in less than 12 hours. CXR may show a widened mediastinum, mediastinal adenopathy, or pleural effusion with infiltrates. Questionable CXR results may be followed with a chest computed tomography (CT). There are no rapid tests available for early disease. However, rapid PCR and immunohistochemical stains are available at reference labs for confirmatory testing.
- Antibiotic therapy is indicated. Ciprofloxacin, doxycycline, or amoxicillin may be used for prophylaxis following suspected exposure. Treatment of anthrax disease includes ciprofloxacin or doxycycline, plus one or two additional antibiotics, including penicillin, rifampin, clindamycin, vancomycin, imipenem, and chloramphenicol. (Refer to antibiotic protocols in Section Four.)
- Mechanical ventilation and PEEP-assisted ventilation may be needed.

- Fluid administration and vasopressors may be needed to treat hypotension.
- Hemodialysis may be necessary in cases involving renal failure.
- All suspected and confirmed cases should be immediately reported to the CDC through your local and state health departments.

SPECIAL CONSIDERATIONS

Noneffective Therapies

- Trimethoprim/sulfamethoxazole, third-generation cephalosporins, and most macrolides.

Infection Control

- Use standard precautions (strict hand washing, gloves, and splash precautions). Cutaneous anthrax may be transmitted from person to person through direct contact with the infected area. However, inhalational anthrax disease is not transmitted person to person. Private rooms or negative-pressure patient rooms are not required. Lab personnel should be notified of suspected anthrax samples and take appropriate precautions. Spores on surfaces may be killed by a 10% hypochlorite solution.

Vaccination

- A licensed, cell-free, effective vaccine exists, but its use is limited. Vaccination consists of an initial 6-dose series (0, 2, and 4 weeks; 6, 12, and 18 months). This is followed by an annual booster. It is not available to the general public. This vaccine is considered as an investigational new drug (IND) for mass prophylaxis during public health emergencies. It may be used in combination with a prophylactic antimicrobial regimen to reduce the time of antibiotic therapy from 60 days to 30 days. This includes a 3-dose vaccine regimen (0, 2, 4 weeks) in combination with 30 days of antimicrobial prophylaxis.

Botulism (*Clostridium botulinum* toxin)

SUBSTANCE IDENTIFICATION

Botulism is caused by a group of neurotoxins produced by the anaerobic, spore-forming bacillus *Clostridium botulinum*. There are three forms of botulism: foodborne, wound, and infant (also called intestinal) botulism. *Foodborne botulism* results from ingesting the preformed toxin in contaminated food. This exposure results in a presynaptic inhibition that affects both muscarinic and nicotinic receptors. This causes descending paralysis that can eventually lead to respiratory failure and death. *Wound botulism* occurs when a wound is contaminated with *C. botulinum*. This form of botulism illness is most commonly associated with injected drug use or traumatic injury. *Infant (intestinal) botulism* occurs with susceptible infants who ingest *C. botulinum* spores that germinate in their intestines. This ingestion results in difficulty feeding, constipation, weakness, and muscle hypotonia ("floppy baby syndrome").

Eight separate toxin types are produced: A, B, C alpha, C beta, D, E, F and G. Types A, B, C2, E, F, and G are know to cause disease in humans. These toxins are regarded as being among the most potent toxic substances known to man. Botulinum toxin could be used to contaminate water or food supplies or could be delivered as an aerosol. If an aerosol release is used, symptoms will be similar to those of food botulism with a delayed onset.

ROUTES OF EXPOSURE

Ingestion
Inhalation
Skin (wound botulism)

TARGET ORGANS

Primary
Nervous system
Skin
Secondary
Cardiovascular system
Respiratory system
Renal system
Gastrointestinal system

LIFE THREAT

Descending paralysis resulting in respiratory failure. Possible direct effect on the heart, resulting in dysrhythmia.

SIGNS AND SYMPTOMS BY SYSTEM

Cardiovascular: Dysrhythmias, tachycardia secondary to hypoxia. Postural hypotension may occur.

CNS: Dizziness, slurred speech, descending bilateral paralysis beginning with the cranial nerves. Progressive descending weakness and paralysis may result in loss of diaphragmatic function and respiratory failure. Paresthesias and depressed or absent deep tendon reflexes. Sensation is usually intact and the patient remains alert and oriented. Seizures are possible. Muscle weakness of striated muscle groups.

Respiratory: Sore throat, tachypnea, dyspnea, and respiratory failure secondary to bulbar paralysis.

Gastrointestinal: Dry mouth, dysphagia (difficulty swallowing), absent gag reflex, nausea, vomiting, constipation, enlarged abdomen.

Eye: Dilated pupils (mydriasis), double vision (diplopia), drooping eyelids (ptosis), photophobia, abnormal extraocular movements, oculomotor nerve paralysis.

Metabolic: Afebrile.

Renal: Urinary retention.

Other: Fatigue and muscle weakness, dysarthria (imperfect speech due to poor muscle control).

INCUBATION PERIOD/SYMPTOM PROGRESSION

The incubation period for botulism varies according to the dose and route of exposure. Food botulism and inhalational botulism typically have an incubation period of 12 to 36 hours. However, symptoms have been reported as early as 3 hours and as long as 16 days after exposure.

Initial presentation of bulbar palsies includes dilated pupils (mydriasis), double vision (diplopia), drooping eyelids (ptosis), photophobia, hoarseness, dysarthric speech. Patients remain afebrile. Symptoms progress to descending, symmetrical skeletal muscle paralysis. Despite the progressing symptoms, patients remain fully awake and aware. The descending weakness may eventually produce a sudden respiratory arrest.

MEDICAL CONDITIONS THAT MAY INCREASE RISK FOLLOWING EXPOSURE

Adults with unusual GI flora caused by bowel problems or antibiotics may be susceptible to intestinal (infant) botulism.

DECONTAMINATION

- If a covert aerosol release is successfully accomplished, patients seen days later will not pose a risk to providers and do not require decontamination. Patient decontamination is warranted only in the immediate aftermath of a known release. Surfaces, bedding, and dressings in contact with body fluids, as well as instruments used for invasive procedures on patients with known or suspected botulism exposure, should be sterilized with a sporicidal agent such as hypochlorite (bleach).
- If a suspected overt release has occurred:

  Wear respiratory protection such as an air-purifying respirator with appropriate cartridges/filters or positive-pressure SCBA. Protective equipment such as gloves, suits, boot covers, and eye protection should be used. A qualified, experienced person should make decisions regarding the type of personal protective equipment necessary.

  Delay entry into the suspected release area until trained personnel and proper protective equipment are available.

Remove patient from contaminated area.
Quickly remove and isolate patient's clothing, jewelry, and shoes.
Gently brush away dry particles and blot excess liquids with absorbent material.
Rinse patient with warm water, 32° C to 35° C (90° F to 95° F), if possible.
Wash patient with a mild liquid soap and large quantities of water.
Refer to decontamination protocol in Section Three.

IMMEDIATE FIRST AID

- For overt releases:

  Ensure that adequate decontamination has been carried out as needed.

  If patient is not breathing, start artificial respiration, preferably with a demand-valve resuscitator, bag-valve-mask device, or pocket mask, as trained. Perform CPR as necessary.

  Immediately flush contaminated eyes with gently flowing water.

  Do not induce vomiting. If vomiting occurs, lean patient forward or place on left side (head-down position, if possible) to maintain an open airway and prevent aspiration.

  Keep patient quiet and maintain normal body temperature.

  Obtain medical attention.

BASIC TREATMENT

- Establish a patent airway (oropharyngeal or nasopharyngeal airway, if needed). Suction if necessary.
- Watch for signs of respiratory insufficiency and assist ventilations if necessary.
- Administer oxygen by nonrebreather mask at 10 to 15 L/min.
- Monitor for shock and treat if necessary (refer to shock protocol in Section Three).
- For eye contamination, flush eyes immediately with water. Irrigate each eye continuously with 0.9% saline (NS) during transport (refer to eye irrigation protocol in Section Three).

ADVANCED TREATMENT

- Consider orotracheal or nasotracheal intubation for airway control in the patient who is unconscious or is in severe respiratory distress.
- Positive-pressure ventilation techniques with a bag-valve-mask device will be needed.
- Monitor cardiac rhythm and treat arrhythmias as necessary (refer to cardiac protocol in Section Three).
- Treat seizures with diazepam (Valium) or lorazepam (Ativan) (refer to diazepam and lorazepam protocols in Section Four and seizure protocol in Section Three).
- Start IV administration of D_5W TKO. Use 0.9% saline (NS) or lactated Ringer's (LR) if signs of hypovolemia are present. For hypotension with signs of hypovolemia, administer fluid cautiously. Watch for signs of fluid overload (refer to shock protocol in Section Three).
- Botulinum antitoxin should be administered to all suspected botulism patients. The antitoxin can halt, but not reverse, the descending paralysis that is present. Potential exists for serious complications from the antitoxin, and recommendations for safe administration of treatment have changed over time. Closely review package insert guidance prior to initiation of antitoxin therapy. DIRECT PHYSICIAN ORDER ONLY.

- Use proparacaine hydrochloride to assist eye irrigation (refer to proparacaine hydrochloride protocol in Section Four).

INITIAL EMERGENCY DEPARTMENT CONSIDERATIONS

- Presumptive diagnosis should be made on signs and symptoms alone in the setting of a known or suspected outbreak. Consider presumptive botulism diagnosis any time a cluster of patients is identified experiencing sudden afebrile weakness and paralysis. A single case of botulism is considered to be a public health emergency and requires immediate investigation by local and state public health authorities. Presumptive diagnosis is made on signs and symptoms but must be confirmed by a reference lab. The toxin can be detected in foods, serum, stool, and gastric fluid. The reference laboratory test is a mouse bioassay. Samples must be refrigerated during storage and transport. Serum samples must be obtained prior to antitoxin treatment. In addition, the laboratory must be notified if the patient has received any anticholinesterase medications.
- The differential diagnosis includes Guillain-Barré syndrome and myasthenia gravis. Both can be ruled out by electromyography (EMG) and response to anticholinesterases. Other useful initial studies include ABGs, pulse oximetry, CBC, electrolytes, urinalysis, and renal function tests. Bedside spirometry to determine forced vital capacity. Obtain chest radiograph.
- Mechanical ventilation may be needed.

SPECIAL CONSIDERATIONS

Noneffective Therapies

- Avoid aminoglycosides and clindamycin. They may worsen paralytic symptoms.

Infection Control

- Standard precautions are necessary. Botulism is not an infectious condition and is not spread person to person.

Vaccination

- There is currently no vaccine available to the general public. Researchers and lab workers potentially exposed to *C. botulinum* or its toxins may be eligible for a pentavalent toxoid vaccine. In addition, a trivalent antitoxin for toxin types A, B, and E can be obtained from the CDC. Optimal results are obtained if given early in the course of the illness. Skin testing for hypersensitivity to horse serum should precede antitoxin administration.
- Dosage (adults and children) is a single 10-ml vial diluted 1:10 in 0.9% saline (NS) solution administered by slow intravenous infusion. Antitoxin is held at CDC quarantine stations throughout the United States. Information can be obtained from the CDC at (404) 639-2206 or (404) 639-2888.

115

Brucellosis (*Brucella abortus, B. canis, B. suis,* and *B. melitensis*)

SUBSTANCE IDENTIFICATION

Brucellosis is a zoonotic disease caused by one of six species of *Brucella*, a family of gram-negative, aerobic coccobacilli. It is nonmotile and does not form spores or capsules. It is commonly found in hoofed animals such as dairy cattle, sheep, and swine but can also be found in other animals. Four *Brucella* species can infect humans: *B. abortus, B. canis, B. suis*, and *B. melitensis*. Humans develop the disease following ingestion or inhalation of *Brucella* organisms. Occupational infections occur in lab workers, veterinarians, and slaughterhouse workers. Brucellosis may also occur as a foodborne illness among those who consume unpasteurized dairy products. Although there are usually fewer than 100 cases annually in the United States, brucellosis is endemic in Asia and the Middle East. It is considered a lower-threat biological weapon because it results in low mortality. However, it is still considered a threat because it has a high morbidity, producing a long, incapacitating illness. *B. suis* and *B. melitensis* have been weaponized as biological agents. The organism is highly infective and can survive for weeks in soil or water.

Human disease is divided into three stages: acute, subacute, and chronic. The *acute stage* (exposure to 2 months) is characterized by a flulike illness with nonspecific symptoms. The *subacute stage* (2 to 12 months) presents with similar symptoms. The *chronic stage* (longer than 12 months) has predominantly neuropsychiatric symptoms. The chronic stage is uncommon with adequate treatment. Mortality is less than 5% in untreated patients. Brucellosis is also known as undulant fever, Malta fever, and Mediterranean fever.

ROUTES OF EXPOSURE

Inhalation
Ingestion
Eye or skin absorption

TARGET ORGANS

Primary

Cardiovascular system
Nervous system
Gastrointestinal system
Renal system
Hepatic system
Eyes
Skin

Secondary
Respiratory system
Blood

LIFE THREAT

Central nervous system disease and endocardial infection.

SIGNS AND SYMPTOMS BY SYSTEM

Cardiovascular: Endocarditis. Rarely occurs but is the most common cause of death.

Respiratory: Pleuritic chest pain, dyspnea, and nonproductive cough. Pneumonia and bronchitis may occur.

CNS: Headache, malaise, and fatigue. Involvement of the central or peripheral nervous system may occur. Meningitis, encephalitis, stroke, or intracerebral hemorrhage may occur. Chronic stage may include neuropsychiatric symptoms.

Gastrointestinal: Anorexia, colitis, abdominal pain, nausea, vomiting, diarrhea, constipation, and mild spleen damage.

Skin: Rash and profuse sweating.

Eye: Eye irritation and possible optic nerve involvement.

Metabolic: Fever.

Blood: Anemia, neutropenia, thrombocytopenia, DIC, and pancytopenia may occur.

Renal: Urinary tract infection symptoms; nephritis may occur.

Hepatic: Hepatic and spleen injury.

Other: Epistaxis, myalgia, back pain, arthralgia, vertebral osteomyelitis, and arthritis. Chronic cases may develop.

INCUBATION PERIOD/SYMPTOM PROGRESSION

The incubation period is 5 to 60 days.

Many patients are initially asymptomatic. Those with symptoms experience nonspecific, flulike illness. GI symptoms are most common, with over 70% reporting nausea, vomiting, diarrhea, constipation, abdominal pain, and anorexia. Osteoarticular complications are also a common complaint; specifically, sacroiliitis, joint pain, and vertebral osteomyelitis are commonly seen. Pleuritic chest pain and nonproductive cough are the most common respiratory symptoms. CXR usually remains normal. Some patients develop CNS disorders that may include meningitis, encephalitis, neuropathies, and at times, severe behavioral changes. The chronic stage (longer than 12 months) has predominantly neuropsychiatric symptoms.

MEDICAL CONDITIONS THAT MAY INCREASE RISK FOLLOWING EXPOSURE

Preexisting cardiovascular or neurological problems.

DECONTAMINATION

- If a covert release is successfully accomplished, patients seen days or weeks later will not pose a risk to providers and do not require decontamination. Patient decontamination is warranted only in the immediate aftermath of a known release. Surfaces, bedding, and dressings in contact with body fluids, as well as instruments used for invasive procedures on patients with known or suspected brucellosis, should be sterilized with a sporicidal agent such as hypochlorite (bleach).
- If a suspected overt release has occurred:

  Wear respiratory protection such as an air-purifying respirator with appropriate cartridges/filters or positive-pressure SCBA. Protective equipment such as gloves, suits, boot covers, and eye protection should be used. A qualified, experienced person should make decisions regarding the type of personal protective equipment necessary.

Delay entry into the suspected release area until trained personnel and proper protective equipment are available.

Remove patient from contaminated area.

Quickly remove and isolate patient's clothing, jewelry, and shoes.

Gently brush away dry particles and blot excess liquids with absorbent material.

Rinse patient with warm water, 32° C to 35° C (90° F to 95° F), if possible.

Wash patient with a mild liquid soap and large quantities of water.

Refer to decontamination protocol in Section Three.

IMMEDIATE FIRST AID

- For overt releases:

  Ensure that adequate decontamination has been carried out as needed.

  If patient is not breathing, start artificial respiration, preferably with a demand-valve resuscitator or bag-valve-mask device as trained. Perform CPR as necessary.

  Immediately flush contaminated eyes with gently flowing water.

  Do not induce vomiting. If vomiting occurs, lean patient forward or place on left side (head-down position, if possible) to maintain an open airway and prevent aspiration.

  Keep patient quiet and maintain normal body temperature.

  Obtain medical attention.

BASIC TREATMENT

- Establish a patent airway (oropharyngeal or nasopharyngeal airway, if needed). Suction if necessary.
- Watch for signs of respiratory insufficiency and assist ventilations if necessary.
- Administer oxygen by nonrebreather mask at 10 to 15 L/min.
- Monitor for shock and treat if necessary (refer to shock protocol in Section Three).
- For eye contamination, flush eyes immediately with water. Irrigate each eye continuously with 0.9% saline (NS) during transport (refer to eye irrigation protocol in Section Three).

ADVANCED TREATMENT

- Consider orotracheal or nasotracheal intubation for airway control in the patient who is unconscious or is in severe respiratory distress.
- Positive-pressure ventilation techniques with a bag-valve-mask device may be beneficial.
- Monitor cardiac rhythm and treat arrhythmias as necessary (refer to cardiac protocol in Section Three).
- Start IV administration of D_5W TKO. Use 0.9% saline (NS) or lactated Ringer's (LR) if signs of hypovolemia are present. For hypotension with signs of hypovolemia, administer fluid cautiously. Consider vasopressors if patient is hypotensive with a normal fluid volume (refer to shock protocol in Section Three).
- Until sensitivities are identified, combination antimicrobial therapy is recommended. Adults should be treated with doxycycline and streptomycin or

rifampin. Children (>8 years old) should be treated with doxycycline and tetracycline or TMP/SMX (trimethoprim/sulfamethoxazole). Alternative therapies include doxycycline and gentamicin; TMP/SMX and gentamicin; and ofloxacin and rifampin. Patients with meningoencephalitis or endocarditis should receive long-term therapy with rifampin, tetracycline, and an aminoglycoside (refer to antibiotic protocols in Section Four).

- Use proparacaine hydrochloride to assist eye irrigation (refer to proparacaine hydrochloride protocol in Section Four).

INITIAL EMERGENCY DEPARTMENT CONSIDERATIONS

- Presumptive diagnosis should be made on signs and symptoms alone in the setting of a known or suspected outbreak. Presumptive laboratory diagnosis is accomplished with ELISA followed by Western blot. Confirmatory tests include serum agglutinin titer (SAT) test to detect antibodies and blood or bone marrow culture (may require >30 days to grow *Brucella*). Other useful studies include ABGs, pulse oximetry, CBC with platelet count (lymphocyte count is often elevated), electrolytes, renal and liver function tests (elevated LDH, alkaline phosphatase, GGT, and aminotransferase levels), and urinalysis. Chest radiograph (CXR). Although the CXR may remain within normal limits, lung abscesses, nodules, and pleural effusions may be seen.
- Combination antibiotic therapy is indicated. Doxycycline, gentamicin, streptomycin, tetracycline, rifampin, and TMP/SMX are antibiotics of choice. (Refer to antibiotic protocols in Section Four.)

SPECIAL CONSIDERATIONS

Infection Control

- Use standard precautions (strict hand washing, gloves, and splash precautions). Person-to-person transmission has been reported following exposure to infected tissue and through sexual contact. However, no transmission has been reported through routine patient care.

Vaccination

- No vaccine for humans is currently available. An animal vaccine is used throughout the United States and is responsible for the low incidence of disease in North America.

116 Crimean-Congo Hemorrhagic Fever (Bunyaviridae, *Nairovirus*)

SUBSTANCE IDENTIFICATION

Crimean-Congo hemorrhagic fever (CCHF) is a severe hemorrhagic fever syndrome resulting from exposure to a Bunyaviridae *Nairovirus*. These organisms exist naturally in livestock, ruminants, hares, birds, and ticks across Eastern Europe, Africa, Asia, and the Middle East. Humans are normally exposed by the bite of an infected tick. Occupational exposures have occurred among butchers of infected animals. Some person-to-person cases have been reported among family members of primary cases, and also some nosocomial infections occur among health care workers exposed to blood and body fluids. Some cases are asymptomatic and mild. However, mortality is approximately 30%. This mortality rate may be increased if cases result from aerosol exposure. The normal incubation period is 7 to 12 days. This incubation period may increase to several weeks or months if the transmission mode is via aerosol exposures. Death normally occurs as a result of massive hemorrhage within 2 weeks of symptom onset.

ROUTES OF EXPOSURE

Inhalation
Skin
Arthropod vector (tickborne)

TARGET ORGANS

Primary
Cardiovascular system
Respiratory system
Secondary
Nervous system
Gastrointestinal system

LIFE THREAT

Cardiovascular collapse and acute respiratory distress syndrome.

SIGNS AND SYMPTOMS BY SYSTEM

Cardiovascular: Tachycardia, bradycardia (not present in children), muffled heart sounds, hypotension, and cardiovascular collapse.

Respiratory: Hemorrhagic pneumonia, acute respiratory distress syndrome, dyspnea.

CNS: Headache, malaise, myalgia, weakness.

Gastrointestinal: Nausea, vomiting, diarrhea, abdominal pain.

Skin: Petechiae, pallor, hematomas.

Metabolic: Fever.

Hepatic: Hepatosplenomegaly, hepatitis, jaundice.

Renal: Proteinuria.

Blood: Leukopenia, excessive bleeding, disseminated intravascular coagulation (DIC).

INCUBATION PERIOD/SYMPTOM PROGRESSION

The initial incubation period is 1 to 2 weeks; may be longer if route of exposure is inhalation. Initial symptoms include sudden onset of flulike symptoms for 2 to 7 days. If illness progresses to fulminant disease, symptoms include hepatosplenomegaly, hepatitis, jaundice, leukopenia, excessive bleeding, disseminated intravascular coagulation (DIC), shock, acute respiratory distress syndrome, and death due to cardiovascular collapse.

MEDICAL CONDITIONS THAT MAY INCREASE RISK FOLLOWING EXPOSURE

Preexisting acute or chronic respiratory disease.

DECONTAMINATION

- If a covert release is successfully accomplished, patients seen days or weeks later will not pose a risk to providers and do not require decontamination. Patient decontamination is warranted only in the immediate aftermath of a known release. Surfaces, bedding, and dressings in contact with body fluids, as well as instruments used for invasive procedures on patients with known or suspected Crimean-Congo hemorrhagic fever, should be sterilized with a sporicidal agent such as hypochlorite (bleach).
- If a suspected overt release has occurred:

  Wear respiratory protection such as an air-purifying respirator with appropriate cartridges/filters or positive-pressure SCBA. Protective equipment such as gloves, suits, boot covers, and eye protection should be used. A qualified, experienced person should make decisions regarding the type of personal protective equipment necessary.

  Delay entry into the suspected release area until trained personnel and proper protective equipment are available.

  Remove patient from contaminated area.

  Quickly remove and isolate patient's clothing, jewelry, and shoes.

  Gently brush away dry particles and blot excess liquids with absorbent material.

  Rinse patient with warm water, 32° C to 35° C (90° F to 95° F), if possible.

  Wash patient with a mild liquid soap and large quantities of water.

  Refer to decontamination protocol in Section Three.

IMMEDIATE FIRST AID

- For overt releases:

  Ensure that adequate decontamination has been carried out as needed.

  If patient is not breathing, start artificial respiration, preferably with a demand-valve resuscitator or bag-valve-mask device or between resuscitator and bag, as trained. Perform CPR as necessary.

  Immediately flush contaminated eyes with gently flowing water.

  Do not induce vomiting. If vomiting occurs, lean patient forward or place on left side (head-down position, if possible) to maintain an open airway and prevent aspiration.

  Keep patient quiet and maintain normal body temperature.

  Obtain medical attention.

BASIC TREATMENT

- Establish a patent airway (oropharyngeal or nasopharyngeal airway, if needed). Suction if necessary.
- Watch for signs of respiratory insufficiency and assist ventilations if necessary.
- Administer oxygen by nonrebreather mask at 10 to 15 L/min.
- Monitor for pulmonary edema and treat if necessary (refer to pulmonary edema protocol in Section Three).
- Monitor for shock and treat if necessary (refer to shock protocol in Section Three).
- For eye contamination, flush eyes immediately with water. Irrigate each eye continuously with 0.9% saline (NS) during transport (refer to eye irrigation protocol in Section Three).

ADVANCED TREATMENT

- Consider orotracheal or nasotracheal intubation for airway control in the patient who is unconscious or is in severe respiratory distress.
- Positive-pressure ventilation techniques with a bag-valve-mask device may be beneficial.
- Monitor cardiac rhythm and treat arrhythmias as necessary (refer to cardiac protocol in Section Three).
- Start IV administration of D_5W TKO. Use 0.9% saline (NS) or lactated Ringer's (LR) if signs of hypovolemia are present. For hypotension with signs of hypovolemia, administer fluid cautiously. Watch for signs of fluid overload (refer to shock protocol in Section Three).
- Ribavirin treatment consists of an initial loading dose followed by 10 days of therapy. Also consider interferon, convalescent human plasma, and supportive treatment, including IV fluids, colloids, and management of coagulopathy. DIRECT PHYSICIAN ORDER ONLY.
- Use proparacaine hydrochloride to assist eye irrigation (refer to proparacaine hydrochloride protocol in Section Four).

INITIAL EMERGENCY DEPARTMENT CONSIDERATIONS

- Presumptive diagnosis should be made on signs and symptoms alone in the setting of a known or suspected outbreak. Useful diagnostics include CBC (demonstrating thrombocytopenia and leukopenia), urinalysis (demonstrating proteinuria and hematuria), blood culture, (which may identify virus during the acute phase of the disease), and ELISA testing (which may be useful for antigen detection or identification of IgM antibodies from blood or CSF).
- Local and state health department must be notified and involved in confirmatory testing.
- Mechanical ventilation and PEEP-assisted ventilation are indicated. Ventilation with small tidal volumes (6 ml/kg) has been associated with decreased mortality in patients with ARDS.
- Cautious fluid administration and vasopressors may be needed to treat hypotension.
- Antibiotic therapy is indicated to treat general infections. (Refer to antibiotic protocols in Section Four.)
- Transfusion of RBCs is indicated to maintain oxygen delivery if hemoglobin levels decrease.

- All suspected and confirmed cases should be immediately reported to the CDC through your local and state health departments.

SPECIAL CONSIDERATIONS

Infection Control

- Use contact precautions including strict hand washing, gloves, gowns, and splash precautions. Person-to-person transmission has been associated with acutely ill individuals, including cases of nosocomial CCHF transmission to health care providers through direct contact with blood or body fluids.

Vaccination

- There is currently no Crimean-Congo hemorrhagic fever vaccine available.

117

Food Safety Threat (*Escherichia coli* O157:H7, Salmonellosis, Shigellosis)

SUBSTANCE IDENTIFICATION

Foodborne illnesses result from microbes or toxins entering the body through the gastrointestinal tract by consumption of contaminated food or beverages. Hundreds of pathogens can cause these illnesses, including bacteria, viruses, toxins, and parasites. More than 200 different foodborne diseases afflict millions each year across the United States. Specific foodborne diseases each pose a variety of different symptoms. Therefore no single syndrome can define foodborne illness. The groups at greatest risk for severe complications from these illnesses include the elderly and small children.

Three foodborne diseases that are considered potential bioterrorism agents are: *Escherichia coli* O157:H7, salmonellosis, and shigellosis. An estimated 73,000 annual cases of *E. coli* O157:H7 infection occur in the United States, resulting in more than 2,000 hospitalizations and about 60 deaths. Salmonellosis is caused by ingestion of *Salmonella* bacilli. More than 2,000 *Salmonella* serotypes cause disease, including an estimated 1.4 million illnesses in the United States and over 500 fatalities. Although there are approximately 14,000 confirmed laboratory cases of shigellosis each year in the United States, actual estimates approach 500,000 cases annually.

Delineating an act of bioterrorism from background illnesses is a daunting task. The key to foodborne bioterrorism preparedness is an increased index of suspicion and an understanding of how to rapidly notify your local and state public health officials when cases arouse suspicion. The investigation that public health officials initiate will often characterize a common exposure, prevent additional cases, and identify responsible parties.

ROUTES OF EXPOSURE

Ingestion

TARGET ORGANS

Primary

Gastrointestinal system

Secondary

Renal system

Hepatic system

Cardiovascular system

Nervous system

Respiratory system

LIFE THREAT

Thrombocytopenia, hemolytic-uremic syndrome (HUS)

Chronic kidney failure

SIGNS AND SYMPTOMS BY SYSTEM

Cardiovascular: Myocardial dysfunction.

Respiratory: Acute respiratory distress syndrome, pleural effusions.

CNS: Headache, malaise, fatigue, seizure, stroke, psychosis, confusion, convulsions, and coma.

Gastrointestinal: Nonbloody or bloody diarrhea, abdominal cramping, hyperactive bowel sounds, nausea, vomiting, pancreatitis, and colonic necrosis.

Skin: Faint maculopapular rash on trunk may occur.

Metabolic: Fever.

Blood: Anemia or thrombocytopenia may occur.

Renal: Permanent renal impairment is possible.

Other: Dehydration.

INCUBATION PERIOD/SYMPTOM PROGRESSION

Incubation period is variable by pathogen and clinical course.
E. coli O157:H7 incubation period is typically 3 days (range of 1 to 8 days).
Salmonellosis incubation period is usually 5 to 21 days for enteric (typhoid or paratyphoid) fever and 6 to 48 hours for nontyphoidal gastroenteritis.
Shigellosis incubation period is 1 to 3 days.
E. coli O157:H7 infection may be asymptomatic. Initial symptoms include abdominal cramps, nausea, vomiting, diarrhea (bloody or non-bloody) and may include fever. These symptoms may progress to hemolytic-uremic syndrome (HUS) in children or thrombocytopenia in adults. Long-term permanent renal or neurological dysfunction is possible.
Typhoid or paratyphoid enteric salmonellosis begins with diarrhea or constipation followed by fever, abdominal tenderness, and flulike symptoms. It may progress to a severe bacteremia infection with high fever, headache, and weakness. This illness may persist for several weeks. In nearly a third of these illnesses, the patients develop a faint rash on the trunk, and a tenth of patients experience confusion and delirium.

Nontyphoidal salmonellosis includes an acute onset of diarrhea, nausea, vomiting, abdominal cramps, myalgias, malaise, chills, and fever. Stools may simply be loose or may be profuse and watery. In a small number of cases, bacteremia may develop. This is a particular risk among elderly or immune compromised patients.

Shigellosis infection begins with abdominal cramps, nausea, fever, and watery diarrhea. Over the following 48 to 72 hours the diarrhea may become bloody mucoid stools and the patient experiences urgency and tenesmus. This may be followed by high fever, hyperactive bowel sounds, abdominal tenderness, and rectal ulcerations. Untreated illness normally lasts about 1 week but may continue for up to 1 month.

MEDICAL CONDITIONS THAT MAY INCREASE RISK FOLLOWING EXPOSURE

Very young or very old age, preexisting chronic disease, immune compromising conditions

DECONTAMINATION

- These pathogens may be delivered via food contamination and do not require decontamination. Standard precautions are warranted. Surfaces, bedding, and dressings in contact with body fluids, as well as instruments used for invasive procedures on patients with known or suspected disease, should be sterilized with a sporicidal agent such as hypochlorite (bleach).

IMMEDIATE FIRST AID

- Do not induce vomiting. If vomiting occurs, lean patient forward or place on left side (head-down position, if possible) to maintain an open airway and prevent aspiration.
- Keep patient quiet and maintain normal body temperature.
- Obtain medical attention.

BASIC TREATMENT

- Establish a patent airway (oropharyngeal or nasopharyngeal airway, if needed). Suction if necessary.
- Watch for signs of respiratory insufficiency and assist ventilations if necessary.
- Administer oxygen by nonrebreather mask at 10 to 15 L/min.
- Monitor for shock and treat if necessary (refer to shock protocol in Section Three).

ADVANCED TREATMENT

- Consider orotracheal or nasotracheal intubation for airway control in the patient who is unconscious or is in severe respiratory distress.
- Positive-pressure ventilation techniques with a bag-valve-mask device may be beneficial.
- Monitor cardiac rhythm and treat arrhythmias as necessary (refer to cardiac protocol in Section Three).
- Start IV administration of D_5W TKO. Use 0.9% saline (NS) or lactated Ringer's (LR) if signs of hypovolemia are present. For hypotension with signs of hypovolemia, administer fluid cautiously. Consider vasopressors if patient is hypotensive with a normal fluid volume. Watch for signs of fluid overload (refer to shock protocol in Section Three).
- Antimicrobial therapy:
  - *E. coli* O157:H7 infection therapy is mostly supportive, with close monitoring for complications in high-risk patients. Antibiotics may increase the risk of HUS and should be avoided. They may reduce competing flora and allow overgrowth of *E. coli* O157:H7. Also avoid antidiarrheals, since they may also increase the risk of HUS. Hemodialysis or peritoneal dialysis may be needed.
  - Typhoid and paratyphoid enteric salmonellosis should be treated with antibiotics. The drugs of choice include ciprofloxacin, ceftriaxime, or imipenem. Alternative therapies include amoxicillin or TMP/SMX. However, some organisms are resistant to these and therapy should be adjusted according to results of sensitivity testing (refer to antibiotic protocols in Section Four).
  - Nontyphoidal salmonellosis requires only supportive therapy. Antibiotics should be avoided.
  - Shigellosis may be treated with antibiotics. The drug of choice is TMP/SMX DS. Alternative therapies include ciprofloxacin, levofloxacin, nalidixic acid (for children), and azithromycin (for drug-resistant organisms).

INITIAL EMERGENCY DEPARTMENT CONSIDERATIONS

- Presumptive diagnosis should be made on clinical presentation and the history of possible exposures. Stool cultures early in the course of illness are essential. Methylene blue staining of stool or rectal mucous samples will detect fecal white blood cells in over half of *E. coli* O157:H7 infections. Direct fluorescent antibody microscopy may be helpful. CBC often shows a left shift in shigellosis cases. Typhoid or paratyphoid enteric salmonellosis can also be diagnosed with cultures of blood, urine, bone marrow, GI secretions, and biopsy of skin rash.

SPECIAL CONSIDERATIONS

Noneffective Therapies

- Avoid antimicrobial therapy for *E. coli* O157:H7 and nontyphoidal salmonellosis.

Infection Control

- Use standard precautions (strict hand washing, gloves, and splash precautions). Person-to-person transmission is unlikely during routine patient care.

Vaccination

- A polyvalent vaccine has recently been developed for *E. coli* O157:H7. Initial tests have shown that it is safe and effectively increases antibody levels in humans. However, it is not widely available. There are also three vaccines for typhoid and paratyphoid enteric salmonellosis. They include a live, attenuated oral vaccine, a Vi capsular polysaccharide vaccine, and a heat-killed organism vaccine.

118

Glanders (*Burkholderia mallei*)

SUBSTANCE IDENTIFICATION

Glanders is primarily an equine disease caused by the aerobic, gram-negative non–spore-forming bacillus *Burkholderia mallei*. It naturally occurs in horses, donkeys, and mules. Human infections are rare but sometimes occur from handling infected animals. It is more common in Asia, the Middle East, and South America and typically occurs in veterinarians, slaughterhouse workers, and others who work with animals.

B. mallei is believed to have been used as a biological weapon against cavalry horses in World War I and on horses and humans during World War II. The occurrence of human cases in the absence of animal cases should raise suspicion of an intentional release. Aside from lab workers contracting glanders from occupational exposures, there have been no cases of human glanders in the United States for decades. In the case of an intentional release, it is expected to cause moderate morbidity and low mortality.

Human disease has been reported in three forms: pulmonary disease, a localized form (mucous membranes), and a rapidly fatal septicemic illness or a chronic disease condition (farcy). Acute infections are often fatal.

ROUTES OF EXPOSURE

Inhalation
Contact with mucous membranes
Compromised skin

TARGET ORGANS

Primary
Respiratory system
Gastrointestinal system
Eyes
Skin

Secondary
Nervous system
Cardiovascular system
Hepatic system
Lymphatic system
Blood

LIFE THREAT

Pneumonia, and septicemia.

SIGNS AND SYMPTOMS BY SYSTEM

Cardiovascular: Tachycardia and hypotension.

Respiratory: Pleuritic chest pain, dyspnea, and pneumonia.

CNS: Headache and fatigue.

Gastrointestinal: Abdominal pain, nausea, diarrhea, and mild splenomegaly.

Skin: Papular rash and profuse sweating. Localized skin infections with nodule formation.

Eye: Photophobia, lacrimation, and severe conjunctivitis.
Metabolic: Fever.
Blood: Mild leukocytosis or leukopenia.
Hepatic: Hepatic and spleen injury.
Other: Myalgia; cervical adenopathy; discharge from eyes, nose, and lips. Chronic infection may result in subcutaneous and intramuscular abscesses and visceral lesions.

INCUBATION PERIOD/SYMPTOM PROGRESSION

Incubation period is 10 to 14 days; it is longer in the chronic form of disease. The disease may present as either acute or chronic illness. The acute form of disease is more likely following an intentional aerosol release.

Following inhalation of organisms, the infection is carried through hematogenous spread. Septicemic symptoms may arise, including acute onset of fever, headache, photophobia, rigors, myalgias, diarrhea, night sweats, pleuritic pain, erythroderma sometimes accompanied by lesions, and leukopenia. Tachycardia, cervical adenopathy, and mild hepatomegaly or splenomegaly may also occur. The pulmonary form of disease may show CXR with miliary lesions, small lung abscesses, or bronchopneumonia. Infection of the mucous membranes may also present with nasal ulcers or nodules that secrete bloody discharge and may also lead to septicemia. The chronic form of the disease may be asymptomatic or include periodic symptoms and remission for years. Cutaneous and intramuscular abscesses on the limbs may also result in regional lymphadenopathy. Osteomyelitis, brain abscesses, or meningitis is also possible. Differential diagnosis for chronic disease may include TB or syphilis.

MEDICAL CONDITIONS THAT MAY INCREASE RISK FOLLOWING EXPOSURE

Chronic respiratory or immune compromising conditions

DECONTAMINATION

- If a covert release is successfully accomplished, patients seen days or weeks later will not pose a risk to providers and do not require decontamination. Patient decontamination is warranted only in the immediate aftermath of a known release. Surfaces, bedding, and dressings in contact with body fluids, as well as instruments used for invasive procedures on patients with known or suspected glanders, should be sterilized with a sporicidal agent such as hypochlorite (bleach).
- If a suspected overt release has occurred:
  - Wear respiratory protection such as an air purifying respirator with appropriate cartridges/filters or positive-pressure SCBA. Protective equipment such as gloves, suits, boot covers, and eye protection should be used. A qualified, experienced person should make decisions regarding the type of personal protective equipment necessary.
  - Delay entry into the suspected release area until trained personnel and proper protective equipment are available.
  - Remove patient from contaminated area.
  - Quickly remove and isolate patient's clothing, jewelry, and shoes.
  - Gently brush away dry particles and blot excess liquids with absorbent material.

- Rinse patient with warm water, 32° C to 35° C (90° F to 95° F), if possible.
- Wash patient with a mild liquid soap and large quantities of water.
- Refer to decontamination protocol in Section Three.

IMMEDIATE FIRST AID

- For overt releases:
  - Ensure that adequate decontamination has been carried out as needed.
  - If patient is not breathing, start artificial respiration, preferably with a demand-valve resuscitator or bag-valve-mask device, as trained. Perform CPR as necessary.
  - Immediately flush contaminated eyes with gently flowing water.
  - Do not induce vomiting. If vomiting occurs, lean patient forward or place on left side (head-down position, if possible) to maintain an open airway and prevent aspiration.
  - Keep patient quiet and maintain normal body temperature.
  - Obtain medical attention.

BASIC TREATMENT

- Establish a patent airway (oropharyngeal or nasopharyngeal airway, if needed). Suction if necessary.
- Watch for signs of respiratory insufficiency and assist ventilations if necessary.
- Administer oxygen by nonrebreather mask at 10 to 15 L/min.
- For eye contamination, flush eyes immediately with water. Irrigate each eye continuously with 0.9% saline (NS) during transport (refer to eye irrigation protocol in Section Three).

ADVANCED TREATMENT

- Consider orotracheal or nasotracheal intubation for airway control in the patient who is unconscious or is in severe respiratory distress.
- Positive-pressure ventilation techniques with a bag-valve-mask device may be beneficial.
- Monitor cardiac rhythm and treat arrhythmias as necessary (refer to cardiac protocol in Section Three).
- Start IV administration of D_5W TKO. Use 0.9% saline (NS) or lactated Ringer's (LR) if signs of hypovolemia are present. For hypotension with signs of hypovolemia, administer fluid cautiously. Consider vasopressors if patient is hypotensive with a normal fluid volume. Watch for signs of fluid overload (refer to shock protocol in Section Three)
- Antimicrobial therapy is indicated. However, efficacy in humans is questionable and sensitivity testing is essential. Severe infections may initially be treated with ceftazidime followed by one of the following: TMP 2 (trimethoprim 2), amoxicillin-clavulanate, or sulfadiazine. Localized infections, including pulmonary disease, are treated with one of the following: amoxicillin-clavulanate, tetracycline, sulfadiazine, or TMP 2. Alternative therapies include fluoroquinolones, doxycycline, and rifampin (refer to antibiotic protocols in Section Four).
- Use proparacaine hydrochloride to assist eye irrigation (refer to proparacaine hydrochloride protocol in Section Four).

INITIAL EMERGENCY DEPARTMENT CONSIDERATIONS

- Presumptive diagnosis should be made on signs and symptoms alone in the setting of a known or suspected outbreak. Chest radiograph may show miliary lesions, small lung abscesses, or bronchopneumonia. Gram stain of lesion exudates may show small gram-negative rods that stain irregularly with methylene blue. Blood cultures may be negative until the patient is moribund. Bacteria must be grown in a special culture media and are dangerous to lab workers.

- Laboratory work with *B. mallei* is designated as biosafety level 3. Complement fixation testing is considered positive when titers are ≥1:20. Other useful initial studies include ABGs, pulse oximetry, CBC with platelet count (mild leukocytosis with shift to the left or leukopenia), electrolytes, renal and liver function tests, and urinalysis.
- Antibiotic therapy is indicated. Amoxicillin-clavulanate, ceftazidime, tetracycline, sulfadiazine, or TMP 2 are effective in adult patients. Tetracycline is not recommended for pregnant women or children younger than 8 years of age. Alternative therapies include fluoroquinolones, doxycycline, and rifampin (refer to antibiotic protocols in Section Four).

SPECIAL CONSIDERATIONS

Infection Control

- Droplet precautions are recommended for patients with pulmonary disease (gloves, gown, mask, splash precautions, and strict hand washing). Contact precautions including gown and gloves are recommended if a patient has only skin lesions. Isolate patients and cohort with other confirmed glanders cases. Mask patients during transport. Sample aerosolization is possible in a lab setting. Biosafety level 3 precautions are required for sample handling

Vaccination

- No vaccine is currently available.

119

Hantavirus

SUBSTANCE IDENTIFICATION

Hantaviruses include several zoonotic viruses with rodents as a natural host. Normally these viruses are shed by rodents, exposing humans in poorly ventilated homes. Dried rodent feces or urine is aerosolized and inhaled by humans, resulting in Hantavirus pulmonary syndrome (HPS). There are at least three pathogenic Hantaviruses. Sin Nombre (no-name) virus is the most common form in North America. The host for Sin Nombre virus is the deer mouse. Other types include Black Creek Canal virus carried by the cotton rat, rice rat, or white-footed mouse and the Andes virus. The inhalational form of Hantavirus causes HPS that presents as a rapid-onset respiratory illness. Other Hantaviruses can affect the kidneys.

Three phases of the disease have been identified. The prodromal phase for HPS disease typically lasts 1 to 5 weeks and is characterized by a rapid onset of flulike symptoms. The cardiopulmonary phase is characterized by often-severe respiratory and cardiovascular complications. That is followed by the convalescent phase, characterized by improved pulmonary and cardiac function.

ROUTES OF EXPOSURE

Inhalation

TARGET ORGANS

Primary

Respiratory system

Secondary

Vascular system

Nervous system

Cardiovascular system

Gastrointestinal system

LIFE THREAT

Acute respiratory distress syndrome (ARDS) and cardiovascular collapse.

SIGNS AND SYMPTOMS BY SYSTEM

Cardiovascular: Tachycardia, dysrhythmias (commonly bradycardia, pulseless electrical activity, ventricular tachycardia, or ventricular fibrillation), hypotension and cardiovascular collapse. Septic shock may occur.

Respiratory: Tachypnea, dyspnea, rales, cough. Capillary leak syndrome leading to pulmonary edema and acute respiratory distress syndrome. CXR may be abnormal.

CNS: Headache, dizziness, malaise, persistent mental status changes.

Gastrointestinal: Nausea, vomiting, diarrhea, abdominal pain.

Skin: Cyanosis, erythemas on trunk and face, and petechiae over the upper trunk and on the soft palate.

Metabolic: Fever.

Hepatic: Liver damage with increased liver enzymes and creatinine.

Renal: Proteinuria without frank renal failure.

Blood: Elevated white blood cell count. Disseminated intravascular coagulation (DIC) may occur in late stages of the illness.
Other: Hyponatremia and metabolic acidosis. Joint and back pain.

INCUBATION PERIOD/SYMPTOM PROGRESSION

The incubation period for Hantavirus pulmonary syndrome is 1 to 5 weeks. Sudden onset of flu-like symptoms for 3 to 5 days, followed by rapid development of acute respiratory distress lasting 2 to 3 days for survivors.

MEDICAL CONDITIONS THAT MAY INCREASE RISK FOLLOWING EXPOSURE

Preexisting acute or chronic respiratory disease.

DECONTAMINATION

- If a covert release is successfully accomplished, patients seen days or weeks later will not pose a risk to providers and do not require decontamination. Patient decontamination is warranted only in the immediate aftermath of a known release.
- If a suspected overt release has occurred:
  - Wear respiratory protection such as an air-purifying respirator with appropriate cartridges/filters or positive-pressure SCBA. Protective equipment such as gloves, suits, boot covers, and eye protection should be used. A qualified, experienced person should make decisions regarding the type of personal protective equipment necessary.
  - Delay entry into the suspected release area until trained personnel and proper protective equipment are available.
  - Remove patient from contaminated area.
  - Quickly remove and isolate patient's clothing, jewelry, and shoes.
  - Gently brush away dry particles and blot excess liquids with absorbent material.
  - Rinse patient with warm water, 32° C to 35° C (90° F to 95° F), if possible.
  - Wash patient with a mild liquid soap and large quantities of water.
  - Refer to decontamination protocol in Section Three.

IMMEDIATE FIRST AID

- For overt releases:
  - Ensure that adequate decontamination has been carried out as needed.
  - If patient is not breathing, start artificial respiration, preferably with a demand-valve resuscitator or bag-valve-mask device, as trained. Perform CPR as necessary.
  - Immediately flush contaminated eyes with gently flowing water.
  - Do not induce vomiting. If vomiting occurs, lean patient forward or place on left side (head-down position, if possible) to maintain an open airway and prevent aspiration.
  - Keep patient quiet and maintain normal body temperature.
  - Obtain medical attention.

BASIC TREATMENT

- Establish a patent airway (oropharyngeal or nasopharyngeal airway, if needed). Suction if necessary.
- Watch for signs of respiratory insufficiency and assist ventilations if necessary.
- Administer oxygen by nonrebreather mask at 10 to 15 L/min.

- Monitor for pulmonary edema and treat if necessary (refer to pulmonary edema protocol in Section Three).
- Monitor for shock and treat if necessary (refer to shock protocol in Section Three).
- For eye contamination, flush eyes immediately with water. Irrigate each eye continuously with 0.9% saline (NS) during transport (refer to eye irrigation protocol in Section Three).

ADVANCED TREATMENT

- Consider orotracheal or nasotracheal intubation for airway control in the patient who is unconscious, has severe pulmonary edema, or is in severe respiratory distress.
- Positive-pressure ventilation techniques with a bag-valve-mask device may be beneficial.
- Monitor cardiac rhythm and treat arrhythmias as necessary (refer to cardiac protocol in Section Three).
- Consider drug therapy for pulmonary edema (refer to pulmonary edema protocol in Section Three).
- Start IV administration of D_5W TKO. Use 0.9% saline (NS) or lactated Ringer's (LR) if signs of hypovolemia are present. For hypotension with signs of hypovolemia, administer fluid cautiously. Consider vasopressors if patient is hypotensive with a normal fluid volume. Watch for signs of fluid overload (refer to shock protocol in Section Three).
- Use proparacaine hydrochloride to assist eye irrigation (refer to proparacaine hydrochloride protocol in Section Four).

INITIAL EMERGENCY DEPARTMENT CONSIDERATIONS

- Presumptive diagnosis should be made on signs and symptoms alone in the setting of a known or suspected outbreak. Useful initial studies include chest radiograph, ABGs, pulse oximetry, urinalysis, CBC (peripheral smear showing triad of thrombocytopenia, leukocytosis with a left shift in myeloid series, and large immunoblastic lymphocytes before hypoxia occurs is unique and characteristic of HPS), electrolytes, renal and liver function tests. Serology, PCR, or immunohistochemistry can confirm cases. A pulmonary artery catheter measuring mixed venous oxygen tension, pulmonary artery wedge pressure, and cardiac output should be used to monitor severely ill patients.
- Mechanical ventilation and PEEP-assisted ventilation are indicated. Ventilation with small tidal volumes (6 ml/kg) has been associated with decreased mortality in patients with ARDS.
- Cautious fluid administration and vasopressors may be needed to treat hypotension.
- Antibiotic therapy is indicated to treat general infections. (Refer to antibiotic protocols in Section Four.)
- Transfusion of RBCs is indicated to maintain oxygen delivery if hemoglobin levels decrease.
- Bradykinin antagonist salvage therapy in critically ill patients is available at the University of New Mexico.
- All suspected and confirmed cases should be immediately reported to the CDC through your local and state health departments. The CDC Hantavirus Task Force telephone number is (404) 639-1510.

SPECIAL CONSIDERATIONS

Noneffective Therapies

- Ribavirin has no clearly positive influence on patient outcome and is no longer included under CDC protocol. It is not effective in HPS.

Infection Control

- Use standard precautions, including strict hand washing, gloves, and splash precautions. Person-to-person transmission has not been associated with HPS cases in the United States. However, person-to-person transmission, including nosocomial transmission of Andes virus, was documented during an outbreak in Argentina and suspected to have occurred to a lesser extent during another outbreak in Chile associated with the same virus.

Vaccination

- There are currently no Hantavirus vaccines available.

120

Melioidosis (*Burkholderia pseudomallei*)

SUBSTANCE IDENTIFICATION

Melioidosis is a rare disease caused by the aerobic, gram-negative bacillus *Burkholderia pseudomallei*. This organism is normally found in soil and water throughout tropical regions. It is endemic in Southeast Asia and northern Australia and is also seen in the South Pacific, Africa, India, and the Middle East. Some isolated cases have occurred in Central and South America, but it is rarely found in North America. Human disease usually results from aspiration or ingestion or from contact of compromised skin with contaminated soil or water.

Many different forms of disease may result from *B. pseudomallei* exposure, including acute localized, pulmonary, septicemic, suppurative, and a range of subclinical infections. If the organism is used as a bioterrorism agent, it is more likely to be aerosolized, resulting in the pulmonary form of disease. However, the incubation period can range from 2 days to several years, making the trends in community illness following a release very difficult to characterize. An outbreak of pulmonary melioidosis may include illnesses ranging from mild bronchitis to severe pneumonia with or without acute lung abscesses.

ROUTES OF EXPOSURE

Inhalation or compromised skin

TARGET ORGANS

Primary

Respiratory system for aerosol exposure

Skin for contact exposure

Secondary

Nervous system

Gastrointestinal system

LIFE THREAT

Severe pneumonia and/or acute lung abscesses, septic shock

SIGNS AND SYMPTOMS BY SYSTEM

Cardiovascular: Tachycardia, dysrhythmias (commonly bradycardia, pulseless electrical activity, ventricular tachycardia or ventricular fibrillation), hypotension, and cardiovascular collapse. Septic shock may occur.

Respiratory: Bronchitis, productive or non-productive cough, dyspnea, pneumonia, acute lung abscesses. CXR may be abnormal with pneumonia, lung abscesses, miliary nodules, or cavitary lesions similar to TB.

CNS: Headache, malaise.

Gastrointestinal: Nausea, diarrhea, abdominal pain.

Skin: Pustules (septicemic disease), localized nodules or pustules (acute localized disease), skin and subcutaneous abscesses (chronic suppurative disease).

Metabolic: Fever.

Hepatic: Liver damage with increased liver enzymes and creatinine (chronic suppurative disease).
Blood: Elevated white blood cell count.
Other: Anorexia.

INCUBATION PERIOD/SYMPTOM PROGRESSION

The incubation period for melioidosis may be as little as 2 days. However, cases have been documented several years following the presumed exposure.

MEDICAL CONDITIONS THAT MAY INCREASE RISK FOLLOWING EXPOSURE

Preexisting acute or chronic respiratory disease.

DECONTAMINATION

- If a covert release is successfully accomplished, patients seen days or weeks later will not pose a risk to providers and do not require decontamination. Patient decontamination is warranted only in the immediate aftermath of a known release.
- If a suspected overt release has occurred:
  - Wear respiratory protection such as an air-purifying respirator with appropriate cartridges/filters or positive-pressure SCBA. Protective equipment such as gloves, suits, boot covers, and eye protection should be used. A qualified, experienced person should make decisions regarding the type of personal protective equipment necessary.
  - Delay entry into the suspected release area until trained personnel and proper protective equipment are available.
  - Remove patient from contaminated area.
  - Quickly remove and isolate patient's clothing, jewelry, and shoes.
  - Gently brush away dry particles and blot excess liquids with absorbent material.
  - Rinse patient with warm water, 32° C to 35° C (90° F to 95° F), if possible.
  - Wash patient with a mild liquid soap and large quantities of water.
  - Refer to decontamination protocol in Section Three.

IMMEDIATE FIRST AID

- For overt releases:
  - Ensure that adequate decontamination has been carried out as needed.
  - If patient is not breathing, start artificial respiration, preferably with a demand-valve resuscitator or bag-valve-mask device, as trained. Perform CPR as necessary.
  - Immediately flush contaminated eyes with gently flowing water.
  - Do not induce vomiting. If vomiting occurs, lean patient forward or place on left side (head-down position, if possible) to maintain an open airway and prevent aspiration.
  - Keep patient quiet and maintain normal body temperature.
  - Obtain medical attention.

BASIC TREATMENT

- Establish a patent airway (oropharyngeal or nasopharyngeal airway, if needed). Suction if necessary.
- Watch for signs of respiratory insufficiency and assist ventilations if necessary.
- Administer oxygen by nonrebreather mask at 10 to 15 L/min.

- Monitor for pulmonary edema and treat if necessary (refer to pulmonary edema protocol in Section Three).
- Monitor for shock and treat if necessary (refer to shock protocol in Section Three).
- For eye contamination, flush eyes immediately with water. Irrigate each eye continuously with 0.9% saline (NS) during transport (refer to eye irrigation protocol in Section Three).

ADVANCED TREATMENT

- Consider orotracheal or nasotracheal intubation for airway control in the patient who is unconscious or is in severe respiratory distress.
- Positive-pressure ventilation techniques with a bag-valve-mask device may be beneficial.
- Monitor cardiac rhythm and treat arrhythmias as necessary (refer to cardiac protocol in Section Three).
- Start IV administration of D_5W TKO. Use 0.9% saline (NS) or lactated Ringer's (LR) if signs of hypovolemia are present. For hypotension with signs of hypovolemia, administer fluid cautiously. Consider vasopressors if patient is hypotensive with a normal fluid volume. Watch for signs of fluid overload (refer to shock protocol in Section Three).
- Consider antimicrobial therapy. Treatment for 60 days may be required. Insufficient data exist describing the efficacy of antibiotic treatment in humans. The primary drugs of choice are ceftazidime-imipenem or amoxicillin-clavulanate. Alternative therapies include penicillin, doxycycline, azlocillin, ticarcillin-clavulanic acid, ceftriaxone, and aztreonam (refer to antibiotic protocols in Section Four).
- Use proparacaine hydrochloride to assist eye irrigation (refer to proparacaine hydrochloride protocol in Section Four).

INITIAL EMERGENCY DEPARTMENT CONSIDERATIONS

- Presumptive diagnosis should be made on clinical suspicion and history of potential exposure. CXR may be abnormal, with pneumonia, lung abscesses, miliary nodules, or cavitary lesions similar to those of TB. Culture blood, urine, or skin lesions.
- Mechanical ventilation and PEEP-assisted ventilation are indicated. Ventilation with small tidal volumes (6 ml/kg) has been associated with decreased mortality in patients with ARDS.
- Cautious fluid administration and vasopressors may be needed to treat hypotension.

SPECIAL CONSIDERATIONS

Infection Control

- Use standard precautions including strict hand washing, gloves, and splash precautions. Person-to-person transmission has not been associated with melioidosis. However, cases have been associated with sexual contact. In addition, aerosol-producing lab procedures may place lab workers at risk.

Vaccination

- There is currently no melioidosis vaccine available.

Plague *(Yersinia pestis)*

SUBSTANCE IDENTIFICATION

Plague is a disease caused by the anaerobic, gram-negative bacterium *Yersinia pestis*. The natural host for this organism is the wild rodent. Approximately 10 human plague cases occur naturally each year in the western United States. Human cases also occur in South America, and portions of Africa, Asia, and Europe. It is transmitted naturally from rodents to humans through flea bites. There are three common syndromes: *bubonic* (75% to 97% of all cases), *pneumonic* (<14% of all cases), and *septicemic* (<20% of all cases). The bubonic form of plague is the most likely form of the disease to be seen from naturally occurring infections. However, a terrorist attack could potentially involve the release of infected fleas, resulting in bubonic cases. Pneumonic plague would most commonly be associated with a bioterrorism attack. Person-to-person transmission is possible through airborne droplets from infected individuals. This potential transmission complicates the management of a large outbreak and poses significant infection control challenges.

Untreated pneumonic plague has a mortality rate approaching 100%. It spreads through the lymph system and may involve multiple organ systems. All forms of plague can progress to the septicemic or pneumonic forms of the disease.

ROUTES OF EXPOSURE

Inhalation
Skin and eye contact
Flea bites
Injection

TARGET ORGANS

Primary
Respiratory system
Secondary
Vascular system
Nervous system
Cardiovascular system
Gastrointestinal system

LIFE THREAT

Septic shock, acute respiratory distress syndrome (ARDS), disseminated intravascular coagulation (DIC), bacterial meningitis, and skin necrosis.

SIGNS AND SYMPTOMS BY SYSTEM

Cardiovascular: Tachycardia and circulatory collapse.

Respiratory: Tachypnea, productive cough, hemoptysis, dyspnea, abnormal breath sounds (rales and rhonchi). Acute respiratory distress syndrome may occur. CXR usually shows patchy bilateral infiltrates and/or consolidation.

CNS: Headache, nervousness, decreased level of consciousness, and coma. Meningitis and seizures may occur.

Gastrointestinal: Vomiting, diarrhea, abdominal pain.

Skin: Cyanosis, mottled skin, and petechiae. Tissue necrosis, especially of the appendages, may occur. Swollen lymph nodes (buboes) may occur with bubonic plague; they are not seen with pneumonic plague.
Metabolic: Fever.
Renal: Hematuria and proteinuria.
Blood: Elevated white blood cell count. Disseminated intravascular coagulation (DIC) may occur in late stages of the illness.
Other: Joint and lower back pain,

INCUBATION PERIOD/SYMPTOM PROGRESSION

Pneumonic Plague

The incubation period for pneumonic plague is 1 to 6 days (average 2 to 4 days)

Disease progresses rapidly from flulike symptoms with cough and hemoptysis to dyspnea, stridor, cyanosis, respiratory failure, circulatory collapse, and death.

MEDICAL CONDITIONS THAT MAY INCREASE RISK FOLLOWING EXPOSURE

Preexisting acute or chronic respiratory disease.

DECONTAMINATION

- If a covert release is successfully accomplished, patients seen days or weeks later will not pose a risk to providers and do not require decontamination. Patient decontamination is warranted only in the immediate aftermath of a known release. Surfaces, bedding, and dressings in contact with body fluids, as well as instruments used for invasive procedures on patients with known or suspected plague, should be sterilized with a sporicidal agent such as hypochlorite (bleach).
- If a suspected overt release has occurred:
  - Wear respiratory protection such as an air-purifying respirator with appropriate cartridges/filters or positive-pressure SCBA. Protective equipment such as gloves, suits, boot covers, and eye protection should be used. A qualified, experienced person should make decisions regarding the type of personal protective equipment necessary.
  - Delay entry into the suspected release area until trained personnel and proper protective equipment are available.
  - Remove patient from contaminated area.
  - Quickly remove and isolate patient's clothing, jewelry, and shoes.
  - Gently brush away dry particles and blot excess liquids with absorbent material.
  - Rinse patient with warm water, 32° C to 35° C (90° F to 95° F), if possible.
  - Wash patient with a mild liquid soap and large quantities of water.
  - Refer to decontamination protocol in Section Three.

IMMEDIATE FIRST AID

- For overt releases:
  - Ensure that adequate decontamination has been carried out as needed.
  - If patient is not breathing, start artificial respiration, preferably with a demand-valve resuscitator or bag-valve-mask device, as trained. Perform CPR as necessary.
  - Immediately flush contaminated eyes with gently flowing water.
  - Do not induce vomiting. If vomiting occurs, lean patient forward or place on left side (head-down position, if possible) to maintain an open airway and prevent aspiration.

- Keep patient quiet and maintain normal body temperature.
- Obtain medical attention.

BASIC TREATMENT

- Establish a patent airway (oropharyngeal or nasopharyngeal airway, if needed). Suction if necessary.
- Watch for signs of respiratory insufficiency and assist ventilations if necessary.
- Administer oxygen by nonrebreather mask at 10 to 15 L/min.
- Monitor for pulmonary edema and treat if necessary (refer to pulmonary edema protocol in Section Three).
- Monitor for shock and treat if necessary (refer to shock protocol in Section Three).
- Anticipate seizures and treat if necessary (refer to seizure protocol in Section Three).
- For eye contamination, flush eyes immediately with water. Irrigate each eye continuously with 0.9% saline (NS) during transport (refer to eye irrigation protocol in Section Three).

ADVANCED TREATMENT

- Consider orotracheal or nasotracheal intubation for airway control in the patient who is unconscious, has severe pulmonary edema, or is in severe respiratory distress.
- Positive-pressure ventilation techniques with a bag-valve-mask device may be beneficial.
- Consider drug therapy for pulmonary edema (refer to pulmonary edema protocol in Section Three).
- Monitor cardiac rhythm and treat arrhythmias as necessary (refer to cardiac protocol in Section Three).
- Start IV administration of D_5W TKO. Use 0.9% saline (NS) or lactated Ringer's (LR) if signs of hypovolemia are present. For hypotension with signs of hypovolemia, administer fluid cautiously. Consider vasopressors if patient is hypotensive with a normal fluid volume. Watch for signs of fluid overload (refer to shock protocol in Section Three).
- Treat seizures with diazepam (Valium) or lorazepam (Ativan) (refer to diazepam and lorazepam protocols in Section Four and seizure protocol in Section Three).
- Use proparacaine hydrochloride to assist eye irrigation (refer to proparacaine hydrochloride protocol in Section Four).

INITIAL EMERGENCY DEPARTMENT CONSIDERATIONS

- Presumptive diagnosis should be made on signs and symptoms alone in the setting of a known or suspected outbreak. Treatment should be initiated any time plague is suspected. Do not delay treatment while waiting on confirmatory testing results. Useful initial studies include chest radiograph, ABGs, pulse oximetry, CBC, electrolytes, renal and liver function tests, blood/sputum Gram stains and cultures (may not be positive for 48 hours), and antibody titer (hemagglutinating antibody titer rises in 8 to 14 days).
- Mechanical ventilation and PEEP-assisted ventilation may be needed.
- Fluid administration and vasopressors may be needed to treat hypotension.
- Antibiotic therapy is indicated. Streptomycin, gentamicin, doxycycline, ciprofloxacin, tetracycline, and chloramphenicol may be used. (Refer to antibiotic protocols in Section Four).

- Hemodialysis may be necessary in cases involving renal failure.
- All suspected and confirmed cases should be immediately reported to the CDC through your local and state health departments.
- Assistance can be obtained from the Center for Disease Control's plague center in Ft. Collins, Colorado: (970) 221-6450 or (970) 221-6418.

SPECIAL CONSIDERATIONS

Noneffective Therapies

- Third-generation cephalosporins.

Infection Control

Pneumonic plague: droplet isolation
Bubonic or septicemic plague: standard precautions

- Pneumonic plague is transmitted through respiratory droplets of infected patients. Management of suspected pneumonic plague patients should include droplet isolation through the use of private rooms, cohorting of confirmed cases, and masking of patients during transport. Isolation may be discontinued 48 hours after initiation of antimicrobial therapy if patient shows clinical improvement.
- Bubonic or septicemic plague: Standard precautions are adequate. Institute contact precautions if bubo is draining. Avoid surgical procedures that produce aerosols.

Vaccination

- Plague vaccine is no longer available in the United States. A killed, whole-cell vaccine was available in the United States until it was discontinued in 1998. It had very little efficacy against pneumonic plague. Research is currently under way exploring the development of a new vaccine.

Psittacosis *(Chlamydia psittaci)*

SUBSTANCE IDENTIFICATION

Psittacosis is an acute chlamydial disease caused by an intracellular pathogen, *Chlamydia psittaci*. The organism exists naturally in birds. Parakeets, parrots, and lovebirds are primary reservoirs but other breeds, including, poultry, pigeons, canaries, and sea birds, can be carriers. Human disease usually results from inhalation of dried droppings, secretions, and dust from the feathers of infected birds. Once inhaled, the organisms enter the blood stream and spread to the reticuloendothelial tissue. The resulting sequelae may include endocarditis, hepatitis, and neurological complications. In addition, severe pneumonia may occur, requiring intensive care support. Over the past decade less than 50 confirmed cases of this disease have been reported in the United States. Many more natural cases have likely occurred but were incorrectly diagnosed. A bioterrorism-related outbreak of psittacosis resulting from the aerosolization of *C. psittaci* would likely produce more severe cases than those observed in natural outbreaks.

ROUTES OF EXPOSURE

Inhalation

TARGET ORGANS

Primary

Respiratory system

Secondary

Nervous system

Gastrointestinal system

Cardiovascular system

Hepatic system

LIFE THREAT

Severe pneumonia, respiratory failure, and collapse; neurological complications such as meningitis, encephalitis, and seizures; endocarditis and hepatitis.

SIGNS AND SYMPTOMS BY SYSTEM

Cardiovascular: Bradycardia, pericarditis, or endocarditis with a negative culture.

Respiratory: Nonproductive cough within the first several days. Cough may become productive, include blood-tinged sputum, and progress to severe pneumonia requiring intensive care. Respiratory failure and collapse is possible. CXR is usually abnormal, with nodular, segmental, or lobular consolidation as well as miliary, patchy, or diffuse infiltrates.

CNS: Headache, malaise. May progress to a variety of abnormalities, including cranial nerve palsies, deafness, confusion, meningitis, encephalitis, and seizures.

Gastrointestinal: Nausea, diarrhea, abdominal pain, constipation (GI symptoms are not common).

Skin: Maculopapular rash referred to as "Horder's spots," with a pink, blanching presentation similar to the rose spots of typhoid fever.

Metabolic: High fever.

Hepatic: Hepatomegaly, hepatitis with jaundice.

Blood: Elevated white blood cell count; culture is possible but may pose particular risks to lab workers.

INCUBATION PERIOD/SYMPTOM PROGRESSION

The incubation period for psittacosis is typically 5 to 15 days.

Initial onset may be slowly progressing flulike symptoms. An initial nonproductive cough may become productive and include blood-tinged sputum. Frequently, bradycardia is present and a maculopapular skin rash may develop. Symptoms may progress to include respiratory failure, pericarditis, endocarditis, hepatitis, and severe neurological abnormalities such as encephalitis.

MEDICAL CONDITIONS THAT MAY INCREASE RISK FOLLOWING EXPOSURE

Preexisting acute or chronic respiratory disease.

DECONTAMINATION

- If a covert release is successfully accomplished, patients seen days or weeks later will not pose a risk to providers and do not require decontamination. Patient decontamination is warranted only in the immediate aftermath of a known release.
- If a suspected overt release has occurred:
  - Wear respiratory protection such as an air-purifying respirator with appropriate cartridges/filters or positive-pressure SCBA. Protective equipment such as gloves, suits, boot covers, and eye protection should be used. A qualified, experienced person should make decisions regarding the type of personal protective equipment necessary.
  - Delay entry into the suspected release area until trained personnel and proper protective equipment are available.
  - Remove patient from contaminated area.
  - Quickly remove and isolate patient's clothing, jewelry, and shoes.
  - Gently brush away dry particles and blot excess liquids with absorbent material.
  - Rinse patient with warm water, 32° C to 35° C (90° F to 95° F), if possible.
  - Wash patient with a mild liquid soap and large quantities of water.
  - Refer to decontamination protocol in Section Three.

IMMEDIATE FIRST AID

- For overt releases:
  - Ensure that adequate decontamination has been carried out as needed.
  - If patient is not breathing, start artificial respiration, preferably with a demand-valve resuscitator or bag-valve-mask device, as trained. Perform CPR as necessary.
  - Immediately flush contaminated eyes with gently flowing water.
  - Do not induce vomiting. If vomiting occurs, lean patient forward or place on left side (head-down position, if possible) to maintain an open airway and prevent aspiration.
  - Keep patient quiet and maintain normal body temperature.
  - Obtain medical attention.

BASIC TREATMENT

- Establish a patent airway (oropharyngeal or nasopharyngeal airway, if needed). Suction if necessary.

- Watch for signs of respiratory insufficiency and assist ventilations if necessary.
- Administer oxygen by nonrebreather mask at 10 to 15 L/min.
- Monitor for shock and treat if necessary (refer to shock protocol in Section Three).
- For eye contamination, flush eyes immediately with water. Irrigate each eye continuously with 0.9% saline (NS) during transport (refer to eye irrigation protocol in Section Three).

ADVANCED TREATMENT

- Consider orotracheal or nasotracheal intubation for airway control in the patient who is unconscious or is in severe respiratory distress.
- Positive-pressure ventilation techniques with a bag-valve-mask device may be beneficial.
- Monitor cardiac rhythm and treat arrhythmias as necessary (refer to cardiac protocol in Section Three).
- Start IV administration of D_5W TKO. Use 0.9% saline (NS) or lactated Ringer's (LR) if signs of hypovolemia are present. For hypotension with signs of hypovolemia, administer fluid cautiously. Consider vasopressors if patient is hypotensive with a normal fluid volume. Watch for signs of fluid overload (refer to shock protocol in Section Three).
- Antimicrobial therapy for psittacosis consists of a 10- to 21-day course of doxycycline or tetracycline. Erythromycin may be used also but is less effective (refer to antibiotic protocols in Section Four).
- Use proparacaine hydrochloride to assist eye irrigation (refer to proparacaine hydrochloride protocol in Section Four).

INITIAL EMERGENCY DEPARTMENT CONSIDERATIONS

- Presumptive diagnosis should be made on clinical suspicion and history of potential exposure. CXR is usually abnormal, with nodular, segmental, or lobular consolidation as well as miliary, patchy, or diffuse infiltrates. Lab tests include IgM microimmunofluorescence (MIF), blood or sputum cultures, and investigational diagnostics such as PCR, direct fluorescent antibody assay, and ELISA testing.
- Mechanical ventilation and PEEP-assisted ventilation are indicated. Ventilation with small tidal volumes (6 ml/kg) has been associated with decreased mortality in patients with ARDS.
- Cautious fluid administration and vasopressors may be needed to treat hypotension.

SPECIAL CONSIDERATIONS

Infection Control

- Use droplet precautions including strict hand washing, gloves, gown, mask, and splash precautions. Suspected psittacosis patients should be isolated and confirmed patients may be cohorted. Person-to-person transmission has been documented. Therefore, patients suspected of having the disease must be isolated and should wear a mask when being transported.

Vaccination

- There is currently no psittacosis vaccine available.

123

Q Fever *(Coxiella burnetii)*

SUBSTANCE IDENTIFICATION

Q fever (query fever) is an acute febrile, zoonotic disease caused by exposure to the rickettsia species *Coxiella burnetii*. It is a ubiquitous organism found on every continent and is a common disease in farm animals (goats, sheep, and cows). It also infects dogs, cats, birds, rodents, and ticks. Animals are frequently asymptomatic carriers and shed large quantities of organisms in placental tissue at parturition. Human Q fever is rare but sometimes occurs in veterinarians, butchers, and farmers. It is transmitted via inhalation of aerosolized particles from body fluids, tissues, or excreta of infected animals, through direct contact with contaminated materials, and through drinking contaminated milk. It also can occur in endemic areas in individuals with no identifiable direct animal contact. Q fever infections can occur as an acute or chronic disease. The incidence is much greater than reported due to the mildness of the self-limiting, flulike illness.

Q fever could be used as a biological weapon and would likely be aerosolized and result in disease similar to naturally occurring cases. Death is rare regardless of treatment. *C. burnetii* organisms can persist in the environment for many years in contaminated dust or aerosols. As little as one organism can cause disease. Person-to-person transmission is rare, but contaminated clothing may pose a risk.

ROUTES OF EXPOSURE

Inhalation
Ingestion
Skin or eye contact
Arthropod vector (tickborne)

TARGET ORGANS

Primary
Respiratory system
Secondary
Cardiovascular system
Gastrointestinal system
Hepatic system
Nervous system
Skin

LIFE THREAT

Q fever is an incapacitating agent that normally presents as a mild flulike illness. However, it can progress to atypical pneumonia and in rare cases lead to hepatitis, endocarditis, meningitis, and osteomyelitis.

SIGNS AND SYMPTOMS BY SYSTEM

Cardiovascular: Bradycardia, myocarditis, pericarditis, endocarditis.

Respiratory: Pleuritic chest pain, nonproductive cough, sore throat, rales, atypical pneumonia.

CNS: Severe headache, malaise, fatigue, confusion, meningitis.

Gastrointestinal: Abdominal pain, nausea, vomiting, diarrhea, constipation,.
Skin: Sweats, no rash.
Eye: Eye irritation, optic neuritis.
Metabolic: Fever.
Renal: Hematuria, renal failure.
Hepatic: Transient liver injury, granulomatous hepatitis, spleen damage.
Other: Weight loss, anorexia, myalgia, placental infection, abortions, premature births, and low-birth-weight infants sometimes reported in women with infections during pregnancy.

INCUBATION PERIOD/SYMPTOM PROGRESSION

The incubation period for inhalational illness is 10 to 40 days (20-day average). This period varies according to the dose received when exposed. Greater exposures can substantially decrease incubation periods.

The initial illness consists of sudden flulike symptoms including headache, high fever, chills, fatigue, malaise, myalgia, and anorexia. These symptoms may progress to atypical pneumonia or less often to hepatitis. By the end of the first week of illness, about one quarter of patients will experience chest pain, cough, and rales. A small proportion of cases may progress to endocarditis, meningitis, encephalitis, or osteomyelitis. Death is a very rare outcome regardless of treatment. Q fever is normally a benign condition that resolves in less than 2 weeks. A chronic postacute Q fever syndrome may last for several years after exposure if it is not treated.
Q fever may also present in a chronic form with or without an initial acute illness. It occurs in approximately 5% of patients.

MEDICAL CONDITIONS THAT MAY INCREASE RISK FOLLOWING EXPOSURE

Preexisting chronic kidney disease or valvular heart disease, history of vascular graft, transplant recipients, cancer patients, and immunocompromised patients such as HIV-infected patients.

DECONTAMINATION

- If a covert release is successfully accomplished, patients seen days or weeks later will not pose a risk to providers and do not require decontamination. Patient decontamination is warranted only in the immediate aftermath of a known release. Surfaces, bedding, and dressings in contact with body fluids, as well as instruments used for invasive procedures on patients with known or suspected Q fever, should be sterilized with a sporicidal agent such as hypochlorite (bleach).
- If a suspected overt release has occurred:
  - Wear respiratory protection such as an air-purifying respirator with appropriate cartridges/filters or positive-pressure SCBA. Protective equipment such as gloves, suits, boot covers, and eye protection should be used. A qualified, experienced person should make decisions regarding the type of personal protective equipment necessary.
  - Delay entry into the suspected release area until trained personnel and proper protective equipment are available.
  - Remove patient from contaminated area.
  - Quickly remove and isolate patient's clothing, jewelry, and shoes.
  - Gently brush away dry particles and blot excess liquids with absorbent material.
  - Rinse patient with warm water, 32° C to 35° C (90° F to 95° F), if possible.

- Wash patient with a mild liquid soap and large quantities of water.
- Refer to decontamination protocol in Section Three.

IMMEDIATE FIRST AID

- For overt releases:
  - Ensure that adequate decontamination has been carried out as needed.
  - If patient is not breathing, start artificial respiration, preferably with a demand-valve resuscitator, bag-valve-mask device, or pocket mask, as trained. Perform CPR as necessary.
  - Immediately flush contaminated eyes with gently flowing water.
  - Do not induce vomiting. If vomiting occurs, lean patient forward or place on left side (head-down position, if possible) to maintain an open airway and prevent aspiration.
  - Keep patient quiet and maintain normal body temperature.
  - Obtain medical attention.

BASIC TREATMENT

- Establish a patent airway (oropharyngeal or nasopharyngeal airway, if needed). Suction if necessary.
- Watch for signs of respiratory insufficiency and assist ventilations if necessary.
- Administer oxygen by nonrebreather mask at 10 to 15 L/min.
- For eye contamination, flush eyes immediately with water. Irrigate each eye continuously with 0.9% saline (NS) during transport (refer to eye irrigation protocol in Section Three).

ADVANCED TREATMENT

- Consider orotracheal or nasotracheal intubation for airway control in the patient who is unconscious or is in severe respiratory distress.
- Positive-pressure ventilation techniques with a bag-valve-mask device may be beneficial.
- Monitor cardiac rhythm and treat arrhythmias as necessary (refer to cardiac protocol in Section Three).
- Start IV administration of D_5W TKO. Use 0.9% saline (NS) or lactated Ringer's (LR) if signs of hypovolemia are present. For hypotension with signs of hypovolemia, administer fluid cautiously. Watch for signs of fluid overload (refer to shock protocol in Section Three).
- Early antibiotic therapy is recommended. Drugs of choice include doxycycline, tetracycline, ciprofloxacin, ofloxacin, and pefloxacin. The course of treatment is normally 2 to 3 weeks. Treatment of Q fever endocarditis includes up to 3 years of drug therapy using doxycycline and either rifampin or ciprofloxacin (refer to antibiotic protocols in Section Four).
- Use proparacaine hydrochloride to assist eye irrigation (refer to proparacaine hydrochloride protocol in Section Four).

INITIAL EMERGENCY DEPARTMENT CONSIDERATIONS

- Presumptive diagnosis should be made on signs and symptoms alone in the setting of a known or suspected outbreak. Differential diagnosis includes *Mycoplasma*, *Legionella*, and *Chlamydia* infection, tularemia, and plague. CXR may show patchy pneumonitis. Acute and convalescent serology can confirm diagnosis. Confirmatory serology is indirect fluorescence antibody (IFA) for detection of IgM antibodies.

- There are two antigenic phases of the disease. During Phase I, the early days of an acute infection, the antibody level may be low. During Phase II of acute infection, usually in the second week of illness, the antibody levels jump by several orders of magnitude. In chronic infection, the reverse is true.
- Do not attempt to culture blood, sputum, or urine.
- Other useful initial studies include ABGs, pulse oximetry, CBC with platelet count, electrolytes, renal and liver function tests, and urinalysis. Laboratory work with *C. burnetii* is designated as biosafety level 3.
- Antibiotic therapy is indicated. Doxycycline, tetracycline, ofloxacin, pefloxacin are effective in adult patients. (Refer to antibiotic protocols in Section Four.)

SPECIAL CONSIDERATIONS

Infection Control

- Use standard precautions (gloves, strict handwashing, etc.). Person-to-person transmission is not known to occur. Barrier nursing techniques should be utilized. However, contaminated clothing is believed to pose a risk as a source of infection and should be appropriately handled. (NOTE: This is not an issue if the exposure is discovered retrospectively.) *C. burnetii* is a highly stable organism and may be resistant to heat and some disinfectants.

Vaccination

- There is currently no Q fever vaccine available.

124

Ricin Toxin

SUBSTANCE IDENTIFICATION

Ricin is a highly potent phytotoxin found in the seeds of the castor bean plant (*Ricinus communis*). Castor beans are grown around the world and are pressed to make castor oil. Ricin is present in the waste "mash" left over from the process. In the body it alters ribosomal RNA-blocking protein synthesis, resulting in the death of infected cells. It has some medical applications in cancer treatment to kill abnormal cells. An accidental exposure to ricin is very unlikely. Any case of ricin poisoning should be assumed to be the result of a deliberate act. Ricin can be processed for delivery as a powder, liquid, pellet, or dissolved in water. It is a very stable substance that is not affected significantly by extreme heat or cold temperatures. Large amounts of agent would be needed to cover a significant area. Patients may be exposed by inhalation, ingestion, injection, or skin absorption. The effects of poisoning depend on the route of exposure.

ROUTES OF EXPOSURE

Inhalation
Ingestion
Injection
Skin absorption if mixed with absorbable solvent

TARGET ORGANS

Dependent on route of exposure

Primary

Respiratory system (inhalation)
Gastrointestinal system (ingestion)
Skin and muscle (injection/absorption)

Secondary

Nervous system
Cardiovascular system
Gastrointestinal system
Renal system
Hepatic system

LIFE THREAT

Necrosis of upper and lower respiratory system, pulmonary edema, cyanosis, and acute respiratory distress syndrome (ARDS) with inhalation exposure. Gastrointestinal damage with fluid loss leading to shock with ingestion exposure. Also, cytotoxic effects on the liver, CNS, kidneys, and adrenal glands may occur. Death usually occurs on the third day or later after exposure.

SIGNS AND SYMPTOMS BY SYSTEM

Cardiovascular: Low blood pressure, cardiovascular collapse, shock.

Respiratory (inhalation exposure): Tightness of the chest, difficulty breathing, upper and lower respiratory inflammation and necrosis, pulmonary edema, acute respiratory distress syndrome (ARDS).

CNS: Headache, hallucinations, seizures, decreased level of consciousness.
Gastrointestinal (ingestion exposure): Gastrointestinal lesions with abdominal pain, nausea, vomiting, GI hemorrhage with hematemesis and hematochezia.
Metabolic: Fever.
Renal (ingestion exposure): Renal failure, kidney necrosis, damage to adrenal glands.
Hepatic (ingestion exposure): Elevation of hepatic enzymes, liver necrosis.
Other: Arthralgias, cyanosis. Redness and pain of skin and eyes, local tissue and muscle necrosis (contact exposure).

INCUBATION PERIOD/SYMPTOM PROGRESSION

For inhalation illness the incubation period is 18 to 24 hours, with acute onset of flulike symptoms in 4 to 8 hours followed by respiratory inflammation and pulmonary edema. ARDS and respiratory failure are likely within 36 to 72 hours. The incubation period for ingestion is about 2 hours after exposure. Initial GI symptoms include abdominal pain, nausea, vomiting, and bloody diarrhea. The patient may then proceed to shock and death or make a temporary recovery for 1 to 5 days before presenting with liver, spleen, kidney, and CNS effects.

MEDICAL CONDITIONS THAT MAY INCREASE RISK FOLLOWING EXPOSURE

Preexisting chronic diseases of any exposed major body system may increase ricin intoxication susceptibility and severity.

DECONTAMINATION

- If a covert release is successfully accomplished, patients seen days later will not pose a risk to providers and do not require decontamination. Patient decontamination is warranted only in the immediate aftermath of a known release. Surfaces, bedding, and dressings in contact with body fluids, as well as instruments used for invasive procedures on patients with known or suspected ricin exposure should be sterilized with a sporicidal agent such as hypochlorite (bleach).
- If a suspected overt release has occurred:
  - Wear respiratory protection such as an air-purifying respirator with appropriate cartridges/filters or positive-pressure SCBA. Protective equipment such as gloves, suits, boot covers, and eye protection should be used. A qualified, experienced person should make decisions regarding the type of personal protective equipment necessary.
  - Delay entry into the suspected release area until trained personnel and proper protective equipment are available.
  - Remove patient from contaminated area.
  - Quickly remove and isolate patient's clothing, jewelry, and shoes.
  - Gently brush away dry particles and blot excess liquids with absorbent material.
  - Rinse patient with warm water, 32° C to 35° C (90° F to 95° F), if possible.
  - Wash patient with a mild liquid soap and large quantities of water.
  - Refer to decontamination protocol in Section Three.

IMMEDIATE FIRST AID

- For overt releases:
  - Ensure that adequate decontamination has been carried out as needed.

- If patient is not breathing, start artificial respiration, preferably with a demand-valve resuscitator, bag-valve-mask device, or pocket mask, as trained. Perform CPR as necessary.
- Immediately flush contaminated eyes with gently flowing water.
- Do not induce vomiting. If vomiting occurs, lean patient forward or place on left side (head-down position, if possible) to maintain an open airway and prevent aspiration.
- Keep patient quiet and maintain normal body temperature.
- Obtain medical attention.

BASIC TREATMENT

- Establish a patent airway (oropharyngeal or nasopharyngeal airway, if needed). Suction if necessary.
- Watch for signs of respiratory insufficiency and assist ventilations if necessary.
- Administer oxygen by nonrebreather mask at 10 to 15 L/min.
- Monitor for pulmonary edema and treat if necessary (refer to pulmonary edema protocol in Section Three).
- Monitor for shock and treat if necessary (refer to shock protocol in Section Three).
- For eye contamination, flush eyes immediately with water. Irrigate each eye continuously with 0.9% saline (NS) during transport (refer to eye irrigation protocol in Section Three).

ADVANCED TREATMENT

- Consider orotracheal or nasotracheal intubation for airway control in the patient who is unconscious, has severe pulmonary edema, or is in severe respiratory distress.
- Positive-pressure ventilation techniques with a bag-valve-mask device may be beneficial.
- Consider drug therapy for pulmonary edema (refer to pulmonary edema protocol in Section Three).
- Monitor cardiac rhythm and treat arrhythmias as necessary (refer to cardiac protocol in Section Three.
- Start IV administration of D_5W TKO. Use 0.9% saline (NS) or lactated Ringer's (LR) if signs of hypovolemia are present. For hypotension with signs of hypovolemia, administer fluid cautiously. Watch for signs of fluid overload (refer to shock protocol in Section Three).
- Treatment is based on route of exposure and is mostly supportive. No antidote exists.
- If route of exposure is ingestion, use activated charcoal, magnesium citrate, and gastric lavage. In addition to suspected ingestion, consider GI decontamination for suspected large aerosol exposures.
- Use proparacaine hydrochloride to assist eye irrigation (refer to proparacaine hydrochloride protocol in Section Four).

INITIAL EMERGENCY DEPARTMENT CONSIDERATIONS

- Presumptive diagnosis should be made on signs and symptoms alone in the setting of a known or suspected outbreak. Lab and radiological test results are not specific. Collect serum and respiratory secretions for antigen detection. ELISA testing for ricin-specific antibodies and PCR testing for castor plant DNA can be performed. Other useful studies include ABGs, pulse oximetry, CXR, CBC with differential, and electrolytes. Renal and liver function tests should be monitored closely.

- Mechanical ventilation and PEEP-assisted ventilation may be needed in cases resulting in pulmonary involvement.

SPECIAL CONSIDERATIONS

Infection Control

- Standard precautions are adequate (strict handwashing, gloves, and splash precautions). Ricin is an intoxicant and is not transmitted from person-to-person.

Vaccination

- No vaccine is currently available.

125 Smallpox (Variola Major, Variola Minor)

SUBSTANCE IDENTIFICATION

Smallpox disease has claimed more lives than any other infectious disease in human history. It is caused by variola viruses, which are members of the Orthopoxvirus family. The only known reservoirs for these organisms are research lab freezers. The disease was eradicated in the 1970s through a WHO-sponsored campaign. However, it still remains a threat as a bioterrorism agent, and a single confirmed case today would be considered an international public health emergency.

There are two forms of this virus: variola major and variola minor. Variola major is the most likely form of the organism to be used as a weapon. It was the most common form seen in historical epidemics and has a mortality of approximately 30%. Variola minor is a less common organism with a very low mortality of <1%. The disease is transmitted person-to-person through inhalation or direct contact with viral particles. Following exposure, there is usually a 2-week asymptomatic incubation period (7 to 17 days). This is followed by a prodromal illness characterized by acute flulike symptoms for 2 to 5 days. At the end of the prodromal period, the patient becomes infectious and the characteristic, centrifugal macular rash develops. It quickly becomes papular, pustular, and then scabs over. The scabs separate in 2 to 3 weeks, signaling the end of the period of communicability. Severe scarring is common. Other complications of the disease may include encephalitis, secondary bacterial infections, conjunctivitis, and blindness. Most deaths occur by the second week as a result of massive inflammation and toxemia.

ROUTES OF EXPOSURE

Inhalation
Contact

TARGET ORGANS

Primary
Respiratory system
Mucosal membranes
Skin
Secondary
Nervous system
Cardiovascular system
Gastrointestinal system

LIFE THREAT

Massive inflammation, toxemia, encephalitis, or secondary bacterial infections

SIGNS AND SYMPTOMS BY SYSTEM

Cardiovascular: Tachycardia and septic shock may occur.

Respiratory: Pharyngitis, occasional cough and bronchitis; pneumonia is rare.

CNS: Headache, malaise, encephalitis, delirium in adults, seizures in children.
Gastrointestinal: Nausea, vomiting, diarrhea, abdominal pain.
Skin: Early erythematous, measles-like rash in 10% of patients; typical smallpox skin rash begins on the forehead and upper arms, spreading to the trunk; rash is centrifugally focused on head, arms, and legs. It is important to note that the palms and soles are not spared from lesions. The lesions are hard and feel like a pellet under the skin. In addition, they are extremely painful. Although they are of different size, the lesions are all in the same stage of development.
Eyes: Conjunctivitis, blindness.
Metabolic: Fever.
Other: The virus is systemic but does not normally involve other organ systems. Symptoms are more severe in the malignant or hemorrhagic form of the disease and include hemorrhages into the skin and mucous membranes.

INCUBATION PERIOD/SYMPTOM PROGRESSION

The incubation period for smallpox is 7 to 17 days (average 12 days). The incubation period is usually symptom free. It is followed by a 2- to 5-day flulike prodromal illness.

Symptoms include fever, malaise, headache, backache, chills, rigors, abdominal pain, vomiting, and diarrhea. At the end of the prodromal period, the patient becomes infectious and the characteristic, centrifugal macular rash develops, which usually begins on the forehead and upper arms, spreading to the trunk. The rash is centrifugally focused on head, arms, and legs. The palms and soles are not spared from lesions. The lesions are hard and feel like a pellet under the skin. They are extremely painful. Although they are different in size, the lesions are all in the same stage of development. Crusting of the lesions begins at day 8 or 9 of the illness. Scabs separate over the following 2 to 3 weeks. When all scabs have separated, infectiousness of the patient ends. Severe scarring and pitting of the skin is common. Other complications of the disease may include encephalitis, secondary bacterial infections, conjunctivitis, and blindness. Most deaths occur by the second week as the result of massive inflammation and toxemia. The presentation described is classical smallpox and accounts for over 90% of smallpox cases. However, there are two less common variants of disease: malignant (flat) and hemorrhagic.

The malignant, or flat, smallpox has a velvety atypical rash. The lesions do not completely develop but are so densely clustered that skin resembles crepe rubber. Bleeding into the skin may also occur. This form of disease has a very high (>90%) mortality. There is also a uniformly fatal, hemorrhagic form of smallpox that is characterized by a diffuse erythematous rash, leading to petechiae and hemorrhages into the skin and mucous membranes. The malignant and hemorrhagic forms of smallpox usually cause death within 1 week.

MEDICAL CONDITIONS THAT MAY INCREASE RISK FOLLOWING EXPOSURE

Preexisting acute or chronic immune compromising conditions.

DECONTAMINATION

- If a covert release is successfully accomplished, patients seen days or weeks later will not pose a risk to providers and do not require decontamination. Patient decontamination is warranted only in the immediate aftermath of a known release. However, isolation of patients with suspected disease is essential.

- If a suspected overt release has occurred or if individuals are identified as recently exposed to infectious patients:
  - Wear respiratory protection such as an air-purifying respirator with appropriate cartridges/filters or positive-pressure SCBA. Protective equipment such as gloves, suits, boot covers, and eye protection should be used. A qualified, experienced person should make decisions regarding the type of personal protective equipment necessary.
  - Delay entry into the suspected release area until trained personnel and proper protective equipment are available.
  - Remove patient from contaminated area.
  - Quickly remove and isolate patient's clothing, jewelry, and shoes. Double-bag soiled clothing or dressings in a clearly labeled leak-proof bag. Material should be carefully handled and stored. Consider autoclaving or incinerating.
  - Gently brush away dry particles and blot excess liquids with absorbent material.
  - Rinse patient with warm water, 32° C to 35° C (90° F to 95° F), if possible.
  - Wash patient with a mild liquid soap and large quantities of water.
  - Refer to decontamination protocol in Section Three.

IMMEDIATE FIRST AID

- For overt releases:
  - Ensure that adequate decontamination has been carried out as needed.
  - If patient is not breathing, start artificial respiration, preferably with a demand-valve resuscitator or bag-valve-mask device, as trained. Perform CPR as necessary.
  - Immediately flush contaminated eyes with gently flowing water.
  - Do not induce vomiting. If vomiting occurs, lean patient forward or place on left side (head-down position, if possible) to maintain an open airway and prevent aspiration.
  - Keep patient quiet and maintain normal body temperature.
  - Obtain medical attention.

BASIC TREATMENT

- Establish a patent airway (oropharyngeal or nasopharyngeal airway, if needed). Suction if necessary.
- Watch for signs of respiratory insufficiency and assist ventilations if necessary.
- Administer oxygen by nonrebreather mask at 10 to 15 L/min.
- Monitor for pulmonary edema and treat if necessary (refer to pulmonary edema protocol in Section Three).
- Monitor for shock and treat if necessary (refer to shock protocol in Section Three).
- For eye contamination, flush eyes immediately with water. Irrigate each eye continuously with 0.9% saline (NS) during transport (refer to eye irrigation protocol in Section Three).

ADVANCED TREATMENT

- Consider orotracheal or nasotracheal intubation for airway control in the patient who is unconscious, has severe pulmonary edema, or is in severe respiratory distress.

- Positive-pressure ventilation techniques with a bag-valve-mask device may be beneficial.
- Consider drug therapy for pulmonary edema (refer to pulmonary edema protocol in Section Three).
- Monitor cardiac rhythm and treat arrhythmias as necessary (refer to cardiac protocol in Section Three).
- Start IV administration of D_5W TKO. Use 0.9% saline (NS) or lactated Ringer's (LR) if signs of hypovolemia are present. For hypotension with signs of hypovolemia, administer fluid cautiously. Consider vasopressors if patient is hypotensive with a normal fluid volume. Watch for signs of fluid overload (refer to shock protocol in Section Three).
- There is no specific treatment for smallpox. Vaccination of exposed individuals within 4 days of exposure may lessen the severity of the illness. Cidofovir has shown some effectiveness against orthopox viruses but has not been used to treat human smallpox. It also has some serious side effects such as renal failure.
- Use proparacaine hydrochloride to assist eye irrigation (refer to proparacaine hydrochloride protocol in Section Four).

INITIAL EMERGENCY DEPARTMENT CONSIDERATIONS

- Presumptive diagnosis should be made on signs and symptoms alone in the setting of a known or suspected outbreak. As quickly as possible, identify and vaccinate everyone exposed to the primary case. This will reduce the severity of illness among those infected. Monitor exposed individuals for 17 days. If fever or rash appears, immediately isolate them until diagnosis is accomplished.
- Suspected cases of smallpox must be strictly isolated, and all specimens should be collected and processed by local or state health department staff. Only recently vaccinated workers should be allowed to acquire and handle samples. The CDC must also be notified and involved.
- Initial testing includes electron microcopy of vesicle fluid at a reference lab. This can quickly rule out non-orthopox viruses. Confirmation of *variola* as the specific virus may be accomplished by polymerase chain reaction (PCR) and by antibody essays.
- Rapid identification and vaccination of exposed individuals, isolation of suspected cases, and strict infection control measures are essential to limit the potential transmission of disease. With no specific treatment available, extensive supportive care may be needed for smallpox patients. Consider antiviral drugs such as cidofovir in confirmed cases.
- Mechanical ventilation and PEEP-assisted ventilation are indicated. Ventilation with small tidal volumes (6 ml/kg) has been associated with decreased mortality in patients with ARDS.
- Cautious fluid administration and vasopressors may be needed to treat hypotension.
- Antibiotic therapy is indicated to treat general infections. (Refer to antibiotic protocols in Section Four.)
- Transfusion of RBCs is indicated to maintain oxygen delivery if hemoglobin levels decrease.
- All suspected and confirmed cases should be immediately reported to the CDC through your local and state health departments.

SPECIAL CONSIDERATIONS

Infection Control

- Use airborne, droplet, and contact precautions, including strict hand washing, gown, gloves, and N-95 respirator or equivalent. Smallpox usually spreads person-to-person via respiratory droplets or direct contact. Airborne exposures may also occur, particularly among smallpox patients with a cough. Maintain strict isolation and cohort patients with confirmed disease in negative-pressure rooms. Take additional precautions when handling contaminated materials such as linens. Consider cremation of deceased smallpox patients.

Vaccination

- Many variants of smallpox vaccine are available. All are attenuated-strain vaccinia viruses administered using a bifurcated needle technique. Throughout history, this vaccine has been fully protective in all age groups when a good "take" is observed. A good take includes the development of a small pustule and scab at the vaccination site. The vaccine also may be used after exposure to reduce the severity of smallpox disease among exposed individuals. However, the vaccine must be given within 3 days of exposure; if given after exposure, it may not prevent disease. Smallpox vaccine has severe side effects among certain populations, including immunocompromised individuals, pregnant women, infants younger than 1 year of age, and those with acute or chronic skin conditions such as eczema.

Staphylococcal Enterotoxin B (*Staphylococcus aureus*)

SUBSTANCE IDENTIFICATION

Staphylococcal enterotoxin B (SEB) is a pyrogenic toxin produced by *Staphylococcus aureus*. It is usually associated with foodborne illnesses that result from improper food handling practices. Ingested SEB can cause a severe, self-limiting illness that includes vomiting, abdominal pain, and diarrhea lasting 6 to 10 hours. If SEB is inhaled, it presents a very different clinical picture of sudden, flulike symptoms, including fever, headache, chills, myalgias, and nonproductive cough. More severe exposures may also include retrosternal chest pain, hypotension, nausea, vomiting, diarrhea, and dehydration. Conjunctivitis may also result from aerosol exposure. The illness resulting from SEB inhalation exposures is incapacitating but seldom lethal. Recovery occurs in less than 2 weeks in >99% of those exposed. SEB is very potent and very stable in the atmosphere. As an aerosolized biological weapon, it could incapacitate large numbers of people throughout a sizable geographic region.

ROUTES OF EXPOSURE

Inhalation
Ingestion

TARGET ORGANS

Primary
Respiratory system
Gastrointestinal system
Nervous system
Eyes

LIFE THREAT

SEB is considered an incapacitating agent. Mortality is estimated to be less than 1%, but severe exposures of vulnerable populations may cause some fatalities due to shock and respiratory involvement.

SIGNS AND SYMPTOMS BY SYSTEM

Cardiovascular: Postural hypotension due to fluid loss.

Respiratory: Nonproductive cough, chest pain, dyspnea, pulmonary edema in severe cases.

CNS: Headache, weakness, dizziness.

Gastrointestinal: Abdominal pain, nausea, vomiting, and diarrhea (oral exposure or inadvertent swallowing of aerosolized toxin).

Eye: Conjunctivitis, conjunctival injection (aerosolized attack).

Metabolic: Fever, chills (aerosolized attack).

Other: Myalgia.

INCUBATION PERIOD/SYMPTOM PROGRESSION

The incubation period following ingestion of SEB is 1 to 6 hours. This illness presents as an acute GI problem including retching, vomiting, abdominal pain, and diarrhea. Patients may also experience headache, dizziness, and weakness. This form of illness is normally limited to less than 24 hours (average 8 hours) before resolution.

The incubation period for inhalation SEB exposure is 3 to 12 hours. Initial symptoms include a sudden onset of fever, chills, headache, myalgia, and nonproductive cough, followed by nausea, vomiting, and diarrhea. Most patients recover from inhalational exposure to SEB in less than 2 weeks. Mortality is less than 1%.

MEDICAL CONDITIONS THAT MAY INCREASE RISK FOLLOWING EXPOSURE

Preexisting acute or chronic respiratory conditions

DECONTAMINATION

- If a covert aerosolized release is successfully accomplished or food is contaminated, patients seen hours later will not pose a risk to providers and do not require decontamination. Patient decontamination is warranted only in the immediate aftermath of a known release. Surfaces, bedding, and dressings in contact with body fluids, as well as instruments used for invasive procedures on patients with known or suspected SEB exposure should be sterilized with a sporicidal agent such as hypochlorite (bleach).
- If a suspected overt release has occurred:
  - Wear respiratory protection such as an air-purifying respirator with appropriate cartridges/filters or positive-pressure SCBA. Protective equipment such as gloves, suits, boot covers, and eye protection should be used. A qualified, experienced person should make decisions regarding the type of personal protective equipment necessary.
  - Delay entry into the suspected release area until trained personnel and proper protective equipment are available.
  - Remove patient from contaminated area.
  - Quickly remove and isolate patient's clothing, jewelry, and shoes.
  - Gently brush away dry particles and blot excess liquids with absorbent material.
  - Rinse patient with warm water, 32° C to 35° C (90° F to 95° F), if possible.
  - Wash patient with a mild liquid soap and large quantities of water.
  - Refer to decontamination protocol in Section Three.

IMMEDIATE FIRST AID

- For overt releases:
  - Ensure that adequate decontamination has been carried out as needed.
  - If patient is not breathing, start artificial respiration, preferably with a demand-valve resuscitator, bag-valve-mask device, or pocket mask, as trained. Perform CPR as necessary.
  - Immediately flush contaminated eyes with gently flowing water.
  - Do not induce vomiting. If vomiting occurs, lean patient forward or place on left side (head-down position, if possible) to maintain an open airway and prevent aspiration.
  - Keep patient quiet and maintain normal body temperature.
  - Obtain medical attention.

BASIC TREATMENT

- Establish a patent airway (oropharyngeal or nasopharyngeal airway, if needed). Suction if necessary.
- Watch for signs of respiratory insufficiency and assist ventilations if necessary.
- Administer oxygen by nonrebreather mask at 10 to 15 L/min.
- Monitor for pulmonary edema and treat if necessary (refer to pulmonary edema protocol in Section Three).
- Monitor for shock and treat if necessary (refer to shock protocol in Section Three).
- For eye contamination, flush eyes immediately with water. Irrigate each eye continuously with 0.9% saline (NS) during transport (refer to eye irrigation protocol in Section Three).

ADVANCED TREATMENT

- Consider orotracheal or nasotracheal intubation for airway control in the patient who is unconscious, has severe pulmonary edema, or is in severe respiratory distress.
- Positive-pressure ventilation techniques with a bag-valve-mask device may be beneficial.
- Consider drug therapy for pulmonary edema (refer to pulmonary edema protocol in Section Three).
- Monitor cardiac rhythm and treat arrhythmias as necessary (refer to cardiac protocol in Section Three).
- Start IV administration of D_5W TKO. Use 0.9% saline (NS) or lactated Ringer's (LR) if signs of hypovolemia are present. For hypotension with signs of hypovolemia, administer fluid cautiously. Watch for signs of fluid overload (refer to shock protocol in Section Three).
- There is no specific antidote for inhalation SEB. Airway management, oxygen, and mechanical ventilation.
- Avoid emetics and purgatives.
- Use proparacaine hydrochloride to assist eye irrigation (refer to proparacaine hydrochloride protocol in Section Four).

INITIAL EMERGENCY DEPARTMENT CONSIDERATIONS

- Presumptive diagnosis should be made on signs and symptoms alone in the setting of a known or suspected outbreak. Consider inhalation SEB in any large cluster of patients with unexplained acute pulmonary symptoms. Differential diagnosis may include chemical exposures, other toxins such as ricin, and other respiratory infections. SEB is difficult to detect in the serum because it has usually dissipated by the time symptoms appear. Conduct urinalysis for SEB as soon as possible. It persists in the urine for several hours. Laboratory findings in general are not useful for diagnosis.
- Patients will develop an antibody response as they recover. Consider convalescent serum tests to retrospectively confirm diagnosis. Other useful initial studies include pulse oximetry, CBC, and electrolytes.
- Antiemetics and antidiarrheals may be indicated.
- Mechanical ventilation and PEEP-assisted ventilation may be needed in severe cases resulting in pulmonary edema.

SPECIAL CONSIDERATIONS

Noneffective Therapies

- Avoid emetics and purgatives.

Infection Control

- Standard precautions are adequate (strict hand washing, gloves, splash precautions). SEB is not transmitted person-to-person.

Vaccination

- No vaccine is currently available.

Tularemia *(Francisella tularensis)*

SUBSTANCE IDENTIFICATION

Francisella tularensis is a hardy, slow-growing, highly infectious, aerobic organism. Exposure to as few as 10 organisms can result in tularemia, also known as "rabbit fever" and "deer fly fever." This disease is almost always rural and has naturally occurred in every state in the United States except Hawaii. Several small outbreaks but no large-scale epidemics have been reported. If human cases are identified in a nonendemic area, in urban areas, or in persons without risk factors, an intentional release of *F. tularensis* as a biological weapon should be suspected. Humans may acquire tularemia in a variety of ways. The route of exposure determines the resulting form of disease.

Types of tularemia include pneumonic, typhoidal, ulceroglandular, glandular, oculoglandular, and oropharyngeal. It is normally transmitted through handling infected small mammals such as rabbits or rodents or through the bites of ticks, deer flies, or mosquitoes that have fed on infected animals. These routes of exposure may result in ulceroglandular or glandular tularemia. If an infected animal is eaten after being inadequately cooked or if contaminated food or water is otherwise ingested, the resulting disease may be oropharyngeal tularemia. It is also possible to directly inoculate the eye, resulting in oculoglandular tularemia. The types of tularemia most likely to result from an aerosol release as a biological weapon include pneumonic and typhoidal tularemia.

Mortality depends on the type of infection. The most common forms of the disease, such as ulceroglandular tularemia (50% to 85% of all cases), have a low mortality (<5%). However, primary pneumonic cases have a much higher mortality of 30% to 60% if not treated.

ROUTES OF EXPOSURE

Inhalation (possible with weaponized agents)
Skin or eye contact
Ingestion
Bites of infected animals or arthropods

TARGET ORGANS

Primary

Respiratory system
Hepatic system
Renal system
Cardiovascular system
Nervous system

LIFE THREAT

Respiratory failure, sepsis, and shock.

SIGNS AND SYMPTOMS BY SYSTEM

Cardiovascular: Cardiovascular collapse and shock.
Respiratory: Dyspnea, productive cough, rales, tracheitis, bronchitis, pleural effusions, pneumonia.
CNS: Myalgias, headache, meningismus (painful irritation of brain and spinal cord).
Gastrointestinal: Abdominal pain, vomiting, bloody diarrhea (gastrointestinal tularemia).
Skin: Erythematous, ulcerative skin lesions (ulceroglandular tularemia).
Eye: Severe conjunctivitis, corneal granulomas or ulcers (oculoglandular tularemia).
Metabolic: High fever, chills.
Renal: Kidney damage.
Hepatic: Liver damage.
Other: Rhabdomyolysis.

INCUBATION PERIOD/SYMPTOM PROGRESSION

The incubation period for tularemia ranges from 1 to 21 days (average 3 to 5 days) following inhalation. Symptoms of typhoidal tularemia include flulike symptoms such as fever, headache, myalgias, malaise, abdominal pain, and meningismus. Symptoms of pneumonic disease include cough, dyspnea, pleural effusions, pneumonia, and lymphadenopathy. If untreated, tularemia may progress to respiratory failure, sepsis, and shock. The mortality rate in untreated patients is about 35%

The other forms of tularemia disease are less likely to result from an aerosol release. These include ulceroglandular disease with ulcerative skin lesions; glandular disease with flulike symptoms similar to those of typhoidal tularemia; oculoglandular disease with severe conjunctivitis; and oropharyngeal disease with pharyngitis and tonsillitis.

MEDICAL CONDITIONS THAT MAY INCREASE RISK FOLLOWING EXPOSURE

Preexisting acute or chronic immune compromising conditions

DECONTAMINATION

- If a covert release is successfully accomplished, patients seen days or weeks later will not pose a risk to providers and do not require decontamination. Patient decontamination is warranted only in the immediate aftermath of a known release. Surfaces, bedding, and dressings in contact with body fluids, as well as instruments used for invasive procedures on patients with known or suspected disease, should be sterilized with a sporicidal agent such as hypochlorite (bleach).
- If a suspected overt release has occurred:
  - Wear respiratory protection such as an air-purifying respirator with appropriate cartridges/filters or positive-pressure SCBA. Protective equipment such as gloves, suits, boot covers, and eye protection should be used. A qualified, experienced person should make decisions regarding the type of personal protective equipment necessary.
  - Delay entry into the suspected release area until trained personnel and proper protective equipment are available.
  - Remove patient from contaminated area.
  - Quickly remove and isolate patient's clothing, jewelry, and shoes.

- Gently brush away dry particles and blot excess liquids with absorbent material.
- Rinse patient with warm water, 32° C to 35° C (90° F to 95° F), if possible.
- Wash patient with a mild liquid soap and large quantities of water.
- Refer to decontamination protocol in Section Three.

IMMEDIATE FIRST AID

- For overt releases:
  - Ensure that adequate decontamination has been carried out as needed.
  - If patient is not breathing, start artificial respiration, preferably with a demand-valve resuscitator, bag-valve-mask device, or pocket mask, as trained. Perform CPR as necessary.
  - Immediately flush contaminated eyes with gently flowing water.
  - Do not induce vomiting. If vomiting occurs, lean patient forward or place on left side (head-down position, if possible) to maintain an open airway and prevent aspiration.
  - Keep patient quiet and maintain normal body temperature.
  - Obtain medical attention.

BASIC TREATMENT

- Establish a patent airway (oropharyngeal or nasopharyngeal airway, if needed). Suction if necessary.
- Watch for signs of respiratory insufficiency and assist ventilations if necessary.
- Administer oxygen by nonrebreather mask at 10 to 15 L/min.
- Monitor for shock and treat if necessary (refer to shock protocol in Section Three).
- For eye contamination, flush eyes immediately with water. Irrigate each eye continuously with 0.9% saline (NS) during transport (refer to eye irrigation protocol in Section Three).

ADVANCED TREATMENT

- Consider orotracheal or nasotracheal intubation for airway control in the patient who is unconscious or is in severe respiratory distress.
- Positive-pressure ventilation techniques with a bag-valve-mask device may be beneficial.
- Monitor cardiac rhythm and treat arrhythmias as necessary (refer to cardiac protocol in Section Three).
- Start IV administration of D_5W TKO. Use 0.9% saline (NS) or lactated Ringer's (LR) if signs of hypovolemia are present. For hypotension with signs of hypovolemia, administer fluid cautiously. Consider vasopressors if patient is hypotensive with a normal fluid volume. Watch for signs of fluid overload (refer to shock protocol in Section Three).
- Antimicrobial therapy is recommended. For prophylactic treatment of individuals with suspect exposures, doxycycline and tetracycline are the primary drugs of choice. Appropriate antimicrobial therapy for treatment of disease includes: streptomycin, gentamicin, ciprofloxacin, doxycycline, and tetracycline. (Refer to antibiotic protocols in Section Four).
- Use proparacaine hydrochloride to assist eye irrigation (refer to proparacaine hydrochloride protocol in Section Four).

INITIAL EMERGENCY DEPARTMENT CONSIDERATIONS

- Presumptive diagnosis should be made on signs and symptoms alone in the setting of a known or suspected outbreak. *F. tularensis* can be cultured from the blood and exudates. However, the sensitivity is low and a specific cystine-enriched media is required. Gram stains may be negative. Agglutination, microagglutination, and ELISA may be useful tests, but it may take up to 2 weeks from the onset of symptoms for antibodies to appear. PCR testing is recommended. Other useful initial studies include ABGs, pulse oximetry, CBC, electrolytes, and renal and liver function tests.
- Antibiotic therapy is indicated. For treatment: streptomycin, gentamicin, ciprofloxacin, doxycycline, and tetracycline. For prophylaxis: doxycycline and tetracycline (refer to antibiotic protocols in Section Four).

SPECIAL CONSIDERATIONS

Noneffective Therapies

- Beta-lactams, including third-generation cephalosporins, and macrolides

Infection Control

- Standard precautions are adequate. (strict hand washing, gloves, splash precautions). Although *F. tularensis* is a very hardy and highly infectious organism, it is not contagious person-to-person. It may be transmitted through direct contact with body fluids or through an insect vector but does not require additional precautions for patient management. However, lab workers should be notified if tularemia is suspected so that they can take appropriate precautions. Routine laboratory specimen handling requires biosafety level 2, and large-volume or aerosol-generating procedures require biosafety level 3.

Vaccination

- A live attenuated vaccine exists. It offers some protection against the pneumonic form of tularemia. However, the use of this vaccine has been very limited and is available only to a small number of high-risk lab workers. Because the vaccine has a delayed protective effect and the disease has a short incubation period, this vaccine is not effective for post-exposure prophylaxis.

Typhus (Rickettsia prowazekii, R. typhi, R. tsutsugamushi)

SUBSTANCE IDENTIFICATION

Typhus is caused by rickettsial, gram-negative, small obligate intracellular coccobacilli that infect the cytoplasm of host cells. It is commonly transmitted from person-to-person in the feces of body lice. Most historical epidemics have occurred during periods of famine or war. There are three types of typhus: epidemic or louse-borne typhus (*Rickettsia prowazekii*); endemic typhus (*Rickettsia typhi*), also known as murine typhus; and scrub typhus (*Rickettsia tsutsugamushi*). Of these, epidemic typhus is the most dangerous and is carried by lice.

Endemic typhus is transmitted to humans through flea bites and is seldom fatal. Scrub typhus is transmitted to humans through chigger bites and may lead to many complications, including death. *R. tsutsugamushi* (scrub typhus) is a delicate organism that cannot be effectively delivered as an aerosol. *R. prowazekii* (epidemic or louse-borne typhus) and *R. typhi* (endemic or murine typhus) are both hardy enough organisms to be used as aerosolized biological weapons. Mortality depends on the type of disease. Without treatment, epidemic typhus has a mortality rate as high as 40%. Scrub typhus is less lethal, with a mortality rate of approximately 30%. The mortality rate of endemic (murine) typhus is less than 5%.

ROUTES OF EXPOSURE

Inhalation
Vectors (lice, fleas, larval mites)

TARGET ORGANS

Primary
Respiratory system
Cardiovascular system
Neurological system
Skin
Eyes
Secondary
Gastrointestinal system
Hepatic system
Renal system

LIFE THREAT

Organ failure, disseminated intravascular coagulation (DIC), vascular collapse leading to shock and death

SIGNS AND SYMPTOMS BY SYSTEM

Cardiovascular: Myocarditis, vasculitis, cardiovascular collapse, shock, arrhythmias, gangrene in distal extremities.

Respiratory: Sore throat, nonproductive cough, respiratory failure, pneumonia, acute respiratory distress syndrome (ARDS).

CNS: Headache, confusion, delirium, meningismus, hallucinations, slurred speech, unsteady gait, cranial nerve dysfunction, cerebral thrombosis, coma, seizures.
Gastrointestinal: Abdominal pain, nausea, vomiting, diarrhea.
Skin: Petechiae and rash prominent on trunk (not found on face, palms, or soles), gangrene in distal extremities.
Eye: Conjunctivitis and photophobia.
Metabolic: Chills and fever. Hyponatremia, hypocalcemia, and metabolic acidosis.
Blood: Thrombocytopenia and disseminated intravascular coagulation (DIC).
Renal: Acute renal failure.
Hepatic: Jaundice and liver damage.
Other: Myalgia, transient deafness, and tinnitus.

INCUBATION PERIOD/SYMPTOM PROGRESSION

The incubation period for epidemic typhus is about 7 days, for endemic typhus 7 to 14 days, and for scrub typhus 6 to 18 days.

All three types of disease have a similar 2-week, flulike prodrome that includes sudden onset of fever, chills, headache, and myalgia. Epidemic typhus usually progresses to a 24- to 73-hour period of malaise, prostration, and respiratory symptoms. Murine or endemic typhus progresses to nausea and GI symptoms. About half of patients will develop a maculopapular or petechial rash. Scrub typhus is characterized by a papule at the inoculation site. It may progress to a black eschar similar to cutaneous anthrax. Other symptoms of scrub typhus may include conjunctivitis, ocular pain, bradycardia, and cough.

All forms of typhus may then progress to CNS symptoms, including delirium, stupor, meningismus, or coma. All forms also have the potential to produce a maculopapular or petechial rash. Illness may lead to organ failure, disseminated intravascular coagulation, and vascular collapse leading to shock and death. The course of recovery for survivors may take months.

MEDICAL CONDITIONS THAT MAY INCREASE RISK FOLLOWING EXPOSURE

Preexisting acute or chronic immune compromising conditions, clotting disorders, liver disease, kidney disease.

DECONTAMINATION

- If a covert release is successfully accomplished, patients seen days or weeks later will not pose a risk to providers and do not require decontamination. Patient decontamination is warranted only in the immediate aftermath of a known release. Surfaces, bedding, and dressings in contact with body fluids, as well as instruments used for invasive procedures on patients with known or suspected typhus, should be sterilized with a sporicidal agent such as hypochlorite (bleach).
- If a suspected overt release has occurred:
  - Wear respiratory protection such as an air-purifying respirator with appropriate cartridges/filters or positive-pressure SCBA. Protective equipment such as gloves, suits, boot covers, and eye protection should be used. A qualified, experienced person should make decisions regarding the type of personal protective equipment necessary.
  - Delay entry into the suspected release area until trained personnel and proper protective equipment are available.
  - Remove patient from contaminated area.

- Quickly remove and isolate patient's clothing, jewelry, and shoes.
- Gently brush away dry particles and blot excess liquids with absorbent material.
- Rinse patient with warm water, 32° C to 35° C (90° F to 95° F), if possible.
- Wash patient with a mild liquid soap and large quantities of water.
- Refer to decontamination protocol in Section Three.

IMMEDIATE FIRST AID

- For overt releases:
  - Ensure that adequate decontamination has been carried out as needed.
  - If patient is not breathing, start artificial respiration, preferably with a demand-valve resuscitator, bag-valve-mask device, or pocket mask, as trained. Perform CPR as necessary.
  - Immediately flush contaminated eyes with gently flowing water.
  - Do not induce vomiting. If vomiting occurs, lean patient forward or place on left side (head-down position, if possible) to maintain an open airway and prevent aspiration.
  - Keep patient quiet and maintain normal body temperature.
  - Obtain medical attention.

BASIC TREATMENT

- Establish a patent airway (oropharyngeal or nasopharyngeal airway, if needed). Suction if necessary.
- Watch for signs of respiratory insufficiency and assist ventilations if necessary.
- Administer oxygen by nonrebreather mask at 10 to 15 L/min.
- Monitor for pulmonary edema and treat if necessary (refer to pulmonary edema protocol in Section Three).
- Monitor for shock and treat if necessary (refer to shock protocol in Section Three).
- Anticipate seizures and treat if necessary (refer to seizure protocol in Section Three).
- For eye contamination, flush eyes immediately with water. Irrigate each eye continuously with 0.9% saline (NS) during transport (refer to eye irrigation protocol in Section Three).

ADVANCED TREATMENT

- Consider orotracheal or nasotracheal intubation for airway control in the patient who is unconscious, has severe pulmonary edema, or is in severe respiratory distress.
- Positive-pressure ventilation techniques with a bag-valve-mask device may be beneficial.
- Consider drug therapy for pulmonary edema (refer to pulmonary edema protocol in Section Three).
- Monitor cardiac rhythm and treat arrhythmias as necessary (refer to cardiac protocol in Section Three).
- Start IV administration of D_5W TKO. Use 0.9% saline (NS) or lactated Ringer's (LR) if signs of hypovolemia are present. For hypotension with signs of hypovolemia, administer fluid cautiously. Consider vasopressors if patient is hypotensive with a normal fluid volume. Watch for signs of fluid overload (refer to shock protocol in Section Three).

- Treat seizures with diazepam (Valium) or lorazepam (Ativan) (refer to diazepam and lorazepam protocols in Section Four and seizure protocol in Section Three).
- Treat fever with aspirin or acetaminophen. Aspirin should only be used for adult patients. Cooling measures (cooling blanket or tepid sponging) may be necessary.
- Antimicrobial therapy is recommended. Primary drugs of choice include doxycycline, tetracycline, and chloramphenicol. Fluoroquinolones such as ciprofloxacin and macrolides such as azithromycin may also be effective. However, there are not sufficient efficacy data for these therapies to recommend them as first-line treatment (refer to antibiotic protocols in Section Four).
- Use proparacaine hydrochloride to assist eye irrigation (refer to proparacaine hydrochloride protocol in Section Four).

INITIAL EMERGENCY DEPARTMENT CONSIDERATIONS

- Presumptive diagnosis should be made on signs and symptoms alone in the setting of a known or suspected outbreak. PCR is the most reliable test for diagnosis. A Weil-Felix test may also be used. In addition, indirect fluorescent antibody titer testing may be accomplished to detect antibodies to specific typhus antigens. Other useful initial studies include ABGs, pulse oximetry, CBC, ESR, coagulation tests and platelets, fluid and electrolyte status, and liver and renal function tests.
- Mechanical ventilation and PEEP-assisted ventilation may be needed.
- Antibiotic therapy is highly effective. Doxycycline, tetracycline, and chloramphenicol are all effective (refer to antibiotic protocols in Section Four).

SPECIAL CONSIDERATIONS

Noneffective Therapies

- Fluoroquinolones such as ciprofloxacin and macrolides such as azithromycin may be useful, but their efficacy is not known.

Infection Control

- Standard precautions are needed (strict hand washing, gloves, splash precautions, etc.).

Vaccination

- A formalin-inactivated vaccine is available for *R. prowazekii* (epidemic typhus) only. There is no effective vaccine for endemic or scrub typhus. Individuals at risk for exposure to these forms of the disease may be prophylactically treated with antimicrobials such as doxycycline.

Viral Encephalitis (Alphaviruses)

Venezuelan equine encephalitis (VEE), eastern equine encephalitis (EEE), and western equine encephalitis (WEE)

SUBSTANCE IDENTIFICATION

Viral encephalitis illnesses such as Venezuelan equine encephalitis (VEE), eastern equine encephalitis (EEE), and western equine encephalitis (WEE) are caused by exposure to alphaviruses that are normally transmitted by mosquitoes. The primary viremic hosts of these organisms are horses, mules, and donkeys (equidae). Human disease has occurred through mosquito vectors and through laboratory exposures. It is possible to weaponize these agents and deliver them as aerosols or through intentional release of infected mosquitoes. In natural human epidemics, severe and sometimes fatal encephalitis in equidae precedes human cases. Therefore, if an outbreak occurs in the winter months or in the absence of equine cases, this may be an initial clue that an intentional release has occurred. *Secondary* spread in a natural outbreak by person-to-person contact occurs at a negligible rate. Because many viral encephalitic diseases produce only an asymptomatic or mild illness, some variants are less desirable as biological weapons.

However, VEE produces nearly 100% symptomatic infections in exposed individuals and was weaponized in the 1950s by the United States. It is likely that other countries have also weaponized this agent. If VEE is released as an aerosol, it will cause a very low mortality rate (<1%) but may result in a significant number of neurological cases.

EEE is a rare disease (about 4 cases per year) that occurs in the eastern United States. It has a high mortality rate (35%) and severe morbidity, with about 35% of survivors experiencing some long-term neurological deficit. This makes EEE one of the most serious mosquito-borne diseases in the United States and a possible bioterrorism threat.

Most WEE infections are asymptomatic or mild, nonspecific illnesses.

ROUTES OF EXPOSURE

Inhalation (as a weaponized agent, not seen to date in human outbreaks)
Skin and eye contact
Mosquito vector

TARGET ORGANS

Primary
Central nervous system
Secondary
Respiratory system

Cardiovascular system
Gastrointestinal system
Hepatic system
Blood

LIFE THREAT

Central nervous system involvement progressing to severe encephalitis. In naturally occurring epidemics, encephalitic cases have a mortality rate of 20% to 35%.

SIGNS AND SYMPTOMS BY SYSTEM

Cardiovascular: Tachycardia.

Respiratory: Sore throat, nonexudative pharyngitis, nonproductive cough; respiratory failure in severe cases.

CNS: Headache, myalgia, delirium, decreased level of consciousness, somnolence, paralysis, cranial nerve palsies, seizures, severe encephalitis.

Gastrointestinal: Nausea, vomiting, diarrhea.

Eye: Photophobia, double vision.

Metabolic: Fever, chills.

Hepatic: Liver damage.

Blood: Leukopenia.

Other: Teratogenic effects: fetal encephalitis may occur.

INCUBATION PERIOD/SYMPTOM PROGRESSION

The incubation period for Venezuelan equine encephalitis (VEE) typically is 2 to 6 days. The incubation may be longer for other viral encephalitic diseases (EEE—5 to 15 days; WEE—1 to 20 days).

Initial symptoms include a sudden onset of flulike symptoms, including fever, rigors, headache, malaise, myalgias, and photophobia. Additional symptoms may quickly ensue, including nausea, vomiting, diarrhea, sore throat, and cough. These initial symptoms last 1 to 3 days, and the illness may completely resolve in less than 2 weeks. However, neurological symptoms may worsen and may include delirium, decreased level of consciousness, somnolence, paralysis, cranial nerve palsies, seizures, and meningismus, and severe encephalitis. Children are at an increased risk for severe neurological symptoms. Permanent neurological sequelae are possible and the mortality rate may be as high as 35%. If an outbreak occurs from an aerosol release, it is likely that illness will be more severe and mortality may be higher.

MEDICAL CONDITIONS THAT MAY INCREASE RISK FOLLOWING EXPOSURE

Preexisting acute or chronic immune compromising conditions

DECONTAMINATION

- If a covert release is successfully accomplished, patients seen days or weeks later will not pose a risk to providers and do not require decontamination. Patient decontamination is warranted only in the immediate aftermath of a known release. Surfaces, bedding, dressings in contact with body fluids, as well as instruments used for invasive procedures on patients with known or suspected viral encephalitis, should be sterilized with a sporicidal agent such as hypochlorite (bleach).
- If a suspected overt release has occurred:
  - Wear respiratory protection such as an air-purifying respirator with appropriate cartridges/filters or positive-pressure SCBA. Protective equipment

such as gloves, suits, boot covers, and eye protection should be used. A qualified, experienced person should make decisions regarding the type of personal protective equipment necessary.
- Delay entry into the suspected release area until trained personnel and proper protective equipment are available.
- Remove patient from contaminated area.
- Quickly remove and isolate patient's clothing, jewelry, and shoes.
- Gently brush away dry particles and blot excess liquids with absorbent material.
- Rinse patient with warm water, 32° C to 35° C (90° F to 95° F), if possible.
- Wash patient with a mild liquid soap and large quantities of water.
- Refer to decontamination protocol in Section Three.

IMMEDIATE FIRST AID

- For overt releases:
  - Ensure that adequate decontamination has been carried out as needed.
  - If patient is not breathing, start artificial respiration, preferably with a demand-valve resuscitator, bag-valve-mask device, or pocket mask, as trained. Perform CPR as necessary.
  - Immediately flush contaminated eyes with gently flowing water.
  - Do not induce vomiting. If vomiting occurs, lean patient forward or place on left side (head-down position, if possible) to maintain an open airway and prevent aspiration.
  - Keep patient quiet and maintain normal body temperature.
  - Obtain medical attention.

BASIC TREATMENT

- Establish a patent airway (oropharyngeal or nasopharyngeal airway, if needed). Suction if necessary.
- Watch for signs of respiratory insufficiency and assist ventilations if necessary.
- Administer oxygen by nonrebreather mask at 10 to 15 L/min.
- Anticipate seizures and treat if necessary (refer to seizure protocol in Section Three).
- For eye contamination, flush eyes immediately with water. Irrigate each eye continuously with 0.9% saline (NS) during transport (refer to eye irrigation protocol in Section Three).

ADVANCED TREATMENT

- Consider orotracheal or nasotracheal intubation for airway control in the patient who is unconscious or is in severe respiratory distress.
- Positive-pressure ventilation techniques with a bag-valve-mask device may be beneficial.
- Monitor cardiac rhythm and treat arrhythmias as necessary (refer to cardiac protocol in Section Three).
- Start IV administration of D_5W TKO. Use 0.9% saline (NS) or lactated Ringer's (LR) if signs of hypovolemia are present. For hypotension with signs of hypovolemia, administer fluid cautiously. Consider vasopressors if patient is hypotensive with a normal fluid volume. Watch for signs of fluid overload (refer to shock protocol in Section Three).
- Treat seizures with diazepam (Valium) or lorazepam (Ativan) (refer to diazepam and lorazepam protocols in Section Four and seizure protocol in Section Three).

- There is no specific treatment. Uncomplicated cases require only supportive care.
- Use proparacaine hydrochloride to assist eye irrigation (refer to proparacaine hydrochloride protocol in Section Four).

INITIAL EMERGENCY DEPARTMENT CONSIDERATIONS

- Presumptive diagnosis should be made on signs and symptoms alone in the setting of a known or suspected outbreak. Serum testing includes ELISA for virus-specific IgM, complement fixation, and neutralizing antibodies. CBC may show leukopenia and lymphopenia. Lumbar puncture may be abnormal, with high opening pressure and high WBC count. Other useful initial studies include ABGs, pulse oximetry, electrolytes, and liver function tests. A cranial CT and lumbar puncture should be obtained for patients with an altered mental status.
- Supportive therapy to ensure adequate ventilation, treat seizure activities, maintain fluid and electrolyte balance, prevent secondary bacterial infections.

SPECIAL CONSIDERATIONS

Infection Control

- Standard precautions are needed (strict hand washing, gloves, splash precautions, etc.). Also institute vector control to prevent secondary infections.

Vaccination

- Effective vaccines are not available for most alphaviruses. An investigational, live, attenuated, cell culture–propagated vaccine (TC-83) is available for high-risk laboratory personnel working with VEE virus. A second investigational vaccine (C-84) is available for nonresponders or for use as a booster to T-83.

Viral Hemorrhagic Fevers

Filoviruses (Ebola, Marburg)
Arenaviruses (Lassa Fever, Machupo)

SUBSTANCE IDENTIFICATION

The term "viral hemorrhagic fevers" (VHFs) describes a severe, multisystem syndrome caused by one of four virus families: arenaviruses, filoviruses, bunyaviruses, and flavivruses. These are all RNA viruses and naturally reside in an animal reservoir host or arthropod vector. Examples of primary host animals include rats and mice. However, the hosts for some agents, such as Ebola and Marburg, remain a mystery. Transmission to humans occurs when infected hosts or vectors expose humans through urine, feces, saliva, blood, or other excretions. This may occur through rodents, arthropod vectors, or exposure to infected animals being cared for or slaughtered. Some of these viruses can also spread from person to person through close contact with infected people or exposure to their body fluids. VHF illness is initially characterized by fever, fatigue, dizziness, muscle aches, and loss of strength. Those symptoms worsen as vascular damage occurs. More severe symptoms include hypotension, facial edema, pulmonary edema, and mucosal hemorrhages. Some patients will show signs of bleeding from body orifices, internal organs and under the skin. Even though the patient may show marked hemorrhage, they rarely die from the blood loss. Death usually results from multi-organ failure and cardiovascular collapse. Mortality for VHFs ranges from 15% to 30% but has been as high as 50% in some outbreaks. Although these agents have not been transmitted to humans via aerosols, it is possible to weaponize them for aerosol delivery. Due to the highly infectious and lethal nature of these organisms, they are considered to be a significant threat as bioterrorism agents.

ROUTES OF EXPOSURE

Inhalation (as a weaponized agent, not seen to date in human outbreaks)
Skin and eye contact
Injection

TARGET ORGANS

Primary
Vascular system
Secondary
Cardiovascular system
Nervous system
Respiratory system
Hepatic system
Renal system
Gastrointestinal system
Eyes

LIFE THREAT

Disseminating intravascular coagulation (DIC), thrombocytopenia, multiorgan failure, and cardiovascular collapse

SIGNS AND SYMPTOMS BY SYSTEM

Cardiovascular: Hypotension, chest pain, hypovolemic shock, cardiovascular collapse.

Respiratory: Sore throat, nonproductive cough, hiccup, tachypnea, pulmonary edema, acute respiratory distress syndrome.

CNS: Headache, myalgia, tinnitus, hearing loss, confusion, delirium.

Gastrointestinal: Vomiting, diarrhea, abdominal pain, gastrointestinal hemorrhage.

Skin: Delayed onset of skin rash, petechiae, hemorrhage, central cyanosis, facial and neck edema.

Eye: Conjunctivitis, unilateral loss of vision, conjunctival hemorrhage.

Metabolic: Fever.

Renal: Hematuria, oliguria, anuria, renal failure.

Hepatic: Nonicteric hepatitis, hepatic enzyme elevation.

Blood: Gastrointestinal bleeding; bleeding from other organs, orifices, mucous membranes. and skin; thrombocytopenia, disseminating intravascular coagulation (DIC).

Other: Joint and lower back pain.

INCUBATION PERIOD/SYMPTOM PROGRESSION

Most VHFs have an initial incubation period ranging from a couple days to a couple of weeks (e.g., Ebola, 2-21 days; Marburg, 3-9 days; Lassa, 3-16 days).

Following the incubation period there is an abrupt onset of flulike symptoms, including fever, headache, joint pain, sore throat, vomiting, abdominal pain, and diarrhea. A skin rash may also develop approximately 1 week later. Around the third day of illness, hemorrhagic complications may develop, including petechiae, facial edema, pulmonary edema, mucosal hemorrhage, frank bleeding from the GI tract or other sites. DIC, thrombocytopenia, high fever, and delirium occur according to the severity of disease. Multiorgan failure and fatal shock are possible. For survivors, recovery may take several weeks.

MEDICAL CONDITIONS THAT MAY INCREASE RISK FOLLOWING EXPOSURE

Preexisting acute or chronic immune compromising conditions, clotting disorders, liver disease, kidney disease

DECONTAMINATION

- If a covert release is successfully accomplished, patients seen days or weeks later will not pose a risk to providers and do not require decontamination. Patient decontamination is warranted only in the immediate aftermath of a known release. Surfaces, bedding, and dressings in contact with body fluids, as well as instruments used for invasive procedures on patients with known or suspected VHF should be sterilized with a sporicidal agent such as hypochlorite (bleach).
- If a suspected overt release has occurred:
  - Wear respiratory protection such as an air-purifying respirator with appropriate cartridges/filters or positive-pressure SCBA. Protective equipment such as gloves, suits, boot covers, and eye protection should be used. A

qualified, experienced person should make decisions regarding the type of personal protective equipment necessary.
- Delay entry into the suspected release area until trained personnel and proper protective equipment are available.
- Remove patient from contaminated area.
- Quickly remove and isolate patient's clothing, jewelry, and shoes.
- Gently brush away dry particles and blot excess liquids with absorbent material.
- Rinse patient with warm water, 32° C to 35° C (90° F to 95° F), if possible.
- Wash patient with a mild liquid soap and large quantities of water.
- Refer to decontamination protocol in Section Three.

IMMEDIATE FIRST AID

- For overt releases:
  - Ensure that adequate decontamination has been carried out as needed.
  - If patient is not breathing, start artificial respiration, preferably with a demand-valve resuscitator or bag-valve-mask device, as trained. Perform CPR as necessary.
  - Immediately flush contaminated eyes with gently flowing water.
  - Do not induce vomiting. If vomiting occurs, lean patient forward or place on left side (head-down position, if possible) to maintain an open airway and prevent aspiration.
  - Keep patient quiet and maintain normal body temperature.
  - Obtain medical attention.

BASIC TREATMENT

- Establish a patent airway (oropharyngeal or nasopharyngeal airway, if needed). Suction if necessary.
- Watch for signs of respiratory insufficiency and assist ventilations if necessary.
- Administer oxygen by nonrebreather mask at 10 to 15 L/min.
- Monitor for pulmonary edema and treat if necessary (refer to pulmonary edema protocol in Section Three).
- Monitor for shock and treat if necessary (refer to shock protocol in Section Three).
- Anticipate seizures and treat if necessary (refer to seizure protocol in Section Three).
- For eye contamination, flush eyes immediately with water. Irrigate each eye continuously with 0.9% saline (NS) during transport (refer to eye irrigation protocol in Section Three).

ADVANCED TREATMENT

- Consider orotracheal or nasotracheal intubation for airway control in the patient who is unconscious, has severe pulmonary edema, or is in severe respiratory distress.
- Positive-pressure ventilation techniques with a bag-valve-mask device may be beneficial.
- Consider drug therapy for pulmonary edema (refer to pulmonary edema protocol in Section Three).
- Monitor cardiac rhythm and treat arrhythmias as necessary (refer to cardiac protocol in Section Three).

- Start IV administration of D_5W TKO. Use 0.9% saline (NS) or lactated Ringer's (LR) if signs of hypovolemia are present. For hypotension with signs of hypovolemia, administer fluid cautiously. Consider vasopressors if patient is hypotensive with a normal fluid volume. Watch for signs of fluid overload (refer to shock protocol in Section Three).
- Treat seizures with diazepam (Valium) or lorazepam (Ativan) (refer to diazepam and lorazepam protocols in Section Four and seizure protocol in Section Three).
- Intensive supportive care is needed. There is no other specific treatment for VHFs. An antiviral drug, ribavirin, has been successful in the treatment of arenaviruses such as Lassa fever when given early in the illness (prior to day 7). In addition, convalescent human plasma has been useful in treating Argentine hemorrhagic fever when given early in the illness. (prior to day 9).
- Use proparacaine hydrochloride to assist eye irrigation (refer to proparacaine hydrochloride protocol in Section Four).

INITIAL EMERGENCY DEPARTMENT CONSIDERATIONS

- Presumptive diagnosis should be made on signs and symptoms alone in the setting of a known or suspected outbreak. In addition to a variety of VHFs, differential diagnosis for these diseases may include typhoid fever, rickettsial infection, leptospirosis, fulminant hepatitis, and meningococcemia. A CBC will usually show thrombocytopenia and leukopenia. Proteinuria and hematuria will be seen. Viral cultures (blood or throat swab) taken during the acute phase of disease will be positive. Also consider CSF, ascites fluid, or pleural fluid as indicated. ELISA (enzyme-linked immunosorbent assay) and immunofluorescence (IFA) tests are available for specific IgM antibodies. Other useful initial studies include arterial blood gases (ABGs), pulse oximetry, electrolytes, and renal and liver function tests. Prothrombin time/international normalized ratio (PT/INR) and partial thromboplastin time (PTT) levels should be monitored. Because these viruses are classified as biosafety level 4 agents, work is limited to selected laboratories such as the CDC in Atlanta.
- Mechanical ventilation and PEEP-assisted ventilation may be needed.
- Transfusions with fresh frozen plasma and packed red cells may be necessary in cases of severe hemorrhage.
- Hemodialysis may be necessary in cases of renal failure.
- Consider antiviral therapy. Ribavirin loading dose of 30 mg/kg of body weight IV followed by 16 mg/kg IV every 6 hours for 4 days, then 8 mg/kg every 8 hours for 6 days in the adult patient.

SPECIAL CONIDERATIONS

Infection Control

- Standard and contact precautions are needed. (patient isolation, strict handwashing, gloves, gown, splash precautions, etc.) In addition, if the patient is hemorrhaging, coughing, vomiting, or experiencing diarrhea, airborne precautions should be instituted including negative-pressure room, respiratory protection (N-95 respirator minimum), and eye protection is required for anyone within 3 feet of the patient.

Vaccination

- No antidote or vaccine is available.

Water Safety Threats

Vibrio cholerae
Cryptosporidium parvum

SUBSTANCE IDENTIFICATION

Waterborne illnesses result from microbes entering the body through the gastrointestinal tract by consumption of contaminated water. Many pathogens can cause waterborne illnesses, including bacteria such as *Vibrio cholerae* and parasites such as *Cryptosporidium parvum.*

V. cholerae is a free-living, gram-negative organism that causes cholera, a severe diarrheal disease. This disease has been the cause of massive fatalities throughout history. However, current water treatment practices easily control this threat. If a terrorist selected this organism as a weapon against a water system, it would take an enormous quantity to overcome chlorination.

Unlike bacteria, some parasites such as *C. parvum* have an outer shell that protects them against chlorine disinfection. It also enables them to survive for long periods outside an animal or human host. These parasites cause cryptosporidiosis, a usually mild diarrheal disease. In healthy individuals, the disease may last 1 to 2 weeks. Although it is mild, it can have considerable economic impact through absenteeism of those affected. In immunocompromised populations, the disease may be severe, long-term, and life-threatening. No effective therapy is available. In recent history, this has become one of the most common waterborne human diseases in the United States.

The key to waterborne bioterrorism preparedness is an increased index of suspicion and an understanding of how to rapidly notify local and state public health officials when cases arouse suspicion. The investigation that public health officials initiate will often characterize a common exposure, prevent additional cases, and identify responsible parties.

ROUTES OF EXPOSURE

Ingestion

TARGET ORGANS

Primary

Gastrointestinal system

Secondary

Cardiovascular system

Renal system

LIFE THREAT

Rapid loss of body fluids leading to circulatory collapse

SIGNS AND SYMPTOMS BY SYSTEM

Cardiovascular: Circulatory collapse.

CNS: Headache, malaise, fatigue.

Gastrointestinal: Abdominal cramping, watery diarrhea among cryptosporidiosis patients, gray-brown (rice water) diarrhea among cholera patients, hyperactive bowel sounds, nausea.

Metabolic: Fever.

Other: Weight loss, dehydration.

INCUBATION PERIOD/SYMPTOM PROGRESSION

The incubation period is variable by pathogen and clinical course.

The incubation period for *cholera* ranges from several hours to 5 days (average 2 to 3 days) depending on the dose of organisms. Initial symptoms consist of sudden onset of headache, abdominal cramping, watery diarrhea, vomiting, fever, and malaise. Symptoms may progress to a "rice water" diarrhea with excessive fluid loss, severe muscle cramps, circulatory collapse, and death in nearly 50% of untreated patients. The disease lasts from 1 day to 1 week.

The incubation period for *cryptosporidiosis* is 2 to 10 days. Initial symptoms include diarrhea, watery stool, abdominal cramps, and mild fever. Some people have no symptoms. Those with normal immune function usually recover within 2 weeks. However, those with compromised immune systems are at a much greater risk of long-term illness and possible death.

MEDICAL CONDITIONS THAT MAY INCREASE RISK FOLLOWING EXPOSURE

Very young or very old age, preexisting chronic disease, immune compromising conditions.

DECONTAMINATION

- These pathogens may be delivered via water contamination and do not require decontamination. Standard precautions are warranted. Surfaces, bedding, and dressings in contact with body fluids, as well as instruments used for invasive procedures on patients with known or suspected disease, should be sterilized with a sporicidal agent such as hypochlorite (bleach).

IMMEDIATE FIRST AID

- If patient is not breathing, start artificial respiration, preferably with a demand-valve resuscitator, bag-valve-mask device, or pocket mask, as trained. Perform CPR as necessary.
- Do not induce vomiting. If vomiting occurs, lean patient forward or place on left side (head-down position, if possible) to maintain an open airway and prevent aspiration.
- Keep patient quiet and maintain normal body temperature.
- Obtain medical attention.

BASIC TREATMENT

- Establish a patent airway (oropharyngeal or nasopharyngeal airway, if needed). Suction if necessary.
- Watch for signs of respiratory insufficiency and assist ventilations if necessary.
- Administer oxygen by nonrebreather mask at 10 to 15 L/min.
- Monitor for shock and treat if necessary (refer to shock protocol in Section Three).

ADVANCED TREATMENT

- Consider orotracheal or nasotracheal intubation for airway control in the patient who is unconscious or is in severe respiratory distress.

- Positive-pressure ventilation techniques with a bag-valve-mask device may be beneficial.
- Monitor cardiac rhythm and treat arrhythmias as necessary (refer to cardiac protocol in Section Three).
- Start IV administration of D_5W TKO. Use 0.9% saline (NS) or lactated Ringer's (LR) if signs of hypovolemia are present. For hypotension with signs of hypovolemia, administer fluids cautiously. Consider vasopressors if patient is hypotensive with a normal fluid volume. Watch for signs of fluid overload (refer to shock protocol in Section Three).
- Primary treatment consists of rapid fluid and electrolyte replacement.
- If a determination is made that the illness is due to a bacterial infection such as cholera, antimicrobial therapy is recommended. Drugs of choice include ciprofloxacin, doxycycline, tetracycline, or erythromycin (refer to antibiotic protocol in Section Four).
- If a parasitic disease is suspected, such as cryptosporidiosis, there is no effective treatment beyond fluid replacement and antidiarrheal medication. Patients with weakened immune systems may require antiretroviral therapy to enhance their immune function and reduce severity of symptoms.
- Use proparacaine hydrochloride to assist eye irrigation (refer to proparacaine hydrochloride protocol in Section Four).

INITIAL EMERGENCY DEPARTMENT CONSIDERATIONS

- The clinical picture as described is an important diagnostic.
- *Vibrio cholerae* can be cultured from stool on a special media. In addition, stool specimens will show no RBCs or WBCs and almost no protein. Phase-contrast microscopy will show a highly motile vibrio.
- *Cryptosporidium parvum* can be identified using an acid-fast or immunofluorescence staining on an unconcentrated fecal smear. Microscopy using immunofluorescence antibody is also very sensitive and fast. PCR testing is also emerging as an effective tool.

SPECIAL CONSIDERATIONS

Infection Control

- Use standard precautions (strict hand washing, gloves, and splash precautions). Person-to-person transmission is unlikely during routine patient care.

Vaccination

- There is a cholera vaccine but it is of limited value in response to bioterrorism because of its delayed protective effects. There is no vaccine for cryptosporidiosis.

132

Blood Agents (Cyanides and Related Compounds)

Hydrogen Cyanide (AC), Cyanogen Chloride (CK), Related Compounds

SUBSTANCE IDENTIFICATION

Hydrogen cyanide (AC) and cyanogen chloride (CK) are extremely toxic materials. The two letter abbreviation following the chemical name is the military designation for the agent. These agents combine with the ferric ions of iron in the cytochrome-oxidase complex in the mitochondria to inhibit the enzyme and prevent intracellular oxygen utilization. Cyanides are often called "blood agents," although this is an antiquated term. When cyanide was first introduced as a warfare agent, other chemical warfare agents caused mainly local effects: riot control agents affected the skin, eyes, and mucous membranes; phosgene and chlorine affected the lungs. Cyanide, on the other hand, was absorbed and distributed throughout the body by the blood and caused systemic effects; hence the term "blood agent."

The main site of action of cyanide is at the cells, not in the blood. Cyanide can be found in liquid, solid, or gaseous form. In solid form it is white, with a faint almond odor (an estimated 20% of the population is genetically unable to detect this odor). It is widely used in industry as a fumigant, in metal treatment, and in the welding/cutting of heat-resistant metals. with over 300,000 tons produced annually in the United States. It is also used in paper manufacturing, photography, electroplating, blueprinting, and engraving.

Cyanide was used in Word War I without notable military success, probably because of the small amount of cyanide used in the munitions and the volatile nature of cyanide. Nazi Germany's use of cyanide in gas chambers demonstrated the brutal efficiency with which cyanide can kill when released in high concentrations in enclosed spaces. Japan allegedly used cyanide against China before and during Word War II, and Iraq may have used cyanide against the Kurds in the 1980s.

ROUTES OF EXPOSURE

Skin and eye contact
Inhalation
Ingestion
Skin absorption

TARGET ORGANS

Primary
Skin
Eyes
Central nervous system
Cardiovascular system

Secondary
Respiratory system
Gastrointestinal system
Hepatic system
Renal system
Metabolism

LIFE THREAT

Death is caused by an inhibitory action on the cytochrome oxidase system, preventing mitochondrial use of oxygen to make adenosine triphosphate (ATP). Cyanide brings cellular respiration to a halt. Cyanogen chloride also has a local irritant effect on the eyes, upper respiratory tract. and lungs.

SIGNS AND SYMPTOMS BY SYSTEM

Cardiovascular: At first, pulse rate decreases and blood pressure rises. As poisoning continues, bradycardia, heart block, ventricular arrhythmias, hypotension, and cardiovascular collapse may occur. Palpitations and tightness of the chest.

Respiratory: May cause immediate respiratory arrest. Initially, respiratory rate and depth are increased. As poisoning progresses, respirations become slow, gasping, and finally apneic. Respiratory tract irritation and pulmonary edema.

CNS: Immediate coma. Early symptoms include anxiety, agitation, vertigo, weakness, paralysis, headache, confusion, and lethargy. Seizures.

Gastrointestinal: Nausea, vomiting, excessive salivation, and hemorrhage.

Eye: Chemical conjunctivitis. Dilated pupils.

Skin: Dermatitis and, in some cases, ulcers. Pale or reddish skin color with diaphoresis. Cyanosis is not always present.

Renal: Kidney damage.

Hepatic: Hepatic damage.

Metabolism: Anion gap metabolic acidosis and rhabdomyolysis.

Other: May be rapidly fatal, without early symptoms.

SYMPTOM ONSET FOR ACUTE EXPOSURE

Immediate

CO-EXPOSURE CONCERNS

Other oxygen excluders
Simple asphyxiants

THERMAL DECOMPOSITION PRODUCTS INCLUDE

Ammonia gases
Carbon monoxide
Hydrogen cyanide
Nitrogen oxides

MEDICAL CONDITIONS THAT MAY INCREASE RISK FOLLOWING EXPOSURE

Central nervous system disorders
Liver disorders
Kidney disorders
Respiratory system disorders
Thyroid gland dysfunction

DECONTAMINATION

- Wear positive-pressure SCBA and protective equipment specified by references such as the *North American Emergency Response Guidebook*. If special chemical protective clothing is required, consult the chemical manufacturer or specific protective clothing compatibility charts. A qualified, experienced person should make decisions regarding the type of personal protective equipment necessary.
- Delay entry until trained personnel and proper protective equipment are available.
- Remove patient from contaminated area.
- Quickly remove and isolate patient's clothing, jewelry, and shoes.
- Gently brush away dry particles and blot excess liquids with absorbent material.
- Rinse patient with warm water, 32° C to 35° C (90° F to 95° F), if possible.
- Wash patient with a mild liquid soap and large quantities of water. Some authorities recommend a dilute hypochlorite (0.5% solution) as a decontaminating agent (refer to decontamination protocol in Section Three).

IMMEDIATE FIRST AID

- Ensure that adequate decontamination has been carried out as needed.
- If patient is not breathing, start artificial respiration, preferably with a demand-valve resuscitator, bag-valve-mask device, or pocket mask, as trained. Perform CPR if necessary.
- Immediately flush contaminated eyes with gently flowing water.
- Do not induce vomiting. If vomiting occurs, lean patient forward or place on left side (head-down position, if possible) to maintain an open airway and prevent aspiration.
- Keep patient quiet and maintain normal body temperature.
- Obtain medical attention.

BASIC TREATMENT

- Establish a patent airway (oropharyngeal or nasopharyngeal airway, if needed). Suction if necessary.
- Watch for signs of respiratory insufficiency and assist ventilations if necessary.
- Administer oxygen by nonrebreather mask at 10 to 15 L/min.
- Administer amyl nitrite ampules as per protocol. DIRECT PHYSICIAN ORDER ONLY (refer to cyanide kit protocol in Section Four).
- Monitor for shock and treat if necessary (refer to shock protocol in Section Three).
- Monitor for pulmonary edema and treat if necessary (refer to pulmonary edema protocol in Section Three).
- Anticipate seizures and treat if necessary (refer to seizure protocol in Section Three).
- For eye contamination, flush eyes immediately with water. Irrigate each eye continuously with 0.9% saline (NS) during transport (refer to eye irrigation protocol in Section Three).
- Do not use emetics. For ingestion, rinse mouth and administer 5 ml/kg up to 200 ml of water for dilution if the patient can swallow, has a strong gag reflex, and does not drool (refer to ingestion protocol in Section Three).

ADVANCED TREATMENT

- Consider orotracheal or nasotracheal intubation for airway control in the patient who is unconscious, has severe pulmonary edema, or is in severe respiratory distress.

- Positive-pressure ventilation techniques with a bag-valve-mask device may be beneficial.
- Consider drug therapy for pulmonary edema (refer to pulmonary edema protocol in Section Three).
- Monitor and treat cardiac arrhythmias if necessary (refer to cardiac protocol in Section Three).
- Start IV administration of D_5W TKO. Use 0.9% saline (NS) or lactated Ringer's (LR) if signs of hypovolemia are present. For hypotension with signs of hypovolemia, administer fluid cautiously. Consider vasopressors if patient is hypotensive with a normal fluid volume. Watch for signs of fluid overload. (refer to shock protocol in Section Three).
- Administer cyanide antidote kit as per protocol. DIRECT PHYSICIAN ORDER ONLY (refer to cyanide antidote kit protocol in Section Four).
- Treat seizures with diazepam (Valium) or lorazepam (Ativan) (refer to seizure protocol in Section Three and diazepam and lorazepam protocols in Section Four).
- Use proparacaine hydrochloride to assist eye irrigation (refer to proparacaine hydrochloride protocol in Section Four).

INITIAL EMERGENCY DEPARTMENT CONSIDERATIONS

- Useful initial laboratory studies include complete blood count, serum electrolytes, blood urea nitrogen (BUN), creatinine, glucose, urinalysis, and baseline biochemical profile, including serum aminotransferases (ALT and AST), calcium, phosphorus, and magnesium. Determination of anion and osmolar gaps may be helpful. Arterial blood gases (ABGs), chest radiograph, and electrocardiogram may be required.
- Whole blood cyanide concentrations may be drawn. Background and postexposure values are extremely variable. Smokers demonstrate higher background concentrations than nonsmokers.
- Treatment should not be withheld pending laboratory cyanide determinations. Treatment must be based on exposure history and clinical presentation.
- Positive end-expiratory pressure (PEEP)-assisted ventilation may be necessary in patients with acute parenchymal injury who develop pulmonary edema or acute respiratory distress syndrome.
- Obtain toxicological consultation as necessary.

SPECIAL CONSIDERATIONS

- Administration of sodium nitrite may cause hypotension.
- Pulse oximetry readings may not be accurate in these exposures.
- Asymptomatic individuals who may have transiently inhaled cyanide vapors are not at risk for delayed systemic symptoms once removed from the contaminated environment, unless they have ingested the product or continue to have skin exposure to liquids or solids.

133

Choking Agents (Pulmonary/Lung-Damaging Agents)

Phosgene (CG), Diphosgene (DP), Chlorine (Cl), Chloropicrin (PS), Related Compounds

SUBSTANCE IDENTIFICATION

Choking agents are chemical agents that can damage lung tissue. Examples include phosgene (CG), diphosgene (DP), chlorine (Cl), and chloropicrin (PS). The two letter abbreviation following the chemical name is the military designation for the agent.

Phosgene (CG)

Phosgene is the prototype of this class of agents. It was first synthesized in 1812 and was widely used on the battlefields of World War I. Phosgene is transported as a liquid. It has a high vapor pressure, and once it is released from its container it will rapidly turn into a vapor that is four times heavier than air. Phosgene has a characteristic odor of sweet, newly mown hay that may be lost after accommodation. It is relatively insoluble in water and most of its action is on the peripheral portion of the lung (the alveoli). It causes damage to the alveolar-capillary membrane resulting in leakage of fluid into the interstitial portions of the lung. Exposure to phosgene usually results in a delayed onset of signs and symptoms.

Chlorine (Cl)

Chlorine is widely used in the manufacture of chemicals, plastics, and paper. It is also used in water purification and in swimming pools. Industrial exposures have produced large numbers of injuries. Because of its widespread use it presents a sizable terrorism threat. Chlorine is transported as a liquid under pressure. Like phosgene it has a high vapor pressure and will rapidly turn into a vapor when released from its container. Chlorine gas is greenish yellow gas with a characteristic odor. The gas is heavier than air.

ROUTES OF EXPOSURE

Skin and eye contact
Inhalation

TARGET ORGANS

Primary
Skin
Eyes
Respiratory system

Secondary
Central nervous system
Cardiovascular system
Gastrointestinal system

LIFE THREAT

Severe respiratory irritants that can cause damage to the alveoli and resultant pulmonary edema.

SIGNS AND SYMPTOMS BY SYSTEM

Cardiovascular: Cardiovascular collapse, hypovolemia, shock, and arrhythmias.

Respiratory: Throat dryness, pharyngitis, with primarily lower respiratory tract mucous membrane irritation, including pneumonitis and pneumonia. Acute or delayed pulmonary edema, dyspnea, and tachypnea. Cough with thick, bloody, foamy sputum. Noncardiac chest pain. Pulmonary damage (bronchitis, emphysema, fibrosis) may be a late sequela. Compounds with increased water solubility will cause upper airway irritation and burns to the mucous membranes and lungs without a delayed onset.

CNS: Headache, CNS depression to coma and seizures.

Gastrointestinal: Nausea, vomiting, and abdominal pain.

Eye: Chemical conjunctivitis, corneal damage, and burns. Lacrimation and spasm of the eyelids (blepharospasm).

Skin: Irritant dermatitis and chemical burns. Cyanosis.

Renal: Kidney damage.

Hepatic: Liver damage.

Metabolism: Metabolic acidosis.

Other: Ability to detect products by smell may be lost after a relatively brief exposure time (olfactory nerve fatigue).

SYMPTOM ONSET FOR ACUTE EXPOSURE

Immediate
Some symptoms, especially pulmonary edema, may be delayed 2 to 24 hours

CO-EXPOSURE CONCERNS

Chlorine active compounds
Corrosive vapors

THERMAL DECOMPOSITION PRODUCTS INCLUDE

Carbon monoxide
Chloride
Hydrochloric acid if moisture or steam is present

MEDICAL CONDITIONS THAT MAY INCREASE RISK FOLLOWING EXPOSURE

Respiratory system disorders

DECONTAMINATION

- Wear positive-pressure SCBA and protective equipment specified by references such as the *North American Emergency Response Guidebook.* If special chemical protective clothing is required, consult the chemical manufacturer or specific protective clothing compatibility charts. A qualified, experienced person should make decisions regarding the type of personal protective equipment necessary.
- Delay entry until trained personnel and proper protective equipment are available.
- Remove patient from contaminated area.

- Quickly remove and isolate patient's clothing, jewelry, and shoes.
- Gently blot excess liquids with absorbent material.
- Rinse patient with warm water, 32° to 35° C (90° to 95° F), if possible.
- Wash patient with a mild liquid soap and large quantities of water. Some authorities recommend a dilute hypochlorite (0.5% solution) as a decontaminating agent. (refer to decontamination protocol in Section Three).
- Refer to decontamination protocol in Section Three.

IMMEDIATE FIRST AID

- Ensure that adequate decontamination has been carried out as needed.
- If patient is not breathing, start artificial respiration, preferably with a demand-valve resuscitator, bag-valve-mask device, or pocket mask, as trained. Perform CPR if necessary.
- Immediately flush contaminated eyes with gently flowing water.
- Do not induce vomiting. If vomiting occurs, lean patient forward or place on left side (head-down position, if possible) to maintain an open airway and prevent aspiration.
- Keep patient quiet and maintain normal body temperature.
- Obtain medical attention.

BASIC TREATMENT

- Establish a patent airway (oropharyngeal or nasopharyngeal airway, if needed). Suction if necessary.
- Watch for signs of respiratory insufficiency and assist ventilations if necessary.
- Administer oxygen by nonrebreather mask at 10 to 15 L/min.
- Monitor for pulmonary edema and treat if necessary (refer to pulmonary edema protocol in Section Three).
- Anticipate seizures and treat if necessary (refer to seizure protocol in Section Three).
- For eye contamination, flush eyes immediately with water. Irrigate each eye continuously with 0.9% saline (NS) during transport (refer to eye irrigation protocol in Section Three).
- Cover skin burns with dry sterile dressings after decontamination (refer to chemical burn protocol in Section Three).

ADVANCED TREATMENT

- Consider orotracheal or nasotracheal intubation for airway control in the patient who is unconscious, has severe pulmonary edema, or is in severe respiratory distress.
- Positive-pressure ventilation techniques with a bag-valve-mask device may be beneficial.
- Consider drug therapy for pulmonary edema (refer to pulmonary edema protocol in Section Three).
- Monitor cardiac rhythm and treat arrhythmias if necessary (refer to cardiac protocol in Section Three).
- Start IV administration of D_5W TKO. Use 0.9% saline (NS) or lactated Ringer's (LR) if signs of hypovolemia are present. For hypotension with signs of hypovolemia, administer fluid cautiously. Watch for signs of fluid overload (refer to shock protocol in Section Three).
- Treat seizures with diazepam (Valium) or lorazepam (Ativan) (refer to seizure protocol in Section Three and diazepam and lorazepam protocols in Section Four).

- Use proparacaine hydrochloride to assist eye irrigation (refer to proparacaine hydrochloride protocol in Section Four).

INITIAL EMERGENCY DEPARTMENT CONSIDERATIONS

- Useful initial laboratory studies include complete blood count, serum electrolytes, blood urea nitrogen (BUN), creatinine, glucose, urinalysis, and baseline biochemical profile, including serum aminotransferases (ALT and AST), calcium, phosphorus, and magnesium. Determination of anion and osmolar gaps may be helpful. Arterial blood gases (ABGs), chest radiograph, and electrocardiogram may be required.
- Obtain serial chest radiographs and monitor ABGs and respiratory function.
- Positive end-expiratory pressure (PEEP)-assisted ventilation may be necessary in patients with acute parenchymal injury who develop pulmonary edema or acute respiratory distress syndrome.
- Products may cause acidosis; hyperventilation and sodium bicarbonate may be beneficial. Bicarbonate therapy should be guided by patient presentation, ABG determination, and serum electrolyte considerations
- Obtain toxicological consultation as necessary.

SPECIAL CONSIDERATIONS

- Chlorine's relatively high water solubility accounts for the early upper airway symptoms.
- Phosgene's poor water solubility limits its effects on the upper airway, allowing most of the product to penetrate into the lower airways. Phosgene reacts with moisture in the lower airways to form hydrochloric acid and carbon dioxide, with resulting pulmonary edema. This is the mechanism for the delayed-onset pulmonary edema.

134

Incapacitating Agents

3-Quinuclidinyl Benzilate (BZ or QBN), Agent 15, d-Lysergic acid (LSD), Psilocybin, Mescaline, Related Compounds

SUBSTANCE IDENTIFICATION

Incapacitating agents are not designed to kill or seriously injure people. They are designed to impair performance, usually through effects on the central nervous system. The official military incapacitating agents include BZ (3-quinuclidinyl benzilate), which the United States weaponized but then demilitarized, and Agent 15, the Iraqi equivalent of BZ. Other possible agents of concern include D-lysergic acid (LSD), psilocybin, and mescaline. The main effects of the incapacitating agents are central nervous system effects that include realistic and concrete hallucinations and illusions. Effects can last for days.

CNS Depressants (Anticholinergics)

BZ and Agent 15 are CNS depressants. They work by causing an anticholinergic syndrome and interfering with transmission of information across central synapses. In the CNS, anticholinergic compounds disrupt the high integrative functions of memory, problem solving, attention, and comprehension. Relatively high doses produce toxic delirium that destroys the ability to perform any complex task. These compounds also affect the peripheral nervous system by inhibiting acetylcholine at muscarinic receptors (similar to atropine). They may be dispersed by smoke-producing munitions/aerosols or by contaminating isolated supplies of food or water.

CNS Stimulants

LSD, psilocybin, and mescaline act as CNS stimulants. They can cause excessive activity, often by boosting or facilitating transmission of impulses across synapses. Essentially they allow too much information to reach the cortex and other regulatory centers. This makes concentration difficult and causes indecisiveness and an inability to act. It is probable that only small quantities of CNS stimulants would be used to contaminate isolated food and water supplies.

ROUTES OF EXPOSURE

Inhalation
Ingestion
Skin absorption

TARGET ORGANS

Primary

Central and peripheral nervous system

Secondary

Cardiovascular system

Respiratory system
Gastrointestinal system
Eyes
Skin
Renal system

LIFE THREAT

The main effects of the incapacitating agents are non–life-threatening central nervous system effects that include realistic and concrete hallucinations and illusions. Hyperthermia, cardiac arrhythmias, and seizures are life threats secondary to exposure to these agents.

SIGNS AND SYMPTOMS BY SYSTEM

Cardiovascular: Tachycardia, moderate hypertension (hypertension or hypotension is possible with CNS stimulant exposure), decreased capillary tone resulting in skin flushing.

Respiratory: Respiratory depression (anticholinergics), tachypnea, and bronchoconstriction (CNS stimulants).

CNS: Psychosis with hallucinations (visual with anticholinergics, visual and rarely auditory with CNS stimulants), impaired perception of color, halos around objects, memory loss. Dystonic reactions, dyskinesia, restlessness, apprehension, abnormal speech, confusion, agitation, tremor, ataxia, stupor, coma, and seizures. Phantom behaviors such as constant picking, plucking, or grasping motions ("woolgathering"). Behavioral lability, with patients swinging back and forth between quiet confusion or self-absorption in hallucinations to frank combativeness (anticholinergics). Mass hysteria and sharing of illusions and hallucinations (anticholinergics). Flashbacks are possible after exposure to LSD. Panic reactions can occur (most often in children).

Gastrointestinal: Decreased gastric motility, decreased bowel sounds, nausea and vomiting, dry mouth (anticholinergics), salivation (CNS stimulants).

Eye: Mydriasis, photophobia, vision impairment, and pain.

Skin: Flushed, warm skin with decreased sweating (anticholinergics), diaphoresis (CNS stimulants).

Renal: Urinary retention and renal failure.

Other: Increased body temperature may occur due to inhibition of sweating and ability to dissipate heat. Marked hyperthermia may occur in warmer climates. Rhabdomyolysis may occur secondary to marked agitation or profound coma.

SYMPTOM ONSET FOR ACUTE EXPOSURE

Clinical effects from ingestion or inhalation of BZ or Agent 15 appear after an asymptomatic period that can range from 30 minutes to 20 hours (mean is 2 hours). Skin absorption can be delayed, depending on the solvent used, and can appear up to 36 hours later.

Time Course of Effects

BZ and Agent 15 (Anticholinergics):

1. Onset or induction: 0 to 4 hours after exposure. Characterized by parasympathetic blockade and mild CNS effects.
2. Second phase: 4 to 20 hours after exposure. Characterized by stupor with ataxia and hyperthermia.

3. Third phase: 20 to 96 hours after exposure. Characterized by full-blown delirium but can fluctuate from moment to moment.
4. Fourth phase or resolution. Characterized by paranoia, deep sleep, reawakening, crawling or climbing automatisms, and eventual reorientation.

LSD:

1. Somatic: 0 to 60 minutes after exposure. Characterized by tension, light-headedness, mydriasis, twitching, flushing, tachycardia, hypertension, and hyperreflexia.
2. Perceptual: 30 to 60 minutes after exposure. Characterized by visual, auditory, and sensory alterations; distortions of color, distance, shape, and time; synesthesias.
3. Psychic: 2 to 12 hours after exposure. Characterized by euphoria, mood swings, depressions, feelings of depersonalization, derealization, loss of body image.

MEDICAL CONDITIONS THAT MAY INCREASE RISK FOLLOWING EXPOSURE

Cardiac disorders

DECONTAMINATION

- Wear positive-pressure SCBA and protective equipment specified by references such as the *North American Emergency Response Guidebook*. If special chemical protective clothing is required, consult the chemical manufacturer or specific protective clothing compatibility charts. A qualified, experienced person should make decisions regarding the type of personal protective equipment necessary.
- Delay entry until trained personnel and proper protective equipment are available.
- Remove patient from contaminated area.
- Quickly remove and isolate patient's clothing, jewelry, and shoes.
- Gently brush away dry particles and blot excess liquids with absorbent material.
- Rinse patient with warm water, 32° C to 35° C (90° F to 95° F), if possible.
- Wash patient with a mild liquid soap and large quantities of water. Some authorities recommend a dilute hypochlorite (0.5% solution) as a decontaminating agent (refer to decontamination protocol in Section Three).

IMMEDIATE FIRST AID

- Ensure that adequate decontamination has been carried out as needed.
- If patient is not breathing, start artificial respiration, preferably with a demand-valve resuscitator, bag-valve-mask device, or pocket mask, as trained. Perform CPR as necessary.
- Immediately flush contaminated eyes with gently flowing water.
- Do not induce vomiting. If vomiting occurs, lean patient forward or place on left side (head-down position, if possible) to maintain an open airway and prevent aspiration.
- Keep patient quiet and maintain normal body temperature.
- Obtain medical attention.

BASIC TREATMENT

- Establish a patent airway (oropharyngeal or nasopharyngeal airway, if needed). Suction if necessary.
- Watch for signs of respiratory insufficiency and assist ventilations if necessary.

- Administer oxygen by nonrebreather mask at 10 to 15 L/min.
- Monitor for shock and treat if necessary (refer to shock protocol in Section Three).
- Anticipate seizures and treat if necessary (refer to seizure protocol in Section Three).
- Demonstrate a friendly attitude and use firm restraint when necessary. All dangerous objects must be removed from the area and anything likely to be swallowed should be kept away from patients, because bizarre delusions may occur.
- For eye contamination, flush eyes immediately with water. Irrigate each eye continuously with 0.9% saline (NS) during transport (refer to eye irrigation protocol in Section Three).
- Use rapid cooling techniques to manage hyperthermia (refer to heat stress protocol in Section Three).
- Do not use emetics. For ingestion, rinse mouth and administer 5 ml/kg up to 200 ml of water for dilution if the patient can swallow, has a strong gag reflex, and does not drool. Administer activated charcoal (refer to ingestion protocol in Section Three and activated charcoal protocol in Section Four).

ADVANCED TREATMENT

- Consider orotracheal or nasotracheal intubation for airway control in the patient who is unconscious, has severe pulmonary edema, or is in severe respiratory distress.
- Positive-pressure ventilation techniques with a bag-valve-mask device may be beneficial.
- Monitor cardiac rhythm and treat arrhythmias if necessary (refer to cardiac protocol in Section Three).
- Start IV administration of 0.9% saline (NS) or lactated Ringer's (LR) TKO. For hypotension with signs of hypovolemia, administer fluid cautiously. Watch for signs of fluid overload (refer to shock protocol in Section Three).
- Treat seizures or sedate LSD patients with diazepam (Valium) or lorazepam (Ativan) (refer to seizure protocol in Section Three and diazepam and lorazepam protocols in Section Four).
- Administer physostigmine for symptomatic BZ or Agent 15 exposure only (refer to physostigmine protocol in Section Four).
- Use proparacaine hydrochloride to assist eye irrigation (refer to proparacaine hydrochloride protocol in Section Four).

INITIAL EMERGENCY DEPARTMENT CONSIDERATIONS

- Useful initial laboratory studies include complete blood count, serum electrolytes, blood urea nitrogen (BUN), creatinine, glucose, urinalysis, and baseline biochemical profile, including serum aminotransferases (ALT and AST), creatinine, and phosphokinase. Arterial blood gases (ABGs), chest radiograph, and electrocardiogram may be required. Plasma and urine LSD levels can be tested.
- Rhabdomyolysis is possible after seizures or prolonged coma. Administer sufficient 0.9% saline or lactated Ringer's solution to maintain urine output of 2 to 3 ml/kg/hour. Monitor input and output, serum electrolytes, CK, and renal

function. Diuretics may be necessary to maintain urine output. Urinary alkalinization may be helpful.

- Obtain toxicological consultation as necessary.

SPECIAL CONSIDERATIONS

- In most cases of mild exposure, symptoms are self-limited and require supportive management only. Treat severe symptomatic exposures as required.

Nerve Agents

Tabun (GA), Sarin (GB), Soman (GD), GF, VX, Related Compounds

SUBSTANCE IDENTIFICATION

Nerve agents are the most toxic of the chemical agents. Nerve agents include tabun (GA), sarin (GB), soman (GD), GF, and VX. The two letter abbreviation following the chemical name is the military designation for the agent. Exposure to these agents can result in death within minutes of exposure. Nerve agents inhibit acetylcholinesterase in tissue, and their effects are caused by the resulting acetylcholine.

The nerve agent attachment to the acetylcholinesterase enzyme is essentially irreversible, unless removed by therapy. After a period of time the bond between the nerve agent and enzyme "ages." Once the bond is aged the enzyme cannot be reactivated. The period of time that it takes a bond to age is dependent on the specific nerve agent. For most agents there is adequate time to reactivate the enzyme using drug therapy. This therapy is usually carried out by treatment with oxime compounds. However, the aging time of the soman (GD) enzyme complex is about 2 minutes. After the bond is aged, the usefulness of treatment with oximes is greatly decreased.

Nerve agents are liquids under temperate conditions. When they are dispersed, the more volatile agents present both a liquid and vapor hazard. The less volatile agents present a hazard as a liquid or when dispersed in a droplet spray or with an explosive device. Nerve agents are related to the organophosphate (OP) insecticides. These commonly used insecticides include malathion, parathion, and disulfotons. Nerve agents and OP insecticides have similar biological effects. However, one major difference between them is the relative lipid insolubility of nerve agents compared to the lipid solubility of OP insecticides. This accounts for the long duration of action of OP insecticides compared with nerve agents,.

G Agents

Tabun (GA) was first synthesized in the late 1930s by a German scientist searching for a more potent insecticide. Shortly thereafter, sarin (GB) was synthesized, followed by soman (GD) and GF. The "G" agents are considered to be volatile agents and are known as nonpersistent by the military. Nonpersistent agents, depending on temperature, can contaminate surfaces for up to 24 hours. Sarin is the most volatile of these agents but it evaporates more slowly than water. Tabun and sarin were probably used by Iraq against Iran in the 1980s. A dilute solution of sarin was used in the Tokyo subway attack in 1995.

VX

VX was developed by Great Britain and the United States after World War II. It is the most toxic of all the nerve agents. It is 100 to 150 times more toxic than sarin when on the skin. Absorption of a pinhead-sized drop of VX can be fatal. VX is considered a persistent agent and can contaminate surfaces for days to weeks, depending on the temperature and weather. It has the consistency of motor oil. VX presents mostly a liquid or droplet spray hazard.

ROUTES OF EXPOSURE

Skin and eye contact
Inhalation
Skin absorption

TARGET ORGANS

Primary
Central nervous system
Cardiovascular system
Respiratory system
Eyes
Secondary
Skin
Gastrointestinal system
Hepatic system
Metabolism

LIFE THREAT

Respiratory failure caused by chemically mediated pulmonary edema and respiratory muscle paralysis. Inhibits acetylcholinesterase, causing overstimulation of the parasympathetic nervous system, striated muscle, sympathetic ganglia, and CNS. Causes bradycardia, hypotension, and pulmonary edema.

SIGNS AND SYMPTOMS BY SYSTEM

Cardiovascular: Bradycardia (tachycardia possible), ventricular arrhythmias, A-V blocks, and hypotension.

Respiratory: Respiratory failure, bronchoconstriction, wheezing, cough, profuse pulmonary secretions (bronchorrhea), acute pulmonary edema, dyspnea, and tightness of the chest.

CNS: CNS depression, coma, anxiety, headache, dizziness, weakness, loss of muscle coordination, muscle fasciculations, seizures, disorientation, confusion, drowsiness, and slurred speech.

Gastrointestinal: Nausea, vomiting, diarrhea, abdominal cramps, excessive salivation, and defecation.

Renal: Excessive urination.

Eye: Lacrimation, blurred vision. Constricted pupils are common; however, dilated pupils may be present.

Skin: Pale, cyanotic skin with excessive diaphoresis.

Hepatic: Liver damage.

Metabolism: Hypoglycemia or hyperglycemia, and acidosis.

Other: Hypothermia may occur. Classic SLUDGE syndrome (*s*alivation, *l*acrimation, *u*rination, *d*efecation, GI pain, and *e*mesis), May range from flu-type symptoms, anxiety, seizures, and coma. Symptoms may be broken down into muscarinic effects (classic SLUDGE syndrome, cardiac effects, constricted pupils, bronchoconstriction, pulmonary edema) and nicotinic symptoms (muscle fasciculations, tachycardia, hypertension, respiratory paralysis). If dermal absorption and nicotinic receptors are the primary sites of stimulation, the SLUDGE syndrome may not be clinically present. Instead, cardiovascular collapse may be the primary clinical manifestation. The combination of pinpoint pupils and muscle twitching is the most reliable clinical evidence of nerve agent poisoning.

Cholinesterase inhibitor exposures may be cumulative.

Symptoms in children may differ from those found in adults. Pediatric signs and symptoms include CNS depression, flaccid muscle tone, dyspnea, and coma.

SYMPTOM ONSET FOR ACUTE EXPOSURE

Absorption of inhaled nerve agent vapor from the respiratory tract occurs within seconds of exposure.

Liquid skin absorption is slower; for example, it may take up to 18 hours for a small droplet of VX to be absorbed.

CO-EXPOSURE CONCERNS

Organophosphate insecticides
Carbamate insecticides

THERMAL DECOMPOSITION PRODUCTS INCLUDE

Carbon monoxide
Nitrogen oxides
Phosphorus oxides
Sulfur oxides

MEDICAL CONDITIONS THAT MAY INCREASE RISK FOLLOWING EXPOSURE

Respiratory disorders
Neurological disorders

DECONTAMINATION

- Wear positive-pressure SCBA and protective equipment specified by references such as the *North American Emergency Response Guidebook*. If special chemical protective clothing is required, consult the chemical manufacturer or specific protective clothing compatibility charts. A qualified, experienced person should make decisions regarding the type of personal protective equipment necessary.
- Delay entry until trained personnel and proper protective equipment are available.
- Remove patient from contaminated area.
- Quickly remove and isolate patient's clothing, jewelry, and shoes.
- Gently blot any excess liquids with absorbent material.
- Rinse patient with warm water, 32° C to 35° C (90° F to 95° F), if possible.
- Wash patient with a mild liquid soap and large quantities of water. Some authorities recommend a dilute hypochlorite (0.5% solution) as a decontaminating agent (refer to decontamination protocol in Section Three).
- Products are highly absorbable, and decontamination is critical.
- Discard all exposed leather products.
- Refer to decontamination protocol in Section Three.

IMMEDIATE FIRST AID

- Ensure that adequate decontamination has been carried out as needed.
- If patient is not breathing, start artificial respiration, preferably with a demand-valve resuscitator, bag-valve-mask device, or pocket mask, as trained. Perform CPR if necessary.

- Immediately flush contaminated eyes with gently flowing water.
- Do not induce vomiting. If vomiting occurs, lean patient forward or place on left side (head-down position, if possible) to maintain an open airway and prevent aspiration.
- Keep patient quiet and maintain normal body temperature.
- Obtain medical attention.

BASIC TREATMENT

- Establish a patent airway (oropharyngeal or nasopharyngeal airway, if needed). Suction if necessary.
- Aggressive airway control may be needed.
- Watch for signs of respiratory insufficiency and assist ventilations if necessary.
- Administer oxygen by nonrebreather mask at 10 to 15 L/min.
- Monitor for pulmonary edema and treat if necessary (refer to pulmonary edema protocol in Section Three).
- Monitor for shock and treat if necessary (refer to shock protocol in Section Three).
- Anticipate seizures and treat if necessary (refer to seizure protocol in Section Three).
- For eye contamination, flush eyes immediately with water. Irrigate each eye continuously with 0.9% saline (NS) during transport (refer to eye irrigation protocol in Section Three).

ADVANCED TREATMENT

- Consider orotracheal or nasotracheal intubation for airway control in the patient who is unconscious, has severe pulmonary edema, or is in severe respiratory distress.
- Positive-pressure ventilation techniques with a bag-valve-mask device may be beneficial. Initial ventilation may be difficult. Airway resistance may be high (50 to 70 cm H_2O) because of secretions and bronchoconstriction. Frequent suctioning may be necessary.
- Monitor cardiac rhythm and treat arrhythmias if necessary (refer to cardiac protocol in Section Three).
- Start IV administration of D_5W TKO. Use 0.9% saline (NS) or lactated Ringer's (LR) if signs of hypovolemia are present. For hypotension with signs of hypovolemia, administer fluid cautiously and consider vasopressors if patient is hypotensive with a normal fluid volume. Watch for signs of fluid overload (refer to shock protocol in Section Three).
- Administer atropine. Correct hypoxia before administration (refer to atropine protocol in Section Four).
- In severely poisoned patients, administer pralidoxime chloride (2-PAM) (refer to pralidoxime chloride protocol in Section Four).
- Treat seizures with adequate atropinization, correction of hypoxia, and diazepam (Valium) or lorazepam as necessary (refer to seizure protocol in Section Three and diazepam and lorazepam protocols in Section Four).
- In mass casualty events the use of auto-injector atropine and 2-PAM is advised. These auto-injectors are known as the Mark I kit. An auto-injector diazepam is also available (refer to Mark I and diazepam protocols in Section Four for detailed information).

- Administer homatropine drops for miosis and eye pain (refer to homatropine protocol in Section Four).
- Use proparacaine hydrochloride to assist eye irrigation (refer to proparacaine hydrochloride protocol in Section Four).

INITIAL EMERGENCY DEPARTMENT CONSIDERATIONS

- Useful initial laboratory studies include complete blood count, serum electrolytes, blood urea nitrogen (BUN), creatinine, glucose, urinalysis, and baseline biochemical profile, including serum aminotransferases (ALT and AST), calcium, phosphorus, and magnesium. Arterial blood gases (ABGs), chest radiograph, and electrocardiogram may be required.
- Both plasma and red blood cell acetylcholinesterase levels should be obtained. Do not delay therapeutic interventions pending laboratory results. Treat symptomatically.
- Positive end-expiratory pressure (PEEP)-assisted ventilation may be necessary in patients with acute parenchymal injury who develop pulmonary edema or acute respiratory distress syndrome.
- Products may cause acidosis; hyperventilation and sodium bicarbonate may be beneficial. Bicarbonate therapy should be guided by patient presentation, ABG determination, and serum electrolyte considerations.
- In cases of skin absorption and primary nicotinic stimulation, atropine may not reverse the respiratory paralysis. Be prepared to assist ventilations and administer 2-PAM. Initial symptoms may be diaphoresis, muscle fasciculations, and respiratory arrest.
- Nerve agents are relatively lipid insoluble compared to the lipid solubility of the OP insecticides. As such, they usually require a much lower dosage of atropine and do not have the long duration of action of the civilian organophosphates.
- Obtain toxicological consultation as necessary.

SPECIAL CONSIDERATIONS

- Succinylcholine, other cholinergic agents, and aminophylline are contraindicated.
- The end point for atropine administration is the drying of pulmonary secretions.

136

Riot Control Agents

Orthochlorobenzylidene malononitrile (CS), Chloracetophenone CN (Mace), Dibenzoxazepine (CR), Oleoresin capsicum or Pepper spray (OC)

SUBSTANCE IDENTIFICATION

Riot control agents are irritants characterized by low toxicity and a short duration of action. They are also known as "tear gas" or lacrimators. They cause transient discomfort and eye closure. Their purpose is to render the patient temporarily incapable of fighting or resisting. They are commonly used by law enforcement agencies for riot and crowd control. Riot control agents have a high lethal dose and a low effective dose and therefore a high safety ratio. They are solids with low vapor pressures and are dispersed as fine particles or in solutions. Dispersion devices include spray cans, spray tanks, "fogging" devices, and grenades.

Similar agents were used by the French police before World War I to dispel rioters, and they were the first chemical agents to be used during that war. They continued to be used until more toxic/effective agents were developed. Today they are used by law enforcement agencies worldwide. CS has superseded CN because of its stronger irritant effects and its lower toxicity.

ROUTES OF EXPOSURE

Skin and eye contact
Inhalation
Ingestion

TARGET ORGANS

Primary
Skin
Eyes
Respiratory system
Secondary
Cardiovascular system
Gastrointestinal system

LIFE THREAT

The main effects of riot control agents are pain, burning, and irritation of exposed skin and mucous membranes. The effect is transient (about 30 minutes after exposure). Agents have a high safety ratio and have not been found to cause permanent lung damage or exacerbate chronic pulmonary diseases. Nevertheless, airway problems should be anticipated in individuals with lung disease, particularly after higher than average exposure concentrations.

SIGNS AND SYMPTOMS BY SYSTEM

Cardiovascular: Transient increase in heart rate and blood pressure.
Respiratory: With most agents, a mild and transient cough is the only symptom at the time of exposure. Symptoms may be self-limited in mild exposures.
Gastrointestinal: Burning of the mucous membranes, nausea, vomiting, and abdominal pain.
Eye: Chemical conjunctivitis.
Skin: Irritation of the skin, especially mucous membranes, pallor, and cyanosis.
Other: Animals given lethal amounts of CS by intravenous or intraperitoneal routes have developed increased blood thiocyanate concentrations. This indicates that the malononitrile portion of CS had been metabolized to cyanide. The cause of death in these animal tests was lung damage, not cyanide toxicity. The cyanide metabolism appears to occur only with IV or IP administration and not with inhalation exposure. Animal tests with lethal doses of CS by inhalation have not shown this result. Patients with inhalation exposure to CS should not need cyanide antidote therapy.

SYMPTOM ONSET FOR ACUTE EXPOSURE

Immediate

MEDICAL CONDITIONS THAT MAY INCREASE RISK FOLLOWING EXPOSURE

Cardiac disorders
Respiratory disorders

DECONTAMINATION

- Wear positive-pressure SCBA or air purifying respirator with appropriate cartridge/filter and protective equipment specified by references such as the *North American Emergency Response Guidebook.* If special chemical protective clothing is required, consult the chemical manufacturer or specific protective clothing compatibility charts. A qualified, experienced person should make decisions regarding the type of personal protective equipment necessary.
- Delay entry until trained personnel and proper protective equipment are available.
- Remove patient from contaminated area.
- Quickly remove and isolate patient's clothing, jewelry, and shoes.
- In most cases, the best decontamination is moving air across the contaminated area, allowing the agent to blow away. In cases of visible gross contamination, water is useful for removing large amounts of agent, but ultimately the remaining agent will not be removed until the water dries and the agent can blow away.
- Use copious amounts of plain water for removing **gross** contamination only. Bleach solutions should not be used. They may react with CS to form a combination that is more irritating to the skin than CS alone.
- Make sure the water flows away from the face. The hair is the next most effective reservoir (after clothes) for contamination. Use particular care that water does not run from the hair to the eyes and dry the hair after use of water for decontamination.
- Several aftermarket decontamination solutions are available for OC agent decontamination. Some authorities suggest milk (of any type) is also an effective solution because of the antagonistic relationship between lactic acid and the active enzyme in OC.

- Use of water on clothing does NOT remove the contaminant; it merely holds it to the clothes until the water dries, and then the agent is released into the air again.

Special Note on Decontaminating Law Enforcement Personnel

- Law enforcement treatment during riots or civil disturbances is usually geared toward getting personnel back to duty. Avoid, if possible, the use of water on their clothing. Visible agents can be physically removed from the clothing. If the officer's head is decontaminated, use the same precautions as above. Pay particular attention to the hair and decontaminate repeatedly to remove as much agent as possible. The officer's helmet will cause sweat on the head, which will tend to carry the agent back into the eyes.

IMMEDIATE FIRST AID

- Ensure that adequate decontamination has been carried out as needed.
- If patient is not breathing, start artificial respiration, preferably with a demand-valve resuscitator, bag-valve-mask device, or pocket mask, as trained. Perform CPR as necessary.
- Immediately flush contaminated eyes with gently flowing water.
- Do not induce vomiting. If vomiting occurs, lean patient forward or place on left side (head-down position, if possible) to maintain an open airway and prevent aspiration.
- Keep patient quiet and maintain normal body temperature.
- Obtain medical attention.

BASIC TREATMENT

- Establish a patent airway (oropharyngeal or nasopharyngeal airway, if needed). Suction if necessary.
- Encourage patient to take deep breaths.
- Watch for signs of respiratory insufficiency and assist ventilations if necessary.
- Administer oxygen by nonrebreather mask at 10 to 15 L/min.
- For eye contamination, flush eyes immediately with water. For CN or CS exposure irrigate each eye continuously with 0.9% saline (NS) during transport. Use only plain water to irrigate eyes exposed to OC. Saline will cause an increase in pain (refer to eye irrigation protocol in Section Three).
- Do not use emetics. For ingestion, rinse mouth and administer 5 ml/kg up to 200 ml of water for dilution if the patient can swallow, has a strong gag reflex, and does not drool (refer to ingestion protocol in Section Three).

ADVANCED TREATMENT

- Consider orotracheal or nasotracheal intubation for airway control in the patient who is unconscious or is in severe respiratory distress. Early intubation at the first sign of upper airway obstruction may be necessary.
- Positive-pressure ventilation techniques with a bag-valve mask device may be beneficial.
- Monitor cardiac rhythm and treat arrhythmias if necessary (refer to cardiac protocol in Section Three).
- Start IV administration of D_5W TKO. Use 0.9% saline (NS) or lactated Ringer's (LR) if signs of hypovolemia are present. For hypotension with signs of hypovolemia, administer fluid cautiously. Watch for signs of fluid overload. (refer to shock protocol in Section Three)

- Treat seizures with diazepam (Valium) or lorazepam (Ativan) (refer to seizure protocol in Section Three and diazepam and lorazepam protocols in Section Four).
- Use proparacaine hydrochloride to assist eye irrigation (refer to proparacaine hydrochloride protocol in Section Four).

INITIAL EMERGENCY DEPARTMENT CONSIDERATIONS

- Useful initial laboratory studies include complete blood count, serum electrolytes, blood urea nitrogen (BUN), creatinine, glucose, urinalysis, and baseline biochemical profile, including serum aminotransferases (ALT and AST), calcium, phosphorus, and magnesium. Determination of anion and osmolar gaps may be helpful. Arterial blood gases (ABGs), chest radiograph, and electrocardiogram may be required.
- These compounds are solids and it is possible for a particle to cause a corneal abrasion or become embedded in the cornea or conjunctiva and cause tissue damage. Patients complaining of continued eye pain post exposure should receive thorough eye decontamination and ophthalmic examination.
- Obtain toxicological consultation as necessary.

SPECIAL CONSIDERATIONS

- In most cases of mild exposure, symptoms are self-limited and require supportive management only. Use of medications such as atropine, epinephrine, expectorants, and sedatives is not indicated and may cause further damage.
- Treat severe symptomatic exposures as required.

Military Smoke Agents

Hexachloroethane Smoke (Zinc Oxide Mixtures) (HC), Chlorosulfonic Acid (CSA), Sulfur Trioxide–Chlorosulfonic Acid (FS), Titanium Tetrachloride (FM), White Phosphorus (WP), Fog Oil (SGF2), Colored Smokes, Related Compounds

SUBSTANCE IDENTIFICATION

Military smoke agents are used to obscure vision and hide troops, equipment, and areas. Chemicals used to produce smokes include hexachloroethane, grained aluminum, and zinc oxide (HC) mixture; special petroleum oils (fog oil [SGF2]); diesel fuel; red phosphorus (RP) in a butyl rubber matrix; and white phosphorus (WP) plasticized or impregnated in wool felt wedges. Burning phosphorus mixtures produce smokes composed of highly concentrated (60% to 80%) polyphosphorous acids. Sulfur trioxide–chlorosulfonic acid solution (FS) and titanium tetrachloride (FM) are older smoke agents that are seldom used in current operations. The letter abbreviation following the chemical name is the military designation for the agent. The chemical composition of the petroleum-based and colored smokes is similar to that of the bulk materials from which they are generated. Most smokes are not hazardous in concentrations that are normally used for obscuring purposes. However, except with oil smoke, high concentrations of smoke accidentally or intentionally generated in closed spaces can be extremely dangerous. Ill effects can also occur in open spaces if the concentration is sufficient or if the exposure is long enough. Smokes can be dispersed by grenades, candles, pots, artillery shells, air bombs, smoke generators, engine exhausts, and aircraft sprayers.

Hexachloroethane Smoke (HC)

Zinc oxide mixture is a combination of hexachloroethane, aluminum powder, and zinc oxide. On burning, the mixture produces zinc chloride, which rapidly absorbs moisture from the air to form a gray-white smoke. HC smoke can elicit nose, throat, and chest irritation and cough and slight nausea in some individuals. At high concentrations, severe respiratory distress may be fatal.

Chlorosulfonic Acid (CSA) and Sulfur Trioxide–Chlorosulfonic Acid (FS)

These agents are heavy, strongly acid liquids that, when dispersed in the air, absorb moisture to form a dense white fog consisting of small droplets of hydrochloric and sulfuric acids. In moderate concentrations, it is highly irritating to the eyes, nose, and skin.

Titanium Tetrachloride (FM)

Titanium tetrachloride is a corrosive compound that decomposes on contact with moist air, yielding a dense white smoke composed of titanium dioxide, titanium oxychloride, and hydrochloric acid.

White Phosphorus (WP)

White phosphorus is a pale yellow waxy solid that ignites spontaneously on contact with air. The flame produces a hot, dense white smoke composed of particles of phosphorus pentoxide, which are converted by moist air into phosphoric acid.

Fog Oil (SGF2)

Fog oil smokes are produced by vaporizing fuel oils in smoke generators or engine exhausts. The generator or engine exhaust vaporizes either SGF2 or diesel fuel and forces it into the air where it condenses into a dense white smoke. Petroleum oil smokes present a low toxicity threat.

Colored Smokes

Colored smokes are produced by explosive dissemination of dyes. There are no reports of ill effects produced by exposure to colored smokes.

ROUTES OF EXPOSURE

Skin and eye contact
Inhalation

TARGET ORGANS

Primary
Skin
Eyes
Respiratory system
Secondary
Central nervous system
Cardiovascular system
Gastrointestinal system

LIFE THREAT

Hyperemia of the larynx, trachea, and large bronchi occur, along with functional narrowing of the smaller air passages. In severe exposures, chemical pneumonia with pulmonary edema is possible. Shock and serious infection may occur.

SIGNS AND SYMPTOMS BY SYSTEM

Cardiovascular: Cardiac arrhythmias, tachycardia, and cardiogenic shock.

Respiratory: Dyspnea, tachypnea, and irritation of the respiratory tract. Retrosternal chest pain. Hyperemia of the larynx, trachea, and large bronchi. Chemical pneumonia and pulmonary edema.

CNS: Headache, dizziness, and malaise.

Gastrointestinal: Abdominal cramps.

Eye: Conjunctivitis, photophobia, corneal damage, chemical burns, and lacrimation,

Skin: Chemical and thermal burns, irritant dermatitis, and cyanosis.

Other: Unburned white phosphorus may remain in the felt wedges in the WP smoke munitions. It will burn spontaneously if the felt wedges are crushed and the white phosphorus is exposed to air. The white phosphorus particles can imbed in the skin and continue to burn.

SYMPTOM ONSET FOR ACUTE EXPOSURE

Immediate
Some symptoms may be delayed up to 48 hours after exposure.

MEDICAL CONDITIONS THAT MAY INCREASE RISK FOLLOWING EXPOSURE

Respiratory disorders

DECONTAMINATION

- Wear positive-pressure SCBA or air purifying respirator with appropriate cartridge/filter and protective equipment specified by references such as the *North American Emergency Response Guidebook*. If special chemical protective clothing is required, consult the chemical manufacturer or specific protective clothing compatibility charts. A qualified, experienced person should make decisions regarding the type of personal protective equipment necessary.
- Delay entry until trained personnel and proper protective equipment are available.
- Remove patient from contaminated area.
- Quickly remove and isolate patient's clothing, jewelry, and shoes.
- Gently brush away dry particles and blot excess liquids with absorbent material.
- If phosphorus particles are embedded in the skin, continuous water irrigation, water immersion, or sterile water-soaked dressings should be applied during transport to the hospital for surgical debridement. Do not use oil for phosphorus exposure because this may promote dermal absorption.
- Rinse patient with cool water.
- Wash patient with a mild liquid soap and large quantities of water (refer to decontamination protocol in Section Three).

IMMEDIATE FIRST AID

- Ensure that adequate decontamination has been carried out as needed.
- If patient is not breathing, start artificial respiration, preferably with a demand-valve resuscitator, bag-valve-mask device, or pocket mask, as trained. Perform CPR if necessary.
- Immediately flush contaminated eyes with gently flowing water.
- Do not induce vomiting. If vomiting occurs, lean patient forward or place on left side (head-down position, if possible) to maintain an open airway and prevent aspiration.
- Keep patient quiet and maintain normal body temperature.
- Obtain medical attention.

BASIC TREATMENT

- Establish a patent airway (oropharyngeal or nasopharyngeal airway, if needed). Suction if necessary.
- Watch for signs of respiratory insufficiency and assist ventilations if necessary.
- Administer oxygen by nonrebreather mask at 10 to 15 L/min.
- Monitor for pulmonary edema and treat if necessary (refer to pulmonary edema protocol in Section Three).
- Monitor for shock and treat if necessary (refer to shock protocol in Section Three).
- For eye contamination, flush eyes immediately with water. Irrigate each eye continuously with 0.9% saline (NS) during transport (refer to eye irrigation protocol in Section Three).

ADVANCED TREATMENT

- Consider orotracheal or nasotracheal intubation for airway control in the patient who is unconscious, has severe pulmonary edema, or is in severe respiratory distress.
- Positive-pressure ventilation techniques with a bag-valve-mask device may be beneficial.

- Consider drug therapy for pulmonary edema (refer to pulmonary edema protocol in Section Three).
- Monitor cardiac rhythm and treat arrhythmias if necessary (refer to cardiac protocol in Section Three).
- Start IV administration of D_5W TKO. Use 0.9% saline (NS) or lactated Ringer's (LR) if signs of hypovolemia are present. For hypotension with signs of hypovolemia, administer fluid cautiously. Watch for signs of fluid overload (refer to shock protocol in Section Three).
- Use proparacaine hydrochloride to assist eye irrigation (refer to proparacaine hydrochloride protocol in Section Four).

INITIAL EMERGENCY DEPARTMENT CONSIDERATIONS

- Useful initial laboratory studies include complete blood count, prothrombin time, serum electrolytes, blood urea nitrogen (BUN), creatinine, glucose, urinalysis, and baseline biochemical profile, including bilirubin, serum aminotransferases (ALT and AST), calcium, phosphorus, and magnesium. Determination of anion and osmolar gaps may be helpful. Arterial blood gases (ABGs), chest radiograph, and electrocardiogram may be required.
- Chest radiographs associated with severe exposure have demonstrated a dense, diffuse infiltrative process present in one or both lung fields. Repeat chest radiographs have shown progression of the infiltrate even though physical examination results of the chest were normal. Final resolution of the infiltrate may be delayed for a month or longer, even though the patient is asymptomatic during this period.
- Positive end-expiratory pressure (PEEP)-assisted ventilation may be necessary in patients with acute parenchymal injury who develop pulmonary edema or acute respiratory distress syndrome.
- Examine the cornea for erosion by staining it with fluorescein. If corneal erosion is severe, transfer the patient to the care of an ophthalmologist.
- Individuals exposed in closed areas should be kept under observation for at least 48 hours. Most individuals recover in a few days. At moderate exposures, some symptoms may persist for 1 to 2 weeks. In severe exposure, survivors may have reduced pulmonary function for some months after exposure.
- Obtain toxicological consultation as necessary.

SPECIAL CONSIDERATIONS

- If white phosphorous solids are embedded in the skin, keep area submerged in water during transport to the hospital for surgical debridement.

138

Toxic Industrial Chemicals

SUBSTANCE IDENTIFICATION

Many commonly used industrial chemicals may be used as weapons of mass destruction. Toxic industrial chemicals have been defined by the United States military as an industrial chemical that has a 50% lethal concentration (LCt_{50}) value of less than 100,000 mg/min/m^3 (approximately the same as that for ammonia) in any mammalian species and is produced in quantities exceeding 30 tons per year at one production facility. Industrial chemicals can present numerous hazards. These hazards include:

- *Explosives*—chemicals or mixtures that cause sudden almost instantaneous release of pressure, gas, and heat when subjected to sudden shock, pressure, or high temperatures
- *Flammable or combustible compounds*—any solids, liquids, or gases that ignite easily or burn rapidly
- *Toxic compounds*—poisons that cause acute or chronic health problems
- *Corrosive compounds*—materials that cause tissue destruction at the site of contact
- *Irritating compounds*—materials that cause reversible inflammation to tissue
- *Pyrophoric compounds*—materials that ignite spontaneously in air at a temperature below 130° F
- *Water-reactive compounds*—materials that react with water to produce a large amount of heat
- *Oxidizers*—substances that yield oxygen readily to stimulate the combustion of organic matter
- *Organic peroxides*—a type of oxidizer that is very reactive, and potentially explosive, as well as a corrosive or flammability hazard
- *Unstable compounds*—substances that tend to undergo decomposition or other unwanted chemical change during storage or handling

High hazard toxic industrial chemicals are those that are produced in large quantities, have a high degree of toxicity by inhalation, and exist in a state that could present an inhalation hazard. This text has specific guidelines for each of these chemical hazards. Following is a list of the toxic chemicals that received a high hazard index ranking and the specific guidelines where information can be found:

- Ammonia—Guideline 21
- Arsine—Guideline 73
- Boron trichloride—Guideline 103
- Boron trifluoride—Guideline 103
- Carbon disulfide—Guideline 93
- Chlorine—Guidelines 98 and 133
- Diborane—Guideline 103
- Ethylene oxide—Guideline 45
- Fluorine—Guideline 99

- Formaldehyde—Guideline 41
- Hydrogen bromide—Guideline 95
- Hydrogen chloride—Guideline 14
- Hydrogen cyanide—Guidelines 90 and 132
- Hydrogen fluoride—Guideline 16
- Hydrogen sulfide—Guideline 91
- Nitric acid, fuming—Guideline 14
- Phosgene—Guidelines 101 and 133
- Phosphorus trichloride—Guidelines 98 and 109
- Sulfur dioxide—Guideline 105
- Sulfuric acid, fuming—Guideline 14
- Tungsten hexafluoride—Guideline 99

139

Blister Agents (Vesicants)

Sulfur Mustard (HD), Nitrogen Mustard (HN), Lewisite (L), Phosgene Oxime (CX), Mixtures and Related Compounds

SUBSTANCE IDENTIFICATION

Vesicants, or blister agents, were one of the most effective military agents used in World War I. Vesicants chemically burn and blister the skin and other body tissues that they contact. Most vesicants (except phosgene oxime [CX]) are relatively persistent and can remain active in the environment from days to weeks, depending on weather conditions. They were used by the military to produce casualties and to force the opposing troops to wear protective equipment, thus reducing their fighting efficiency. Because of the persistent nature of these agents, they were often used to contaminate terrain, ships, vehicles, etc.

There are three major families of vesicants: sulfur mustard (HD) and nitrogen mustard (HN); arsenical vesicants such as lewisite (L); and halogenated oximes such as phosgene oxime (CX). The letter/s abbreviation following the chemical name is the military designation for the agent.

Mustard (H)

Sulfur mustard (H) was first synthesized in the early 1800s. It was not used as a warfare agent until World War I. Mustard agent made by a distillation process is almost pure and is known as distilled mustard (HD). Nitrogen mustards (HN1, HN2, and HN3) were synthesized in the 1930s but were never produced in large quantities for warfare purposes. Mustard is very persistent in cold and temperate climates and is primarily a liquid hazard. It is less persistent in warmer temperatures and will produce more vapor. At 100° F or above, mustard presents a definite vapor hazard. Its persistence is sometimes enhanced by dissolving it in nonvolatile solvents. Because mustard freezes at about 57° F and is difficult to disperse as a solid, it is sometimes mixed with other agents to lower its freezing point. Common mixtures include mustard and lewisite (HL) and mustard mixed with Agent T (a closely related vesicant), known as HT. Mustard mixed with newer thickening agents is also widely known as HT. Mustard can remain active in stagnant water for several months.

Mustard agents are known for their delayed onset of signs and symptoms. Mustard agents produced the most casualties in World War I, although it had a mortality rate of less than 5%. It has been used numerous times since World War I. In 1930, Italy used mustard against Abyssinia, and in the 1960s Egypt used mustard against Yemen. In the 1980s, mustard was used by Iraq against both Iran and the Kurds. Mustard is still stockpiled as a warfare agent by many European and third world countries.

Lewisite (L)

Lewisite (L) is an arsenical vesicant that damages the skin, eyes, and other body tissues on contact. Lewisite is an oily, colorless liquid. It has an odor of geraniums; the ability to recognize the odor may be lost after accommodation (olfactory nerve fatigue).Unlike the mustard agents, exposure to lewisite causes immediate pain or irritation. Lewisite can be mixed with mustard to lower its freezing point, making it easier to use for ground dispersal or aerial spraying. Lewisite was first synthesized in 1918 by Dr. Wilfred Lee Lewis. Because of production time delays, it was not used in World War I. Lewisite may still be stockpiled by some nations.

Phosgene Oxime (CX)

Phosgene oxime (CX) is an urticant or nettle agent that can cause corrosive-type skin damage. Unlike mustard and lewisite, it does not cause blisters. Both the vapor and liquid cause immediate skin damage on contact. Phosgene oxime is a solid below 95° F. The solid form has a high enough vapor pressure to produce symptoms. Its odor has been described as a pepperish odor that may be lost after accommodation. Phosgene oxime is rapidly absorbed, and systemic distribution to most organs and tissue is rapid. Exposure causes extreme pain in exposed tissue.

ROUTES OF EXPOSURE

Skin and eye contact
Inhalation
Ingestion
Skin absorption

TARGET ORGANS

Primary
Skin
Eyes
Respiratory system
Gastrointestinal system
Blood
Secondary
Central nervous system
Cardiovascular system
Hepatic system
Renal system

LIFE THREAT

Vesicants burn and blister the skin or other body tissues on contact. They act on the eyes, skin, mucous membranes, lungs, and blood-forming organs. Mustard poisoning is believed to result in DNA alkylation and cross-linking in rapidly dividing cells, such as basal keratinocytes, mucosal epithelium, and bone marrow precursor cells. This can lead to cell death and inflammatory reaction. The cause of death in mustard poisoning is often respiratory failure. Severe bronchiolar damage leads to mucosal necrosis and damage to the airway musculature. Airway obstruction and laryngospasm are common causes of death in the first 24 hours. Hemorrhagic pulmonary edema may result. Damage to the precursor cells of the bone marrow leads to pancytopenia and increased susceptibility to infection. Ingestion can cause vomiting and diarrhea. In the skin, there is protease digestion of anchoring filaments at the epidermal-dermal junction and the formation of blisters. Mustard agents bind irreversibly to the tissue within minutes after contact. Mustard poisoning usually results in a delayed onset of signs and symptoms that may extend for up to 48 hours.

Lewisite causes immediate damage to the eyes, skin, and airways. After absorption, lewisite causes an increase in capillary permeability and can result in hypovolemia, shock, and organ damage. Exposure to lewisite cause an immediate onset of pain and irritation. Lesions may require hours to become full-blown.

Phosgene oxime causes immediate corrosive-like damage to the tissues it contacts. It is rapidly absorbed and can cause systemic poisoning. Inhalation and skin exposure can result in pulmonary edema. Exposure causes immediate onset of extreme pain.

SIGNS AND SYMPTOMS BY SYSTEM

Cardiovascular: Hypovolemic shock and circulatory collapse. Tachycardia.

Respiratory: Irritation of the upper airway, sore throat, nonproductive cough changing to productive cough over 1 to 3 days, hoarseness, laryngitis with voice change, laryngospasm, and dyspnea. Pulmonary edema with lewisite and phosgene oxime exposure (mustard agents rarely cause hemorrhagic pulmonary edema). Mustard exposure results in delayed signs and symptoms.

CNS: Seizures, anxiety, apathy, and lethargy

Gastrointestinal: Pain, nausea, and vomiting; both diarrhea and constipation have been reported.

Eye: Irritation, reddening of the eyes, severe conjunctivitis, photophobia, miosis, blepharospasm, edema of the lids and conjunctivae, pain, and corneal damage. Can lead to perforation of the cornea. During World War I, only 1% of casualties from mustard exposure had permanent corneal damage. Lewisite and phosgene oxime cause similar signs and symptoms with a more rapid onset.

Skin: Erythema, with burning, stinging pain usually delayed for 2 to 48 hours after exposure. Small vesicles develop that form into large blisters. The blister fluid is not a vesicant and will not cause any further skin damage. Lewisite exposure causes immediate pain. Erythema and blister formation quickly follow. Full blister formation may take 12 to 18 hours. Phosgene oxime exposure results in immediate onset of extreme pain and erythema, followed by a wheal in approximately 30 minutes without blister formation.

Hepatic: Necrosis after lewisite exposure.

Renal: Necrosis after lewisite exposure.

Blood: Bone marrow suppression (pancytopenia).

SYMPTOM ONSET FOR ACUTE EXPOSURE

Mustard—signs and symptoms can be delayed for 2 to 48 hours
Lewisite and phosgene oxime—immediate

THERMAL DECOMPOSITION PRODUCTS INCLUDE

Sulfur mustard—carbon disulfide, hydrogen sulfide, and sulfur dioxide
Lewisite—metal oxide fumes and arsenic trioxide

MEDICAL CONDITIONS THAT MAY INCREASE RISK FOLLOWING EXPOSURE

Skin disorders
Respiratory disorders
Bone marrow disorders

DECONTAMINATION

- Wear positive-pressure SCBA and protective equipment specified by references such as the *North American Emergency Response Guidebook.* If special chemical protective clothing is required, consult the chemical manufacturer or specific protective clothing compatibility charts. A qualified, experienced person should make decisions regarding the type of personal protective equipment necessary.
- Delay entry until trained personnel and proper protective equipment are available.
- Remove patient from contaminated area.
- Quickly remove and isolate patient's clothing, jewelry, and shoes.
- Gently blot any excess liquids with absorbent material.
- Rinse patient with warm water, 32° C to 35° C (90° F to 95° F), if possible.
- Wash patient with a mild liquid soap and large quantities of water. Some authorities recommend a dilute hypochlorite (0.5% solution) as a decontaminating agent (refer to decontamination protocol in Section Three).
- Immediate decontamination is critical. These products bind with cells within minutes. Immediate decontamination will prevent tissue damage. Later decontamination will prevent further damage, absorption, and the spread of the agent.
- Discard all exposed leather products.
- Refer to decontamination protocol in Section Three.

IMMEDIATE FIRST AID

- Ensure that adequate decontamination has been carried out as needed.
- If patient is not breathing, start artificial respiration, preferably with a demand-valve resuscitator, bag-valve-mask device, or pocket mask, as trained. Perform CPR if necessary.
- Immediately flush contaminated eyes with gently flowing water.
- Do not induce vomiting. If vomiting occurs, lean patient forward or place on left side (head-down position, if possible) to maintain an open airway and prevent aspiration.
- Keep patient quiet and maintain normal body temperature.
- Obtain medical attention.

BASIC TREATMENT

- Establish a patent airway (oropharyngeal or nasopharyngeal airway, if needed). Suction if necessary.
- Aggressive airway control may be needed.
- Watch for signs of respiratory insufficiency and assist ventilations if necessary.
- Administer oxygen by nonrebreather mask at 10 to 15 L/min.
- Monitor for pulmonary edema and treat if necessary (refer to pulmonary edema protocol in Section Three).
- Monitor for shock and treat if necessary (refer to shock protocol in Section Three).
- Anticipate seizures and treat if necessary (refer to seizure protocol in Section Three).
- For eye contamination, flush eyes immediately with water. Irrigate each eye continuously with 0.9% saline (NS) during transport (refer to eye irrigation protocol in Section Three).

ADVANCED TREATMENT

- Consider orotracheal or nasotracheal intubation for airway control in the patient who is unconscious, has severe pulmonary edema, or is in severe respiratory distress. Early intubation at the first sign of upper airway obstruction may be necessary.
- Positive-pressure ventilation techniques with a bag-valve-mask device may be beneficial.
- Consider drug therapy for pulmonary edema (refer to pulmonary edema protocol in Section Three).
- Monitor cardiac rhythm and treat arrhythmias if necessary (refer to cardiac protocol in Section Three).
- Start IV administration of D_5W TKO. Use 0.9% saline (NS) or lactated Ringer's (LR) if signs of hypovolemia are present. For hypotension with signs of hypovolemia, administer fluid cautiously. Watch for signs of fluid overload. (refer to shock protocol in Section Three).
- Treat seizures with diazepam (Valium) or lorazepam (Ativan) (refer to seizure protocol in Section Three and diazepam and lorazepam protocols in Section Four).
- Use proparacaine hydrochloride to assist eye irrigation (refer to proparacaine hydrochloride protocol in Section Four).

INITIAL EMERGENCY DEPARTMENT CONSIDERATIONS

- Useful initial laboratory studies include complete blood count, serum electrolytes, blood urea nitrogen (BUN), creatinine, glucose, urinalysis, coagulation profile, and baseline biochemical profile, including serum aminotransferases (AST and ALT), calcium, phosphorus, and magnesium. Determination of anion and osmolar gaps may be helpful. Arterial blood gases (ABGs), chest radiograph, and electrocardiogram may be required.
- If mustard systemic absorption is large, leukocytes in the blood will decrease beginning on day 3 to 5; this decrease indicates damage to precursor cells in the blood-forming organs. The decrease may be precipitate (e.g., 5,000 to 10,000 cells a day). If marrow damage is severe, erythrocytes and thrombocytes may later decrease.
- Blood and urine arsenic determinations should be done in cases of lewisite poisoning. Treatment should not be delayed in the symptomatic patient, because results may take several days to obtain.
- Positive end-expiratory pressure (PEEP)-assisted ventilation may be necessary in patients with acute parenchymal injury who develop pulmonary edema or acute respiratory distress syndrome.
- Closely monitor hydration state and urinary output and maintain if necessary.
- Urine alkalinization and chelation therapy with BAL or D-penicillamine may be beneficial in symptomatic patients. Therapy should be guided by patient presentation and renal test values.
- Hemodialysis may be required in cases of acute renal failure.
- Obtain toxicological consultation as necessary.

Vomiting Agents

Diphenylchlorarsine (DA), Diphenylaminearsine Chloride (Adamsite [DM]), Diphenylcyanoarsine (DC), Related Compounds

SUBSTANCE IDENTIFICATION

Vomiting agents produce a strong pepper-like irritation in the upper respiratory tract, with irritation of the eyes, and lacrimation. They cause nausea, vomiting, and uncontrollable coughing and sneezing. The principal agents in this group are diphenylchloroarsine (DA), diphenylaminearsine (Adamsite [DM]), and diphenylcyanoarsine (DC). The letter abbreviation following the chemical name is the military designation for the agent. These are solid agents that are dispersed as aerosols. When concentrated, DM smoke is canary yellow; DA and DC smokes are white. All are colorless at lower concentrations in air. These chemicals have a low effective dose and they may not be detectable by colors or visible smoke clouds. They produce their effects by inhalation or direct action on the eyes. Once the particles fall to the ground after dispersion, they are virtually ineffective unless they are resuspended. Symptoms reach their peak within 5 to 10 minutes and disappear 1 to 2 hours after exposure is terminated.

ROUTES OF EXPOSURE

Eye contact
Inhalation

TARGET ORGANS

Primary
Respiratory system
Gastrointestinal system
Eyes
Secondary
Central nervous system

LIFE THREAT

Agents cause uncontrollable coughing and sneezing accompanied by nausea, vomiting, and a general feeling of discomfort. Asthma-like respiratory symptoms may occur after prolonged exposure, and high-concentration exposure in confined spaces has resulted in severe pulmonary tract injury. An obstructed airway secondary to vomiting is possible.

SIGNS AND SYMPTOMS BY SYSTEM

Respiratory: Respiratory tract pain and irritation, uncontrollable coughing and violent sneezing, rhinorrhea, and a sense of fullness in the nose and sinuses. Retrosternal pain, dyspnea, and asthma-like symptoms may appear with prolonged exposure. Severe pulmonary tract injury may occur after high-concentration exposures in confined spaces.

CNS: Severe headache and mental depression.
Gastrointestinal: Excessive salivation; nausea and vomiting.
Eye: Irritation and lacrimation.

SYMPTOM ONSET FOR ACUTE EXPOSURE

May be delayed for several minutes after exposure.
Symptoms usually resolve within 1 to 2 hours after exposure termination.

MEDICAL CONDITIONS THAT MAY INCREASE RISK FOLLOWING EXPOSURE

Respiratory system disorders

DECONTAMINATION

- Wear positive-pressure SCBA and protective equipment specified by references such as the *North American Emergency Response Guidebook.* If special chemical protective clothing is required, consult the chemical manufacturer or specific protective clothing compatibility charts. A qualified, experienced person should make decisions regarding the type of personal protective equipment necessary.
- Delay entry until trained personnel and proper protective equipment are available.
- Remove patient from contaminated area.
- Quickly remove and isolate patient's clothing, jewelry, and shoes.
- Gently brush away dry particles and blot excess liquids with absorbent material.
- Rinse patient with warm water, 32° C to 35° C (90° F to 95° F), if possible.
- Wash patient with a mild liquid soap and large quantities of water. Some authorities recommend a dilute hypochlorite (0.5% solution) as a decontaminating agent (refer to decontamination protocol in Section Three).

IMMEDIATE FIRST AID

- Ensure that adequate decontamination has been carried out as needed.
- If patient is not breathing, start artificial respiration, preferably with a demand-valve resuscitator, bag-valve-mask device, or pocket mask, as trained. Perform CPR as necessary.
- Immediately flush contaminated eyes with gently flowing water.
- Do not induce vomiting. If vomiting occurs, lean patient forward or place on left side (head-down position, if possible) to maintain an open airway and prevent aspiration.
- Keep patient quiet and maintain normal body temperature.
- Obtain medical attention.

BASIC TREATMENT

- Establish a patent airway (oropharyngeal or nasopharyngeal airway, if needed). Suction if necessary.
- Watch for signs of respiratory insufficiency and assist ventilations if necessary.
- Administer oxygen by nonrebreather mask at 10 to 15 L/min.
- For eye contamination, flush eyes immediately with water. Irrigate each eye continuously with 0.9% saline (NS) during transport (refer to eye irrigation protocol in Section Three).
- Rinse mouth with water but do not swallow (refer to ingestion protocol in Section Three).

ADVANCED TREATMENT

- Consider orotracheal or nasotracheal intubation for airway control in the patient who is unconscious, has severe pulmonary edema, or is in severe respiratory distress.

- Positive-pressure ventilation techniques with a bag-valve-mask device may be beneficial.
- Start IV administration of 0.9% saline (NS) or lactated Ringer's (LR) TKO. For hypotension with signs of hypovolemia, administer fluid cautiously. Watch for signs of fluid overload (refer to shock protocol in Section Three).
- Consider the use of ondansetron hydrochloride (Zofran) for symptomatic relief of nausea and vomiting (refer to ondansetron hydrochloride protocol in Section Four).
- Use proparacaine hydrochloride to assist eye irrigation (refer to proparacaine hydrochloride protocol in Section Four).

INITIAL EMERGENCY DEPARTMENT CONSIDERATIONS

- Useful initial laboratory studies include complete blood count, serum electrolytes, blood urea nitrogen (BUN), creatinine, glucose, urinalysis, and baseline biochemical profile, including serum aminotransferases (ALT and AST), calcium, phosphorus, and magnesium. Determination of anion and osmolar gaps may be helpful. Arterial blood gases (ABGs), chest radiograph, and electrocardiogram may be required.
- Obtain toxicological consultation as necessary.

SPECIAL CONSIDERATIONS

- In most cases of mild exposure, symptoms are self-limited and require supportive management only. Treat severe symptomatic exposures as required.

Section Three

TREATMENT PROTOCOLS

Unless otherwise stated, all treatment modalities and drug dosages in this section are based on the adult patient. For pediatric patients, consult the drug protocol section and your medical advisor.

To the best of our knowledge, drug indications, dosages, and precautions contained in these protocols are correct and current as of the time of publication. The reader is urged to review standard pharmacology references and the manufacturer's recommendations for additional details.

These protocols contain suggested treatment. Operating protocols and standing and verbal orders should be established by the local medical advisor. Consult with your medical control physician concerning local treatment protocols.

Inhalation Exposure

MECHANISM OF INJURY

Most hazardous material exposures are via inhalation. Inhalation exposures have five major acute life threat poisoning possibilities:

1. Hypoxia, asphyxiation
2. Direct respiratory system injury
3. Cardiovascular collapse
4. Central nervous system toxicity
5. Systemic poisoning

Examples include chlorine gas, which causes direct pulmonary injury and subsequent pulmonary edema; cyanide gas, which precipitates cardiovascular collapse; and trichloroethylene-induced CNS depression and/or cardiac arrhythmias. In general, water solubility of the material largely influences respiratory tract site and onset of symptoms. Highly water-soluble compounds such as chlorine easily react with water in the upper airway to produce rapid onset of symptoms, whereas phosgene ($COCl_2$) has a much lower solubility, allowing it to reach the lower respiratory tract before it reacts with the respiratory mucosa to produce irritation and possible pulmonary edema.

Remember that water solubility is only one exposure parameter to be considered when predicting health effects. Air concentration, particle size, and duration of exposure before victim evacuation must also be considered. Prolonged exposure to even relatively water-soluble substances may produce pulmonary edema; conversely, low–water-soluble compounds may cause upper airway signs and symptoms as well. Inhaled particle size also dictates lung injury site. Particles measuring 5 to 30 μm are usually deposited in the upper airway. To reach the alveoli, particulates must measure 1 μm or less.

Fire/explosion inhalation victims should always be evaluated for carbon monoxide and/or cyanide poisoning.

SIGNS AND SYMPTOMS

Respiratory—Respiratory tract irritation, coughing, choking, hoarseness, rhinitis, laryngeal spasm, stridor, upper airway obstruction, tracheobronchitis, aspiration pneumonitis, pneumonia, alveolitis, reactive airways dysfunction syndrome (RADS), and pulmonary edema/ acute respiratory distress syndrome (ARDS).

BASIC TREATMENT

- Ensure that patient is decontaminated. Remove all clothing, shoes, and jewelry. Wash the patient with soap and water.
- Ensure an open airway and support respirations if necessary.
- Aggressive airway management may be necessary.
- Administer oxygen by nonrebreather mask at 10 to 15 L/min.
- Monitor for pulmonary edema/ARDS and treat if necessary (refer to pulmonary edema protocol in this section).

ADVANCED TREATMENT

- Consider orotracheal or nasotracheal intubation for airway control in the patient who is unconscious, has severe pulmonary edema, or is in respiratory arrest. Early intubation at the first sign of upper airway obstruction may be necessary.
- Positive-pressure ventilation techniques with a bag-valve-mask device may be beneficial.
- Administer 100% oxygen if carbon monoxide poisoning is suspected. Hyperbaric oxygen therapy should be considered if CNS or cardiac symptoms are present and/or the carboxyhemoglobin concentration is greater than 30%.
- Start IV administration of D_5W TKO. Use lactated Ringer's if signs of hypovolemia are present. Watch for signs of fluid overload.
- Consider drug therapy for pulmonary edema (refer to pulmonary edema protocol in this section).

SPECIAL CONSIDERATIONS

- Systemic toxicity may result from inhalation exposure. Refer to specific guidelines for chemical(s) in question for more detailed information.
- Hospitalized patients may require the following baseline laboratory studies: complete blood count (CBC), platelet count, coagulation profile, serum electrolytes, blood urea nitrogen (BUN), creatinine, glucose, anion gap, and baseline biochemistry panel including serum aminotransferases (ALT and AST), alkaline phosphatase, lactic dehydrogenase, calcium, phosphorus, and magnesium. Additional useful tests, depending on the history of the exposure, include blood cyanide concentration, ethanol, heavy metal(s), and specific poison determinations.
- Measurement of arterial blood gases (ABGs) with measured carboxyhemoglobin, methemoglobin, and percent oxygen saturation determinations is necessary.
- Baseline chest radiograph.
- Measurement of peak flow rates (PFRs) may be helpful.
- Positive end-expiratory pressure (PEEP)–assisted ventilation may be necessary in patients with acute parenchymal injury who develop pulmonary edema or ARDS.
- Some products may cause early olfactory fatigue and therefore have poor warning properties.
- Refer to decontamination protocol in this section.

Dermal Exposure

MECHANISM OF INJURY

Although inhalation exposures occur most frequently, the balance of most hazardous material exposures are via the dermal or ocular route. Dermal exposures have three major acute life threat poisoning possibilities:

1. Local skin irritation, blistering, chemical burns, irritant dermatitis, allergic dermatitis, and allergic reactions.
2. Systemic absorption resulting in cardiovascular collapse, pulmonary toxicity, systemic toxicity, and metabolic acidosis.
3. CNS toxicity, seizures, altered level of consciousness, and coma.

Examples include corrosive dermal injury, ranging from irritation to chemical burns; organophosphate dermal exposure poisoning that produces cardiovascular collapse; and hydrofluoric acid, which causes local burns or systemic fluorosis, hypocalcemia, and hypomagnesemia. Concentration of product, duration of exposure, and skin surface disruption influence rate of absorption and magnitude/expression of symptoms.

SIGNS AND SYMPTOMS

Skin—Irritation, redness, vesicle formation, rash, and partial- and full-thickness burns. Some chemicals may cause burns as deep as and including bone.

BASIC TREATMENT

- Ensure that patient is decontaminated. Remove all clothing, shoes, and jewelry. Wash the patient with soap and water.
- Ensure an open airway and support respirations if necessary.
- Check for singed nasal hair, presence of carbon particles, and oral burns.
- Administer oxygen by nonrebreather mask at 10 to15 L/min.
- Assess and treat any other injuries.
- Estimate body surface area (BSA) of the burn: Rule of nines: BSA is divided into 11 areas of 9% each plus the perineum at 1%; or use Lund and Browder chart (BSA map that corrects for age).
- Cover burned areas with dry sterile dressings.
- Maintain body temperature with blankets. Do not apply external heat.
- Evaluate for systemic toxicity and, if substance is known, treat by specific guideline.

ADVANCED TREATMENT

- Consider orotracheal or nasotracheal intubation at earliest indicated moment if signs of stridor or respiratory distress are present.
- Start IV administration of lactated Ringer's or normal saline TKO.
- Depending on the surface area of the burn and the hemodynamic state of the patient, administer fluids according to the Parkland formula (4ml/kg/% BSA burn), administering half of the estimated IV fluid volume required during the first 8 hours. Consult medical control. See chemical burn protocol in this section.

SPECIAL CONSIDERATIONS

- Systemic toxicity may result from dermal exposure. Refer to chemical burn protocol and specific guidelines for chemical(s) in question for more detailed information.
- Hospitalized patients may require the following baseline laboratory studies: complete blood count (CBC), platelet count, coagulation profile, serum electrolytes, BUN, creatinine, glucose, anion gap, baseline biochemistry panel to include serum aminotransferases (ALT and AST), alkaline phosphatase, lactic dehydrogenase, calcium, phosphorus, and magnesium. Additional useful tests, depending on the history of exposure, include blood cyanide concentration, ethanol, heavy metal(s), and specific poison determinations.
- Measurement of arterial blood gases (ABGs) with measured carboxyhemoglobin, methemoglobin, and percent oxygen saturation determinations may be necessary.
- Baseline chest radiograph.
- Positive end-expiratory pressure (PEEP)–assisted ventilation may be necessary in patients with acute parenchymal injury who develop pulmonary edema or acute respiratory distress syndrome (ARDS).
- Ascertain identification of specific poison. Refer to appropriate guideline.
- Refer to decontamination protocol in this section.

Ingestion Exposure

MECHANISM OF INJURY

Ingestion exposures have six major acute life threat poisoning possibilities:

1. Cardiovascular collapse
2. Pulmonary toxicity
3. CNS toxicity
4. GI tract injury
5. Metabolic poisoning effects
6. Systemic toxicity

Examples include sodium hydroxide ingestion, which causes GI hemorrhage and ulceration with subsequent stricture formation; potassium cyanide ingestion, which produces cardiovascular collapse; and ethylene glycol ingestion, which induces CNS depression and/or cardiac arrhythmias, metabolic acidosis, and renal failure. Symptoms may be delayed, depending on the rate of absorption of the poison.

SIGNS AND SYMPTOMS

Gastrointestinal—Nausea, vomiting, drooling, intestinal obstruction, abdominal pain, hemorrhage, ulceration, perforation, and diarrhea.

BASIC TREATMENT

- Ensure that patient is decontaminated. Remove all clothing, shoes, and jewelry. Wash the patient with soap and water.
- Ensure an open airway and support respirations if necessary.
- For ingestion, rinse mouth and administer 5 ml/kg up to 200 ml of water for dilution if the patient can swallow, has a good gag reflex, and does not drool. Administer activated charcoal (refer to activated charcoal protocol in Section Four).
- Do not use emetics. Toxic effects from many compounds may be delayed, depending on the rate of GI absorption. GI absorption rate may be influenced by a variety of factors, including time of last meal, amount ingested, and lipid solubility of the compound. Because it may take 30 minutes or more for syrup of ipecac to work, vomiting may begin about the time the patient begins to experience symptoms such as loss of consciousness, gag reflex, and/or seizures.

ADVANCED TREATMENT

- Consider orotracheal or nasotracheal intubation for airway control in the patient who is unconscious, has severe pulmonary edema, or is in respiratory arrest. Early intubation at the first sign of upper airway obstruction may be necessary.
- Positive-pressure ventilation techniques with a bag-valve-mask device may be beneficial.
- Administer 100% oxygen if carbon monoxide poisoning is suspected. Hyperbaric oxygen therapy should be considered if CNS or cardiac symptoms are present and/or the carboxyhemoglobin concentration is greater than 30%.
- Monitor cardiac rhythm and treat arrhythmias if necessary (refer to cardiac protocol in this section).

- Start IV administration of D_5W TKO. Use lactated Ringer's if signs of hypovolemia are present. Watch for signs of fluid overload.
- Consider drug therapy for pulmonary edema (refer to pulmonary edema protocol in this section).
- In-hospital gastric lavage may be useful in some ingestion exposure situations. If indicated, gastric lavage should be instituted within the first 4 hours after ingestion, preferably in the first hour after ingestion. Usual contraindications include ingestion of strong corrosives, hemorrhage with coagulation abnormalities, and relatively nontoxic ingestions.

Technique of Gastric Lavage

1. Orogastric tube selection
   a. Use a large-bore orogastric tube (nasogastric tubes except for GI decompression are not indicated). Appropriate sizes are: Adult—30 to 40 French; pediatric—16 to 28 French.
2. Orogastric tube placement
   a. If the patient is unconscious, endotracheal or nasotracheal intubation to protect the airway is indicated before passage of the orogastric tube.
   b. Conscious patients with intact gag reflex may be lavaged without airway intubation. These patients require continuous observation to prevent aspiration.
   c. Maintain the patient in the head-down left lateral decubitus position to prevent aspiration.
   d. Once the tube is passed, continuous patient monitoring is required. To confirm tube placement, use a stethoscope to listen over the stomach for the sound of air as it is instilled via syringe into the orogastric tube. If the patient is endotracheally intubated and resistance to orogastric tube passage is encountered, cautious deflation of the endotracheal tube cuff may be required for orogastric tube passage. Reinflate the endotracheal cuff once the orogastric tube is passed.
   e. Abdominal or chest radiograph may be necessary to confirm tube placement.
3. Gastric Lavage Procedure
   a. Gastric lavage is best accomplished with warmed saline to prevent hypothermia. The appropriate lavage fluid dose aliquot is: Adult—200 to 250 ml; child: 50 to 100 ml.
   b. Leave aliquot in place for about 30 to 60 seconds. Allow gravity to drain. Repeat until clear or at least approximately 2 L have been used in the adult.
   c. Once the lavage is complete, leave tube in place for administration of activated charcoal or multiple-dose activated charcoal dose and cathartics (refer to activated charcoal protocol in Section Four).

SPECIAL CONSIDERATIONS

- Gastric lavage should be considered an in-hospital procedure.
- Systemic poisoning may result from ingestion exposure. Refer to specific guidelines for chemicals in question for more detailed information.
- Hospitalized patients may require the following baseline laboratory studies: complete blood count (CBC), platelet count, coagulation profile, serum electrolytes, BUN, creatinine, glucose, anion gap, baseline biochemistry panel including serum aminotransferases (ALT and AST), alkaline phosphatase, lactic dehydrogenase, calcium, phosphorus, and magnesium. Additional useful tests,

depending on the history of ingestion, include blood cyanide concentration, ethanol, osmolar gap, ethylene glycol, methanol, heavy metal(s), and ingestion-specific poison determinations.

- Measurement of arterial blood gases (ABGs) with measured carboxyhemoglobin, methemoglobin, and percent oxygen saturation determinations may also be necessary.
- Baseline chest radiograph.
- Positive end-expiratory pressure (PEEP)–assisted ventilation may be necessary in patients with acute parenchymal injury who develop pulmonary edema or acute respiratory distress syndrome (ARDS).
- Ascertain identification of specific poison. Refer to appropriate guideline.

Hazardous Materials Absorbed by Activated Charcoal

Alcohol	Mercuric chloride
Antimony	Nicotine
Arsenic	Oxalates
Camphor	Parathion
Chlordane	Phenolphthalein
2,4-Dichlorophenoxyacetic acid (2,4-D)	Phosphorus
Hexachlorophene	Potassium
Iodine	Selenium
Kerosene	Silver
Malathion	Strychnine

Hazardous Materials Not Well Absorbed by Activated Charcoal

Alkalis	Lithium
Boric acid	*N*-Methyl carbamate
Cyanide	Potassium hydroxide
DDT	Sodium hydroxide
Ferrous sulfate	Sodium metasilicate
Mineral acids	

Courtesy Marcel Dekker, Inc. New York.
Adapted from Mofenson et al: Gastrointestinal dialysis with activated charcoal and cathartic in the treatment of adolescent intoxications. Clin Pediatr 24(12):681-684, 1985.

Cardiac Treatment/Advanced Cardiac Life Support Algorithms

Specific information for chemically induced pulmonary edema and shock conditions can be found in the pulmonary edema and shock protocols found in this section.

Specific treatment protocols should be established by local medical control.

Pulseless Ventricular Tachycardia (VT)/ Ventricular Fibrillation (VF)

Basic Life Support

Perform Primary ABCD Survey
(Correct critical problems IMMEDIATELY as they are identified)
Assess responsiveness
Call for help/call for defibrillator
Airway—open the airway
Breathing—deliver two slow breaths, administer oxygen as soon as it is available
Circulation—perform chest compressions
Ensure availability of monitor/**D**efibrillator
On arrival of AED/monitor/defibrillator, evaluate cardiac rhythm

If PEA or asystole, continue CPR and go to appropriate algorithm.
If pulseless VT/VF, shock up to three times (200 J, 200 to 300 J, 360 J, or equivalent biphasic energy).

Perform Primary ABCD Survey
(Correct critical problems IMMEDIATELY as they are identified)
Assess responsiveness
Call for help/call for defibrillator
Airway—open the airway
Breathing—deliver two slow breaths, administer oxygen as soon as it is available

Circulation—perform chest compressions
Ensure availability of monitor/**D**efibrillator
On arrival of AED/monitor/ defibrillator, evaluate cardiac rhythm

If PEA or asystole, continue CPR and go to appropriate algorithm

If pulseless VT/VF, shock up to three times (200 J, 200 to 300 J, 360 J, or equivalent biphasic energy).

Advanced Life Support

Perform Secondary ABCD Survey (ADVANCED) *A*IRWAY
Reassess effectiveness of initial airway maneuvers and interventions
Perform invasive airway management

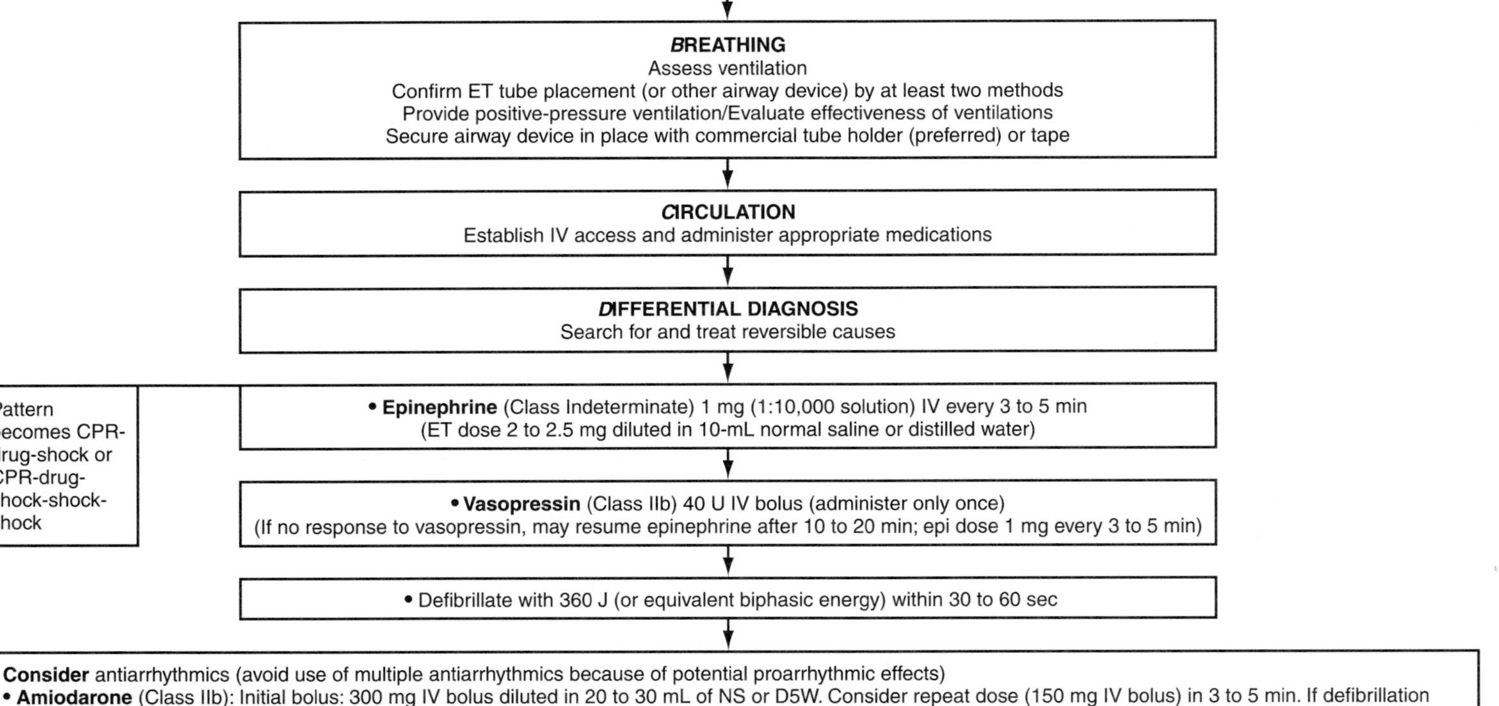

Aehlert B: ACLS Quick Review Study Guide, 2e, St. Louis, 2002, Mosby.

Asystole

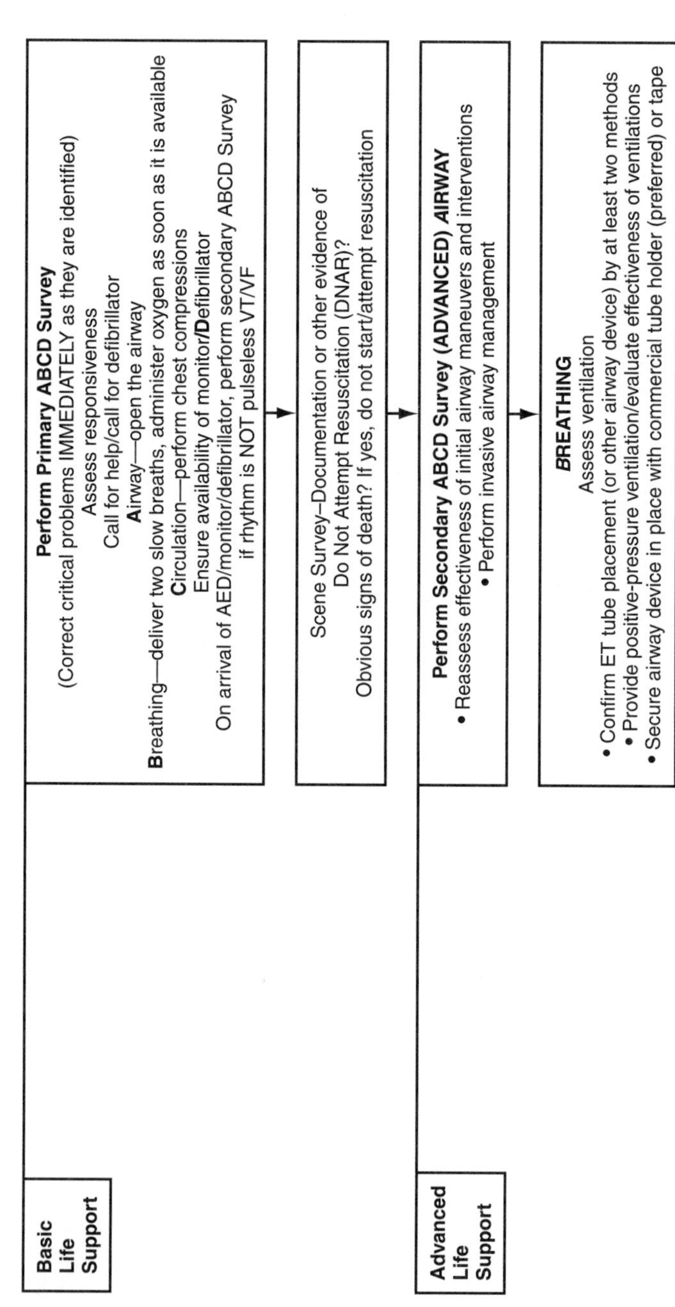

Basic Life Support
Perform Primary ABCD Survey
(Correct critical problems IMMEDIATELY as they are identified)
Assess responsiveness
Call for help/call for defibrillator
Airway—open the airway
Breathing—deliver two slow breaths, administer oxygen as soon as it is available
Circulation—perform chest compressions
Ensure availability of monitor/Defibrillator
On arrival of AED/monitor/defibrillator, perform secondary ABCD Survey
if rhythm is NOT pulseless VT/VF
Scene Survey–Documentation or other evidence of
Do Not Attempt Resuscitation (DNAR)?
Obvious signs of death? If yes, do not start/attempt resuscitation
Advanced Life Support
Perform Secondary ABCD Survey (ADVANCED) AIRWAY
• Reassess effectiveness of initial airway maneuvers and interventions
• Perform invasive airway management
BREATHING
Assess ventilation
• Confirm ET tube placement (or other airway device) by at least two methods
• Provide positive-pressure ventilation/evaluate effectiveness of ventilations
• Secure airway device in place with commercial tube holder (preferred) or tape

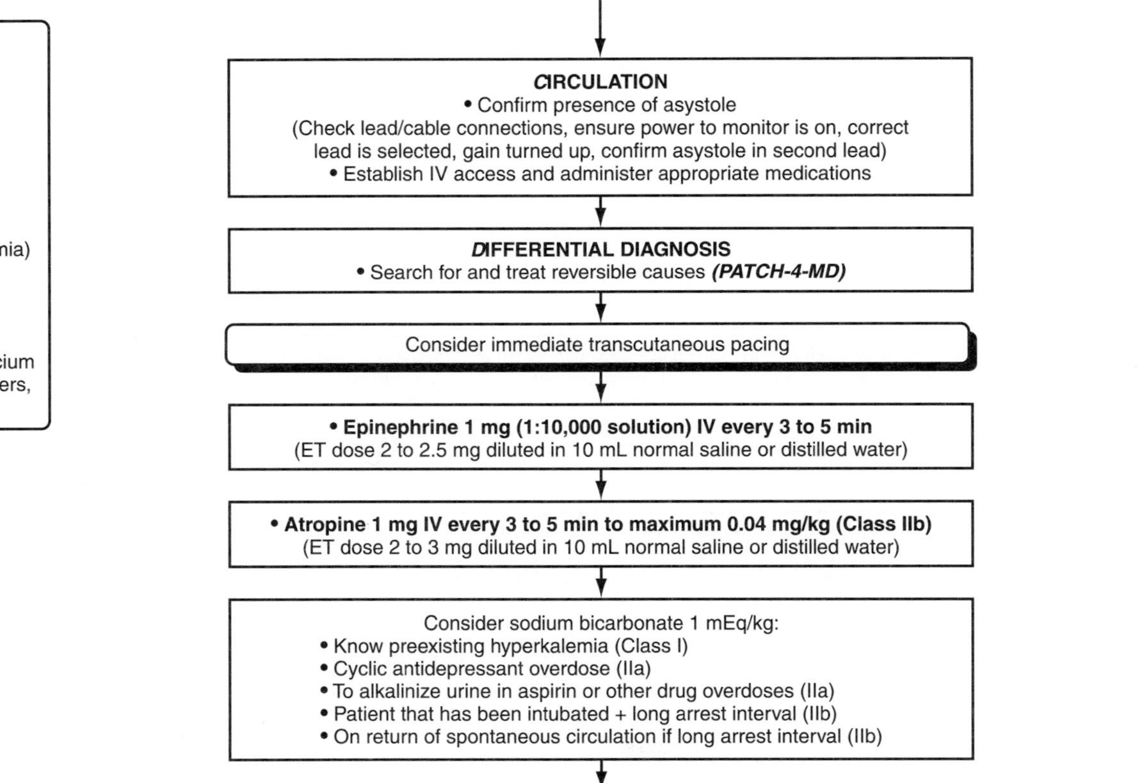

Possible causes of asystole:
PATCH-4-MD

- **P**ulmonary embolism
- **A**cidosis
- **T**ension pneumothorax
- **C**ardiac tamponade
- **H**ypovolemia
- **H**ypoxia
- **H**eat/cold (hypo-/ hyperthermia)
- **H**ypo-/hyperkalemia (and other electrolytes)
- **M**yocardial infarction
- **D**rug overdose accidents (cyclic anti-depressants, calcium channel blockers beta- blockers, digitalis)

Aehlert B: ACLS Quick Review Study Guide, 2e, St. Louis, 2002, Mosby.

Pulseless Electrical Activity (PEA)

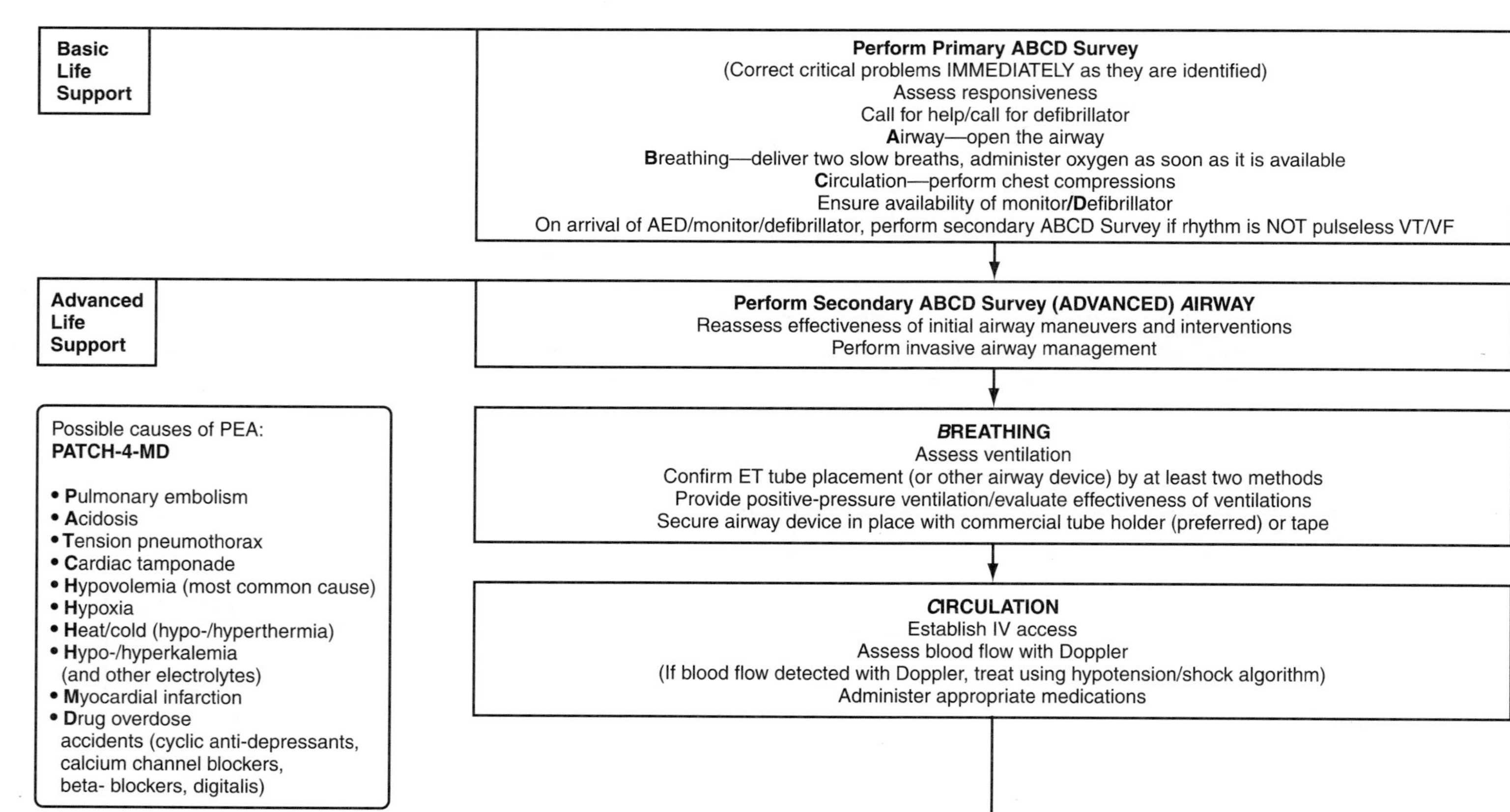

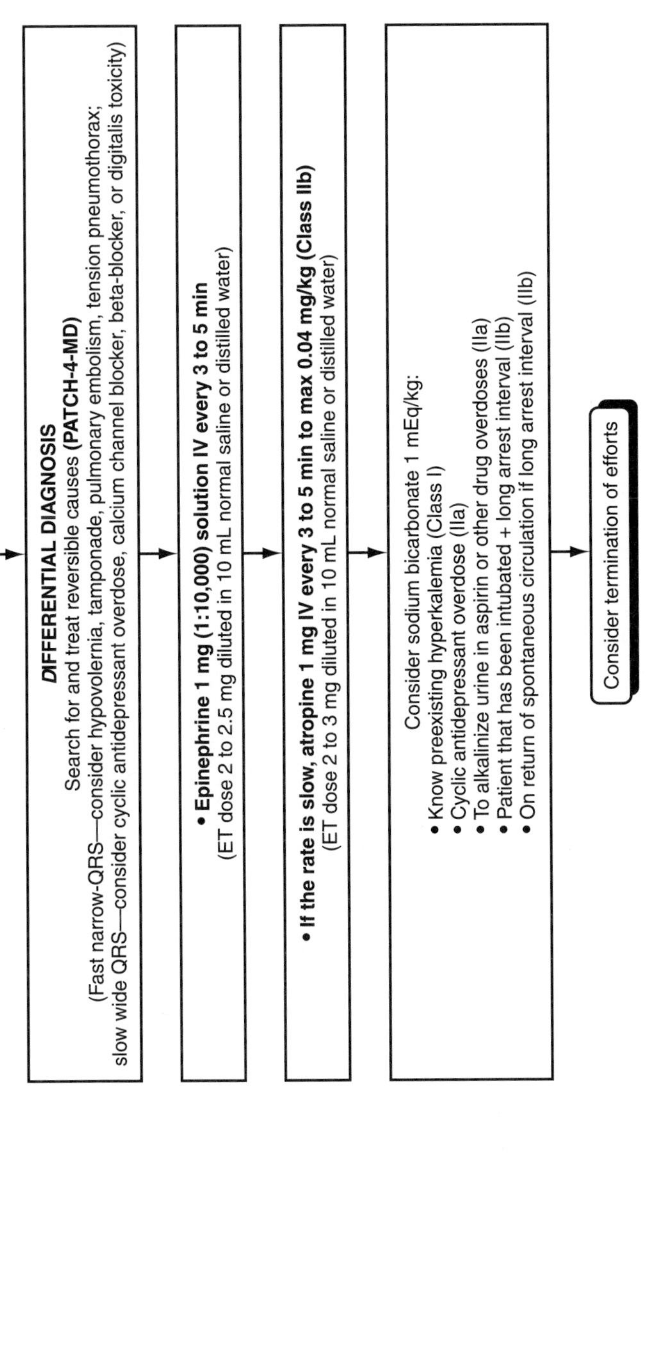

Aehlert B: ACLS Quick Review Study Guide, 2e, St. Louis, 2002, Mosby.

Narrow QRS Tachycardia

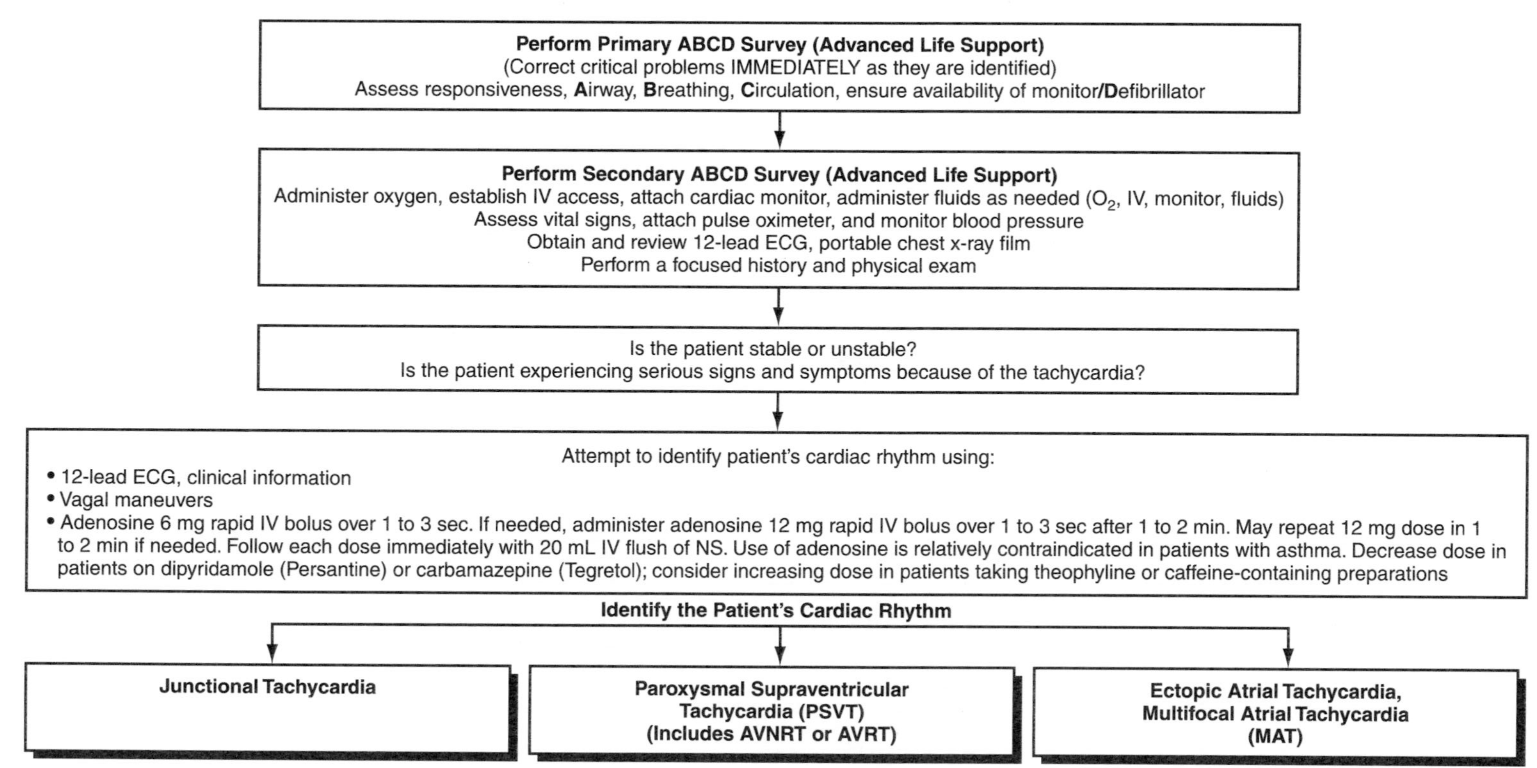

Stable Patient		Stable Patient		Stable Patient	
Normal Cardiac Function	**Impaired Cardiac Function***	**Normal Cardiac Function**	**Impaired Cardiac Function***	**Normal Cardiac Function**	**Impaired Cardiac Function***
Amiodarone (IIb) **or** Beta-blocker (Indeterminate) or Ca++ channel blocker (Indeterminate)	Amiodarone (IIb)	*Priority order:* Ca++ channel blocker (Class I) Beta-blocker (Class I) Digoxin (IIb) Sync cardio-version	*Priority order:* Sync cardio-version Digoxin (IIb) Amiodarone (IIb) Diltiazem (IIb)	Ca++ channel blocker (IIb) **or** Beta-blocker (IIb) **or** Amiodarone (IIb) **or** Flecainide (IIb) or Propafenone (IIb) **or** Digoxin (Indeterminate) **Cardioversion ineffective**	Amiodarone (IIb) **or** Diltiazen (IIb) **or** Digoxin (Indeterminate) **Cardioversion ineffective**

UNSTABLE PATIENT

If hemodynamically unstable PSVT, perform synchronized cardioversion: 50 J, 100 J, 200 J, 300 J, 360 J, (or equivalent biphasic energy)

*Impaired cardiac function = ejection fraction <40% or CHF.

Medication Dosing

Amiodarone—150 mg IV over 10 min, followed by an infusion of 1 mg/min for 6 hours and then a maintenance infusion of 0.5 mg/min. Repeat supplementary infusions of 150 mg as necessary for recurrent or resistant dysrhythmias. Maximum total dially dose 2.0 g

Beta-blockers—*Esmolol:* 0.5 mg/kg over 1 min, followed by a maintenance infusion at 50 mcg/kg/min for 40 min. If inadequate response, administer a second bolus of 0.5 mg/kg over 1 min and increase maintenance infusion to 100 mcg/kg/min. The bolus dose (0.5 mg/kg) and titration of the maintenance infusion (addition of 50 mcg/kg/min) can be repeated every 4 min to a maximum infusion of 300 mcg/kg/min. *Metoprolol:* 5 mg slow IV push over 5 min × 3 as needed to a total dose of 15 mg over 15 min.

Calcium channel blockers: *Diltiazem*—0.25 mg/kg over 2 min (e.g., 15 to 20 mg). If ineffective, 0.35 mg/kg over 2 min (e.g., 20 to 25 mg) in 15 min. Maintenance infusion 5 to 15 mg/hr, titrated to heart rate if chemical conversion successful. Calcium chloride (2 to 4 mg/kg) may be given **slow** IV push if borderline hypotension exists before diltiazem administration. *Verapamil*—2.5 to 5.0 mg slow IV push over 2 min. May repeat with 5 to 10 mg in 15 to 30 min. Maximum dose 20 mg

Digoxin—loading dose 10 to 15 mcg/kg lean body weight

Flecainide, propafenone—IV form not currently approved for use in the United States

Aehlert B: ACLS Quick Review Study Guide, 2e, St. Louis, 2002, Mosby.

Atrial Fibrillation/Atrial Flutter

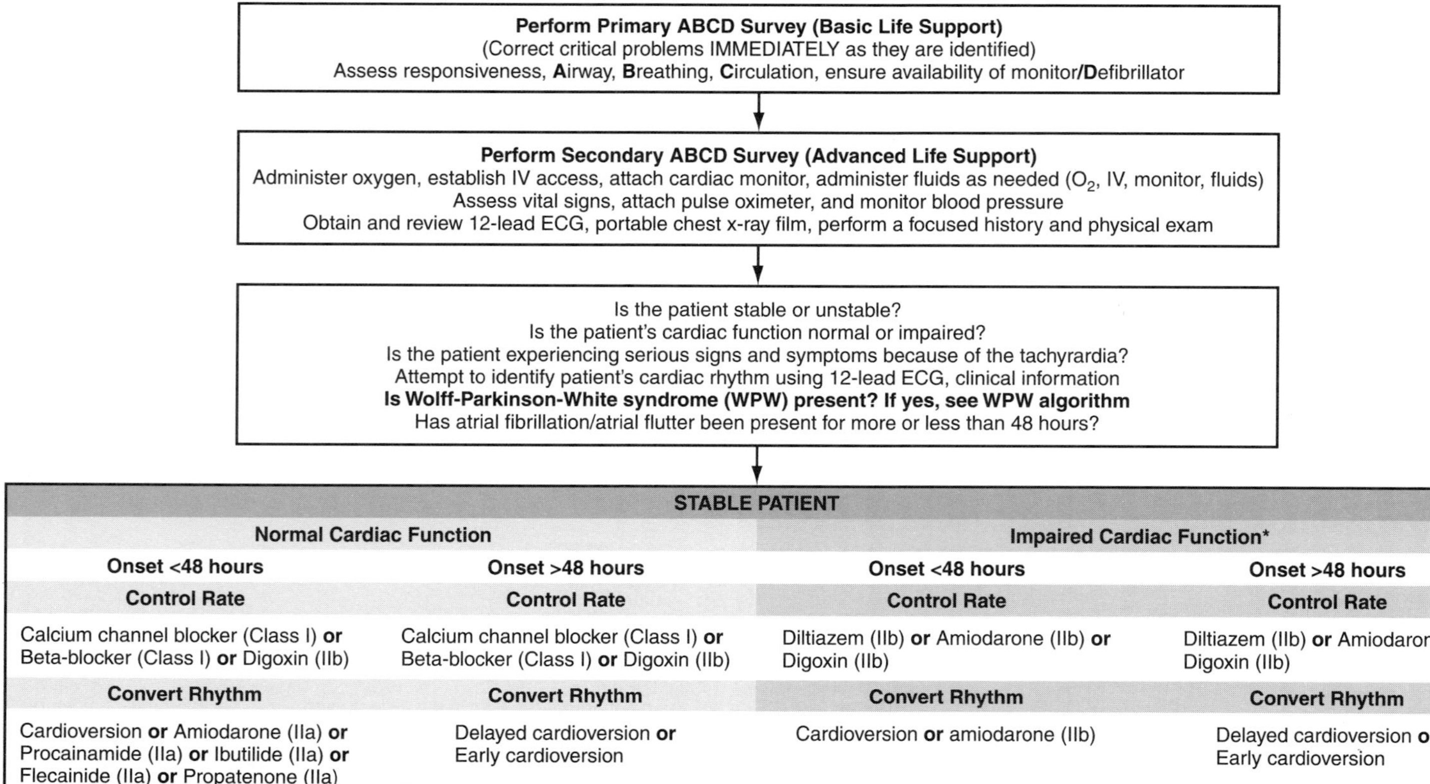

STABLE PATIENT			
Normal Cardiac Function		**Impaired Cardiac Function***	
Onset <48 hours	**Onset >48 hours**	**Onset <48 hours**	**Onset >48 hours**
Control Rate	**Control Rate**	**Control Rate**	**Control Rate**
Calcium channel blocker (Class I) **or** Beta-blocker (Class I) **or** Digoxin (IIb)	Calcium channel blocker (Class I) **or** Beta-blocker (Class I) **or** Digoxin (IIb)	Diltiazem (IIb) **or** Amiodarone (IIb) **or** Digoxin (IIb)	Diltiazem (IIb) **or** Amiodarone **or** Digoxin (IIb)
Convert Rhythm	**Convert Rhythm**	**Convert Rhythm**	**Convert Rhythm**
Cardioversion **or** Amiodarone (IIa) **or** Procainamide (IIa) **or** Ibutilide (IIa) **or** Flecainide (IIa) **or** Propatenone (IIa)	Delayed cardioversion **or** Early cardioversion	Cardioversion **or** amiodarone (IIb)	Delayed cardioversion **or** Early cardioversion

Delayed cardioversion: anticoagulation therapy for 3 weeks before cardioversion, for at least 48 hours in conjunction with cardioversion, and for at least 4 weeks after successful cardioversion.
Early cardioversion: IV heparin immediately, transesophageal echocardiography (TEE) to rule out atrial thrombus, cardioversion within 24 hr, anticoagulation × 4 wks

Unstable patient
If hemodynamically unstable, perform synchronized cardioversion: Atrial fibrillation: 100 J, 200 J, 300 J, 360 J, or equivalent biphasic energy. Atrial flutter: 50 J, 100 J, 200 J, 300 J, 360 J, or equivalent biphasic energy

Medication Dosing
Amiodarone—150 mg IV bolus over 10 min followed by an infusion of 1 mg/min for 6 hours and then a maintenance infusion of 0.5 mg/min. Repeat supplementary infusions of 150 mg as necessary for recurrent or resistant dysrhythmias. Maximum total dially dose 2.0 g **Beta-blockers**—*Esmolol:* 0.5 mg/kg over 1 min followed by a maintenance infusion at 50 mcg/kg/min for 4 min. If inadequate response, administer a second bolus of 0.5 mg/kg over 1 min and increase maintenance infusion to 100 mcg/kg/min. The bolus dose (0.5 mg/kg) and titration of the maintenance infusion (addition of 50 mcg/kg/min) can be repeated every 4 min to a maximum infusion of 300 mcg/kg/min. *Metoprolol:* 5 mg slow IV push over 5 min × 3 as needed to a total dose of 15 mg over 15 min. *Propranolol:* 0.1 mg/kg slow IV push divided in 3 equal doses at 2 to 3 min intervals. Do not exceed 1 mg/min. Repeat after 2 min, if necessary. *Atenolol:* 5 mg slow IV (over 5 min). Wait 10 min, then give second dose of 5 mg slow IV (over 5 min) **Calcium channel blockers:** *Diltiazem*—0.25 mg/kg over 2 min (e.g., 15 to 20 mg). If ineffective, 0.35 mg/kg over 2 min (e.g., 20 to 25 mg) in 15 min. Maintenance infusion 5 to 15 mg/hr, titrated to heart rate if chemical conversion successful. Calcium chloride (2 to 4 mg/kg) may be given **slow** IV push if borderline hypotension exists before diltiazem administration. *Verapamil*—2.5 to 5.0 mg slow IV push over 2 min. May repeat with 5 to 10 mg in 15 to 30 min. Maximum dose 20 mg **Ibutilide**—Adults ≥60 kg: 1 mg (10 mL) over 10 min. May repeat × 1 in 10 min. Adults <60 kg: 0.01mg/kg IV over 10 min **Procainamide:**—100 mg over 5 min (20 mg/min). Maximum total dose 17 mg/kg. Maintenance infusion 1 to 4 mg/min Flecainide, propafenone—IV form not currently approved for use in the United States **Sotalol**—1 to 1.5 mg/kg IV slowly at a rate 10 mg/min

*Impaired cardiac function = ejection fraction <40% or CHF

Aehlert B: ACLS Quick Review Study Guide, 2e, St. Louis, 2002, Mosby.

Wolff-Parkinson-White (WPW) Syndrome

Perform Primary ABCD Survey (Basic Life Support)
(Correct critical problems IMMEDIATELY as they are identified)
Assess responsiveness, **A**irway, **B**reathing, **C**irculation, ensure availability of monitor/**D**efibrillator

↓

Perform Secondary ABCD Survey (Advanced Life Support)
Administer oxygen, establish IV access, attach cardiac monitor, administer fluids as needed (O_2, IV, monitor, fluids)
Assess vital signs, attach pulse oximeter, and monitor blood pressure
Obtain and review 12-lead ECG, portable chest x-ray film, perform a focused history and physical exam

↓

Is the patient stable or unstable?
Is the patient experiencing serious signs and symptoms because of the tachycardia?
Is the patient's cardiac function normal or impaired?
Attempt to identify patient's cardiac rhythm using 12-lead ECG, clinical information
Is Wolff-Parkinson-White syndrome (WPW) present? (e.g., young patient, HR >300, ECG: short PR interval, wide QRS, delta wave)
Has WPW been present for more or less than 48 hours?

↓

Normal Cardiac Function		Impaired Cardiac Function*	
Onset <48 hours	**Onset >48 hours**	**Onset <48 hours**	**Onset >48 hours**
Control Rate	**Control Rate**	**Control Rate**	**Control Rate**
Cardioversion **or** Amiodarone (IIb) **or** Procainamide (IIb) **or** Flecainide (IIb) **or** Propatenone (IIb) **or** Sotalol (IIb)	Use antiarrhythmics with extreme caution because of embolic risk	Cardioversion **or** Amiodarone (IIb)	Use antiarrhythmics with extreme caution because of embolic risk
Convert Rhythm	**Convert Rhythm**	**Convert Rhythm**	**Convert Rhythm**
Cardioversion **or** Amiodarone (IIb) **or** Procainamide (IIb) **or** Flecainide (IIb) **or** Propatenone (IIb) **or** Sotalol (IIb)	Delayed cardioversion **or** Early cardioversion	Cardioversion	Delayed cardioversion **or** Early cardioversion

Delayed cardioversion: Anticoagulation tharapy for 3 weeks before cardioversion for at least 48 hours in conjunction with cardioversion and for at least 4 weeks after successful cardioversion.
Early cardioversion: IV heparin immediately, transesophageal echocardiography (TEE) to rule out atrial thrombus, cardioversion within 24 hr, anticoagulation × 4 weeks

Medication Dosing
Amiodarone—150 mg IV bolus over 10 min followed by an infusion of 1 mg/min for 6 hours and then a maintenance infusion of 0.5 mg/min. Repeat supplementary infusions of 150 mg as necessary for recurrent or resistant dysrhythmias. Maximum total dially dose 2.0 g **Procainamide**—100 mg over 5 min (20 mg/min). Maximum total dose 17 mg/kg. Maintenance infusion 1 to 4 mg/min **Flecainide, propafenone**—IV form not currently approved for use in the United States **Sotalol**—1 to 1.5 mg/kg IV slowly at a rate 10 mg/min

*Impaired cardiac function = ejection fraction <40% or CHF.

Aehlert B: ACLS Quick Review Study Guide, 2e, St. Louis, 2002, Mosby.

Symptomatic Bradycardia

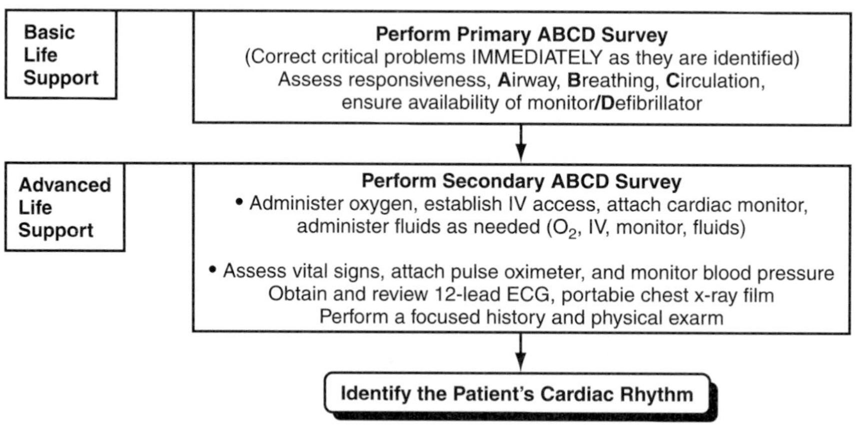

Is the patient experiencing serious signs and symptoms because of the bradycardia?

SIGNS	SYMPTOMS
Low blood pressure, shock, pulmonary congestion, congestive heart failure, angina, acute MI, ventricular ectopy	Chest pain, weakness, fatigue, dizziness, lightheadedness, shortness of breath, exercise intolerance, decreased level of responsiveness

- If no serious signs and symptoms, observe
- If serious signs and symptoms are present, further intervention depending on the cardiac rhythm identified

NARROW QRS BRADYCARDIA

- **Sinus bradycardia**
- **Junctional rhythm**
- **Second-degree AV block, type I**
- **Third-degree (complete) AV block**

- **Atropine 0.5 to 1.0 mg IV:** May repeat every 3 to 5 min to a total dose of 2.5 mg (0.03 to 0.04 mg/kg). Total cumulative dose should not exceed 2.5 mg over 2.5 hours
- **Transcutaneous pacemaker (TCP):** Pacing should not be delayed while waiting for IV access or for atropine to take effect
- **Dopamine infusion:** 5 to 20 mcg/kg/min
- **Epinephrine infusion:** 2 to 10 mcg/min
- **Isoproterenol infusion:** 2 to 10 mcg/min (low doses)

WIDE QRS BRADYCARDIA

- **Second-degree AV block, type II**
- **Third-degree (complete) AV block**
- **Ventricular escape (idioventricular) rhythm**

- **Transcutaneous pacemaker:** As an interim device until transvenous pacing can be accomplished
- **Dopamine infusion:** 5 to 20 mcg/kg/min
- **Epinephrine infusion:** 5 to 10 mcg/min
- **Isoproterenol infusion:** 2 to 10 mcg/min (low doses)

Aehlert B: ACLS Quick Review Study Guide, 2e, St. Louis, 2002, Mosby.

Sustained Monomorphic Ventricular Tachycardia

Perform Primary ABCD Survey (Basic Life Support)
(Correct critical problems IMMEDIATELY as they are identified)
Assess responsiveness, **A**irway, **B**reathing, **C**irculation, ensure availability of monitor/**D**efibrillator

↓

Perform Secondary ABCD Survey (Advanced Life Support)
Administer oxygen, establish IV access, attach cardiac monitor, administer fluids as needed (O_2, IV, monitor, fluids)
Assess vital signs, attach pulse oximeter, and monitor blood pressure
Obtain and review 12-lead ECG, portable chest x-ray film, perform a focused history and physical exam

↓

Is the patient stable or unstable?
Is the patient experiencing serious signs and symptoms because of the tachycardia?
Determine if the rhythm is monomorphic or polymorphic VT and determine patient's QT interval

↓

Stable Patient	
Normal Cardiac Function	**Impaired Cardiac Function***
May proceed directly to synchronized cardioversion or use **one** of the following:	
• Procainamide (IIa) • Sotalol (IIa) • Amiodarone (IIb) • Lidocaine (IIb)	• Amiodarone (IIb) • Lidocaine (Indeterminate)

If medication therapy ineffective, perform synchronized cardioversion

Unstable VI with a Pulse

If hemodynamically unstable, sync 100 J, 200 J, 300 J, and 360 J (or equivalent biphasic energy)
If hypotensive (systolic BP <90), unresponsive, or if severe pulmonary edema exists, defibrillate with same energy

Medication Dosing

Amiodarone: 150 mg IV bolus over 10 min. If chemical conversion successful, follow with IV infusion of 1 mg/min for 6 hours and then a maintenance infusion of 0.5 mg/min. Repeat supplementary infusions of 150 mg as necessary for recurrent or resistant dysrhythmias. Maximum total dialy dose 2.0 g
Lidocaine: 1 to 1.5 mg/kg initial dose. Repeat dose is half the initial dose every 5 to 10 min. Maximum total dose 3 mg/kg. If chemical conversion successful, maintenance infusion 1 to 4 mg/min. If impaired cardiac function dose = 0.5-0.75 mg/kg IV push. May repeat every 5 to 10 min. Maximum total dose 3 mg/kg. If chemical conversion successful, maintenance infusion 1 to 4 mg/min
Procainamide: 100 mg over 5 min (20 mg/min). Maximum total dose 17 mg/kg. If chemical conversion successful, maintenance infusion 1 to 4 mg/min
Sotalol: 1 to 1.5 mg/kg IV slowly at a rate 10 mg/min

*Impaired cardiac function = ejection fraction <40% or CHF.

Aehlert B: ACLS Quick Review Study Guide, 2e, St. Louis, 2002, Mosby.

Polymorphic Ventricular Tachycardia

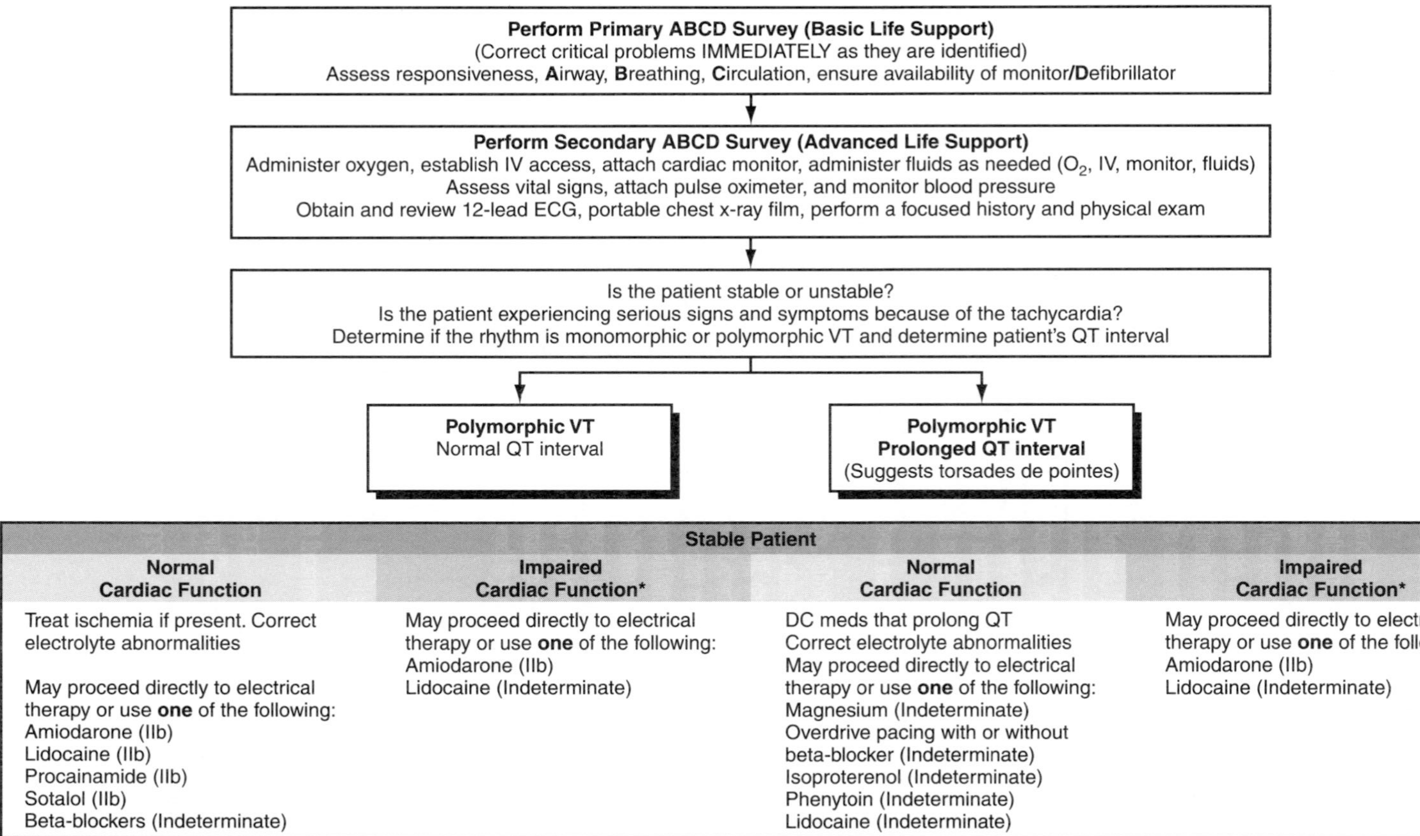

Stable Patient			
Normal Cardiac Function	**Impaired Cardiac Function***	**Normal Cardiac Function**	**Impaired Cardiac Function***
Treat ischemia if present. Correct electrolyte abnormalities May proceed directly to electrical therapy or use **one** of the following: Amiodarone (IIb) Lidocaine (IIb) Procainamide (IIb) Sotalol (IIb) Beta-blockers (Indeterminate)	May proceed directly to electrical therapy or use **one** of the following: Amiodarone (IIb) Lidocaine (Indeterminate)	DC meds that prolong QT Correct electrolyte abnormalities May proceed directly to electrical therapy or use **one** of the following: Magnesium (Indeterminate) Overdrive pacing with or without beta-blocker (Indeterminate) Isoproterenol (Indeterminate) Phenytoin (Indeterminate) Lidocaine (Indeterminate)	May proceed directly to electrical therapy or use **one** of the following: Amiodarone (IIb) Lidocaine (Indeterminate)

If medication therapy ineffective, use electrical therapy

Unstable patient
Sustained (>30 sec or causing hemodynamic collapse) polymorphic VT should be treated with an unsynchronized shock, using an initial energy of 200 J; if unsuccessful, a second shock of 200 to 300 J should be given and, if necessary, a third shock of 360 J

Medication Dosing
Amiodarone—150 mg IV bolus over 10 min. If chemical conversion successful, follow with IV infusion of 1 mg/min for 6 hours and then a maintenance infusion of 0.5 mg/min. Repeat supplementary infusions of 150 mg as necessary for recurrent or resistant dysrhythmias. Maximum total daily dose 2.0 g **Beta-blockers**—*Esmolol:* 0.5 mg/kg over 1 min followed by a maintenance infusion at 50 mcg/kg/min for 4 min. If inadequate response, administer a second bolus of 0.5 mg/kg over 1 min and increase maintenance infusion to 100 mcg/kg/min. The bolus dose (0.5 mg/kg) and titration of the maintenance infusion (addition of 50 mcg/kg/min) can be repeated every 4 min to a maximum infusion of 300 mcg/kg/min. *Metoprolol:* 5 mg slow IV push over 5 min × 3 as needed to a total dose of 15 mg over 15 min. *Atenolol:* 5 mg slow IV (over 5 min). Wait 10 min, then give second dose of 5 mg slow IV (over 5 min) **Isoproterenol**—Can be used as a temporizing measure until overdrive pacing can be instituted if no evidence of coronary artery disease, ischemic syndromes, or other contraindications. 2 to 10 mcg/min. Mix 1 mg in 500 mL NS or D5W **Lidocaine:**—1 to 1.5 mg/kg initial dose. Repeat dose (half the initial dose) every 5 to 10 min. Maximum total dose 3 mg/kg. If chemical conversion successful, maintenance infusion 1 to 4 mg/min. If impaired cardiac function, dose = 0.5 to 0.75 mg/kg IV push. May repeat every 5 to 10 min. Maximum total dose 3 mg/kg. If chemical conversion successful, maintenance infusion 1 to 4 mg/min **Magnesium:**—Loading dose of 1 to 2 g mixed in 50 to 100 mL over 5 to 60 min IV. If chemical conversion successful, follow with 0.5 to 1.0 g.hr IV infusion **Phenytoin:**—250 mg IV at a rate of 25 to 50 mg/min in NS using a central vein **Procainamide:**—100 mg over 5 min (20 mg/min). Maximum total dose 17 mg/kg. If chemical conversion successful, maintenance infusion 1 to 4 mg/min **Sotalol**—1 to 1.5 mg/kg IV slowly at a rate 10 mg/min

*Impaired cardiac function = ejection fraction <40% or CHF.

Aehlert B: ACLS Quick Review Study Guide, 2e, St. Louis, 2002, Mosby.

Wide QRS Tachycardia of Unknown Origin

Perform Primary ABCD Survey (Basic Life Support)
(Correct critical problems IMMEDIATELY as they are identified)
Assess responsiveness, **A**irway, **B**reathing, **C**irculation, ensure availability of monitor/**D**efibrillator

↓

Perform Secondary ABCD Survey (Advanced Life Support)
Administer oxygen, establish IV access, attach cardiac monitor, administer fluids as needed (O_2, IV, monitor, fluids)
Assess vital signs, attach pulse oximeter, and monitor blood pressure
Obtain and review 12-lead ECG, portable chest x-ray film, perform a focused history and physical exam

↓

Is the patient stable or unstable?
Is the patient experiencing serious signs and symptoms because of the tachycardia?
Use 12-lead ECG/clinical information to help clarify rhythm diagnosis

↓

Rhythm confirmed as SVT Go to narrow-QRS tachycardia algorithm

Wide-Complex Tachycardia of Unknown Origin Stable Patient

Rhythm confirmed as VT Go to VT algorithm

Normal Cardiac Function	Impaired Cardiac Function*
Sync cardioversion **or** Procainamide (IIb) **or** Amiodarone (IIb)	Sync cardioversion **or** Amiodarone (IIb)

If medication therapy ineffective, perform synchronized cardioversion

Unstable Patient

If hemodynamically unstable, sync 100 J, 200 J, 300 J, and 360 J, or equivalent biphasic energy. If hypotensive (systolic BP<90), unresponsive, or if severe pulmonary edema exists, defibrillate with same energy

Medication Dosing

Amiodarone—150 mg IV bolus over 10 min. If chemical conversion successful, follow with IV infusion of 1 mg/min for 6 hours and then a maintenance infusion of 0.5 mg/min. Repeat supplementary infusions of 150 mg as necessary for recurrent or resistant dysrhythmias. Maximum total daily dose 2.0 g
Procainamide—100 mg over 5 min (20 mg/min). Maximum total dose 17 mg/kg. If chemical conversion successful, maintenance infusion 1 to 4 mg/min

*Impaired cardiac function = ejection fraction <40% or CHF.

Aehlert B: ACLS Quick Review Study Guide, 2e, St. Louis, 2002, Mosby.

Chemical Burns

MECHANISM OF INJURY

Various chemicals, corrosives (acids and alkalies) can cause tissue damage ranging from skin irritation to severe burns. The liquefaction necrosis effect of alkalies (depending on concentration and other factors) generally produces more tissue damage than acids. Hydrofluoric (HF) acid is an exception.

SIGNS AND SYMPTOMS

Skin—Irritation, redness, vesicle formation, rash, and partial- and full-thickness burns may result. Some chemicals (e.g., HF acid) may cause burns to all layers of tissue, including bone.

BASIC TREATMENT

- Ensure that patient is decontaminated. Remove all clothing, shoes, and jewelry. Wash the patient with soap and water.
- Ensure an open airway and support respirations if necessary.
- Check for singed nasal hair, presence of carbon particles, and oral burns.
- Administer oxygen by nonrebreather mask at 10 to 15 L/min.
- Assess and treat any other injuries.
- Estimate body surface area (BSA) of the burn: Rule of nines: BSA is divided into 11 areas of 9% each plus the perineum at 1%; or use Lund and Browder Chart, which is a BSA map that corrects for age.
- Cover burned areas with dry sterile dressings.
- Maintain body temperature with blankets. Do not apply external heat.
- Evaluate for systemic toxicity and, if substance is known, treat by specific guideline.

ADVANCED TREATMENT

- Consider orotracheal or nasotracheal intubation at earliest indicated moment if signs of stridor or respiratory distress are present.
- Start IV administration of lactated Ringer's or normal saline TKO.
- Depending on the surface area of the burn and the hemodynamic state of the patient, administer fluids according to the Parkland formula (4 ml/kg/% BSA burn), administering ½ of the estimated IV fluid volume required during the first 8 hours; consult medical control.
- If no respiratory distress or trauma, consider the administration of morphine sulfate as an analgesic. DIRECT PHYSICIAN ORDER ONLY (refer to morphine sulfate protocol in Section Four).

SPECIAL CONSIDERATIONS

- For ocular burns, refer to eye irrigation protocol in this section.
- Refer to calcium gluconate gel protocol in Section Four for treatment of HF acid burns.
- Cover imbedded fragments of water-reactive metals such as sodium, lithium, and magnesium with a light cooking oil to help reduce possible tissue reaction.

- Immerse imbedded fragments of phosphorus in water or cover with moist sterile dressings during transport.
- Do not use any topical antibiotic or anesthetic ointments on burn area.
- Routine use of prophylactic antibiotics is not recommended.
- Refer to decontamination protocol in this section.

Decontamination

INDICATIONS

- Limit tissue damage and absorption and prevent systemic poisoning.
- Confine contamination to a specified area.
- Prevent secondary contamination of emergency medical services (EMS) and hospital personnel.

DECONTAMINATION DECISIONS

- Consider:
    - Potential toxicity
    - Nature of chemical
    - State of matter
    - Concentration of the product
    - Route of exposure
    - Duration of the exposure
    - Potential for secondary contamination
- Examples of agents with low risk of secondary contamination:
    - Gases (simple asphyxiants, carbon monoxide): Some gas exposures may react with skin moisture and create acid or alkali conditions (e.g., chlorine, anhydrous ammonia) and need to be decontaminated for the care of the patient.
    - Inhalation only: exposure to volatile liquid or vapor. Be aware of any concurrent liquid or solid exposures.
- Examples of agents with high risk of secondary contamination:
    - Corrosive products
    - Asbestos
    - Highly toxic products (cyanide salts)
    - Methemoglobin formers (nitrates, nitrites)
    - Pesticides/herbicides
    - High-viscosity liquids (phenols)
    - Oily or adherent products
    - Dusts and powders
    - Radioactive liquids and dusts
- Exposure considerations:
    - Over 14 million chemicals are listed in the Chemical Abstract Service (CAS)
    - Large amount of product
    - Continuing effect on patient
    - Flammable products may cause fire hazards
    - If any visible product or odor remains on patient

WHEN IN DOUBT, DECONTAMINATE!

PREHOSPITAL DECONTAMINATION CONCEPTS

- Decontaminate in the warm zone, before transport, with simultaneous patient care by protected responders.

- Emergency medical decontamination is usually considered as a primary procedure to stop the chemical action on the patient and allow for safe care and transport. In other words, the purpose of emergency decontamination is to get the patient as clean as reasonably possible, depending on scene conditions and patient presentation. If time, patient presentation, and scene conditions permit, a secondary, detailed decontamination procedure should be carried out. This secondary process may be better carried out at a prepared and properly equipped hospital receiving emergency department.
- Many departments/agencies now have, or have access to, specially designed decontamination trailers, tents, and equipment. Primary emergency medical decontamination should not be delayed while these are set up. However, this equipment is ideal for secondary, detailed decontamination.
- Hospitals are poor choices for primary decontamination. The chemical continues to affect the patient during transport. Transport vehicles and personnel may also become contaminated.
- In inclement weather, use the inside of a cargo truck/trailer or a specially prepared stationary ambulance (walls and floor covered by plastic sheeting, nonessential equipment removed) for decontamination. Other shelters (e.g., local facilities such as schools, firehouses, garages, and indoor car wash areas) may be used after the initial rinse at scene for thorough decontamination. Remember that transport personnel, vehicles, and the facility used are contaminated. Another problem associated with indoor facility use is containment of runoff. Consult with local water authorities for assistance.
- Because of the high probability of hypothermia, have sheets and blankets available to cover nonambulatory patients. Supply blankets, disposable clothes or scrubs, and footwear for ambulatory patients after decontamination.
- Decontaminated patients should be transferred to a clean backboard or scoop stretcher to triage or to a non-contaminated transport team in the cold zone.
- Proper protective equipment is necessary for patient care during decontamination operations. Responders should not attempt to use protective equipment without proper training and fit testing as required. Equipment selection should be performed by an informed, knowledgeable individual using appropriate reference materials.
- Equipment and the transport ambulance should be isolated until complete decontamination can be ensured. All potentially contaminated articles should be isolated for proper disposal according to local, state, and federal regulations. See transportation procedure in Section Five for further guidance on transportation concerns.

HOSPITAL/CLINIC DECONTAMINATION CONCEPTS

- Emergency departments should have decontamination capability. Contaminated patients may arrive at the emergency department without going through EMS channels. Contamination may be missed initially, or a secondary, detailed decontamination may be necessary.
- Hospital decontamination can be conducted outside the emergency department using portable equipment. An alternative to outside decontamination is a specially designed room with a separate entrance, contained drains, and separate ventilation system.

- Decontaminated patients should be passed to non-contaminated personnel on a clean backboard, scoop stretcher, or bed.
- Protective equipment should be used in conjunction with adequate ventilation that moves contaminates away from responders' breathing zone.
- In cases of secondary decontamination procedures, a lesser degree of protective equipment may be adequate. This decision should be made by a knowledgeable individual and based on the nature of the chemical threat and available ventilation.
- The equipment and room should be isolated until complete decontamination can be ensured. All potentially contaminated articles should be isolated for proper disposal according to local, state, and federal regulations.

DECONTAMINATION PROCEDURE

PREPARATION

- Identify the product, life threat, and route of exposure.
- Establish a controlled access system with an entry and exit point.
- Establish at a minimum a two-stage decontamination area that is upwind and uphill from the contaminated area and away from environmentally sensitive areas. Take into consideration the distance from contaminated area; if distance is great, transportation may be required (e.g., a pickup truck).
- The first decontamination stage is clothing removal/water rinse. The second stage consists of a soap and water wash and rinse (if a more extensive decontamination process is necessary, refer to resource data sources and on-scene specialists).

AMBULATORY PATIENT DECONTAMINATION

- Have patients exit the contaminated area.
- Provide shelter and assist patients if necessary in quickly removing clothing, jewelry, and shoes. Isolate these items. If assisting, wear positive-pressure SCBA, air-purifier respirator with appropriate cartridge/filter, and protective equipment specified by references such as the *North American Emergency Response Guidebook.* If special chemical protective clothing is required, consult the chemical manufacturer or specific protective clothing compatibility charts.
- Have patient carry out the following procedures (properly protected responders should assist if necessary):
  - Gently brush off solid or particulate contaminants as completely as possible before washing to reduce the likelihood of a chemical reaction with water. Blot visible liquid contaminants from the body with absorbent material before washing. Use care not to cause any tissue damage.
  - Rinse patient with copious amounts of water. If possible, use warm water, 32° C to 35° C (90° F to 95° F) so that extensive washing can be accomplished. There is a high risk of hypothermia if cold water is used. Never use hot water. Use low water pressure and a gentle spray to avoid aggravating any soft tissue injuries. Avoid overspray and splashing.
  - Use gentle running water from midline to lateral face for eye decontamination. Remove contact lenses if possible. For removal of contact lens and emergency eye care, refer to eye irrigation protocol in this section.
  - Wash patient with baby shampoo or a mild liquid soap. Some authorities suggest using a dilute (0.5%) hypochlorite solution for pesticides, biological agents, and chemical warfare agents. Standard bleach solution is 5%

hypochlorite solution. Bleach can be diluted 1 part bleach to 10 parts water to make the decontamination solution. Fresh bleach should be used. If hypochlorite solution is used, care should be taken to avoid open wounds and the patient's eyes. There is some evidence that skin damage from certain chemical agents (mustard) can be exacerbated by the use of even a dilute hypochlorite solution. Because of these limitations many teams are using baby shampoo or a mild soap.

  - Pay special attention to hair, nail beds, and skin folds. Soft brushes and sponges may be used. Be careful not to abrade the skin, and use extra caution over bruised or broken skin areas. Damaged skin areas can enhance the dermal absorption of toxic products.
  - Rinse patient with copious amounts of water.
  - Contain runoff if possible and feasible. Small children's wading pools, commercially manufactured units/tables, draft tanks, or improvised plastic/frame units may be useful. If no containers are immediately available, try to channel runoff to a containment area. Patient decontamination should not be delayed to obtain containment pools. Local and state water officials should be notified as soon as possible if the runoff cannot be contained.
  - Protect patient from hypothermia.
- Ambulatory patient self-decontamination should be supervised by EMS personnel to ensure adequate decontamination.

NONAMBULATORY PATIENT DECONTAMINATION

- Wear positive-pressure SCBA, air-purifying respirator with appropriate cartridge/filter, and protective equipment specified by references such as the *North American Emergency Response Guidebook.* If special chemical protective clothing is required, consult the chemical manufacturer or specific protective clothing compatibility charts. A qualified, experienced person should make decisions regarding the type of personal protective equipment needed.
- Delay entry until equipment is available.
- Remove patient from contaminated area.
- Quickly remove and isolate patient's clothing, jewelry, and shoes.
- Brush off solid or particulate contaminants as completely as possible before washing to reduce the likelihood of a chemical reaction with water. Blot visible liquid contaminants from the body with absorbent material before washing. Use care not to damage skin.
- Rinse patient with copious amounts of water. If possible, use warm water, 32° C to 35° C (90° F to 95° F) , so that extensive washing can be accomplished. There is a high risk of hypothermia if cold water is used. Never use hot water. Use low water pressure on hose lines to control the spray and avoid aggravating any soft tissue injuries. Avoid overspray and splashing.
- Use gentle running water from midline to lateral face for eye decontamination. Remove contact lenses if possible. For removal of contact lens and emergency eye care, refer to the eye irrigation protocol in this section.
- Wash patient with baby shampoo or a mild liquid soap. Some authorities suggest using a dilute (0.5%) hypochlorite solution for pesticides, biological agents, and chemical warfare agents. Standard bleach solution is 5% hypochlorite solution. Bleach can be diluted 1 part bleach to 10 parts water to make the

decontamination solution. Fresh bleach should be used. If hypochlorite solution is used, care should be taken to avoid open wounds and the patient's eyes. There is some evidence that skin damage from certain chemical agents (mustard) can be exacerbated by the use of even a dilute hypochlorite solution. Because of these limitations many teams are using baby shampoo or a mild soap.

- Pay special attention to hair, nail beds, and skin folds. Soft brushes and sponges may be used. Be careful not to abrade the skin, and use extra caution over bruised or broken skin areas. Damaged skin areas can enhance the dermal absorption of toxic products.
- Rinse patient with copious amounts of water..
- Contain runoff if possible and feasible. Small children's wading pools, commercially manufactured units/tables, draft tanks, or improvised plastic/frame units may be useful. If no containers are immediately available, try to channel runoff to a retention area. Patient decontamination should not be delayed to obtain containment pools. Local and state water officials should be notified as soon as possible if the runoff cannot be contained.
- Protect patient from hypothermia.

DECONTAMINATION ORDER

- For nonambulatory patients, decontaminate the head and face first. Brush or blot visible contaminants away from mouth and nose, and then soap/rinse in the same manner. Isolate patient's airway with oxygen mask, bag-valve mask, or SCBA as soon as possible.
- Decontaminate areas of skin damage or gross contamination next.
- Take care not to allow contamination into areas of tissue damage. Gently covering areas of tissue damage with a plastic cover/wrap help prevent this.
- Decontaminate rest of body as necessary.

SPECIAL CONSIDERATIONS

MASS CASUALTY DECONTAMINATION PROCEDURE

Mass decontamination remains one of the significant bottlenecks in mass casualty incidents or weapons of mass destruction response. Some agencies are using a procedure known as the "drench drill." This procedure uses fire department apparatus or hoses to decontaminate extremely large numbers of patients in a very short period of time. There are many different ways to establish a "drench drill" operation:

- The simplest way to establish this system uses one fire department engine. One $1\frac{1}{2}$ inch fire hose is deployed to spray water from one side and a second nozzle is placed on a discharge gate to provide water spray from two directions.
- A less manpower-intensive system can be rapidly established by parking two fire department engines side by side approximately 25 feet apart. This establishes a decontamination corridor and a focal point for victims to move toward. Hose nozzles are placed on the engine's discharge gates so that water from each engine sprays to the center of the corridor. Patients then are directed to walk though the water spray. Consider shutting the motors on the engines off and using a third engine to supply the pressure. This will reduce exhaust emissions in the decontamination area.

- The engines can be parked closer together with ladders bridging the tops. Hoses are run over the top of the ladders with nozzles pointing down. This will establish a more conventional overhead shower spray. If time permits, tarps can be placed over the ladders to allow male/female separation and some privacy.
- If aerial apparatus (ladder, platform, squirt, etc.) are available, they can be deployed to provide the overhead spray. An engine can be used to provide a side spray in addition to the overhead spray.
- Many departments have started to use Class A foam sprayed from a hose line or discharge gate as a surfactant.
- In all cases a hose line can be deployed to ensure an adequate final rinse.
- Blankets, extra clothing, and Tyvek (disposable paper) suits should be available.

While this procedure does move a lot of people through the decontamination process, there are concerns that must be addressed:

- Because cold water is used, hypothermia is a major concern even in temperate weather.
- If clothes are left on during the “drench drill” operation, contamination could be driven to the skin; therefore, patients should disrobe before going through the decontamination process.
- Many patients will be unwilling to disrobe without some form of privacy. Adding to this concern is the probable presence of media at the incident site. If time allows, tarps and ladders can be used to provide some privacy.
- This procedure is not very effective with nonambulatory patients. Since they must be carried through the water spray, only the front of the patient is cleaned, and patient care during the process is next to impossible.
    - The Incident Commander should weigh the need for and consequence of using this type of emergency decontamination.

Because of these concerns many teams are using decontamination trailers or special, rapidly deployed tents. These systems are easy to setup and provide shelter and privacy during the decontamination process. Water heater/decontamination solution mixer units are available to supply heated decontamination and rinse water through fixed shower nozzles to improve decontamination efficiency and reduce the effects of hypothermia. Air heaters can be used to warm the structures during cold weather. Patient roller systems or carts can be used to increase the efficiency and the throughput of the decontamination process. If these systems are not immediately available at the scene, they can be used for a more thorough decontamination after the “Drench Drill” technique has been used for emergency decontamination.

AMBULATORY PATIENT PROCESS

- Ambulatory patients should undress and isolate their clothes and personal possessions in plastic bags marked to identify the patient.
- They should then move through a minimum two-stage decontamination process. The first stage should consist of a decontamination solution spray followed by the second stage water rinse. If possible, warm water should be used. Water heater/decontamination solution mixer units are available to supply heated decontamination and rinse water through fixed shower nozzles to improve decontamination efficiency and reduce the effects of hypothermia.
- Speaker systems with recorded messages can be used to instruct patients on decontamination procedures as they progress through the system.

- Patients should be checked for residual contamination using monitoring equipment and then should redress in disposable clothing.
- As much privacy as possible should be maintained during the decontamination process.

NONAMBULATORY PATIENT PROCESS

- Nonambulatory patients should be moved from the contaminated area to the decontamination area. Some teams use special patient roller systems or stretcher carts to more effectively move patients through the decontamination process.
- The patient's clothes should be removed and isolated in plastic bags marked to identify the patient.
- As in the ambulatory system, water heater/decontamination solution mixer units can be used to supply heated solution and rinse water to spray nozzles. Patients are sprayed with decontamination solution and washed with sponges or soft brushes. They are then rinsed with warm water.
- Finally, patients are checked for contamination using monitoring equipment.
- Trained and properly protected medical personnel should provide essential medical care during the decontamination process.
- Adequate blankets should be available to reduce the effects of hypothermia.

As in standard decontamination operations, runoff should be collected if possible. Due to the amount of runoff associated with mass decontamination operations, this may be an extremely difficult task. Patient decontamination should not be delayed to allow for runoff containment. Local and state water officials should be notified as soon as possible if runoff cannot be contained. The EPA has published a position paper stating that patient care comes first. First responders will not be held liable for environment regulations if runoff water cannot be contained during a mass casualty decontamination operation. If possible, runoff should be contained but it should not delay the implementation of decontamination operations. Proper authorities must be notified if the water is allowed to run from the site. In all cases, runoff must not be allowed to run into patient treatment and responder staging areas.

Some weapons of mass destruction decontamination teams use video cameras to photograph both ambulatory and nonambulatory patients' faces as they leave the decontamination area. The videotape is then given to local or federal law enforcement agencies to document the identity of the patients who were decontaminated.

RADIATION INCIDENT CONCERNS

- Transportation incidents where radioactive materials are the only significant hazard may present a special decontamination concern.
- Packages for large-quantity shipments are designed to withstand accident conditions and as such are unlikely to release their contents. Small-quantity shipments (such as a medical imaging isotope) are more likely to be involved in a radiation release. Life-threatening conditions from the radioactive material released in these situations is unlikely. Trauma is a much greater risk.
- Prolonged field decontamination of patients with life-threatening injuries may delay needed trauma care.
- Effective, complete decontamination may require radiological monitoring equipment that may not be available in the field.

- Most important, improper decontamination methods may facilitate internalization by transferring contamination to areas of tissue damage or by converting contaminants to a form that could be more readily absorbed through the skin.
- Decontamination for victims of transportation accidents where releases of small quantities of radioactive materials are the only significant hazard should include:
  - Patients with electromagnetic radiation (gamma) exposure, when removed from the area of contamination, require no further decontamination. For patients with particle or liquid exposure, follow the remainder of this section.
  - Quickly remove and isolate patient's clothing, jewelry, and shoes.
  - Package the patient using reverse isolation procedures such as transportation bags, plastic, and blankets. This helps prevent the spread of contamination during transport.
  - Provide adequate ambulance ventilation (properly operating intake and exhaust fans of proper size).
  - Use adequate EMS personnel protective equipment if available. See EMS/hazardous materials equipment procedure in Section Five.
  - Notify the emergency department that a potentially contaminated patient is en route and supply personnel with all available information concerning the identity and nature of the contaminant.
  - Complete decontamination should be carried out at the emergency department, guided by radiological monitoring devices and under the direction of a physician and/or health physicist.
  - Exercise extreme care to keep contaminants away from areas of tissue damage and body cavity openings.
  - Assistance and advice on patient decontamination and management concerns may be obtained from the Oak Ridge Radiation Emergency Assistance Center and Training Site, 24 hours a day by calling (615) 576-3131 or (615) 481-1000 and asking for Reacts Team.
  - In transportation incidents involving a large-quantity shipment that has sustained a container breech, a large release at a fixed facility, if other chemical contaminants besides radioactive materials are suspected, or in cases involving large numbers of patients (e.g., radiological dispersion device) standard field and emergency department decontamination guidelines should be followed.
  - In cases involving mass causalities, the transportation of contaminated patients may quickly overwhelm the EMS and hospital systems. In these cases patient decontamination should take place prior to transport to the hospital.

Eye Irrigation

MECHANISM OF INJURY

Chemical exposure may cause damage to the eyes, ranging from chemical conjunctivitis to severe burns.

SIGNS AND SYMPTOMS

Eyes—Local pain, visual disturbances, lacrimation, edema, corneal abrasion, corneal lacerations, and redness.

BASIC TREATMENT

- Flush with water. Use a low-pressure flow from a hose, or pour water from a container to irrigate.
- Remove contact lenses with a lens removal suction bulb. Gently place bulb cup end against the contact lens; then pull the bulb away from the eye in a straight line. Be sure not to touch the cornea with the suction bulb, because permanent damage may be caused. If you encounter difficulty, slide the lens onto the sclera and continue irrigation. Save each lens in a separate, labeled sterile container filled with sterile saline solution.
- In adults, if globe and lid are intact and without edema, an eye irrigation lens (e.g., Morgan Therapeutic Lens) may be used. Flush each eye continuously during transport with a minimum of 1000 ml of normal saline. Do not force lens; if unable to insert easily, do not use.

Irrigation Lens Insertion

- Have advanced personnel instill topical anesthetic.
- Attach IV tubing to lens.
- Start irrigation fluid flow.
- Have patient look down; insert lens under upper lid.
- Have patient look up; retract lower lid and gently lower lens into place.

Irrigation Lens Removal

- Have patient look up; retract lower lid below the inferior border of the lens and hold that position.
- Have patient look down; retract the upper lid, and the lens will be extruded.
- Use caution not to flush chemical into other eye. Flush from the medial canthus of the eye to the lateral aspect of the globe.

ALTERNATIVE EYE IRRIGATION METHODS

- If unable to use lens, irrigate each eye continuously during transport with a minimum of 1000 ml of normal saline, using large-bore IV tubing.
- Use caution not to flush chemical into other eye. Flush from the medial canthus of the eye to the lateral aspect of the globe.
- A nasal cannula taped to the bridge of the nose may be used for simultaneous hands-free irrigation of both eyes. IV tubing from a 1000-ml bag of normal saline is connected to the cannula tubing to deliver the irrigation fluid.

EYE IRRIGATION IN CHILDREN

- Irrigate each eye continuously during transport with a minimum of 1000 ml of normal saline, using large-bore IV tubing.

- Use caution not to flush chemical into other eye. Flush from the medial canthus of the eye to the lateral aspect of the globe.

ADVANCED TREATMENT

- Check for allergies to "-caine" drugs. If no contraindications, administer 1 to 2 drops of proparacaine hydrochloride in each eye to facilitate the use of irrigation lens.

SPECIAL CONSIDERATIONS

- In cases of exposure to the riot control agent OC (pepper spray), only plain water should be used for eye irrigation. The use of saline solutions will result in an increase in pain.
- Advise patient not to rub eyes.
- Do not force irrigation lens; if difficulty is encountered inserting lenses, do not use them.
- Remember, rapid ocular decontamination is essential.
- Continue to irrigate during transport.
- Conjunctival sac pH is usually measured at 10-minute intervals during irrigation. The target range for conjunctival sac pH is between 7 and 8. With effective irrigation, most pH paper shows a pH of approximately 8 when touched to the area of the lower conjunctival fornix. In cases of concentrated acid or alkali burns, eye irrigation may need to be continued for up to 2 hours or more in an attempt to normalize the pH of the anterior chamber.
- Obtain ophthalmological consultation as required.

Frostbite

MECHANISM OF INJURY

Frostbite can be caused by contact with leaking compressed gas or cryogenic cylinders.

SIGNS AND SYMPTOMS

Superficial frostbite to the skin presents with a red color followed by gray, white, or mottled coloring. Patients report stinging, burning, or paresthesia. The affected area is stiff to the touch, but underlying tissues remain soft.

Deep frostbite presents with a white, yellow-white, or mottled, bluish-white colored skin that is hard, cold, and insensitive to the touch.

BASIC TREATMENT

- Ensure that patient is decontaminated. Remove all clothing, shoes, and jewelry. Wash the patient with soap and water.
- Ensure an open airway and support respirations if necessary.
- Administer oxygen by nonrebreather mask at 10 to15 L/min.
- Handle the affected area gently and protect it from friction and pressure.
- For superficial frostbite, rewarm with body heat. Do not use dry or radiant heat.
- For deep frostbite or frozen skin areas with extensive transport times to the hospital, warm the affected area in a water bath at a temperature of 37.8° to 40.6° C (100° to 105° F). Monitor the temperature of the bath and ensure that it remains constant. Keep area immersed until it is completely flushed in color, is warm to the touch, blanches with tactile pressure, and stays flushed when removed from the bath. Do not use dry or radiant heat.
- Prolonged rewarming may be necessary, and the procedure may be very painful. Rewarming may be best accomplished in the hospital setting, unless transport times are long.
- Check neurovascular status before and after warming.
- Place sterile cotton between affected digits.
- Apply soft, sterile dressings lightly over affected parts.
- Maintain body temperature with blankets. Do not apply external heat.
- Assess and treat any other injuries.

ADVANCED TREATMENT

- Consider administering morphine sulfate as an analgesic if no respiratory distress or other trauma is present. DIRECT PHYSICIAN ORDER ONLY (refer to morphine sulfate protocol in Section Four).

SPECIAL CONSIDERATIONS

- Do not remove clothes that are frozen to the area until after the area is warmed.
- Do not allow area to refreeze.
- Do not apply antibiotic or anesthetic ointments.
- Do not rupture blisters.

Heat Stress

MECHANISM OF INJURY

The ability of the body to regulate heat may be impaired by chemical exposure and by wearing personal protective equipment. This overloads an individual's thermal response mechanism and at the same time increases an individual's heat production by adding bulk and weight, which increases the work necessary to perform required activities. Certain chemical exposures (e.g., pentachlorophenol, dinitrophenol, 2,4-D/2,4,5-T, and sodium azide) may also cause an increased risk of heat exposure.

HEAT STRESS FACTORS

Environmental temperature
Radiant heat
Humidity
Workload
Personal protective equipment

PREDISPOSING FACTORS

Lack of physical fitness
Lack of heat acclimatization
Age
Dehydration
Obesity
Alcohol and drug use
Infection
Sunburn
Diarrhea
Chronic disease

PERSONAL PROTECTIVE EQUIPMENT

Adds weight and bulk
Impairs the body's normal heat exchange mechanisms (evaporation, convection, radiation)
Increases energy expenditure

TYPES OF HEAT STRESS

Heat Fatigue

Common effect of prolonged heat exposure
Loss of coordination and alertness
Heat rash, edema, and fatigue

Heat Cramps

Physically fit individual but poorly acclimatized
Occurs during or after work
Affects most major muscle groups
Cause unknown

Heat Syncope

Self-limited in nature

Probably vasovagal in origin
Increased risk with conditions causing dehydration

Heat Exhaustion

Ill-defined precursor of heatstroke
Caused by excessive loss of fluid and/or electrolytes through perspiration
Patient shows postural vital sign changes
Nausea and vomiting
Confusion
Elevated core temperature up to 40° C (104° F)

SUSPECT HEAT STROKE!

Heat Stroke

The body's heat-regulatory process fails, and the sweating mechanism stops. Heat stroke is a life-threatening condition. Recent studies have shown that there are two types of heat stroke. Classic heat stroke occurs when the patient has been exposed to high temperatures over a long period of time (days to weeks). Hot, red, and dry skin are the hallmark signs of classic heatstroke. Exertional heat stroke occurs when too much fluid has been lost to the sweating mechanism and the body's cooling mechanism is overwhelmed. Athletes, firefighters, and responders in chemical PPE with heat stress will suffer from the exertional type. Exertional heat stroke is often misdiagnosed as heat exhaustion because the skin will still be wet in the initial stages. Level of consciousness should be used to determine if the patient is suffering from heat exhaustion or heat stroke.

Decreased level of consciousness, seizures, and coma. Mental status abnormalities are the most important indicators of heat stroke.
Tachycardia
Hyperventilation
Usually skin is dry, but in the initial stages of occupational heat stroke the skin may be wet.
Temperature core elevated greater than 40° C (104° F).
T-wave ECG changes may be seen.

TREATMENT (BASIC AND ADVANCED AS APPROPRIATE)

Heat Fatigue

- Rest.
- Remove from direct sunlight and place in a cool climate.
- Fluid replacement.
- Transport to hospital if necessary.

Heat Cramps

- Rest.
- Remove from direct sunlight and place in a cool climate.
- Oral fluid replacement.
- Do not use hot packs.
- Do not massage the cramping area.
- Transport to hospital if necessary.

Heat Syncope

- ABCs (airway, breathing, circulation).
- Place patient in supine position.
- Raise legs 6 to 8 inches.

- Rule out other causes.
- Oral fluid replacement if no airway compromise.
- Assess for toxic exposure or other causes.
- Transport to hospital as necessary.

Heat Exhaustion

- ABCs.
- Administer oxygen by nonrebreather mask at 10 to 15 L/min.
- Remove from exposure.
- Rapid cooling (see Heat Stroke).
- Cardiac monitoring. Treat arrhythmias if necessary (refer to cardiac protocol in this section)
- Start IV administration of normal saline or lactated Ringer's titrated to maintain adequate blood pressure.
- Assess for toxic exposure or other causes.
- Transport to appropriate medical facility.

Heat Stroke

- ABCs; intubate if necessary.
- Administer oxygen by nonrebreather mask at 10 to 15 L/min.
- Start IV administration of normal saline or lactated Ringer's, titrated to maintain adequate blood pressure.
- Cardiac monitoring. Treat arrhythmias if necessary (refer to cardiac protocol in this section).
- Measures for rapid cooling include:
  - Ice packs in areas where blood vessels are close to skin surface.
  - Water mist, to allow for evaporation on skin and maximum cooling effect.
  - Large fans.
  - Cold water–soaked sheets or towels placed over body.
  - Cold water poured over patient (not as effective as water mist unless in high-humidity atmosphere).
  - Submersion in cold water (very difficult to care for patient).
- Treat hypotension (refer to shock protocol in this section).
- Treat seizures (refer to seizure protocol in this section).
- To avoid overcooling and hypothermia, slow or modify cooling measures when temperature reaches 37.8° C to 38.9° C (100° F to 102° F).
- Assess for toxic exposure or other causes.
- Rapid transport to appropriate medical facility.

SPECIAL CONSIDERATIONS

- Condition may be aggravated by certain drugs (atropine, belladonna, antihistamines, diuretics, thyroid hormone, acetylsalicylic acid).
- Exposure to compounds such as sodium azide, pentachlorophenol, dinitrophenols, 2,4-D and 2,4,5-T may cause disturbances in body temperature regulation and exacerbate heat stress conditions.
- Exposures above 39° C (102.2° F) for extended periods of time in the first trimester of pregnancy may increase the risk of birth defects.
- Refer to hazardous materials team medical support protocol in Section Five for prevention and monitoring guidelines.

Hypothermia

MECHANISM OF INJURY

Body core temperature below 35° C (95° F) caused by prolonged exposure to cold environments or abnormal thermoregulation:

Core Temperature	Symptoms
32° C to 35° C (89.6° F to 95° F)	Mild symptoms
32° C (89.6° F)	Moderate symptoms
30° C (86° F) or below	Profound hypothermia; high mortality rate

Patients may develop hypothermia while undergoing decontamination procedures in cold environments. Removing protective equipment in cool environments may lead to rapid cooling as a result of evaporation from moist skin.

SIGNS AND SYMPTOMS

Cardiovascular—Bradycardia, arrhythmias (atrioventricular [AV] block, nodal tachycardia, atrial fibrillation [AF] and ventricular fibrillation [VF], increased QT interval, premature ventricular contractions [PVCs], and Osborne J waves), and hypotension.

Respiratory—Decreased rate and depth.

CNS—Decreased level of consciousness, confusion, lethargy, stupor, and withdrawn or combative behavior. Paresthesias and pain in the extremities. Shivering may occur in an attempt to raise body temperature.

Skin—Pale and cool.

Other—Shivering stops at a core temperature of 30° C (86° F). Mild hypothermia may present with an uncoordinated, staggering gait. Severe hypothermia may present with stiffness, rigor, and an inability to walk.

GENERAL TREATMENT

- Ensure adequate decontamination.
- Ensure an open airway and assist ventilations if necessary.
- Administer oxygen by nonrebreather mask at 10 to 15 L/min.
- Remove wet clothing and protect against wind chill.
- Place patient in horizontal position.
- Cover with warm blankets.
- Avoid rough movement and excessive activity.
- Monitor cardiac rhythm if equipped and qualified.
- Monitor core temperature.

SPECIFIC TREATMENT (AS QUALIFIED)

If pulse and breathing are present and core temperature is 34° C to 36° C (93.2° F to 96.8° F):

- Continue passive rewarming (dry clothing and blankets).
- Perform active external rewarming (warm baths, hot packs, radiant heat).

If pulse and breathing are present and core temperature is 30° C to 34° C (86° F to 93.2° F):

- Continue passive rewarming.
- Perform active external rewarming of truncal areas only.

If pulse and breathing are present and core temperature is <30° C (86° F):

- Perform active internal rewarming:
  - Warm IV fluids at 43° C (109° F).
  - Warm humidified oxygen at 42° C (108° F).
  - Peritoneal lavage (KCl-free fluid).
  - Extracorporeal rewarming.
  - Esophageal rewarming tubes.
- Continue active internal rewarming until:
  - Core temperature is >95° F (>35° C).
  - Spontaneous circulation returns.
  - Resuscitation efforts cease.

If pulseless/apneic:

- Start CPR.
- Defibrillate for ventricular tachycardia (VT)/VF with up to a total of three shocks (200 J, 300 J, 360 J).
- Intubate.
- Ventilate with warm, humidified oxygen at 42° C to 46° C (108° F to 115° F).
- Establish IV line.
- Infuse with warm normal saline at 43° C (109° F).

If pulseless/apneic and core temperature is <30° C (86° F):

- Continue CPR.
- Withhold IV medications.
- Limit shocks for VT/VF to a maximum of three defibrillations.
- Transport to hospital.
- Follow internal active rewarming sequence detailed in previous paragraphs.

If pulseless/apneic and core temperature is >30° C (86° F):

- Continue CPR.
- Give IV medications as indicated but at longer than standard intervals.
- Repeat defibrillation for VT/VF, which may occur as core temperature rises.
- Follow internal active rewarming sequence detailed above.

SPECIAL CONSIDERATIONS

- Rough handling, including intubation, may precipitate VF.
- All active internal and active external rewarming procedures are better carried out in-hospital. This includes the use of warmed IV fluids and warm, humidified oxygen ventilation.
- Decontamination efforts during weather extremes should be carried out with warm water or in heated areas whenever possible. This minimizes the risk of hypothermia. Warm blankets should be available to cover patients immediately after decontamination.
- Tympanic membrane or rectal temperatures should be used to guide treatment.

Patient Evaluation

ROUTES OF EXPOSURE

- Inhalation
- Skin absorption
- Skin and eye contact
- Ingestion
- Injection

POTENTIAL CHEMICAL HAZARDS

- Flammables
- Corrosives
- Poisons
- Sensitizers (allergens)
- Radiation

POTENTIAL PHYSICAL HAZARDS

- Fire
- Heat
- Cold
- Mechanical trauma
- Explosion

EVENT HISTORY

- Nature of accident
- Substance(s) involved
- Route of exposure
- Duration of exposure
- Number of patients
- Associated trauma
- Past medical history
- Allergies and medications
- Examination findings and vital signs
- Initial signs and symptoms
- Signs and symptoms at initial EMS evaluation
- Treatment administered
- Signs and symptoms now
- Compatibility of signs and symptoms with poisoning and exposure pattern

PATIENT EXAMINATION

- Primary examination (ABCDE):
  - Airway
  - Breathing
  - Circulation/C-spine
  - Decontamination needs
  - Evaluate for systemic toxicity
  - Skin color and condition

- Secondary examination:
  - Vital signs
  - Confirm history of exposure
- Take pertinent medical history:
  - Current medications
  - Allergies to medications
  - Serious illnesses/operations
  - Previous exposures
- Complete physical examination with special attention to:
  - Mental status/neurobehavioral assessment
  - Skin and eyes
  - Airway
  - Pulmonary system
  - Cardiovascular system
  - Gastrointestinal system
  - Neurological system

POSSIBLE DIAGNOSTIC TESTS

- Complete blood count
- Reticulocyte count
- Platelet count
- Coagulation profile
- Serum electrolytes (sodium, potassium, chloride, bicarbonate)
- Determination of anion and osmolar gaps
- Blood urea nitrogen (BUN)
- Glucose
- Biochemical profile to include
  - Baseline liver survey
    Alkaline phosphatase
    Alanine aminotransferase (ALT)
    Aspartate aminotransferase (AST)
    Lactate dehydrogenase (LDH)
    Total bilirubin
  - Calcium
  - Creatinine
  - Phosphorus
  - Magnesium
  - Cholesterol
  - Triglycerides
- Arterial blood gases (ABGs)
  - With measured percent oxygen saturation
- Carboxyhemoglobin
- Methemoglobin
- Specific toxicology tests
  - Serum ethanol
  - Serum methanol
  - Serum ethylene glycol
  - Whole blood cyanide

- Metals
  - Arsenic (blood/urine)
  - Cadmium (blood/urine)
  - Copper (serum/blood)
  - Iron (serum)
  - Lead (blood/urine)
  - Lithium (serum)
  - Magnesium (plasma)
  - Mercury (blood/urine)
- Beryllium lymphocyte transformation test
- Total iron-binding capacity (TIBC)
- Free erythrocyte protoporphyrin (FEP) or zinc protoporphyrin (ZPP)
- Plasma cholinesterase
- Red blood cell cholinesterase

- Other toxicology tests as indicated by specific exposure
- Urinalysis
- Chest radiograph
- Pulmonary function studies
- Electrocardiogram (ECG)

Pulmonary Edema

MECHANISM OF INJURY

Fluid leaking from the pulmonary capillaries into the alveoli can be caused by circulatory overload, cardiac failure, and toxic inhalations that cause either cardiac failure or direct damage to the alveolar basement membranes. Twenty percent of lung weight is fluid. With acute pulmonary edema, fluid content can reach 1000 times normal. Acute pulmonary edema usually has a rapid onset. Toxic exposures may exhibit a delayed onset of pulmonary edema from hours to days.

SIGNS AND SYMPTOMS

Cardiovascular—Increased heart rate and jugular venous distention.

Respiratory—Dyspnea, cough, Cheyne-Stokes respirations, orthopnea, moist breath sounds (rales and rhonchi), and, in severe cases, pink (blood-tinged) frothy sputum.

CNS—Anxiety, decreased level of consciousness, and coma.

Other—The cause, either cardiac or direct lung damage, must be determined.

BASIC TREATMENT

- Ensure an open airway; suction if necessary.
- Support respirations if necessary.
- Administer oxygen by nonrebreather mask at 10 to 15 L/min.
- Position patient in a sitting position to increase gas exchange.
- Place arms and legs in a dependent position if possible.

ADVANCED TREATMENT

- Consider orotracheal or nasotracheal intubation for airway control.
- Consider positive-pressure ventilation.
- Monitor cardiac rhythm and treat arrhythmias if necessary.
- Start IV administration of 5% dextrose in water (D_5W) TKO.
- Administer furosemide (Lasix) if patient is not hypotensive. DIRECT PHYSICIAN ORDER ONLY (refer to furosemide protocol in Section Four).
- Consider the use of albuterol to decrease reversible bronchospasm if wheezes are present. DIRECT PHYSICIAN ORDER ONLY (refer to albuterol protocol in Section Four).

If pulmonary edema is due to cardiac (pump) failure:

- Administer morphine sulfate. DIRECT PHYSICIAN ORDER ONLY (refer to morphine sulfate protocol in Section Four).
- Refer to Cardiac Treatment protocol in this section.

Seizures

MECHANISM OF INJURY

Many metabolic disturbances can result from toxic exposures, including hypocapnia, cerebral anoxia, water intoxication, and hypoglycemia. Seizures can occur as the result of any of these abnormalities. Certain compounds such as strychnine, picrotoxin, pentylenetetrazol, camphor, DDT, chlorinated insecticides, parathion and other organophosphates, and fluoroacetates may cause seizures.

SIGNS AND SYMPTOMS

CNS—Focal, grand mal seizures, and/or status epilepticus.

Other—Increased temperature, fractures, dislocations, trauma to the tongue, and incontinence of urine and stool.

BASIC TREATMENT

- Ensure an open airway and support ventilations if necessary.
- Administer oxygen by nonrebreather mask at 10 to 15 L/min.
- Do not force anything between the teeth.
- Protect patient from injury. Do not restrain.
- Reassess patient following seizure.

ADVANCED TREATMENT

- Consider orotracheal or nasotracheal intubation for airway control in unconscious patients or patients with status epilepticus.
- Monitor cardiac rhythm and treat arrhythmias if necessary.
- Start IV administration of lactated Ringer's or normal saline TKO and draw blood for later laboratory analysis.
- Monitor for signs of hypoglycemia (decreased level of consciousness, tachycardia, pallor, dilated pupils, and diaphoresis).
- If signs of hypoglycemia and/or low blood glucose (<50 mg/dl) are present, administer 50% dextrose if necessary. Draw blood sample for glucose determination before administration (refer to 50% dextrose protocol in Section Four).
- If patient is actively convulsing, administer diazepam (Valium) or lorazepam (Ativan) (refer to diazepam and lorazepam protocol in Section Four).

SPECIAL CONSIDERATIONS

- Diazepam and lorazepam may depress respiratory drive; be prepared to assist respirations.
- Reduce external stimuli as much as possible.

Shock

HYPOVOLEMIC SHOCK

MECHANISM OF INJURY

Chemical exposure can cause increased permeability of the blood vessel walls, with resultant leakage of plasma (water) across cell membranes out of the vascular system, causing hypovolemia. Hemorrhage caused by trauma may also occur.

SIGNS AND SYMPTOMS

Cardiovascular—Usually pulse rate is >120 beats/min and weak (bradycardia or normal rate may be observed). Blood pressure <90 torr systolic with jugular venous pressure decreased. Positive orthostatic changes are present (pulse rate increase of 20 or more or blood pressure decrease of 20 torr or more, or a combination of 20 or more when the patient is moved from supine to standing position).

Respiratory—Increased rate with shallow respirations.

CNS—Anxiety, restlessness, confusion, decreased level of consciousness, and coma.

Skin—Pale, diaphoretic, cool or, in cases of dehydration, warm and dry.

BASIC TREATMENT

- Ensure an open airway and support ventilations if necessary.
- Administer oxygen by nonrebreather mask at 10 to 15 L/min.
- Control any external bleeding.
- Elevate legs 10 to 12 inches.
- Splint fractures.
- Maintain body temperature.
- Monitor vital signs every 5 minutes.

ADVANCED TREATMENT

- Consider orotracheal or nasotracheal intubation for airway control.
- Start IV administration of lactated Ringer's or normal saline. Administer a fluid bolus of 250 to 500 ml in the adult patient, 20 ml/kg in the pediatric patient (may be repeated up to three times). Titrate IV flow to maintain an adequate blood pressure. If no response, consider the use of sympathomimetics (DIRECT PHYSICIAN ORDER ONLY).

SPECIAL CONSIDERATIONS

- Use of the pneumatic antishock garment is controversial but may be useful in certain circumstances. Consult your local medical advisor.
- Hypotension is a late sign. Be prepared to institute treatment before the blood pressure falls.
- After IV fluids are started during initial resuscitation efforts, watch for signs of fluid overload and cerebral and/or pulmonary edema.
- The elderly and patients with chronic hypertension may be hypovolemic, with vital signs that appear normal.
- Look for cardiac signs with traumatic shock: cardiac tamponade and tension pneumothorax.

- Rapid transport to an appropriate treatment center is essential; do not waste time on scene.

CARDIOGENIC SHOCK

MECHANISM OF INJURY

Chemical agents may impair the cardiovascular system by reducing the circulation by direct cardiotoxicity. Many types of cardiac problems, including electrical conduction deficits and loss of contractility, may be seen.

SIGNS AND SYMPTOMS

Cardiovascular—Chest pain or a heavy pressure sensation in the chest. Blood pressure <90 torr systolic; pulse rate normal, fast, or slow and possibly irregular. Jugular venous pressure is increased, but may be normal in the initial stages.

Respiratory—Increased rate with shallow respirations. Signs of pulmonary edema.

CNS—Anxiety, restlessness, confusion, decreased level of consciousness, and coma.

Skin—Cyanotic, cool, and diaphoretic.

BASIC TREATMENT

- Ensure an open airway and support ventilations if necessary.
- Administer oxygen by nonrebreather mask at 10 to 15 L/min.
- Ensure complete rest and position of comfort.

ADVANCED TREATMENT

- Consider orotracheal or nasotracheal intubation for airway control.
- Monitor cardiac rhythm and treat arrhythmias if necessary.
- Start IV administration of D_5W TKO.
- Administer norepinephrine or dopamine (Intropin). Titrate to a systolic blood pressure of 90 to 100 torr. DIRECT PHYSICIAN ORDER ONLY (refer to specific drug protocols in Section Four).
- Treat pulmonary edema symptoms if necessary.
- Use a cautious fluid challenge of 250 ml of lactated Ringer's or normal saline if signs of hypovolemia are present. DIRECT PHYSICIAN ORDER ONLY .

SPECIAL CONSIDERATIONS

- Rapid transport is essential.
- Refer to Cardiac Treatment protocol in this section for further information

ANAPHYLACTIC SHOCK

MECHANISM OF INJURY

In severe allergic reactions, the body reacts to a foreign substance by releasing histamine and other chemical mediators of anaphylaxis. These may cause bronchial spasm and dilation of peripheral blood vessels and alter the permeability of the cell membranes, allowing fluid to leak from the vascular space into the interstitial spaces.

SIGNS AND SYMPTOMS

Cardiovascular—Increased pulse rate with blood pressure <90 torr systolic. A tight feeling may be present in the chest.

Respiratory—Cough and stridor, possibly indicating an upper airway obstruction. Dyspnea and diffuse wheezing.

CNS—Headache, anxiety, restlessness, decreased level of consciousness, and coma.
Skin—Facial edema and a flushed appearance with rash, redness, and itching.

BASIC TREATMENT

- Ensure an open airway and support ventilations if necessary.
- Administer oxygen by nonrebreather mask at 10 to 15 L/min.

ADVANCED TREATMENT

- Consider orotracheal or nasotracheal intubation for airway control. Intubation may be necessary at the first indication of upper airway obstruction.
- Monitor cardiac rhythm and treat arrhythmias if necessary.
- Start IV administration of lactated Ringer's or normal saline TKO.
- Administer epinephrine subcutaneously (SQ) or, if symptoms are severe, by IV push. By direct physician order or standing order protocol (refer to epinephrine protocol in Section Four).
- Consider the use of albuterol to decrease reversible bronchospasm. DIRECT PHYSICIAN ORDER ONLY (refer to albuterol protocol in Section Four).

SPECIAL CONSIDERATIONS

- Rapid transport is essential.
- Use epinephrine with caution in children and elderly patients.

VASOGENIC SHOCK

MECHANISM OF INJURY

Chemical agents may cause a defect in the responsiveness of vascular smooth muscles to neural or hormonal stimuli or depress vasomotor center activity in the brain stem. In either case, widespread vasodilation without primary loss of volume causes hypotension.

SIGNS AND SYMPTOMS

Cardiovascular—Usually pulse rate is >120 beats/min and weak (bradycardia or normal pulse rate possible). Blood pressure >90 torr systolic and jugular venous pressure is decreased. Positive orthostatic changes.
Respiratory—Increased rate with shallow respirations.
CNS—Anxiety, restlessness, confusion, decreased level of consciousness, and coma.
Skin—Warm, dry, and flushed.

BASIC TREATMENT

- Ensure an open airway and support ventilations if necessary.
- Administer oxygen by nonrebreather mask at 10 to 15 L/min.
- Elevate legs 6 to 12 inches.

ADVANCED TREATMENT

- Consider orotracheal or nasotracheal intubation for airway control.
- Start IV administration of lactated Ringer's or normal saline TKO.
- Administer dopamine (Intropin) or norepinephrine (Levophed). Titrate to a systolic blood pressure of 90 to 100 mm Hg. DIRECT PHYSICIAN ORDER ONLY (refer to specific drug protocols in Section Four).

SPECIAL CONSIDERATIONS

- Rapid transport is essential.

Section Four

DRUG PROTOCOLS

SPECIFIC PHYSIOLOGIC ANTAGONISTS

With the exception of ethanol, fomepizole, and the chelating agents, most of these medications can be used in the prehospital setting. Antibiotic therapy is usually not considered "pre-hospital therapy" but may be administered in a mass prophylaxis program. Prehospital use varies according to local jurisdiction. Consult your state EMS regulations and local medical control protocols for further information.

Unless otherwise stated, all treatment modalities and drug dosages in this section are based on the adult patient. For pediatric patients, consult the drug protocol section and your medical advisor. Medication use in pregnant patients should be guided by physician control.

To the best of our knowledge, drug indications, dosages, and precautions contained in these protocols are correct and current as of the time of publication. The reader is urged to review standard pharmacology references and the manufacturer's recommendations for additional details.

These protocols contain suggested treatment. Operating protocols and standing and verbal orders should be established by the local medical advisor. Consult with your medical control physician concerning local medication protocols.

Adenosine (Adenocard)

MAJOR ACTIONS

- A naturally occurring purine nucleoside that acts on the atrioventricular (AV) node to slow conduction and inhibit anterograde and retrograde reentry pathways.
- Therapeutic half-life is less than 5 seconds.
- Shortens cardiac cell action potential.
- Decreases atrial contractility.
- Decreases cyclic adenosine monophosphate (cAMP) concentration and reduces norepinephrine release.

INDICATIONS

- Conversion of narrow complex paroxysmal supraventricular tachycardia (PSVT) to sinus rhythm.

DOSAGE

- Adult: 6 mg rapid IV push over 1 to 3 seconds, using the injection port nearest the nub of the IV catheter. The dose should be followed by a 20-ml saline flush. If no response is observed within 1 to 2 minutes, a 12-mg repeat dose may be administered. A third dose of 12 mg may be given if no conversion has occurred. Maximum dose is 30 mg.
- Pediatric: 100 μg/kg rapid IV push. Maximum single dose is 12 mg. If no response, the repeat dose is 100 to 200 μg/kg rapid IV push. Consult medical control.

PRECAUTIONS

- Continuous electrocardiography (ECG) monitoring is essential.
- Contraindicated in patients with second- or third-degree heart block, with sick sinus syndrome unless a pacemaker is in place, and with known hypersensitivity to the drug, asthma, poison, or drug-induced tachycardia.
- In atrial fibrillation (AF), atrial flutter, and ventricular tachycardia (VT), adenosine will not terminate the arrhythmia but may produce a transient block which may aid in diagnosis.
- May cause flushing, coughing/dyspnea, hypotension, headache, chest pain, back pain, neck pain, palpitations, nausea, syncope, shortness of breath, bradycardia, and a metallic taste.
- Effects of adenosine are antagonized by xanthines such as theophylline and caffeine.
- Adenosine is potentiated by dipyridamole (Persantine). Effects are prolonged in patients on carbamazepine (Tegretol).
- Transient heart blocks have been noted to occur, as well as transient (6 to 12 sec) episodes of asystole. Temporary bronchospasm and hypotension have also occurred.
- May cause coronary vasodilation in low doses and peripheral vasodilation at higher doses.
- Use with caution in pregnancy.

HOW SUPPLIED

- 2-ml/6 mg vials (3 mg/ml).

Amiodarone Hydrochloride (Cordarone)

MAJOR ACTIONS

- Possesses electrophysiologic characteristics of all four classes of antiarrhythmics, by inhibiting sympathetic stimulation; blocks potassium channels as well as calcium channels.
- Inhibits alpha and beta receptors and possesses both vagolytic and calcium channel blocking properties
- At the sinoatrial (SA) node it slows the heart rate, slows conduction at the AV junction, and decreases ventricular response.
- Hemodynamically vasodilates coronary and peripheral vasculature, suppresses SA node function, and prolongs PR, QRS, and QT intervals.

INDICATIONS

- Shock-refractory pulseless ventricular tachycardia/ventricular fibrillation .
- Polymorphic VT, wide-complex tachycardia of uncertain origin.
- Stable VT when cardioversion is unsuccessful.
- Adjunct to electrical cardioversion of SVT/PSVT and atrial tachycardia (AT).
- Ectopic or multifocal atrial tachycardia (MAT) with normal left ventricular (LV) function.
- Pharmacologic conversion of atrial fibrillation and rate control of atrial fibrillation or flutter when other therapies ineffective.

DOSAGE

- Cardiac arrest—pulseless VT/VF (adult): Initial bolus 300 mg IV bolus diluted in 20 to 30 ml of NS or D_5W. Initial infusion rate should not exceed 30 mg/min.
  - Consider IV repeat dose of 150 mg every 3 to 5 minutes.
  - If defibrillation successful, follow with IV infusion of 1 mg/min for 6 hours (mix 900 mg in 500 ml NS). Then decrease IV infusion rate to 0.5 mg/min for 18 hours.
- Wide-complex tachycardia (stable): Rapid IV infusion of 150 mg over first 10 minutes. May repeat rapid infusion every 10 minutes as needed.
  - Maximum daily dose 2.0 g IV/24 hours.

PRECAUTIONS

- Hypotension, bradycardia, and AV block require slowing or discontinuing of medication.
- Contraindications are hypersensitivity, sinus node dysfunction, marked sinus bradycardia, second- and third-degree block, and syncope with bradycardia. Use with caution in patients with electrolyte abnormalities.
- Infusions lasting longer than 2 hours require polyolefin or glass bottles containing D_5W and polyvinyl chloride tubing.
- Drug should be stored at room temperature of 15° C to 25° C (59° F to 77° F).

- Has additive effect with other medications that prolong the QT interval and impairs metabolism of digoxin, theophylline and warfarin.
- Terminal elimination is extremely long; half life lasts up to 40 days or more.

HOW SUPPLIED

- 50-mg/ml vial.

Lidocaine (Xylocaine)

MAJOR ACTIONS

- Inhibits the influx of sodium through the fast channels of the myocardial cell membrane and decreases conduction in ischemic cardiac tissue without adversely affecting normal conduction.
- Elevates fibrillation threshold by reducing myocardial excitability.
- Suppresses ventricular arrhythmias.
- Block or infiltration anesthetic agent.

INDICATIONS

- Monomorphic VT, polymorphic VT with normal QT interval.
- Pulseless VT/VF that persists after defibrillation and epinephrine.
- Control of hemodynamically compromising premature ventricular contractions (PVCs).
- Preintubation in head injuries. Minimizes rise in intracranial pressure associated with intubation.

DOSAGE

- Adult: 1 to 1.5 mg/kg IV bolus over 2 to 3 minutes initially, with repeat bolus of 0.5 to 0.75 mg/kg every 5 to 10 minutes if needed, to a maximal total loading dose of 3 mg/kg.
- Pediatric: 1 mg/kg IV bolus.
- NOTE: Many administration methods exist for lidocaine. We believe that this method is most applicable for prehospital use. For hospital use, continuous infusion rates, and other dose regimens, consult current ACLS guidelines.

PRECAUTIONS

- Excessive doses may cause myocardial and circulatory depression.
- May cause CNS disturbances such as dizziness, disorientation, sleepiness, confusion, and seizures, as well as visual and auditory disturbances.
- May increase ventricular rate if used in the presence of atrial fibrillation.
- May cause complete AV block.
- Contraindicated with idioventricular or escape rhythms and Wolff-Parkinson-White (WPW) syndrome.
- Use with caution in patients with impaired liver function, shock, conduction deficits, and pulmonary edema.

HOW SUPPLIED

- Lidocaine hydrochloride.
- 100-mg/5 ml preloaded syringe (20 mg/ml) 2%.
- 100-mg/10 ml preloaded syringe (10 mg/ml) 1%.
- NOTE: Do not use dilution-strength syringes (1 and 2 g) for IV push use.

Magnesium Sulfate

MAJOR ACTIONS

- Magnesium deficiency is associated with cardiac arrhythmias and sudden cardiac death.
- Hypomagnesemia can precipitate refractory ventricular fibrillation.
- Hypomagnesemia can inhibit the replenishment of intracellular potassium.

INDICATIONS

- Hypomagnesemia with ventricular tachycardia or ventricular fibrillation.
- Torsades de pointes.
- Hypomagnesemia caused by systemic poisoning from hydrofluoric acid or fluoride exposure.

DOSAGE

- Adult: Loading dose of 1 to 2 g (8 to 16 mEq) mixed in 50 to 100 ml of D_5W and administered intravenously over 5 to 60 minutes. Actual infusion rate depends on clinical symptoms and severity of hypomagnesemia. A maintenance infusion of 0.5 to 1 g (4 to 8 mEq)/hour should follow for up to 24 hours.
- For torsades de pointes (adult): Administer 1 to 2 g intravenously over 1 to 2 minutes. Follow with same amount infused over 60 minutes.
- For pediatric doses and dosage for other hypomagnesemia conditions, refer to medical control and/or pharmacology texts.

PRECAUTIONS

- Use with caution in patients with decreased renal function. Maintain an adequate urine flow.
- Contraindicated in patients with known heart block, myocardial damage, respiratory depression, and renal failure.
- Weak or absent deep tendon reflexes, flaccid paralysis, hypothermia, drowsiness, hypocalcemia, hypotension, and respiratory paralysis may be seen with use.
- May cause hypokalemia. Monitor serum potassium concentration.

HOW SUPPLIED

- 10%, 12.5%, 25%, 50%; in 2-ml, 5-ml, 10-ml, 20-ml, and 30-ml ampules, vials, and prefilled syringes.

Procainamide (Pronestyl)

MAJOR ACTIONS

- Suppresses PVCs and recurrent VT.
- Has negative chronotropic, dromotropic effects and mild negative inotropic effects.
- Causes peripheral vasodilation.

INDICATIONS

- Ventricular arrhythmias, especially PVCs and VT in suspected myocardial infarction or cardiac contusion.
- Recommended when lidocaine is contraindicated or has failed to suppress ventricular ectopy.
- Wide-complex tachycardias that cannot be distinguished from VT.

DOSAGE

- Adult: 20 mg/min until arrhythmia is suppressed, hypotension ensues, or the QRS complex is widened by 50% of its original width or until a total of 17 mg/kg is reached (1.2 g for a 70-kg patient). In urgent situations up to 30 mg/min may be administered up to a total dose of 17 mg/kg. The maintenance infusion rate is 1 to 4 mg/min.
- Pediatric: Safety and efficacy are not well established. Consult local medical control.

PRECAUTIONS

- Maintenance dose should be reduced if patient has renal insufficiency.
- Blood concentrations should be monitored in renal failure and if the patient is receiving a constant infusion of more than 3 mg/min for more than 24 hours.
- Should be avoided in patients with preexisting QT prolongation, torsades de pointes, third-degree blocks, digitalis toxicity, tricyclic antidepressant–induced arrhythmias, and myasthenia gravis.
- Use with caution in patients with acute myocardial infarction or cardiac, hepatic, or renal insufficiency.
- May increase ventricular rate in atrial fibrillation and atrial flutter.
- May cause bradycardia, reflex tachycardia, hypotension, atrioventricular block, widened QRS, prolongation of PR or QT interval ventricular arrhythmias, seizures, and CNS depression.
- In cardiac arrest, use bolus therapy only. Consider maintenance infusion following resuscitation.
- Hypersensitivity reactions have been reported.

HOW SUPPLIED

- Procainamide hydrochloride.
- 1-g/10 ml vial (100 mg/ml).

Antibiotics

OVERVIEW

The following pages include recommendations for use of antibiotics, also known as antimicrobial drugs, in response to biological events. The usefulness of these drugs is limited to fighting infections caused by bacteria. The focus here is on the primary drugs of choice. Some alternative antimicrobial therapies are not described here in detail. The decision concerning which pharmaceuticals to use during a crisis must be made in cooperation with local public health agencies. This decision may also be influenced by sensitivity testing results of the specific threat organism.

Specific information on antitoxins, antivirals, and vaccines can be obtained from your local or state public health authorities based on the product availability and distribution planning in your region. If you need to identify the availability of a specific product and cannot contact local or state public health representatives, the CDC Emergency Response Hotline (24 hours) is 770-488-7100.

Before providing any described treatments to a patient, review drug insert information and discuss potential drug sensitivities and history of previous reactions with the patient

Aminoglycosides

MAJOR ACTIONS

- Aminoglycosides bind to the 30S subunit of bacterial ribosomes and block the attachment of the 50S subunit to the initiation complex.

EXAMPLES

- Amikacin
- Gentamicin
- Netilmicin
- Streptomycin
- Tobramycin

INDICATIONS

- Treatment of disease resulting from gram-negative bacteria.
- Can be used against some gram-positive bacteria (not typically employed because other antibiotics are more effective with fewer side effects).
- Prophylaxis of individuals with suspected exposure to susceptible gram-positive or gram-negative organisms.

DOSAGE

Dosage recommendations are based on the diagnosis or suspected exposure.

- For all patients, substitute oral antibiotics for IV antibiotics as soon as the clinical condition improves.

Gentamicin dosages include:

- Adult treatment

  Neurobrucellosis: 2 mg/kg IV loading dose, 1.7 mg/kg IV every 8 hours or 5 to 7 mg/kg IV once daily for 2 to 4 weeks (plus doxycycline or cotrimoxazole and rifampin for 8 to 12 weeks).

  Brucellosis (uncomplicated): 2 mg/kg IV loading dose, 1.7 mg/kg IV every 8 hours or 5 mg/kg IV once daily for 7 to 10 days (plus doxycycline or cotrimoxazole for 6 weeks).

  Plague: 5 mg/kg IV or IM once daily, or 2 mg/kg loading dose and 1.7 mg/kg IV or IM every 8 hours for 10 days.

  Tularemia: 5 mg/kg IV or IM once daily for 10 days.

- Pediatric treatment

  Neurobrucellosis: 2 mg/kg IV every 8 hours for 2 to 4 weeks (plus doxycycline, if over 8 years of age or cotrimoxazole and rifampin if under 8 years of age) for 8 to 12 weeks.

  Brucellosis (uncomplicated): 2 mg/kg IV every 8 hours for 7 to 10 days (plus doxycycline, if over 8 years of age, or cotrimoxazole) for 6 weeks.

  Plague: 2.5 mg/kg IV every 8 hours for 10 days.

  Neonate plague: 2.5 mg/kg IV or IM every 12 hours for 10 days.

  Tularemia: 2.5 mg/kg IV or IM every 8 hours for 10 days.

Streptomycin dosages include:

- Adult treatment

Anthrax: 30 mg/kg/day IM or IV (alternative treatment used with penicillin).

Neurobrucellosis: 1 g IM daily for 2 to 4 weeks (plus rifampin for 8 to 12 weeks plus either doxycycline or cotrimoxazole for 8 to 12 weeks).

Brucellosis (uncomplicated): 1 g IM daily for 10 to 14 days (plus doxycycline for 6 weeks).

Plague: 1 g IM twice daily for 10 days.

Tularemia: 1 g IM twice daily for 10 days.

- Pediatric treatment

  Brucellosis (uncomplicated) (over 8 years of age): 20 to 30 mg/kg/day IM divided every 12 hours or every day for 10 to 14 days (plus doxycycline for 6 weeks).

  Plague: 15 mg/kg IM twice daily, not to exceed 2 g daily.

  Tularemia: 15 mg/kg IM twice daily, not to exceed 2 g daily.

PRECAUTIONS

- Hypersensitivity to aminoglycosides such as gentamicin or streptomycin.
- Hypersensitivity to sulfites.
- May cause fever, rash, nausea, vomiting, or vertigo.
- Side effects include nephrotoxicity (kidney damage) and ototoxicity (hearing loss).

HOW SUPPLIED

- Gentamicin: Solution for injection: 10 mg/ml, 40 mg/ml.
- Streptomycin: Lyophilized powder: 1 g.

Chloramphenicol

MAJOR ACTIONS

- Primarily bacteriostatic.
- Binds to the 50S subunit of the ribosome and inhibits bacterial protein synthesis.

INDICATIONS

- Primary treatment for typhus.
- Alternative treatment for anthrax, glanders, plague, and tularemia.

DOSAGE

- Adults and children: 50 mg/kg/day PO or IV in divided doses every 6 hours.
- Newborns: ≤ 1 month old should not be given >25 mg/kg/day initially.
- Adjust doses to result in serum levels of 10 to 30 μg/ml (31 to 93 μmol/L) in order to avoid toxicity, especially in newborns, premature infants, and patients with hepatic disease.

PRECAUTIONS

- Use should be restricted to serious infections when other drugs are not as effective or are more toxic. In rare cases may cause irreversible, lethal aplastic anemia.
- Gray baby syndrome (infants).
- Myelosuppression.
- Nausea and vomiting.
- Rash.

HOW SUPPLIED

- Injection: 1 g.

Fluoroquinolones

MAJOR ACTIONS

- Gram-negative activity: Inhibits DNA gyrase resulting in dsDNA fragmentation.
- Gram-positive activity: Inhibits DNA type IV topoisomerase.

EXAMPLES

- Ciprofloxacin: The generic name for the antibiotic manufactured and sold by Bayer Pharmaceuticals under the brand name Cipro.
- Ofloxacin, sold under the brand name Floxin.

INDICATIONS

- Treatment of disease resulting from gram-negative infections such as pneumonic plague and tularemia.
- Treatment of disease resulting from gram-positive infections including inhalational or cutaneous anthrax.
- Prophylaxis of individuals with suspected exposure to susceptible gram-positive or negative organisms.

DOSAGE

Dosage recommendations are based on the diagnosis or suspected exposure.

- For all patients, substitute oral antibiotics for IV antibiotics as soon as the clinical condition improves.

For example, ciprofloxacin dosages include:

- Adult treatment
  Inhalational anthrax: 400 mg IV every 12 hours for 60 days.
  Cutaneous anthrax: 500 mg PO every 12 hours for 60 days.
  Food poisoning: 500 mg PO twice daily for 5 to 7 days.
  Plague: 400 mg IV every 12 hours for 10 days or 500 mg PO twice daily for 10 days.
  Typhus: 500 mg PO twice daily.
  Tularemia: 400 mg IV every 12 hours for 10 days or 500 mg PO twice daily for 14 days.
- Adult prophylaxis
  Anthrax: 500 mg PO twice daily for 60 days.
  Plague: 500 mg PO twice daily for 7 days.
  Tularemia: 500 mg PO twice daily for 14 days.
- Pediatric treatment (do not exceed 1 g per day in children)
  Inhalational anthrax: 20 to 30 mg/kg/day IV divided every 12 hours for 60 days.
  Cutaneous anthrax: 20 to 30 mg/kg/day PO divided twice daily for 60 days.
  Plague: 15 mg/kg IV every 12 hours for 10 days or 20 mg/kg PO twice daily for 10 days.
  Tularemia: 15 mg/kg IV every 12 hours for 10 days or 15 mg/kg PO twice daily for 14 days.

- Pediatric prophylaxis (do not exceed 1 g per day in children)
  Anthrax: 20 to 30 mg/kg/day PO divided twice daily for 60 days.
  Plague: 20 mg/kg PO twice daily for 7 days.
  Tularemia: 15 mg/kg PO twice daily for 14 days.

PRECAUTIONS

- Safety and effectiveness in children and adolescents below the age of 18 years have not been established.
- Use with caution in pregnant and nursing mothers.
- May cause nausea, diarrhea, taste disturbance, photosensitivity, dermatitis, and neurological effects such as seizures, headache, dizziness, and tremors.

HOW SUPPLIED

- Ciprofloxacin:
  Powder for suspension: 250 mg/5 ml, 500 mg/5 ml.
  Solution for injection: 200 mg, 400 mg.
  Tablets of 250 mg, 500 mg, 750 mg.
- Ofloxacin:
  Single use vials: Concentrated solution equivalent of 400 mg.
  Pre-mixed in flexible containers: Single-use, pre-mixed solution in 50 ml and 100 ml flexible containers. Each contains a dilute solution with the equivalent of 200 mg or 400 mg, respectively, in 5% dextrose (D_5W).
  Tablets of 200 mg, 300 mg, and 400 mg.

Macrolides

MAJOR ACTIONS

- The macrolides bind reversibly to the 50S subunit and inhibit elongation of the protein by blocking the translocation of the ribosome to the next codon on the mRNA.

EXAMPLES

- Azithromycin (Zithromax).
- Clarithromycin (Biaxin).
- Dirithromycin (Dynabac).
- Erythromycin oral (EES, EryPed, Ery-Tab, PCE Dispertab, Pediazole).
- Erythromycin lactobionate.
- Troleandomycin (Tao).

INDICATIONS

- Treatment of disease resulting from aerobic and anaerobic gram-positive cocci, with the exception of enterococci.
- Treatment of disease resulting from gram-negative anaerobes.
- Prophylaxis of individuals with suspected exposure to susceptible gram-positive or gram-negative organisms.

DOSAGE

Dosage recommendations are based on the diagnosis or suspected exposure.

- For all patients, substitute oral antibiotics for IV antibiotics as soon as the clinical condition improves.

Erythromycin dosages include:

- Adult treatment

  Anthrax (alternative treatment): 15 to 20 mg/kg/day IV divided every 6 hours (maximum of 4 g/day), 250 mg PO every 6 hours.

  Q Fever: 500 mg PO four times a day for 10 days.

- Pediatric treatment

  Anthrax (alternative treatment): 20 to 40 mg/kg/day IV divided every 6 hours (1 to 2 hour infusion), 40 mg/kg/day PO divided every 6 hours.

  Q Fever: 40 mg/kg/day PO in 4 divided doses for 10 days.

PRECAUTIONS

- Hypersensitivity to macrolides such as erythromycin products.
- Concomitant therapy with astemizole, terfenadine, or cisapride.
- Contraindicated in individuals with liver disease.
- May cause GI tract disturbances, including nausea, vomiting, and diarrhea.

HOW SUPPLIED

- Erythromycin:

  Solution for injection (erythromycin lactobionate): 500 mg vial, 1 g/vial.

  Capsules of 250 mg.

  Chewable tablets of 200 mg.

  Tablets of 250 mg, 333 mg, 400 mg, 500 mg.

Oral suspension: 100 mg/2.5ml, 200 mg/5 ml, 400 mg/5 ml

- Azithromycin:
  Capsules of 250 mg.
  Oral suspension: 100 mg/5 ml and 200 mg/5 ml.

Penicillin (and Penicillin Derivatives)

MAJOR ACTIONS

- Inhibits bacteria/cell wall synthesis.
- Penetrates outer membrane of some gram-negative organisms.
- Clavulanic acid and sulbactam bind beta-lactamases.

PENICILLIN CATEGORIES

- Natural penicillins
  Penicillin G
  Procaine penicillin G
  Penicillin V
  Benzathine
- Aminopenicillins
  Ampicillin or amoxicillin
  Augmentin or Unasyn
- Extended spectrum penicillin
  Ticarcillin
  Piperacillin
  Carbenicillin
  Timentin
- Penicillinase-resistant semisynthetic penicillin
  Cloxacillin
  Dicloxacillin
  Methicillin
  Nafcillin
  Oxacillin

INDICATIONS

- Penicillin and penicillin derivatives are often alternative or supplemental treatment for some emerging biological threats. Susceptibility of the organism must be confirmed before using it as a primary therapy.
- Penicillin and penicillin derivatives should not be used as single drug therapy for inhalational anthrax.

DOSAGE

- Amoxicillin:
  Adult anthrax treatment (alternative): 500 mg PO every 8 hours for 60 days.
  Pediatric anthrax treatment (alternative): 80 mg/kg/day divided PO in three doses taken every 8 hours for 60 days.
- Penicillin G:
  Adult inhaled anthrax treatment (adjunct): 4 million units IV every 4 hours for 60 days.

Pediatric inhaled anthrax treatment (adjunct): Less than 12 years of age: 50,000 units/kg IV every 6 hours for 60 days. Older than 12 years: adult dosage.

- Penicillin V:
  Adult inhaled anthrax treatment (adjunct): 200 to 500 mg PO QID
  Pediatric inhaled anthrax treatment (adjunct): 25 to 50 mg/kg/day PO in divided doses twice daily or four times a day.

PRECAUTIONS

- Potential adverse effects include anaphylaxis and other hypersensitivity reactions including nephritis, hyperkalemia, and seizures.
- Common adverse effects include diarrhea, nausea, vomiting, maculopapular rash.

HOW SUPPLIED

- Amoxicillin:
  Capsules of 250 mg, 500 mg.
  Chewable tablets of 125 mg, 200 mg, 250 mg, 400 mg.
  Oral suspension: 125 mg/5 ml, 200 mg/5 ml, 250 mg/5 ml, 400 mg/5 ml.
  Tablets of 500 mg, 875 mg.
- Penicillin G:
  Powder for injection: 1 million IU.
- Penicillin V:
  Powder for oral suspension: 125 mg/5 ml, 250 mg/5 ml.
  Tablets of 250 mg, 500 mg.

Rifampin

MAJOR ACTIONS

- Interferes with the activity of enzymes needed for the replication of RNA (ribonucleic acid) in bacterial cells, preventing the bacteria from reproducing.

INDICATIONS

- Primary treatment for neurobrucellosis; sometimes used in combination with doxycycline and gentamicin.
- Alternative treatment for anthrax, plague, and tularemia.

DOSAGE (Brucellosis Treatment Example)

- Adult treatment

  Neurobrucellosis: 600 to 900 mg PO daily (plus doxycycline and gentamicin) for 8 to 12 weeks.

  Brucellosis (uncomplicated): 600 to 900 mg PO daily (plus doxycycline) for 6 weeks.
- Pediatric treatment

  Neurobrucellosis: 20 mg/kg PO daily (plus gentamicin and doxycycline, if over 8 years of age or cotrimoxazole if under 8 years of age) for 8 to 12 weeks.

  Brucellosis (uncomplicated): 20 mg/kg PO daily (plus doxycycline) for 6 weeks.

PRECAUTIONS

- Hypersensitivity to rifampin.
- May cause elevated LFTs, heartburn, nausea, vomiting, thrombocytopenia.

HOW SUPPLIED

- Capsules of 150 mg, 300 mg.
- Powder for injection: 600 mg.

Tetracyclines

MAJOR ACTIONS

- Tetracycline antimicrobials block bacterial translation by binding reversibly to the 30S subunit and distorting it in such a way that the anticodons of the charged tRNAs cannot align properly with the codons of the mRNA.

EXAMPLES

- Doxycycline: The generic name for the antibiotic sold under the brand names Doryx, Doxy 100, Vibramycin, Vibra-tabs.
- Tetracycline under the brand name Achromycin V, Panmycin, Robitet, Robicaps, Sumycin, Tetracap, Topicycline.

INDICATIONS

- Treatment of disease resulting from gram-negative infections such as pneumonic plague and tularemia.
- Treatment of disease resulting from gram-positive infections including inhalational or cutaneous anthrax.
- Prophylaxis of individuals with suspected exposure to susceptible gram-positive or gram-negative organisms.

DOSAGE

Dosage recommendations are based on the diagnosis or suspected exposure.

- For all patients, substitute oral antibiotics for IV antibiotics as soon as the clinical condition improves.

Doxycycline dosages include (*Children older than 8 years or greater than 45 kg should follow adult dosing*):

- Adult treatment
  Inhalational anthrax: 100 mg IV every 12 hours for 60 days.
  Cutaneous anthrax: 100 mg PO every 12 hours for 60 days.
  Plague: 100 mg IV every 12 hours for 10 days or 200 mg IV every day for 10 days.
  Tularemia: 100 mg IV twice daily for 14 to 21 days or 100 mg PO twice daily for 14 days.
- Adult prophylaxis
  Anthrax: 100 mg PO twice daily for 60 days.
  Plague: 100 mg PO twice daily for 7 days.
  Tularemia: 100 mg PO twice daily for 14 days.
- Pediatric treatment
  Inhalational anthrax: 2.2 mg/kg IV or PO every 12 hours for 60 days.
  Plague: 2.2 mg/kg IV every 12 hours for 10 days or 2.2 mg/kg PO every 12 hours for 10 days.
  Tularemia: 2.2 mg/kg IV every 12 hours for 14 to 21 days or 2.2 mg/kg PO every 12 hours for 14 days.
- Pediatric prophylaxis
  Anthrax: 2.2 mg/kg PO every 12 hours for 60 days.

Plague: 2.2 mg/kg PO every 12 hours for 7 days.
Tularemia: 2.2 mg/kg PO every 12 hours for 14 days.

PRECAUTIONS

- Limit use of tetracyclines in children under 8 years of age; can cause staining of teeth, hypoplasia of dental enamel, and abnormal bone growth in children.
- Should be avoided after the first trimester of pregnancy.
- Hypersensitivity to doxycycline products or tetracyclines.
- GI adverse reactions, such as nausea, vomiting, and diarrhea.
- May cause photosensitivity.

HOW SUPPLIED

- Doxycycline:
  Powder for injection: 100 mg.
  Powder for oral suspension: 25 mg/5 ml.
  Capsules of 50 mg, 100 mg.
  Tablets of 100 mg.
  Syrup: 50 mg/5 ml.
- Tetracycline:
  Powder: 25 g, 100 g, 500 g.
  Capsules of 250 mg, 500 mg.
  Tablets of 250 mg, 500 mg.
  Syrup: 125 mg/5 ml.

Trimethoprim-Sulfamethoxazole (TMP-SMX)

MAJOR ACTIONS

- Trimethoprim-sulfamethoxazole (TMP-SMX) is a combination (1:5) of the two drugs and both drugs block the folic acid metabolism cycle of bacteria. They are much more active together than either drug is alone. Sulfamethoxazole is a competitive inhibitor of the incorporation of *p*-aminobenzoic acid. Trimethoprim prevents reduction of dihydrofolate to tetrahydrofolate.

INDICATIONS

- TMP-SMX is active against most gram-positive and gram-negative organisms but is inactive against anaerobes.

DOSAGE

- Adult dose: 160 mg TMP and 800 mg SMX (either with two regular-strength tablets: each tablet contains 80 mg TMP and 400 mg SMX; or one double-strength tablet PO twice daily).
- Pediatric dose: 8 mg/kg TMP and 40 mg/kg SMX PO twice daily.
- IV dosage in both adults and children: 8 to 12 mg/kg TMP and 40 to 60 mg/kg SMX daily in four divided doses.

PRECAUTIONS

- May cause nausea, vomiting, loss of appetite, and allergic skin reactions (rashes).
- Can cause neutropenia (low level of neutrophils).
- May also cause folate deficiency (resulting in macrocytic anemia).

HOW SUPPLIED

- Tablets of 160 mg TMP/800 mg SMX, or 80 mg TMP/400 mg SMX.
- Also available IV or in liquid form for babies and young children.
- There are several brand names for TMP-SMX, including Bactrim, Septra, and Cotrim.

Diazepam (Valium)

MAJOR ACTIONS

- Benzodiazepine antianxiety agent.
- Anticonvulsant. Raises seizure threshold in the motor cortex.
- Produces sedation.
- Acts as a skeletal muscle relaxant.
- Duration of action after IV anticonvulsant administration is 15 minutes to 1 hour.

INDICATIONS

- Patients with active seizure activity.
- Status epilepticus. Any seizure lasting longer than 5 minutes, or two seizures without regaining consciousness.
- Nerve agent exposure.
- Diazepam should only be administered to a patient who is actively seizing except in cases of nerve agent exposure.

DOSAGE

- Adult: 2 to 10 mg in 2-mg increments by slow IV push—10 mg via IM autoinjector for cases of nerve agent exposure.
- Pediatric: 0.2 mg/kg slow IV push. Maximum dose 2 to 5 mg.

PRECAUTIONS

- May cause respiratory depression and/or arrest.
- May cause hypotension and reflex tachycardia.
- Effect is intensified in patients with other CNS depressants or alcohol on board.
- Contraindicated in patients with known hypersensitivity to the drug or with angle-closure glaucoma and in comatose patients.
- Use with caution in patients with psychoses, myasthenia gravis, Parkinson's disease, impaired hepatic function, and impaired respiratory function (COPD).

HOW SUPPLIED

- 20-mg/2 ml ampule, preloaded syringes (10 mg/ml).
- 10-mg/2 ml ampule, preloaded syringes (5 mg/ml).
- 10-mg/2 ml autoinjector.

Lorazepam (Ativan)

MAJOR ACTIONS

- Antianxiety agent.
- Anticonvulsant with rapid onset of action.
- Depresses the CNS at the limbic and subcortical levels of the brain.
- Duration of action after IV anticonvulsant administration is 12 to 24 hours.

INDICATIONS

- As an alternative to diazepam (Valium) in patients with active seizure activity.
- As an alternative to diazepam in status epilepticus (any seizure lasting more than 5 minutes, or two seizures without regaining consciousness).
- Lorazepam has a prolonged duration of action relative to diazepam.
- Lorazepam should not be administered prophylactically for seizure control.

DOSAGE

- Adult: 2-mg incremental doses, slow IV push. Maximum total dose 4 to 8 mg (0.1 mg/kg).

PRECAUTIONS

- May cause respiratory depression and arrest.
- Contraindicated in patients with known hypersensitivity to the drug or with angle-closure glaucoma and in comatose patients.
- Use with caution in patients with psychoses, myasthenia gravis, Parkinson's disease, impaired hepatic function, and impaired respiratory function (COPD).
- May cause hypotension and reflex tachycardia.
- Effect is intensified in patients with other CNS depressants or alcohol on board.

HOW SUPPLIED

- 2-mg/ml ampule, preloaded syringe.
- 4-mg/ml ampule, preloaded syringe.

Dobutamine (Dobutrex)

MAJOR ACTIONS

- A synthetic catecholamine with potent positive inotropic effects.
- Predominant beta-adrenergic agonist increases myocardial contractility and stroke volume resulting in increased cardiac output.
- May produce reflex peripheral vasodilation.

INDICATIONS

- Low cardiac output from decreased myocardial function.
- Cardiogenic shock.

DOSAGE

- Adult: Add 500 mg to 250 ml of D_5W (2000 μg/ml) and administer intravenously at 2 to 20 μg/kg/min titrated to maintain an adequate blood pressure.
- Pediatric: Same as adult.

PRECAUTIONS

- May increase myocardial oxygen demand.
- Replenish volume first when used for hypovolemia.
- Use with caution in atrial fibrillation. Increases AV conduction.
- Accurate titration is difficult without hemodynamic monitoring.
- Contains sodium bisulfite, which may trigger an allergic reaction in patients with sulfite sensitivity.
- May cause headache, tachycardia, hypertension, ventricular arrhythmias, chest pain, nausea, vomiting, and shortness of breath.
- Decreases renal and hepatic function.
- May be inactivated by alkaline solutions.

HOW SUPPLIED

- Dobutamine hydrochloride.
- 250-mg (white powder)/20 ml vial. Reconstitute with 10 to 20 ml of normal saline or sterile water.

Dopamine (Intropin)

MAJOR ACTIONS

- Endogenous catecholamine; metabolic precursor of norepinephrine.
- Has alpha- and $beta_1$-adrenergic and dopaminergic agonist properties.
- Stimulates $beta_1$-adrenergic receptor sites. Releases stored norepinephrine. Minimal $beta_2$-adrenergic effects.
- Effects are dose-dependent.
- At low doses: $Beta_1$ effects include positive inotropic effects with increased cardiac output (increased myocardial contractility and stroke volume) and dopaminergic receptor–agonist effects, producing vasodilation in renal, mesenteric, coronary, and intracerebral vasculature.
- At high doses, alpha-adrenergic effects predominate, causing increased peripheral resistance and renal vasoconstriction.
- At higher doses, actions are very similar to those of norepinephrine (Levophed).
- 1 to 2 μg/kg/min—causes a dilation of mesenteric and renal blood vessels.
- 2 to 10 μg/kg/min—shows beta effects on heart that usually result in increased cardiac output without increasing rate or blood pressure.
- 10 to 20 μg/kg/min—shows alpha effects that cause peripheral vasoconstriction.
- 20 to 40 μg/kg/min—the alpha effects reverse the dilation of the mesenteric and renal blood vessels.

INDICATIONS

- Hypotension without hypovolemia (especially of cardiogenic cause). Secondary use in neurogenic shock.

DOSAGE

- Adult: Mix 800 mg in 500 ml of D_5W or 400 mg in 250 ml of D_5W (1600 μg/ml). Start IV administration at 2.5 to 5 μg/kg/min and titrate to effect. A final dosage range of 5 to 20 μg/kg/min is recommended.
- Pediatric: 6 × body weight (kg) equals milligrams added to diluent to make 100 ml. Then 1 ml/min delivers 1 μg/kg/min. Start at 2 to 5 μg/kg/min and titrate to effect. IV Infusion may be increased to 10 to 20 μg/kg/min to improve blood pressure, perfusion, and urine output.
- NOTE: Microdrip use only. See chart for additional information on adult dosage.

PRECAUTIONS

- Contraindicated in hypovolemic shock.
- May cause tachyarrhythmias and ectopic beats.
- May be deactivated by sodium bicarbonate.
- Can increase myocardial oxygen demand.
- May cause hypertensive crisis.
- May cause nausea and vomiting.
- Tissue infiltration may cause necrosis and sloughing.
- Therapy should not be discontinued abruptly but tapered gradually.

- Norepinephrine or dobutamine should be used if more than 20 μg/kg/min of dopamine is needed to maintain an adequate blood pressure.
- Because dopamine hydrochloride is light sensitive, protect from light.

HOW SUPPLIED

- Dopamine hydrochloride.
- 200-mg/5 ml ampule, preloaded syringe (40 mg/ml).
- 400-mg/5 ml vial (80 mg/ml).

Dopamine Infusions (Adult)*

(infusion rate in drops/minute† or ml/hour)

kg/lb	2	3	4	5	6	7	8	9	10	15	20	30	40	50
40/88	3	5	6	8	9	11	12	14	15	23	30	45	60	75
45/99	3	5	7	8	10	11	14	15	17	25	34	51	68	84
50/110	4	6	8	9	11	13	15	17	19	28	38	56	75	94
55/121	4	6	8	10	12	14	17	19	21	31	41	62	83	103
60/132	5	7	9	11	14	16	18	20	23	34	45	68	90	112
65/143	5	7	10	12	15	17	20	22	24	37	49	73	98	122
70/154	5	8	11	13	16	18	21	24	26	39	53	79	105	131
75/165	6	8	11	14	17	20	23	25	28	42	56	84	113	141
80/176	6	9	12	15	18	21	24	27	30	45	60	90	120	150
85/187	6	10	13	16	19	22	26	29	32	48	64	96	128	159
90/198	7	10	14	17	20	24	27	30	34	51	68	101	135	169
95/209	7	11	14	18	21	25	29	32	36	53	71	107	143	178
100/220	8	11	15	19	23	26	30	34	38	56	75	113	150	188

*Infusion of 400 mg dopamine in 250 ml D_5 W (concentration = 1600 µg/ml).
†Microdrip set = 60 drops/ml.
Courtesy DuPont Critical Care, Waukegan, Ill, a division of E.I. du Pont de Nemours & Co.

Epinephrine (Adrenaline)

MAJOR ACTIONS

- Acts as a catecholamine with both alpha- and beta-adrenergic effects.
- Increases heart rate, contractility, AV conduction, automaticity, and myocardial irritability.
- Produces bronchodilation.
- Produces vasoconstriction and increases arterial blood pressure.
- Inhibits histamine release.

INDICATIONS

- Cardiac resuscitation.
- Anaphylaxis.
- Asthma attacks.
- Bronchoconstriction, bronchospasm.

DOSAGE

- Adult: Cardiac resuscitation: 1 mg of 1:10,000 solution IV push. Epinephrine may be given via endotracheal tube, but 2 to 2.5 times the IV dose may be required for optimal effect. Repeat every 3 to 5 minutes during resuscitation. Each IV dose should be followed by a 20-ml flush of IV fluid to ensure delivery to the central circulation. High-dose epinephrine, up to 5 mg or approximately 0.1 mg/kg, may be considered after the 1-mg dose has failed.
  - Anaphylaxis (with laryngeal edema or severe respiratory distress): 0.1 to 0.5 mg of 1:10,000 solution IV push; repeat in 10 minutes (do not exceed 0.5 mg in 10 minutes).
  - Allergic reaction or asthma: 0.1 to 0.5 mg of 1:1000 solution administered subcutaneously (SQ).
- Pediatric: Cardiac resuscitation: 0.01 mg/kg (0.1 ml/kg of 1:10,000 solution) IV push or intraosseous (IO). Epinephrine may be given by endotracheal tube; the recommended dose is 0.1 mg/kg (0.1 ml/kg of a 1:1000 solution). Second and subsequent doses for unresponsive asystolic and pulseless arrest should be 0.1 mg/kg (0.1 ml/kg of 1:1000 solution) IV or IO. This higher dose should be administered within 3 to 5 minutes following the initial dose and should be repeated every 3 to 5 minutes during resuscitation.
  - Anaphylaxis (with laryngeal edema or severe respiratory distress): 0.01 mg/kg of 1:10,000 solution by slow IV push
  - Allergic reaction or asthma: 0.01 mg/kg of 1:1,000 solution SQ.

PRECAUTIONS

- Correct acidosis before administration.
- Incompatible with alkaline solutions (flush IV line after administering sodium bicarbonate).
- Contraindicated in hypertension.
- May cause supraventricular tachycardia or ventricular irritability.
- Increases myocardial oxygen demand.

- Use with caution for allergic reactions and asthma in patients over 35 years of age.

HOW SUPPLIED

- Epinephrine hydrochloride.
- 1:10,000 1-mg/10 ml preloaded syringes (0.1 mg/ml).
- 1:1000 1-mg/1 mL ampule, preloaded syringes (1 mg/ml).

Isoproterenol (Isuprel)

MAJOR ACTIONS

- Acts as a cardiac stimulant (beta agonist, both chronotropic and inotropic).
- Improves cardiac conduction.
- Produces bronchodilation.
- Produces peripheral vasodilation.
- Increases myocardial oxygen demand.

INDICATIONS

- Hemodynamically unstable bradycardia that is refractory to other drug therapy (see ACLS bradycardia algorithm on p. 644).
- Refractory torsades de pointes.
- Not indicated for cardiac arrest or hypotension.

DOSAGE

- Adult: Mix 1 mg in 500 ml of D_5W (2 μg /ml) and administer as an IV drip at 2 to 10 μg/min. Titrate to heart rate of 60/min.
- Pediatric: Mix 1 mg in 500 ml of D_5W (2 μg/ml) and administer as an IV drip, starting at 0.1 μg/kg/min. Titrate to heart rate and blood pressure. Maximum 1 μg/kg/min.

PRECAUTIONS

- May be harmful at high doses.
- Increases myocardial oxygen demand, which may increase infarct size.
- May cause arrhythmias. Use with caution in patients with ventricular ectopia or tachyarrhythmia.
- Use with caution in patients taking digitalis or in patients with hypokalemia (patients on diuretics).
- Isuprel is a vasodilator and may cause hypotension.
- Isuprel has an additive effect with epinephrine.
- Hepatic or renal insufficiency.
- May be inactivated by alkaline solutions.

HOW SUPPLIED

- 1-mg/5 ml ampules, preloaded syringes (0.2 mg/ml).
- 2-mg/10 ml preloaded syringes (0.2 mg/ml).

Norepinephrine

MAJOR ACTIONS

- Endogenous catecholamine that stimulates $beta_1$ (heart)–and $beta_2$ (bronchial or peripheral vasculature)–adrenergic receptors.
- Alpha-adrenergic receptor agonist that causes an increase in total peripheral resistance and systolic blood pressure.
- Increases force of myocardial contraction.
- Dilates coronary arteries.

INDICATIONS

- Severe hypotension (systolic blood pressure <70 torr) and low total peripheral resistance.

DOSAGE

- Adult: Mix 4 mg in 250 ml of D_5W (yielding 16 μg/ml) and administer as an IV drip. Start at 0.5 to 1 μg/min and titrate to maintain systolic blood pressure between 90 and 100. Patients with refractory shock may require 8 to 30 μg/min.
- Titrate to effect and do not allow systolic blood pressure to rise above 110 torr.
- Pediatric: Not indicated in pediatric patients.

PRECAUTIONS

- May induce renal and mesenteric vasoconstriction.
- May increase myocardial oxygen demand.
- Can cause severe hypertension.
- Can cause bradycardia.
- Administer into large vein to avoid potential extravasation.
- Tissue necrosis occurs if solution extravasates.
- Replace fluid volume before using.
- Alkaline solutions may inactivate norepinephrine.

HOW SUPPLIED

- Norepinephrine.
- 4-mg/4 ml ampules.

Vasopressin (Pitressin)

MAJOR ACTIONS

- Antidiuretic hormone
- Acts at the tissue level by binding to specific receptors, producing potent vasoconstrictor and antidiuretic effects.
- Exerts a greater vasoconstrictive effect under conditions of hypoxia and acidosis than does epinephrine, and the effects of vasopressin last longer.

INDICATIONS

- Alternative pressor to epinephrine in the treatment of adult shock-refractory pulseless VT/VF.
- Hemodynamic support in vasodilatory shock.

DOSAGE

- Adult for cardiac arrest caused by VT/VF: IV/IO: 40 units IV push (one time dose; if no response, epinephrine may be used after 10 to 20 minutes).
- Pediatric use is not recommend at this time.

PRECAUTIONS

- Can precipitate angina or myocardial infarction, not recommended in responsive patients; acute pulmonary edema has been reported.

HOW SUPPLIED

- 20 units/ml injection.

Deferoxamine (Desferal Mesylate)

MAJOR ACTIONS

- Chelates iron by binding ferric (Fe^{+2}) ions.
- Forms soluble feroxamine complex (reddish-colored), which is excreted in urine giving it a vin rosé color.
- 1 gram of deferoxamine binds 85 mg of iron (as ferric ions).

INDICATIONS

- Hospital therapy for acute iron intoxication.

DOSAGE

Iron Chelation Dose

- IM Dose: 90 mg/kg every 8 hours until urine clears.
  - Adult: Maximum 2 g/dose.
  - Pediatric: Maximum 1 g/dose.
- IV Dose: 15 mg/kg/hour until urine clears.
  - Maximum daily dose (adults and children): 6 to 8 g.
  - IV administration route preferred.
- Continue chelation until symptoms remit and/or vin rosé urine color clears.
- Monitor CBC, serum iron, and total iron-binding capacity (TIBC).
  - TIBC may be falsely increased in acute iron toxicity.
  - Serum iron concentration may exhibit rebound effect after chelation.

PRECAUTIONS

- Adverse reactions include skin flushing, generalized erythema, urticaria, hypotension, shock, allergic reactions, anaphylactoid reactions, injection site pain, nausea, vomiting, fever, diarrhea, and blurred vision.
- Maintain adequate renal output.

HOW SUPPLIED

- Parenteral sterile lyophilized powder for injection, 500 mg/ml. Reconstitute with 2 ml of sterile water to yield 250 mg/ml solution.
- For IM use, the 250-mg/ml solution may be administered undiluted.
- For IV use, add to 0.9% saline and administer at rate of 15 mg/kg/hr.

Dimercaprol (British Anti-Lewisite [BAL])

MAJOR ACTIONS

- Dithiol heavy metal chelating agent: arsenic, mercury, gold.
- Developed as a treatment for arsenic-containing chemical warfare agent lewisite.

INDICATIONS

- Hospital therapy for lead, gold, and mercury poisoning.
- Useful adjunctive therapy when used in combination with edetate calcium disodium ($CaNa_2EDTA$) for lead poisoning.
- Acute lead encephalopathy or blood lead >100 μg/ml.
- Asymptomatic patients with blood lead levels >70 μg/ml.
- Chelating agent for acute arsenic, gold, or mercury poisoning; not effective for monoalkyl mercury toxicity, alkyl lead (e.g., tetraethyl lead) poisoning, or chronic elemental mercury poisoning.
- Not effective for arsine (AsH_3) poisoning.

DOSAGE

Severe Arsenic Or Gold Poisoning (Adults And Children)

- 3 mg/kg deep IM every 4 hours for 2 days, four times a day on third day and twice a day thereafter for 10 days.
- Clinical course determines duration of therapy.
- Ensure adequate renal flow before second dose.

Mercury Poisoning (Adults And Children)

- 5 mg/kg IM initially and then 2.5 mg/kg every 12 or 24 hours.
- Clinical course determines duration of therapy.
- Ensure adequate renal flow before second dose.

Acrodynia (Mercury Poisoning: Infants And Children)

- 3 mg/kg deep IM every 4 hours for 48 hours, every 6 hours for the next 24 hours, and then every 12 hours for 7 to 8 days.
- Clinical course determines duration of therapy.
- Ensure adequate renal flow before second dose.

Lead Poisoning

- Refer to Edetate Calcium Disodium ($CaNa_2EDTA$) protocol in this section.

PRECAUTIONS

- Dose-related systolic blood pressure rise and tachycardia usually occurring 15 to 30 minutes after injection.
- Although less likely to cause essential trace metal deficiency syndromes than other chelators, will increase copper excretion.
- Causes increased urinary excretion of zinc.
- Allergic reactions: generalized pruritic, erythematous, maculopapular rash.
- Adverse reactions include nausea, vomiting, abdominal pain, diaphoresis, throat pain, chest pain, hand pain, anxiety, muscular aches and spasms, injection site

pain, and burning sensation in lips, mouth, and throat. Red blood cell hemolysis in patients with glucose-6-phosphate deficiency (G-6-PD) may also occur.

- Interferes with thyroid iodine accumulation.
- Toxic interaction with iron, cadmium, selenium, or uranium.
- Maintain alkaline urine to reduce likelihood of complex dissociation.
- Compound may be nephrotoxic.
- Relatively contraindicated in liver dysfunction.
- Contraindicated in patients allergic to peanuts.
- Obtain toxicologic consultation.

HOW SUPPLIED

- For deep IM injection only: 100 mg/ml of BAL in Oil with 200 mg/ml of benzyl benzoate and 700 mg/ml of peanut oil.

Edetate Calcium Disodium (Calcium Disodium Edetate—$CaNa_2EDTA$, Calcium Disodium Versenate)

MAJOR ACTIONS

- Calcium chelate of edetate disodium: chelating agent for lead and other heavy metals.

INDICATIONS

- Hospital therapy for specific heavy metal exposure.
- Used alone or in combination with dimercaprol (BAL) for lead poisoning.
- May be useful for plutonium, thorium, uranium, yttrium, chromium, manganese, nickel, zinc, and vanadium.
- Not effective for mercury, gold, or arsenic poisoning.
- Combination therapy with BAL for acute lead encephalopathy or blood lead levels greater than 100 μg/dl.
- Combination therapy with BAL for asymptomatic patients with blood lead levels greater than 70 μg/dl.

DOSAGE

- *Acute lead encephalopathy and/or blood lead levels >100 μg/dl with or without symptoms (adults and children):*
  - Dimercaprol: 4 mg/kg (450 mg/m^2/day) IM every 4 hours for 5 days.
  - After 4 hours and when adequate urine output is established, begin infusion of edetate calcium disodium, 250 mg/every 4 hours (1500 mg/m^2/day) for 5 days. IM and IV doses are the same. Continuous IV infusion (1 to 4 mg/ml in normal saline or D_5W) is less painful and preferred.
- *Symptomatic lead poisoning; blood lead levels >70 μg/dl (adults and children):*
  - Dimercaprol: IM infusion, 2.7 mg/kg (300 mg/m^2/day) every 4 hours for 5 days.
  - After 4 hours and when adequate urine output is established, begin continuous infusion of edetate calcium disodium, 1000 mg/m^2/day 5 days.
  - Monitor blood lead concentrations. If blood lead levels decrease to >50 μg/dl, BAL may be stopped.
- *Asymptomatic adults with blood lead levels 56 to 69 μg/dl:*
  - Continuous infusion of edetate calcium disodium, 1000 mg/m^2/day for 5 days. Monitor blood lead concentrations.
- *Asymptomatic children or mildly symptomatic children:*
  - Without nausea and vomiting, children with blood lead levels >45 μg/dl should receive therapy with succimer (see Succimer protocol in this section).

- *If adult blood lead concentration is between 25 and 55 μg/dL, then consider:*
  - Edetate calcium disodium edetate provocative challenge test; adult dose: IV infusion of 500 mg/m^2 (maximum dose 1 g) given over 1 hour. Collect 24-hour urine specimens for lead levels starting with initiation of IV dose. Calculate ratio of micrograms of lead excreted per milligram of edetate calcium disodium. If ratio is greater than 1, the test is positive for total body lead burden, and chelation therapy is indicated.

PRECAUTIONS

- Adverse reactions include renal tubular necrosis, proteinuria, hematuria, glycosuria, thrombophlebitis, IM injection site pain, anorexia, nausea, vomiting, fever, cheilosis, tremors, headache, paresthesias, myalgias, arthralgias, rash, hypercalcemia, dysrhythmias, and bone marrow depression.
- May cause elevations of serum transaminases.
- Contraindicated in hepatitis, severe renal failure, or anuria.
- Maintain adequate urine output to avoid renal toxicity.
- Monitor serum electrolytes, blood urea nitrogen (BUN), glucose, and liver enzymes daily.

HOW SUPPLIED

- Parenteral concentrate for slow IV injection, 200 mg in 5-ml ampules; dilute with 5% dextrose or 0.9% sodium chloride to a concentration of 2 to 4 mg/ml (0.2% to 0.4%).

Penicillamine (D-Penicillamine, Cuprimine, Depen, Titratabs)

MAJOR ACTIONS

- Monothiol chelating agent for copper, iron, mercury, and lead.
- Forms stable soluble complexes that are excreted in the urine.

INDICATIONS

- Hospital or outpatient therapy for heavy metal exposure.
- Treatment of moderate asymptomatic lead poisoning.
- Follow-up oral chelator after treatment with edetate calcium disodium/ dimercaprol (BAL).
- Used for provocative lead chelation test.
- Copper chelating agent for Wilson's disease.
- Penicillamine is used to reduce cystine excretion to prevent renal stone formation.
- Treatment of adult active rheumatoid arthritis.
- May be useful for mercury toxicity.

DOSAGE

- *Moderate asymptomatic lead poisoning:*
  - Adults: 250 to 500 mg/dose every 8 to 12 hours until blood level is < 60 mg/dl.
  - Pediatric: 25 to 40 mg/kg/day in 3 divided doses (refer to Succimer protocol in this section for other treatment options in children).
  - Repeat courses if necessary with 1-week rest intervals in between. Continuous chelation removes trace essential metals including zinc and copper.

Provocative Lead Chelation Test

- Administer D-penicillamine for four doses over 24 hours. Collect 24-hour urine for lead or mercury during that time period.
- *Instructions to patient:*
  - Day 1: On arising, discard 1st void. Begin D-penicillamine regimen (four doses). Begin collection of 24-hour urine specimen in lab provided container.
  - Day 2: On arising save first void. Send 24-hour specimen to lab.

PRECAUTIONS

- Contraindicated in patients allergic to penicillin.
- Allergic skin reactions occur in one third of patients. Allergic reaction are usually manifested by generalized pruritic, erythematous, maculopapular rash. Late (usually after 6 months of therapy)–occurring, pruritic, scaly drug rash also possible.
- Prolonged use may cause iron deficiency anemia.

- Causes increased urinary excretion of zinc and iron.
- Adverse reactions include pruritic scaly rash, proteinuria, hematuria, leukopenia, thrombocytopenia, eosinophilia, bone marrow depression, anemia, ecchymoses with skin friability at pressure sites, oral ulcers, nausea, vomiting, epigastric pain, obliterative bronchiolitis, and hepatic dysfunction.
- May cause elevation in serum aminotransferases.
- May promote lead absorption from GI tract.

HOW SUPPLIED

- Capsules of 125 and 250 mg.

Succimer (Meso 2,3-Dimercaptosuccinic Acid, Chemet)

MAJOR ACTIONS

- Heavy metal chelating agent.
- Forms stable water-soluble complexes with lead.
- Increases urinary excretion of lead.
- May prove useful for mercury and arsenic chelation.
- In therapeutic doses does not deplete essential metals including calcium, iron, and magnesium.
- Structurally related to dimercaprol (BAL).

INDICATIONS

- Hospital or outpatient treatment of lead poisoning in children with blood lead concentrations >45 μg/dl.
- Currently not approved by the Federal Drug Administration (FDA) for use in adults.

DOSAGE

- Pediatric: 10 mg/kg or 350 mg/m^2 every 8 hours for 5 days; then reduce dose frequency to every 12 hours for an additional 14 days of treatment.
- An initial treatment course of 19 days is recommended.

Succimer Dosage Regimen*

Weight			
lbs	**kg**	**Dose (mg)**	**No. of Capsules**
18-35	8-15	100	1
36-55	16-23	200	2
56-75	24-34	300	3
76-100	35-44	400	4
>100	>45	500	5

*An initial treament course of 19 days is recommended.
Courtesy McNeil Consumer Products Co., Fort Washington, PA.

PRECAUTIONS

- A minimum of 2 weeks between treatment courses is recommended. Repeated courses may be needed, depending on blood lead measurements.
- Concomitant administration to patients receiving edetate calcium disodium and/or BAL is not recommended at this time. Patients who have received edetate

calcium disodium and/or BAL may receive succimer, if indicated, after a 4-week interval.

- Adverse reactions include nausea, vomiting, diarrhea, appetite loss, and skin rash.
- May cause elevation in serum transaminases.
- Monitor serum transaminases at baseline and weekly during therapy.

HOW SUPPLIED

- Opaque white gelatin capsules of medicated beads of 100 mg.

50% Dextrose ($D_{50}W$)

MAJOR ACTIONS

- Reverses hypoglycemia by providing free glucose for quick absorption and use.
- Acts as an osmotic diuretic.

INDICATIONS

- Any altered mental state or illness in a patient with known diabetes that might be caused by hypoglycemia.
- Diagnostic tool in an unconscious patient when a reliable history is not available.
- Seizure patients, if history is not available.
- Hypothermia.
- Certain toxic exposures (see Guidelines).

DOSAGE

- Adult: 12.5 to 25 g D_{50} slow IV push. Repeat one time as needed.
- Pediatric: 0.5 to 1 g/kg D_{25} (or D_{50} diluted 1:1) slow IV push.

PRECAUTIONS

- Draw a blood sample in a red-top tube for glucose determination before administration.
- Infiltration causes tissue necrosis.
- May precipitate Wernicke's encephalopathy in thiamine-deficient patients (e.g., alcoholics). Can be prevented with prior IV administration of thiamine (100 mg).
- Suspected intracranial hemorrhage.

HOW SUPPLIED

- D_{50}—25-g/50 ml preloaded syringe (500 mg/ml).
- D_{50}—12.5-g/50 ml preloaded syringe (250 mg/ml).

Furosemide (Lasix)

MAJOR ACTIONS

- Acts as a potent, rapid-acting, loop diuretic that inhibits the resorption of sodium.
- Has a direct effect on the venous system, producing decreased vascular resistance and increased peripheral venous capacitance (venous pooling).
- Decreases renal vascular resistance and produces transiently increased glomerular filtration rate (GFR).
- Works in 5 to 10 minutes, with maximum effect in 30 minutes.

INDICATIONS

- Used to treat acute pulmonary edema.

DOSAGE

- Adult: 0.5 to 1 mg/kg (20 to 40 mg) slow IV push as an initial dose; repeat every 30 minutes up to 2 mg/kg if indicated.
- Pediatric: 0.5 to 1 mg/kg slow IV push; repeat as needed every 30 minutes to a maximum of 2 mg/kg.

PRECAUTIONS

- May cause hypovolemia and circulatory collapse. Do not use in the presence of hypotension or if signs of hypovolemia are present.
- Use in children and pregnant women (DIRECT PHYSICIAN ORDER ONLY).
- Can cause profound diarrhea.
- Can cause hypokalemia and hyponatremia leading to cardiac arrhythmias.
- May cause an allergic reaction in patients who are sensitive to sulfonamides.
- Renal insufficiency.
- Patient should be catheterized if possible to monitor renal output.

HOW SUPPLIED

- 20-mg/2 ml ampule, preloaded syringe (10 mg/ml).
- 40-mg/4 ml ampule, preloaded syringe (10 mg/ml).
- 100-mg/10 ml ampule, preloaded syringe (10 mg/ml).

Homatropine Hydrobromide (Isopto) 2% Ophthalmic Solution

MAJOR ACTIONS

- Blocks the responses of the sphincter muscle of the iris and the accommodative muscle of the ciliary body to cholinergic stimulation. It produces papillary dilation and paralysis of accommodation.

INDICATIONS

- Relief of pain and miosis secondary to nerve agent exposure.

DOSAGE

- Adult and pediatric: 1 drop in each affected eye.

PRECAUTIONS

- Use with extreme caution in infants, small children, and geriatric patients.
- Excessive use may produce systemic atropine poisoning.
- To avoid excessive systemic absorption, the lacrimal sac should be compressed by digital pressure for 2 to 3 minutes after administration.
- Contraindicated in persons with primary glaucoma. Increase in intraocular pressure may occur.
- Patient may experience sensitivity to light.
- Prolonged use may produce local irritation characterized by conjunctivitis, vascular congestion, edema, exudates, and an eczematoid dermatitis.

HOW SUPPLIED

- Homatropine hydrobromide (Isopto) 2%.
- 2% solution in 2-ml dispenser.

Morphine Sulfate

MAJOR ACTIONS

- Acts as a narcotic analgesic that alters the perception of pain and elevates the pain threshold.
- Relaxes respiratory effort and decreases ventilatory rate and tidal volume.
- Causes peripheral vasodilatation, thereby decreasing venous return to the heart.
- Increases vagal tone.
- Relieves pulmonary congestion caused by cardiogenic pulmonary edema.
- Decreases myocardial oxygen demand.
- Causes constriction of the pupil (miosis).
- Maximum effect is seen within 20 minutes.

INDICATIONS

- Cardiac chest pain.
- Cardiogenic pulmonary edema.
- Isolated fractures with on scene/transport time delays and without signs of other trauma.
- Burns without signs of trauma.
- Severe frostbite without signs of trauma during rewarming.

DOSAGE

- Adult: 1 to 3 mg slow IV push; repeat every 5 minutes as necessary. Do not exceed 0.2 mg/kg.
- Pediatric: 0.1 to 0.2 mg/kg slow IV push over 3 to 5 minutes.

PRECAUTIONS

- May cause hypotension; use with caution in patients with hypotension before administration.
- May cause respiratory depression and arrest.
- Contraindicated in patients with hypovolemia.
- Contraindicated in patients with head injuries, abdominal pain, or multiple trauma.
- Contraindicated in patients with respiratory difficulties (except pulmonary edema).
- May cause nausea and vomiting.
- Hepatic or renal insufficiency.
- If used, have naloxone (Narcan) and resuscitation equipment available.

HOW SUPPLIED

- Morphine sulfate.
- 1-mg/1 ml ampule (1 mg/ml).
- 2-mg/1 ml ampule (2 mg/ml).
- 10-mg/1 ml ampule, Tubex (10 mg/ml).
- 10-mg/10 ml preloaded syringe (1 mg/ml).

Proparacaine Hydrochloride Ophthalmic Solution(Alcaine, Kainair, Ocu-Caine, Ophthaine, Ophthetic)

MAJOR ACTIONS

- Stabilizes the neuronal membrane and prevents the initiation and transmission of nerve impulses.
- NOTE: Proparacaine hydrochloride is a short-acting topical anesthetic; the effects begin within 20 to 30 seconds of application. Duration of action is about 15 minutes.

INDICATIONS

- Pain relief to assist eye irrigation and the use of Morgan Therapeutic Eye Irrigation lens.

DOSAGE

- Adult and pediatric: 1 to 2 drops of 0.5% solution in affected eye.
- For longer transports, 1 to 2 drops every 5 to 15 minutes, up to a maximum of 3 doses.

PRECAUTIONS

- Transient signs and symptoms: stinging, burning, and conjunctival redness may occur.
- Severe allergic reactions may occur. Check for allergies to "-caine" anesthetics before administration.
- Warn patient not to rub or touch eyes.
- Do not use discolored solution.
- Store in tight, light-resistant container at room temperature until opened. Store in a tight container under refrigeration after opened.
- Use with caution in patients with cardiac problems or hyperthyroidism.
- For short-term use only. Long-term use may cause corneal opacification.

HOW SUPPLIED

- Proparacaine hydrochloride.
- 0.5% solution in 15-ml dispenser.

Ondansetron Hydrochloride (Zofran)

MAJOR ACTIONS

- Selective receptor antagonism for preventing nausea/vomiting.

INDICATIONS

- Prevention and treatment of nausea and vomiting.

DOSAGE

- Adult (IM/IV infusion): 4 mg to 8 mg undiluted, over 2 to 5 minutes.
- Pediatric: <40 kg: 0.1 mg/kg; >40 kg: 4 mg undiluted, over 2 to 5 minutes.

PRECAUTIONS

- None significant. Unknown whether drug crosses placenta or is distributed in breast milk.
- May occasionally cause anxiety, dizziness, headache, hypoxia, urinary retention, abdominal pain, and blurred vision.

HOW SUPPLIED

- Oral tablets (4-, 8-, and 24-mg); oral solution (4 mg/5 ml); injection (2 mg/ml).

Sodium Bicarbonate

MAJOR ACTIONS

- Acts as an alkalinizing agent and main component of bicarbonate–carbonic acid buffer system.
- Dissociates to yield free bicarbonate ions.
- Bicarbonate ions combine with hydrogen ions produced by metabolic acidosis or hypoxia-induced anaerobic metabolism to maintain acid-base balance.

INDICATIONS

- Cardiac arrest (if indications of preexisting metabolic acidosis and only after other treatments have been used).
- Metabolic acidosis.
- Severe hypercalcemia.
- Hyperkalemia.
- Certain toxic exposures (see specific guideline).

DOSAGE

- Adult—IV: 1 mEq/kg (1 ml/kg of 8.4% solution) as an initial dose; then 0.5 mEq/kg every 10 minutes.
- Pediatric—IV or IO: 1 mEq/kg (1 ml/kg of 8.4% solution) over 1 minute as an initial dose; then 0.5 mEq/kg every 10 minutes. A dilute solution 4.2% (0.5 mEq/ml) may be used in neonates.
- *Whenever possible, any usage should be guided by blood gas determination.*
- NOTE: In cardiac arrest, sodium bicarbonate therapy should be considered only after confirmed interventions such as defibrillation, cardiac compression, intubation, ventilation, and more than one trial of epinephrine have been used.

PRECAUTIONS

- May cause alkalosis, which can cause as many problems as acidosis.
- May increase intravascular volume and increase cardiac workload.
- May increase cerebral acidosis if patient is not being adequately ventilated.
- Precipitates if given with calcium chloride.
- Deactivates catecholamines if given in same line without adequate flushing.

HOW SUPPLIED

- 10-mEq/10 ml preloaded syringe (1 mEq/ml) 8.4%.
- 50-mEq/50 ml preloaded syringe (1 mEq/ml) 8.4%.
- 44.6-mEq/50 ml preloaded syringe (0.9 mEq/ml) 7.5%.
- 5-mEq/10 ml vial (0.5 mEq/ml) 4.2%.

Albuterol (Salbutamol, Proventil, Ventolin)

MAJOR ACTIONS

- Relaxation of bronchial smooth muscle by stimulating $beta_2$-adrenergic receptors.
- May cause some vasodilation.

INDICATIONS

- Pulmonary edema from toxic exposure accompanied by auscultatable wheezes.
- Reversible bronchospasm.
- Asthma.
- Bronchospasm that occurs in association with bronchitis and emphysema.

DOSAGE

- Adult: Nebulized—2.5 mg in 3 to 4 ml NS. Dose may be repeated every 1 to 4 hours as needed. Higher doses (up to 2.5 mg every 15 minutes as needed) may be used for acute attacks (limited by cardiac and other adverse effects).
- Pediatric: Nebulized—0.15 mg (0.03 ml)/kg to a maximum of 2.5 mg in 3 to 4 ml NS. Dose may be repeated every 1 to 4 hours as needed.

PRECAUTIONS

- Contraindicated in patients with cardiac arrhythmias associated with tachycardia.
- Administer with caution in patients with hypertension, hyperthyroidism, diabetes, hypokalemia, congestive heart failure, coronary artery disease, renal insufficiency, hepatic insufficiency, or sensitivity to sympathomimetic amines.
- May cause tachycardia, hypertension, palpitations, nervousness, tremor, nausea, vomiting, muscle cramps, hypotension and hypokalemia, and hyperglycemia.
- May cause paradoxical bronchospasm as a result of repeated excessive use.
- Store in light-resistant containers.

HOW SUPPLIED

- Albuterol sulfate.
- 50-mg/10 ml bottle, nebulizer solution (5 mg/ml 0.5% solution).
- 2.5-mg/2.5 ml ampule, nebulizer solution (1 mg/ml).

Aminophylline (Theophylline Derivative)

MAJOR ACTIONS

- Competitive blocker of phosphodiesterase. Increases active levels of 3′,5′-adenosine monophosphate (cAMP).
- Releases free theophylline.
- Acts as a smooth muscle relaxant.
- Produces bronchodilation.
- Produces vasodilation.
- Acts as a mild diuretic.
- CNS stimulation.
- Stimulates the cardiovascular system and increases cardiac output.
- Stimulates the respiratory drive.
- Increases contractility of the diaphragm.

INDICATIONS

- Bronchospasm.
- Pulmonary edema with associated wheezing.
- Asthma, anaphylaxis, or chronic obstructive pulmonary disease (COPD) with wheezing.

DOSAGE

- Adult: Loading dose 4 to 6 mg/kg in 50 to 250 ml of D_5W administered through a Volutrol over a minimum of 30 minutes.
- Pediatric: Loading dose 4 to 6 mg/kg in 50 to 250 ml of D_5W administered through a Volutrol over a minimum of 30 minutes.
- NOTE: These dosages are used only if patient is not taking theophylline compounds; otherwise, dose should be determined by medical control.
- Anhydrous aminophylline is only 85% theophylline.
- Theophylline has a low therapeutic index; therefore serum concentration monitoring is essential.
- A maintenance dose to maintain serum theophylline concentration in the 10- to 20-μg/ml range should follow the loading dose. Dose should be determined by medical control.
- The maintenance dose must be properly adjusted for children; smokers; and adults with cor pulmonale, congestive heart failure (CHF), COPD, and liver disease. Dose should be determined by medical control.

PRECAUTIONS

- May cause atrial and ventricular ectopy. Also may cause tachycardias. Place patient on monitor before administration.
- May cause hypotension.
- May cause nausea, vomiting, and headache.
- May cause seizures.

- Use with extreme caution in patients with severe hypoxia.
- Use with caution in children.
- Contraindicated if patient is allergic to xanthine compounds.
- Reduce dose if patient is taking theophylline preparations.
- If possible, draw blood sample for theophylline serum concentration prior to administration.

HOW SUPPLIED

- Aminophylline (hydrous).
- 500-mg/10 ml ampule (50 mg/ml).
- 500-mg/20 ml ampule, preloaded syringes (25 mg/ml).
- 250-mg/10 ml ampule, preloaded syringes (25 mg/ml).

Metaproterenol Sulfate (Alupent)

MAJOR ACTIONS

- Synthetic sympathomimetic amine with similar structure and action to that of isoproterenol.
- Acts as a potent beta-adrenergic receptor ($beta_1$ and $beta_2$) stimulator. Almost no alpha-adrenergic effect.
- Inhalant solution has a rapid onset of action.
- Decreases reversible bronchospasm. Increases FEV_1.

INDICATIONS

- Pulmonary edema from toxic exposure accompanied by auscultatable wheezes.
- Reversible bronchospasm.
- Bronchial asthma.
- Bronchospasm that occurs in association with bronchitis and emphysema.

DOSAGE

- Adult: one unit dose vial of 0.6% solution per nebulization treatment. If 5% solution is used, dilute 0.3 ml of solution to 2.5 ml with normal saline. Should not be repeated for 4 hours.
- Pediatric: Inhalant solution is not recommended for use in children under 12 years of age.

PRECAUTIONS

- Administered via nebulizer.
- Contraindicated in patients with cardiac arrhythmias associated with tachycardia.
- Do not administer with another sympathomimetic agent.
- Administer with caution in patients with hypertension, hyperthyroidism, diabetes, CHF, or coronary artery disease.
- May cause tachycardia, hypertension, palpitations, nervousness, tremor, nausea, and vomiting.
- May cause paradoxical bronchospasm from repeated excessive use.
- Do not use if solution is brown in color or has precipitated.
- Store in 15° C to 25° C (59° F to 77° F) environment and protect from light.

HOW SUPPLIED

- Metaproterenol sulfate.
- Inhalant solution; 0.4% or 0.6% unit-dose vials containing 2.5 ml solution.
- Inhalant solution; 5% in of 10-ml or 30-ml bottles with accompanying calibrated dropper.

Oxygen

MAJOR ACTIONS

- Oxygen administration elevates arterial oxygen tension, increases arterial oxygen content, and improves tissue oxygenation.

INDICATIONS

- Suspected hypoxemia from any cause.
- Respiratory distress.
- Shock.
- Suspected myocardial infarction.
- Toxic exposures resulting in respiratory depression, acidosis, or decreased levels of consciousness.
- Coma or altered state of consciousness.
- Cardiac or respiratory arrest.

DOSAGE

- Refer to Oxygen Adjuncts table.

Administration Sets		Delivery Flow Rate (L/Min)	%O_2 (ul)
Nasal cannula (NC)		1-6	25-45
Simple face mask (SFM)		6-12	35-55
Partial rebreather (PRB)		10-15	55-70
Nonrebreather (NRB)		10-15	90
Pocket face mask (PFM)		10	50
Bag-valve-mask	(BVM)	10-15	100 (with reservoir)
	(BVM)	10-15	50% (without reservoir)
	(BVM)	Room air	21%
SFM at 10 L/min + NC at 6 L/min			75%

Formula for Calculating Duration of Oxygen Cylinder Flow

$$\frac{\text{(Actual Gauge Pressure (in psi)} - \text{Safe residual pressure [200]} \times \text{constant}}{\text{Desired flow rate (L/min)}} = \text{Duration of flow (min)}$$

Constants used for various-sized cylinders

Cylinder	D	E	G	H	K	M
Constant	0.16	0.28	2.41	3.14	3.14	1.56

PRECAUTIONS

- Support ventilations as needed.
- May cause respiratory depression in a small percentage of COPD patients. Start out oxygen with a low flow if possible (2 L/min via nasal cannula). Do not withhold oxygen. Be prepared to assist ventilations.
- Drying and irritating to mucous membranes if delivery system is not humidified.
- Never deliver less than 6 L/min by mask. Expired air can accumulate and be rebreathed, thus increasing carbon dioxide levels.

Activated Charcoal

MAJOR ACTIONS

- Nonspecific adsorbent for variety of chemicals and drugs.
- By definition, commercial preparations (1 g) must adsorb 100 mg of strychnine in 50 ml of water to meet USP standards.
- Does not adsorb cyanide, ethanol, methanol, ferrous sulfate, caustics, lithium, mineral acids or hydrocarbon solvents.

INDICATIONS

- Poisoning with chemicals/drugs adsorbable by activated charcoal.
- Useful for drugs that exhibit enterohepatic recirculation.
- Multiple-dose activated charcoal has proved useful for phenobarbital, theophylline, carbamazepine, and digitalis poisonings.
- Refer to specific guideline for use indications.

DOSAGE

- Oral or orogastric tube:
  - Adults: 30 to 100 g.
  - Pediatric: 30 to 50 g or 1 g/kg.
- Sorbitol:
  - Activated charcoal is usually given with the osmotic laxative agent sorbitol to decrease GI transit time. Use with caution in cases of GI obstruction..
  - Adult dose: 100 g (150 ml of 70% solution).
  - Pediatric dose: 1 to 2 ml/kg of 70% solution.

PRECAUTIONS

- Contraindicated in altered level of consciousness with inability to protect the airway.
- Contraindicated in ingestions of caustics, alcohols, and heavy metals.
- Use with caution if there is decreased bowel activity or intestinal obstruction.
- Adsorbed chemical/drug may be released into the GI tract for resorption.
- Administration of activated charcoal followed by GI tract perforation and charcoal peritoneum has been reported.

HOW SUPPLIED

- Powder for suspension:
  - 30 g: Acta-Char.
  - 50 g: Acta-Char.
- Suspension:
  - 0.625 g/5 ml (15, 30 g) in aqueous or sorbitol solution: Acta-Char, Insta-Char.
  - 0.7 g/ml (50 g) in sorbitol solution: Acta-Char Liquid.
  - 1 g/5 ml (12.5, 25, 30, 40, 50 g) in 70% sorbitol solution: Actidose, Charcoaid.
- Also in aqueous solution: Actidose-Aqua, Activated Charcoal Liquid, Insta-Char, Liqui-Char.

Atropine Sulfate

MAJOR ACTIONS

- Antimuscarinic (blocks parasympathetic muscarinic receptor sites); inhibits acetylcholine (postganglionic cholinergic nerve-blocking agent).
- Inhibits parasympathetic nervous system.
- Blocks cholinergic-mediated neuromuscular junctions.
- Increases heart rate by blocking vagal stimulation.
- Increases conduction through the AV node.
- Reduces tone and motility of the GI tract.
- Inhibits salivary, bronchial, and sweat gland secretions.
- Dilates pupils (mydriasis).

INDICATIONS

- Sinus bradycardia or ventricular rates with hypotension.
- Asystole and high-degree blocks with slow ventricular rates.
- Specific physiologic antagonist for toxic exposures of organophosphates, carbamates, and nerve agents.

DOSAGE

- Adult:
  - *Bradycardia:* 0.5 to 1 mg IV push; repeat every 3 to 5 minutes as needed, up to a maximum of 0.04 mg/kg. A total dose of 3 mg (0.04 mg/kg) results in full vagal blockade (cardiac) in humans.
  - *Asystole:* A 1-mg bolus should be given initially and repeated in 3 to 5 minutes.
  - *Symptomatic toxic exposure to organophosphates, carbamates, or similar acting nerve agents:* Initial dose—IV push: 2 mg, repeated every 3 to 5 minutes as needed. Initial dose—IM via autoinjector: 2 to 6 mg, based on level of severity. Repeat 2-mg every 3 to 5 minutes as needed (refer to Mark I antidote kit protocol in this section). Atropine should be given until the lungs are clear to auscultation.
- Pediatric:
  - *Cardiac arrhythmias:* 0.02 mg/kg IV push, with a minimum dose of 0.1 mg and a maximum single dose of 0.5 mg in a child (<12 years) and 1 mg in an adolescent (12 to18 years). The dose may be repeated in 5 minutes, to a maximum total dose of 1 mg in a child and 2 mg in an adolescent.
  - *Symptomatic toxic exposure to organophosphates, carbamates, or similar acting nerve agents:* Initial dose 0.05 to 0.1 mg/kg IV push, up to maximum of 2 mg. Repeat this dose every 3 to 5 minutes as needed. Atropine should be given until the lungs are clear to auscultation.
- NOTE: Initial atropine dose may be given by IM injection or via endotracheal (ET) tube, because the required dosage may be very large; switch to IV route as soon as possible.
- For severely poisoned patients, a continuous infusion at 0.01 to 0.03 mg/kg/min may be required.

PRECAUTIONS

- Severely poisoned patients are relatively atropine resistant. They do not respond to the drug as do patients with cardiac instability. Large amounts may be necessary.
- Adequate oxygenation and ventilation should be assessed before atropine administration.
- Smaller doses of atropine may produce paradoxical bradycardia.
- Do not treat bradycardia (heart rate <60) unless signs of inadequate perfusion (hypotension) are present. In acute myocardial infarction, infarct size may be enlarged by increasing myocardial oxygen demand.
- Increases intraocular pressure.
- Dilates the pupils.
- Hepatic or renal insufficiency.
- If large doses are necessary, preservative-free preparations should be used.

HOW SUPPLIED

- Atropine sulfate.
- 1-mg/10 ml preloaded syringes (0.1 mg/ml).
- 0.5-mg/5 ml preloaded syringes (0.1 mg/ml).
- 1-mg/1 ml ampule (1 mg/ml).
- In multidose vials of 8 mg/20 ml (0.4 mg/ml).
- 2-mg/1 ml autoinjector as part of Mark I antidote kit.

Calcium Gluconate

MAJOR ACTIONS

- Used to treat hydrofluoric acid (HF) and fluoride toxicity.
- Binds the fluoride ion, preventing tissue and systemic injury.
- Depending on the type and extent of exposure, calcium gluconate may be administered via several routes. Calcium gluconate gel may be administered topically. Subcutaneous (SQ) injections or intraarterial (IA) infusion may be used for definitive treatment of local injuries. IV therapy may be needed for systemic signs and symptoms.
- For local injury, the end point of therapy is the elimination of pain.
- For systemic poisoning, therapy should be guided by clinical presentation and laboratory values.

Calcium Gluconate Gel

INDICATIONS

- Mild to moderate skin burns resulting from exposure to HF.

DOSAGE

- No commercial formulation is currently approved in the United States.
- The product may be mixed using calcium gluconate powder and a water-soluble lubricant.
- To make 2.5% w/v gel: mix 3.5 g of USP calcium gluconate powder in 5 oz of water-soluble lubricant (KY or Surgilube) and apply over painful areas. Cover with sterile dressings. For hand and finger exposure, the gel can be placed in a large surgical glove to maximize contact with the hand.

PRECAUTIONS

- Skin surface may look normal; burn is in lower skin layers.
- Bone tissue may be involved.
- Severe burns may require SQ or IA injections; thus, rapid transport to medical facility is essential.
- Consider hand surgeon consult for any hand or finger exposure.
- Watch for systemic poisoning signs and symptoms.

Subcutaneous Injections

INDICATIONS

- Moderate to severe local tissue damage resulting from exposure to HF.
- Patients with no significant pain relief after 45 minutes of topical treatment.

DOSAGE

- Calcium gluconate 10% is infiltrated into the subcutaneous tissue using a 30-gauge needle.
- Injected volume should not exceed 0.5 ml/cm^2.

- Nail removal may be necessary, but some evidence suggests that nail removal may not be necessary if the patient was exposed to less than 10% HF.

PRECAUTIONS

- Small surface area exposure to dilute solutions of HF may not require SQ injections.
- Extremely painful procedure. Local anesthesia should not be used because the therapeutic end point is pain reduction.
- Should only be performed by a physician experienced in this procedure.
- Calcium chloride is irritating to the tissues and should not be used.
- Excessive administration may result in vascular compromise.
- Burn symptoms may be delayed for several hours. Treatment should be guided by history and clinical presentation.
- Consider hand surgeon consult for any hand or finger exposure.
- Watch for systemic poisoning signs and symptoms.

Intraarterial Injections

INDICATIONS

- Moderate to severe extremity tissue damage resulting from exposure to HF.
- Patients with no significant pain relief after 45 minutes of topical treatment.

DOSAGE

- Perform an arteriogram to determine which artery supplies the affected tissue.
- Mix 10 ml of calcium gluconate with 50 ml of 5% dextrose solution and administer over a 4-hour period intraarterially using a parenteral infusion pump.
- Repeat if pain recurs.
- If patient does not experience pain relief, repeat arteriogram to ensure correct artery selection.

PRECAUTIONS

- Small surface area exposure to dilute solutions of HF may not require IA injections.
- An invasive procedure requiring hospital administration.
- Should be performed by an experienced physician.
- Ensure adequate tissue perfusion.
- Burns may be delayed for several hours. Treatment should be guided by history and clinical presentation.
- Consider hand surgeon consult for any hand or finger exposure.
- Watch for systemic poisoning signs and symptoms.

Intravenous Injections

INDICATIONS

- Systemic poisoning resulting from exposure to HF.
- Hypocalcemia secondary to HF exposure.
- If serum calcium concentration cannot be determined rapidly: when there is a history of HF exposure, patient is symptomatic, and has ECG changes consistent with hypocalcemia (prolonged QT interval).

DOSAGE

- Administer 0.1 to 0.2 ml/kg IV up to 10 ml. Repeat dose as necessary.

- Larger than usual doses may be necessary.
- Therapy should be guided by serum calcium and serum potassium determinations.

PRECAUTIONS

- Closely monitor ECG and serum calcium and serum potassium concentrations during therapy.
- Hypotension, bradycardia, and arrhythmias may occur.
- Contraindicated in patients with digitalis toxicity.

Cyanide Antidote Kit

MAJOR ACTIONS

- Amyl nitrite (AN) reacts with hemoglobin (HB) to form an approximate 5% methemoglobin (MHB).
- Sodium nitrite ($NaNO_2$) reacts with hemoglobin to form an approximate 20% to 30% MHB. MHB attracts cyanide (CN) ions from tissue and binds with them to become cyanmethemoglobin (CNMHB).
- Sodium thiosulfate ($Na_2S_2O_3$) converts CNMHB to thiocyanate (HSCN), which is excreted by the kidneys.
- Chemical reaction:
  AN + HB = MHB
  $NaNO_2$ + HB = MHB
  CN + MHB = CNMHB
  $Na_2S_2O_3$ + CNMHB + O_2 = HSCN
- Amyl nitrite, sodium nitrite, and sodium thiosulfate, administered in that order, are the only therapy against cyanide and hydrocyanic acid poisoning currently approved for use in the United States by the FDA.

INDICATIONS

- Treatment of poisoning from cyanide-releasing compounds.
- Treatment of poisoning from cyanide metabolites.
- Use of amyl nitrite and sodium nitrite for hydrogen sulfide poisoning.

DOSAGE

- Adult:
  - Aspirols of amyl nitrite should be broken and held, one at a time, in front of patient's nose. They should be left in place for 15 seconds, followed by a 15-second rest, and repeated until sodium nitrite can be administered. This produces an approximate 5% MHB. The use of amyl nitrite should not delay prompt respiratory support. In case of respiratory arrest, place aspirol inside bag-valve-mask and ventilate (remove after 15 seconds, ventilate for 15 seconds, and repeat) until sodium nitrite can be administered.
  - Stop amyl nitrite administration and administer 300 mg of sodium nitrite (10 ml of 3% solution) by IV push over 5 minutes. This produces a theoretical 20% to 30% MHB.
  - Immediately follow sodium nitrite with 12.5 g of sodium thiosulfate (50 ml of a 25% solution) by IV push over 5 minutes.
  - If toxic signs reappear, repeat both sodium nitrite and sodium thiosulfate at one half the original dose.
- Pediatric:
  - Aspirols of amyl nitrite should be broken and held, one at a time, in front of patient's nose. They should be left in place for 15 seconds, followed by a 15-second rest, and repeated until sodium nitrite can be administered.

This produces an approximate 5% MHB. The use of amyl nitrite should not delay prompt respiratory support. In case of respiratory arrest, place aspirol inside bag-valve-mask and ventilate (remove after 15 seconds, ventilate for 15 seconds, and repeat) until sodium nitrite can be administered.

- *Sodium nitrite dose (IV):* Must be based on child's hemoglobin concentration or body surface area (BSA) or weight. The hemoglobin-based dose is preferred. In most cases, the hemoglobin concentration will not be readily available. The normal hemoglobin for a child is approximately 12 g. **Failure to dose according to one of these dosing parameters may lead to a fatal overdose of sodium nitrite.**

  a. Sodium nitrite based on hemoglobin concentration:

Hemoglobin in grams	Initial IV dose
8	0.22 ml (6.6 mg)/kg
10	0.27 ml (8.7 mg)/kg
12	0.33 ml (10 mg)/kg
14	0.39 ml (11.6 mg)/kg

Do not exceed 10 ml or 300 mg.

  b. Sodium nitrite dose based on BSA:
  6 to 8 ml/m³ or approximately 0.2 ml/kg.
  Do not exceed 10 ml or 300 mg.

  c. Sodium nitrite dose based on body weight estimation: If a child weighs less than 25 kg and it is not possible to obtain a hemoglobin determination rapidly, administer:
  10 mg/kg (0.33 ml/kg).
  Do not exceed 10 ml or 300 mg.

- *Sodium thiosulfate dose (IV):* Calculate dosage on hemoglobin concentration, BSA, or child's weight.

  a. Sodium thiosulfate dose based on hemoglobin concentration:

Hemoglobin in grams	Initial IV dose
8	1.10 ml/kg
10	1.35 ml/kg
12	1.65 ml/kg
14	1.95 ml/kg

Do not exceed 12.5 g.

  b. Sodium thiosulfate dose based on BSA:
  7 g /m³.
  Do not exceed 12.5 g.

  c. Sodium thiosulfate dose based on body weight: If a child weighs less than 25 kg and it is not possible to obtain a hemoglobin determination rapidly, administer:
  1.65 ml/kg of the 25% solution.
  Do not exceed 12.5 g.

- If toxic signs reappear, repeat administration of both sodium nitrite and sodium thiosulfate at one half the original dose.

PRECAUTIONS

- If signs of methemoglobinemia occur (i.e., severe cyanosis, vomiting, coma, and shock), administration of 1% methylene blue is controversial because bound cyanide may be released. Give only under DIRECT MEDICAL CONTROL PHYSICIAN VERBAL ORDER (refer to methylene blue protocol in this section).
- Both sodium nitrite and amyl nitrite in excessive doses can induce a dangerous methemoglobinemia and can be fatal. Monitor MHB concentrations.
- Sodium nitrite can cause hypotension.
- Drug therapy should be in addition to ventilation, oxygen therapy, and rapid transport.

HOW SUPPLIED

- Cyanide Antidote Package.

SPECIAL CONSIDERATIONS

- Other cyanide treatments:
  - 4-dimethylaminophenol (DMAP) is used in Europe as an MHB-generating agent.
  - Hydroxocobalamin (vitamin B_{12a}) is widely used in Europe and is under investigation in the United States. Hydroxocobalamin works by reacting with cyanide to form cyanocobalamin (vitamin B_{12}), which is excreted in the urine.
  - Dicobalt edetate (Kelocyanor) is currently used in Europe. It acts by chelating cyanide to form stable cobalticyanide, which is excreted in the urine.
- Hyperbaric therapy may increase the efficiency of the cyanide antidote kit.

Ethanol (Ethyl Alcohol)

MAJOR ACTIONS

- Hepatic alcohol dehydrogenase has preferential affinity for ethanol.
- Administration of ethanol saturates alcohol dehydrogenase and blocks the breakdown of both methanol and ethylene glycol into toxic by-products. Methanol and ethylene glycol are therefore excreted unchanged.

INDICATIONS

- In-hospital treatment for poisoning with methanol or ethylene glycol.

DOSAGE

- Adult: IV loading dose of 0.7 to 0.8 g/kg. Administer 10 ml/kg of a 10% ethanol solution (0.75 g/10 ml). A maintenance dose of 0.1 g/kg/hr (1.4 ml/kg/hr of 10% ethanol) should be established to maintain a serum ethanol concentration of 100 to 125 mg/dl.

PRECAUTIONS

- Because a 10% solution is the highest concentration that can be administered safely by the IV route, a large amount of solution may be needed. An 80-kg patient requires an 800-ml loading dose. Monitor for pulmonary edema during administration.
- The maintenance dose must be adjusted in chronic alcoholics and during dialysis to maintain a serum alcohol level of 100 to 125 mg/dl.
- Maintenance therapy should be guided by determination of serum ethanol concentrations.
- May cause CNS depression, respiratory depression, hypothermia, hypotension, nausea, vomiting.
- Hypoglycemia may occur after prolonged therapy.
- Therapy should be started as soon as possible after exposure.
- Ethanol therapy is of limited value, as it may take several days to excrete the methanol or ethylene glycol. Definitive treatment is hemodialysis. Ethanol treatment is therefore used to block alcohol dehydrogenase metabolism while preparations are made for hemodialysis.

HOW SUPPLIED

- Absolute ethanol (95%) must be diluted to 10% v/v for IV administration.
- 10% Ethanol and 5% dextrose for injection.
- 5% Ethanol and 5% dextrose for injection.

ANION GAP/OSMOL GAP

- Calculation of the anion gap is a useful way to assess the acid-base status of the patient poisoned by ethylene glycol or methanol.
- The formula for normal anion gap (AG) calculation is:

$$[Na^+] + [K^+] - ([Cl^-] + [HCO_3^-]) = AG$$

Normal range is 8 to 13 mEq/L.

- The normal anion gap is caused by serum phosphates, sulfates, and various organic acids.
- In cases of metabolic acidosis such as in ethylene glycol and methanol poisoning, the anion gap is increased, thus providing a clue to the presence of excess anions.
- Determination of the difference between the measure of serum osmolality and calculated osmolality may be useful in the diagnosis of ethylene glycol, methanol, and isopropyl alcohol poisoning.
- The formula for calculating serum osmolality is:

$$\text{mOsm/kg } H_2O_{calc} = 2(Na^+) + \text{Glucose}/18 + \text{BUN}/2.8$$

- Normal value for the osmolar gap (OG) is 10 mOsm/kg H_2O. Values greater than this may indicate the presence of other low-molecular-weight molecules such as ethylene glycol, methanol, or isopropyl alcohol. Because of the many inherent sources of error in the estimation of the OG, low to normal OG values do not necessarily rule out poisoning.

Flumazenil (Romazicon, 1,4-Imidazodiazepine)

MAJOR ACTIONS

- Benzodiazepine CNS antagonist.
- Blocks benzodiazepine receptor sites.
- Duration of action is 15 to 140 minutes.
- Shorter duration of action than most benzodiazepines. Half-life: 60 minutes.

INDICATIONS

- Complete or partial reversal of benzodiazepine-induced sedation for general anesthesia or diagnostic procedures.
- May be useful in cases of overdoses from benzodiazepines.

DOSAGE

- Adults (not recommended for children under 18 years old):
  - Reversal of benzodiazepine sedation:
    Administer 0.2 mg intravenously over 15 seconds. If desired consciousness level not achieved after 45 seconds, up to four additional doses may be given at 1-minute intervals up to a maximum dose of 1 mg over the 5-minute period. If sedation recurs, follow initial dose regimen up to 1-mg total dose over a 20-minute period. May be repeated twice for a 3-mg total dose over the 1-hour period.
  - Suspected benzodiazepine overdosage:
    Administer 0.2 mg intravenously over 30 seconds. If desired response not obtained after waiting 30 seconds, administer 0.3 mg over 30 seconds. If still suboptimal response, additional doses of 0.5 mg may be given over 30 seconds at 1-minute intervals up to a cumulative dose of 3 mg. Rarely, patients exhibiting a partial response may require additional 0.5-mg doses for a cumulative dose of 5 mg. If symptoms return, 1 mg divided into 0.5-mg doses at 1-minute intervals may be given every 20 minutes up to a maximum total dose of 3 mg/hr.
- NOTE: Only a few patients have been reported to require a total dose of 5 mg.

PRECAUTIONS

- Flumazenil should not be considered as a replacement for adequate airway, ventilatory management, and supportive care in cases of benzodiazepine oversedation or overdosage. Respiratory depression is not always reversed with flumazenil.
- May cause seizures. Do not use in overdoses likely to cause seizures.
- Do not use for mixed benzodiazepine and cyclic antidepressant overdoses.
- May precipitate withdrawal symptoms in patients with physical dependence on benzodiazepines or patients using benzodiazepines for seizure control.
- May cause cardiac arrhythmias.

HOW SUPPLIED

- Parenteral injection for IV use only: 0.1 mg/ml.

Fomepizole (4-methylpyrazole)

MAJOR ACTIONS

- Competitive inhibitor of alcohol dehydrogenase, the first enzyme in the metabolism of ethanol and other alcohols. Prevents the formation of toxic metabolites secondary to methanol or ethylene glycol ingestion.

INDICATIONS

- In-hospital treatment for poisoning with methanol or ethylene glycol.
- Indications are similar to those for ethanol (refer to ethanol in this section).

DOSAGE

- Adult:

  Loading dose: 15 mg/kg up to 1 g. Dilute in at least 100 ml of 0.9% saline (NS) or D_5W and slowly infuse over 30 minutes. Time interval between loading and maintenance doses is 12 hours.

  Maintenance dose: 10 mg/kg every 12 hours for 4 doses. Increase to 15 mg/kg until methanol or ethylene glycol serum levels are <20 mg/dl.

  During hemodialysis: Increase frequency of dosing to every 4 hours.

PRECAUTIONS

- Contraindicated with history of allergy to this medication or other pyrazoles.
- Can cause headache, nausea, and dizziness.
- Transient non–dose dependent hepatic transaminase elevation has been reported after multiple doses.
- Safety and effectiveness in children has not been established.

HOW SUPPLIED

- 1 g/ml in 1.5 ml vials prepackaged in tray packs containing four vials

ANION GAP/OSMOL GAP

- Calculation of the anion gap is a useful way to assess the acid-base status of the patient poisoned by ethylene glycol or methanol.
- The formula for normal anion gap (AG) calculation is:

$$[Na+] + [K+] - ([CL-] + [HCO_3^-]) = AG$$

Normal range is 8 to 13 mEq/L.

- The normal anion gap is caused by serum phosphates, sulfates, and various organic acids.
- In cases of metabolic acidosis such as in ethylene glycol or methanol poisoning, the anion gap is increased, thus providing a clue to the presence of excess anions.
- Determination of the difference between the measure of serum osmolality and calculated osmolality may be useful in the diagnosis of ethylene glycol, methanol, or isopropyl alcohol poisoning.

- The formula for calculating serum osmolality is:

$$mOsm/kg\ H_2O_{calc} = 2(Na^+) + Glucose/18 + BUN/2.8$$

- Normal value for the osmolar gap (OG) is 10 mOsm/kg H_2O. Values greater than this may indicate the presence of other low-molecular-weight molecules such as ethylene glycol, methanol, or isopropyl alcohol. Because of the many inherent sources of error in the estimation of the OG, low to normal OG values do not necessarily rule out poisoning.

Mark I Antidote Kit

In mass casualty events, the use of autoinjector atropine and pralidoxime chloride (2-PAM) is advised. These autoinjectors are known as the Mark I Kit.

Atropine Sulfate

MAJOR ACTIONS

- Antimuscarinic (blocks parasympathetic muscarinic receptor sites); inhibits acetylcholine (postganglionic cholinergic nerve-blocking agent).
- Inhibits parasympathetic nervous system.
- Blocks cholinergic-mediated neuromuscular junctions.
- Increases heart rate by blocking vagal stimulation.
- Increases conduction through the AV node.
- Reduces tone and motility of the GI tract.
- Inhibits salivary, bronchial, and sweat gland secretions.
- Dilates pupils (mydriasis).

Pralidoxime Chloride

MAJOR ACTIONS

- Quaternary ammonium oxime acting as a cholinesterase reactivator.
- Binds with organophosphate (OP), removing it from cholinesterase and restoring cholinesterase function.
- Acts at nicotinic and muscarinic cholinergic receptor sites.
- Synergistic with atropine. Nicotinic site activity relieves paralysis of the respiratory muscles.
- NOTE: Administer as soon as possible after cholinesterase poisoning—preferably within the first 24 hours, before enzyme-OP complex "ages" (covalently bonds). The nerve agent soman (GD) "ages" the enzyme-OP complex within minutes of exposure. Rapid administration is vital. Once covalent bonding occurs, the cholinesterase moiety is irreversibly inactivated. Consider administration even 48 hours or more after exposure if patient is symptomatic.
- Must be used with atropine.
- Relatively slow-acting.

INDICATIONS

- Treatment of symptomatic nerve agent or pesticide/chemicals of the OP class that have anticholinesterase activity exposure. Direct physician order or standing order based on local protocol.

SYMPTOMS AND DOSAGE

Adult Vapor Exposure

- *Mild exposure:*
  - Miosis, dim vision, headache.

  - Rhinorrhea.
  - Salivation.
  - Dyspnea.
  - *Time of onset:* Seconds to minutes after exposure.
  - *Initial Dosage*: 1 Mark I kit; repeat if symptoms recur up to maximum of 3 Mark I kits; then atropine autoinjectors only for continued or recurrent symptoms.
- *Severe exposure:*
  - All of the above symptoms.
  - Severe dyspnea or apnea.
  - Generalized muscular twitching, weakness, or paralysis.
  - Seizures.
  - Loss of consciousness
  - Loss or bladder and/or bowel control.
  - *Time of onset:* Seconds to minutes after exposure.
  - *Initial dosage:* 3 Mark I kits and diazepam (refer to diazepam protocol in this section); repeat with atropine autoinjectors only for continued or recurrent symptoms.

Adult Liquid Exposure

- *Mild/moderate exposure:*
  - Muscle twitching at site of exposure.
  - Sweating at site of exposure.
  - Nausea, vomiting.
  - Feeling of weakness.
  - *Time of onset*: 10 minutes to 18 hours after exposure.
  - *Initial Dosage:* 1 or 2 Mark I kits; repeat if symptoms reoccur up to maximum of 3 Mark I kits; then atropine autoinjectors only for continued or recurrent symptoms.
  - Diazepam may be necessary (refer to diazepam protocol in this section).
- *Severe exposure:*
  - All of the above symptoms.
  - Severe dyspnea or apnea.
  - Generalized muscular twitching, weakness, or paralysis.
  - Seizures.
  - Loss of consciousness.
  - Loss or bladder and/or bowel control.
  - *Time of onset:* Seconds to minutes after exposure.
  - *Initial dosage:* 3 Mark I kits and diazepam (refer to diazepam protocol in this section); repeat with atropine autoinjectors only for continued or recurrent symptoms.

PRECAUTIONS

- Severely poisoned patients are relatively atropine resistant. They do not respond to the drug as do patients with cardiac instability. Large amounts may be necessary.
- Adequate oxygenation and ventilation should be addressed along with antidote administration.
- Atropine will increases intraocular pressure.

- Tachycardia, laryngospasm, and muscle rigidity have been reported with pralidoxime chloride administration.
- Dizziness, blurred vision, diplopia, headache, drowsiness, nausea, hyperventilation, and muscle weakness have been reported with pralidoxime chloride administration.
- Use with caution in patients with hepatic or renal insufficiency.
- A pediatric-size Mark I antidote kit is currently under development.

HOW SUPPLIED

- Mark I antidote kit consisting of:
  - 2-mg/ml—Atropine autoinjector.
  - 600-mg/2 ml—Pralidoxime chloride autoinjector.

Methylene Blue 1%

MAJOR ACTIONS

- Methylene blue is a thiazine dye.
- Two opposite actions on hemoglobin:
  - Low doses of methylene blue reduce methemoglobin to hemoglobin.
  - High doses oxidize hemoglobin iron in the ferrous state (Fe^{+2}) to ferric iron (Fe^{+3}), forming methemoglobin. Only iron in the ferrous state can bind with oxygen.

INDICATIONS

- Poisoning causing methemoglobinemia greater than 30%.
- Methemoglobinemia with signs/symptoms of hypoxia.

DOSAGE

- Adult: 1 to 2 mg/kg (0.1 to 0.2 ml/kg) of a 1% solution given slow IV push over 5 minutes. Repeat as necessary up to total dose of 7 mg/kg.
- Pediatric: Same as adult.

PRECAUTIONS

- For IV use only.
- Must be injected slowly over a period of 5 minutes to prevent local high concentration of the compound from producing additional methemoglobin.
- Do not exceed recommended dosage.
- Large doses may produce nausea, chest and abdominal pain, dizziness, headache, profuse sweating, mental confusion, and the formation of methemoglobin.
- Tissue infiltration may cause necrotic abscesses.
- Contraindicated in patients with glucose-6-phosphate deficiency (G6PD).
- Provides reversible oxidation-reduction by red blood cell methemoglobin reductase to its colorless form, leukomethylene blue. Leukomethylene blue reduces methemoglobin to hemoglobin. Reaction may go both ways.
- Gives urine, feces, and glandular secretions blue-green color.
- May stain skin.
- Do not use in renal failure.

HOW SUPPLIED

- 10-mg/1 ml ampule.
- 10-mg/10 ml ampule.

Naloxone (Narcan)

MAJOR ACTIONS

- Acts as a narcotic (opiate) antagonist.
- Rapid onset of actions.

INDICATIONS

- Used to reverse narcotic effects, especially respiratory depression.
- A diagnostic tool in coma or seizures without a reliable history.

DOSAGE

- Adult: 0.1 to 2 mg slow IV
- Pediatric: 0.01 mg/kg slow IV
- NOTE: Doses may be repeated at 2- to 3-minute intervals if necessary.
- May be given via ET or IM routes.

PRECAUTIONS

- May precipitate opiate withdrawal symptoms. Withdrawal can be violent; try to titrate dose to reverse respiratory depression only.
- May cause hypertension and tachycardia.
- If no response in adult after a total dose of 10 mg, continued administration is probably of no value.
- Because the half-life of Narcan is shorter than that of many narcotics, symptoms may recur. Repeated doses may be necessary.

HOW SUPPLIED

- 0.4-mg/1 ml ampule, preloaded syringe (0.4 mg/ml).
- 1-mg/1 ml ampule, preloaded syringe (1 mg/ml).
- 2-mg/2 ml ampule, preloaded syringe (1 mg/ml).
- 0.04-mg/2 ml ampule (0.02 mg/ml) neonatal.

Pralidoxime Chloride (Protopam Chloride, 2-PAM Chloride, 2-Pyridine Aldoxime Methochloride)

MAJOR ACTIONS

- Quaternary ammonium oxime acting as a cholinesterase reactivator.
- Binds with organophosphate (OP), removing it from cholinesterase, restoring cholinesterase function.
- Acts at nicotinic and muscarinic cholinergic receptor sites.
- Synergistic with atropine. Nicotinic site activity relieves paralysis of the respiratory muscles.
- NOTE: Administer as soon as possible after cholinesterase poisoning—preferably within the first 24 hours, before enzyme-OP complex "ages" (covalently bonds). Once covalent bonding occurs, the cholinesterase moiety is irreversibly inactivated. Consider administration even 48 hours or more after exposure if patient is symptomatic.
- Must be used with atropine.
- Relatively slow-acting.

INDICATIONS

- Treatment of poisoning caused by the pesticides and chemicals of the OP class that have anticholinesterase activity. Controversial use with carbaryl (Sevin), a carbamate-type insecticide, if symptoms are severe. May be useful with other carbamate insecticide poisonings. DIRECT PHYSICIAN ORDER ONLY.

DOSAGE

- Adult: 1 to 2 g of pralidoxime chloride IV drip in 100 ml of normal saline (NS) over 15 to 30 minutes. Dose may be repeated in 1 hour if symptoms are still present. The dose can then be repeated every 6 to 8 hours as necessary for 24 to 48 hours. Symptomatic patients may require extended treatment after 48 hours.
    - For symptomatic nerve agent exposure in the adult patient: 600 mg IM autoinjector up to maximum of 1800 mg (refer to Mark I antidote kit protocol in this section).
- Pediatric: 20 to 40 mg/kg to a maximum dosage of 1 g of pralidoxime chloride IV drip in 100 ml of NS over 15 to 30 minutes. Dose may be repeated in 1 hour if symptoms are still present. The dose can than be repeated every 6 to 8 hours as necessary for 24 to 48 hours. Symptomatic patients may require extended treatment after 48 hours.
- If nicotinic effects persist, a continuous infusion of pralidoxime chloride may be used. A 2.5% concentration can be given at up to 0.5 g/hr. The continuous

infusion may be more beneficial than repetitive, single-dose therapy. Treatment end point is dictated by clinical response.

PRECAUTIONS

- Tachycardia, laryngospasm, and muscle rigidity have been reported as a result of a too-rapid infusion rate.
- Dizziness, blurred vision, diplopia, headache, drowsiness, nausea, hyperventilation, and muscle weakness have been reported.
- Impaired renal function.
- Use pralidoxime chloride with caution when treating OP overdose in cases of myasthenia gravis, because it may precipitate a myasthenic crisis.
- Atropine and pralidoxime chloride are synergistic and should be used together; the signs of atropinization may occur earlier than might be expected when atropine is used alone.
- Pralidoxime chloride is not effective in the treatment of poisoning caused by phosphorus, inorganic phosphates, or OPs that do not have anticholinesterase activity.
- Pralidoxime chloride is not generally recommended to treat intoxication from the carbamate class of insecticides, especially carbaryl. The carbamate/cholinesterase bond is not permanent and will allow the cholinesterase to spontaneously reactivate.

HOW SUPPLIED

- 20-ml vial containing 1 g of sterile pralidoxime chloride (white to off-white porous cake) and one 20-ml ampule of sterile water for injection to be used as a diluent.
- 600-mg/2 ml autoinjector as part of Mark I antidote kit.

Section **Five**

EMS/HAZARDOUS MATERIALS OPERATING PROCEDURES

Unless otherwise stated, all treatment modalities and drug dosages in this section are based on the adult patient. For pediatric patients, consult the drug protocol section and your medical advisor. Medication use in pregnant patients should be guided by physician control.

To the best of our knowledge, drug indications, dosages, and precautions contained in these protocols are correct and current as of the time of publication. The reader is urged to review standard pharmacology references and the manufacturer's recommendations for additional details.

These protocols contain suggested treatment. Operating protocols and standing and verbal orders should be established by the local medical advisor. Consult with your medical control physician concerning local medication protocols.

Preplanning Concerns

HEALTH STATUS OF THE MEDICAL RESPONDER

- Previous poisoning exposure.
- Preexisting medical conditions.
- Reproductive hazard exposure concerns (e.g., lead).

PREPLANNING QUESTIONS

- Who has jurisdiction?
- What is the local type of incident command system (ICS) structure? How does EMS fit in?
- Capabilities of local responders:
  - Fire.
  - Hazmat.
  - Police.
  - Health department.
  - Public utilities.
- Responder response time?
- Local hospital capabilities?
  - Decontamination capabilities.
  - Medical toxicology support.
  - Special drug/equipment availability (e.g., physiologic antagonists, hyperbaric chamber).
- Types of area hazards?
- Types of hazards transported through area?
- From whom is decontamination advice available?

INFORMATION SOURCES

- Local/state Emergency Management Agency.
- Local Emergency Planning Committee (LEPC).
- SARA Title III reports.
- Fire department inspections.
- Fire department reports (previous product releases and problems).
- Police or state patrol records.
- Local industry representatives.

EQUIPMENT

- Compatible with area hazards.
- Protective equipment.
- Disposable equipment.
- Resources.
- Physiologic antagonists and special treatment protocols.
- Location of extra supplies.
- Inventory checklists.

OPERATING PROCEDURES

- Response procedures and checklists.
- Treatment protocols.
- Destination protocols.
- Decontamination protocols.

Scene Operations and Response

SCENE MANAGEMENT

- Advance cautiously at the first indication that hazardous materials are involved; make sure that your approach is from an upwind and uphill direction. Stop a safe distance from the contaminated or potentially contaminated area.
- Isolate the hazard area and secure from unauthorized personnel entry.
- Establish a safe zone that is upwind and uphill (if possible). Avoid low-lying areas. Keep unnecessary people away (including nonessential emergency response personnel).
- Consider establishing scene security if there is any indication of an intentional release. Make sure area is free of secondary devices.
- Isolation and evacuation distances vary depending on chemical/product, weather, and situation. Suggested evacuation distances can be found in the *North American Emergency Response Guidebook.*
- Do not assume that the scene is safe because the substance does not have any apparent odor or obvious color.
- Call for help from local authorities (e.g., police, fire, hazmat team, local or state health department).
- Attempt to identify the products involved by occupancy/location, container shape, markings/color, placards/labels, UN/NA/PIN number, or on-scene personnel. Do not attempt to recover manifest or bill of lading unless wearing proper protective equipment.
- Wear positive-pressure SCBA and protective equipment specified by references such as the *North American Emergency Response Guidebook.* If special chemical protective clothing is required, consult the chemical manufacturer or specific protective clothing compatibility charts. Equipment must be appropriate and compatible with the chemical(s) involved. Selection should be made by a knowledgeable person using appropriate reference materials. **Do not enter hazardous environments, even to perform rescue or carry out decontamination procedures, without proper protective equipment. Responders should never attempt to wear protective equipment without proper training and fit testing as required.**
- If protective equipment is not available or responders are not trained in proper use, limit response activities to scene isolation.
- Consult the *North American Emergency Response Guidebook*; CHEMTREC at 1-800-424-9300; and your local poison center for more complete information.
- Under new transport regulations, all hazardous material shipping papers must include an emergency response telephone number.
- Divide the incident into response zones (hot, warm, cold) to ensure responder and citizen safety.

Hot Zone/Exclusion Zone

- Definition: Area of contamination.
- Entrance requires:
  - Proper training.
  - Appropriate protective equipment.
  - Buddy system.
- EMS involvement depends on your area needs, standard operating procedures, training (preplanning concerns), and specific incident considerations.
- Care of trapped patients may require EMS involvement.
- Triage activities may be required in mass casualty incidents.
- Patient care activities:
  - Rapid patient removal with attention to possible spine injuries.
  - If patient is trapped or pinned, medical/trauma stabilization care may be required (medical procedures must be carried out by qualified personnel).
  - Airway control.
  - Isolate spontaneously breathing patient's airway with an escape mask or self-contained breathing apparatus (SCBA).
  - Ventilatory support with demand valve or bag-valve-mask with reservoir and oxygen as needed.
  - Spine immobilization.
  - Rapid removal when extrication procedures are complete.
- Any activity, including rescue, requires proper preplanning, training, and protective equipment.

Warm Zone/Contamination Reduction Zone

- Definition: Area surrounding hot zone.
- Safety buffer area.
- Decontamination area.
- Access and egress to and from hot zone.
- Entrance requires:
  - Proper training.
  - Proper personal protective equipment (PPE).
  - Buddy system.
- EMS involvement depends on your area needs, standard operating procedures, training (preplanning concerns), and specific incident considerations. As a preplanning concern, identify personnel (either hazmat team/fire with medical training or EMS responder with PPE training) to be available to perform the following:
  - Patient decontamination and medical care during the decontamination process.
  - Supervising ambulatory patient self-decontamination.
  - Triage activities as patients are removed from the hot zone.
  - Immediate care of injured team members during the decontamination process.
  - Patient care activities:

    Medical care during decontamination

    ABCDE:

    Airway

    Breathing

    Circulation (hemorrhage control)/**C**-spine stabilization

Decontamination
Evaluation for systemic toxicity
Spine immobilization
Oxygen administration
Limited invasive procedures
CPR as necessary

- **Any activity in this area will require proper preplanning, training, and protective equipment.**

Cold Zone/Support Zone

- Definition: Safe area, isolated from contamination.
- Command Post/Staging Area/Treatment Area location parameters:
  - Upwind.
  - Uphill.
  - Upstream if necessary.
  - Easy and safe access.
- Staging area for vehicles and equipment.
- EMS involvement depends on your area needs, standard operating procedures, training (preplanning concerns), and incident specific considerations.
- Advise incident commander or planning section chief on potential toxicological, physical, and /or environmental health concerns.
- Establishment of triage and patient care areas.
- Triage of "clean patients."
- Patient destination planning.
- Care and transportation of "clean patients."
- Medical monitoring and care of response team members (refer to Hazardous Materials Response Team Medical Support protocol in this section).
- Patient care activities:
  - Ensure that adequate decontamination has been performed.
  - Transfer patient from decontamination personnel to medical care givers to limit contamination spread.
  - Patient should be on clean backboard or scoop stretcher.
  - Basic and advanced life support functions as required.
- Basic life support:
  - Secure and monitor airway.
  - Ensure adequate C-spine precautions.
  - Administer oxygen.
  - Evaluate pulmonary status and treat respiratory conditions.
  - Evaluate hemodynamic state and treat shock.
  - Treat soft tissue injuries and fractures.
  - Initiate eye irrigation as necessary.
  - Other treatment as required for specific exposure.
- Advanced life support:
  - Ensure patent airway (advanced airway maneuvers).
  - Evaluate for and treat respiratory conditions.
  - Consider the use of pulse oximetry in the exposed patient.
  - Monitor cardiac rhythm.
  - Treat arrhythmias as necessary.

    - Follow and record any changes in level of consciousness.
    - Establish IV line.
    - Shock management.
    - Treat seizures.
    - Specific physiologic antagonists (antidotes) as indicated.
    - Treat chemical irritation, burns, and frostbite.
    - Other treatment as required for specific exposure problems.
- **Any activity in this area requires proper preplanning, training, and minimal protective equipment.**

SPECIAL CONSIDERATIONS

- **All treatment modalities must be carried out under protocol and be approved by local medical control.**

Evidence Preservation

PURPOSE

- An incident involving the release of a weapon of mass destruction becomes a hazardous materials response, a mass casualty incident, and a crime scene all in one. The terrorists responsible for the attack may be mixed in with the victims. Victims will be bringing valuable evidence with them on their clothes and in personal items. Although it is too late to prevent this incident from occurring, law enforcement personnel may be able to prevent the next one by capturing and prosecuting the terrorists. Paramount to this concern is the collection and preservation of evidence.

PROCEDURE

- Medical personnel should have a basic knowledge of this subject. All items removed from patients should be isolated in plastic bags and marked with the information that will link them with the patient. Many triage tags have a tear-off strip that matches the triage tag number. This strip is placed in the bag with the patient's clothing. As much as possible, these bags must be isolated and a proper chain of custody followed. If time and patient numbers permit, clothes and personal items should be placed in paper bags and then isolated in plastic bags. Paper bags will assist in the preservation of evidence.
- Some mass causality decontamination teams use digital or video cameras to photograph patients. The best use of this practice is probably to place video cameras to capture footage as patients approach the decontamination area. This practice will document the patients and the clothing they were wearing as they entered the decontamination area. This may help to match patients to their clothing and effects. It will also eliminate problems encountered if patients are photographed while disrobing. Photographic records should be turned over to proper law enforcement agencies.
- Local law enforcement agencies can assist medical responders in developing proper procedures and training programs.

Chemical Exposure and Triage

TRIAGE CONSIDERATIONS

- Hazardous material exposure may influence triage decisions in a number of ways. Patient access and emergency treatment may be delayed because of scene conditions and decontamination time. Chemicals may modify how the body responds to trauma by amplifying signs and symptoms. Many chemicals may not cause immediate symptoms, and possible delayed symptom onset must be considered to make appropriate triage decisions.

EXPOSURE PATTERNS

- Not all exposed victims are contaminated.
- Chemical(s) involved (toxic, corrosive, reactive, flammable).
- State of matter (solid, liquid, gas).
- Route(s) of exposure.
- Initial symptoms.
- Present symptoms.
- Expected symptoms.
- Associated trauma.
- Potential complications from preexisting medical conditions.
- Risk of secondary contamination.

FACTORS CAUSING DELAY IN PATIENT ACCESS

- Scene contamination.
- Potential secondary devices.
- Extensive isolation areas required.
- Lack of proper protective equipment.
- Multiple patients.
- Time requirements for decontamination.

EXPOSURE EFFECTS ON HUMAN PROTECTIVE RESPONSES

- CNS depression.
- Cardiovascular system (rate changes, myocardial irritability).
- Respiratory system (depression, paralysis, pulmonary edema).

CHEMICAL ASPHYXIATION AND SHOCK

- Effect on available hemoglobin (hemolysis, carboxyhemoglobinemia, methemoglobinemia).
- Depression of cardiac contractility.
- Arrhythmias.
- Effect on vasomotor center.
- Direct effect on blood vessels (increased permeability, vasoconstriction, vasodilatation).

EXAMPLES OF CHEMICALS WITH IMMEDIATE SYMPTOM ONSET

- Highly soluble corrosive vapors/gases (chlorine, ammonia).
- Incapacitating agents/vomiting agents/riot control agents
- Corrosive liquids (hydrochloric acid, sulfuric acid).

- Simple asphyxiants (methane, nitrogen).
- Chemical asphyxiants /"blood agents" (hydrogen sulfide, cyanide).
- Organophosphates (diazinon, malathion, parathion), nerve agents (G agents and VX).
- Methemoglobin formers (nitrates, nitrites).
- Lewisite.

EXAMPLES OF CHEMICALS WITH DELAYED SYMPTOM ONSET

- Biological agents.
- Radiological agents.
- Mustard agents.
- Low-solubility corrosive vapors/gases (nitric acid, phosgene).
- Hydrocarbon solvents.
- Hydrofluoric acid.

EXAMPLES OF CHEMICALS WITH LONG-TERM SEQUELAE

- Carcinogens.
- Reproductive toxicants (mutagens, teratogens).
- Asbestos.
- Allergens/sensitizers (phthalates, glutaraldehyde).
- Heavy metals (lead, mercury, arsenic).

COMPLICATIONS

- Many chemicals may cause both immediate and delayed symptoms, depending on level of exposure and individual reactions:
  - Organophosphates and methemoglobin formers may have immediate or delayed onset.
  - Corrosive vapors may have immediate or delayed, depending on water solubility.
  - Toxic decomposition and metabolic products. The initial chemical encountered may not be the actual poison. Many chemicals produce thermal decomposition products that are more poisonous than the parent compound. Alternatively, some compounds undergo a metabolic process of lethal synthesis (e.g., methylene chloride is partially metabolized to carbon monoxide).
- The chemicals listed above represent only limited examples. Each exposure must be evaluated for its individual toxicity and symptom pattern.

SPECIAL PATIENT POPULATION CONCERNS

- Preexisting medical conditions associated with exposures that cause respiratory, cardiovascular, and/or neurological compromise.
- *Pregnant:* Simple and chemical asphyxiants (especially carbon monoxide) may cause prolonged fetal hypoxia. Chemicals that depress cardiac function may also increase fetal hypoxia. Teratogenic agents may damage the developing fetus.
- *Pediatric:* Lower exposure dose usually needed to cause toxic response.
- *Geriatric:* Preexisting medical conditions, decreased pulmonary/cardiovascular reserve, and decreased immune system function limit physiologic reserve. This patient population may be symptomatic at lower exposure levels than young, healthy adults.

Hazardous Materials Response Team Medical Support

PURPOSE

- To ensure safety of the response team during emergency hazardous materials response and remediation operations.
- To prevent heat- or cold-related injuries.
- To limit chemical exposure health effects on team members.
- To provide toxicologic information to the incident commander.

IMPLEMENTATION

- Incidents involving potential chemical exposure.
- Large incidents.
- Prolonged-duration incidents.
- Climatic or environmental conditions with high or low temperature extremes.

PREENTRY EVALUATION

- Baseline vital signs:
  - Pulse.
  - Blood pressure.
  - Respiratory rate.
  - Temperature.
  - Body weight (if long-duration event is expected).
- Physical evaluation:
  - Breath sounds.
  - Dermatitis, sunburn, or areas of skin damage.
  - ECG rhythm strip if indicated.
  - Mental status evaluation..
- History:
  - Medical history.
  - Recent history of illness, fever, vomiting, or diarrhea.
  - Recent chemical exposures.
  - Recent alcohol consumption.
  - Prescription and over-the-counter (OTC) medications.
- Deny entry if:
  - Altered mental or physical behavior.
  - Pulse irregular (without prior history or previous medical clearance).
  - Pulse greater than 70% maximum heart rate (MHR = 220 – age).
  - Temperature greater than 37.5° C (99.5° F) (oral), 38° C (100.5° F) (core) or less than 36.1° C (97° F) (oral), 36.6° C (98° F) (core).
  - Diastolic blood pressure greater than 105 (consider the stress caused by the incident when using this criterion).

- Respiratory rate greater than 24/min.
- Abnormal lung sounds (wheezing, rales, or rhonchi).
- Recent onset of medical problems.
- Recent history of heat illness, fever, vomiting, diarrhea, or dehydration.
- Heavy alcohol consumption in last 24 hours or any alcohol consumption in last 6 hours.
- Skin lesions, large rash, or significant sunburn.
- New prescription medications (not cleared by medical advisor) or OTC medication use.
- Pregnancy.

- Clear any questionable physical findings or medication questions with medical control.
- Hydration:
  - Each responder should drink 16 oz of water or electrolyte solution diluted 3:1 immediately before entry.
  - Fluids should be cooled to 4.4° C (40° F).
  - Avoid alcohol, caffeinated or carbonated beverages.
- Pre-entrance briefing:
  - Review signs and symptoms of heat stress.
  - Ascertain identity of chemical(s) and evaluate with appropriate resources.
  - Inform all response team members of possible signs and symptoms of chemical exposure.
- Contingency planning:
  - Arrange for medical transportation.
  - Notify hospital to ensure adequate preparation to receive injured.
  - Ensure that patient decontamination is set up and that appropriate medical equipment is available.

POSTEXIT EVALUATION

- Responders should be evaluated (post-decontamination) for signs of heat stress and/or chemical exposure.
- Information obtained during evaluation should be recorded on standard forms.
- If signs of chemical exposure are present, the responder should be treated per appropriate protocol and transported for further care and/or medical follow-up.
- If the age-adjusted heart rate (220 – age × 0.7) is exceeded or if the heart rate does not return to within 10% of baseline by the end of a rest period, heat stress is indicated. The responder should not be allowed to return to service until the heart rate is reduced below 110 beats per minute. The next work period should be shortened by one third. Fluid loss must be replaced.
- If the oral temperature rises 0.8° C (1.5° F) above baseline, the next work period should be decreased by one third. Fluids should be replaced. Responders should not be allowed to work in impermeable clothing if their temperature exceeds. 37.5° C (99.5° F) (oral), 38° C (100.5° F) (core).
- If body water loss (BWL) exceeds 1.5% of total body weight, the responder should increase his or her oral fluid intake.

FLUID REPLACEMENT

- Fluid replacement plays a vital part in preventing heat stress.
- Thirst is not an effective indicator of heat stress.

- Aggressive fluid replenishment is necessary. During hot weather response activities, the responder should consume at least 1 liter of water per hour.
- Fluid replacement is also needed in cold weather. Heat stress and fluid loss occur even when protective equipment is worn.
- Cool water (4.4° C (40° F) is recommended. Carbonated, caffeinated, and alcoholic drinks should be avoided. Fruit juices and electrolyte drinks should be diluted with water (3 parts water to 1 part electrolyte drink).
- Fluid replenishment starts during suit-up, before first entry.

COOLING DEVICES

- Cooling vests and other personal cooling devices may be useful to reduce heat stress; however, their use may add bulk/weight and contribute to heat stress. Use of cooling devices should be carefully evaluated by knowledgeable personnel.
- Fixed-line cooling units are cumbersome for emergency response operations.

CHEMICAL EXPOSURE CONCERNS

- The medical responder can supply information to the incident commander and hazmat team on expected toxicologic health effects, including signs and symptoms, onset times, and required treatment.
- The response team should be evaluated for chemical exposure effects and treated/transported as necessary.
- The response team should be debriefed on expected signs and symptoms of exposure.

SUPPORT LOCATION

- Safe location in the "cold zone."
- Protection from prevailing environmental conditions: cool, shaded area in warm weather; warm, dry area in cold environments.
- Easily reached from the decontamination area.
- Easily accessible by EMS units.
- Large enough for multiple personnel.
- May be a structure or large vehicle (bus, truck) located in the "cold zone."
- Open area may be adequate with appropriate preparations for environmental conditions.

EQUIPMENT

- Fluids for oral replenishment (cool water, electrolyte solutions). Carbonated, caffeinated, or alcoholic beverages should be avoided.
- Food, if long-duration incident (more than 3 hours). Fruit, stew, soup, and broth are digested faster than solid food such as sandwiches. Fats and salty foods should be avoided.
- Medical equipment (oxygen, blood pressure cuffs, thermometers, stethoscopes, cardiac monitors, IV fluids/administration sets, ACLS medications and specific physiologic antagonists).
- Salt tablets are contraindicated.
- Tarps and awnings for shade.
- Fans (warm weather); heaters (cold weather).
- Lights.
- Extra clothing.

ADVANCED CONCEPTS: ENVIRONMENTAL TEMPERATURE MONITORING

- The following may be used as general environmental management information for work in all levels of protection: level A (encapsulated suit and SCBA), level B (protective suit and SCBA), and level C (protective suit and air purifying respirator). Temperature cut-offs are intended for level C environments. Level A and B protection generates more heat build-up and physical stress than level C. The use of these higher levels of protection mandates more conservative ambient temperature limits and heat stress medical monitoring procedures.
- Heat stress monitoring and prevention should be instituted when the adjusted temperature or the wet bulb globe temperature (WBGT) reaches 23.9° C (75° F) (level C work environments). Some authorities have suggested 21° C (70° F) for levels A and B. These measurements take into account the ambient temperature, humidity, and cloud cover (solar load). Both temperatures should be considered, and the higher value used.

Calculation Of Adjusted And Wet Bulb Globe Temperature

- *Adjusted temperature* = dry bulb temperature + 13 (% cloud cover factor)
  - Cloud cover factor:
    No clouds = 1.00
    25% clouds = 0.75
    50% clouds = 0.50
    75% clouds = 0.25
    100% clouds = 0.00
- Wet bulb globe temperature (WBGT) = 0.7 (wet bulb temperature) + 0.2 (black globe temperature) + 0.1 (dry bulb temperature).
- If the WBGT is not available, it can be calculated using the following equation:
  $\text{WBGT} = (0.567T_{db}) + (0.393_{Pa})$
  (T_{db} = dry bulb temperature; P_a = water vapor pressure)
- Cold procedures (warm area, dry clothing, warm food) should be instituted when the wind chill index is below –12° C (10° F).
- The WBGT or wind chill index should be available from local weather stations.

Responder Heat Stress Monitoring

- Heart rate is an excellent indicator of body heat stress. Heat stress is indicated when the age adjusted heart rate is exceeded:
  Age-adjusted heart rate = 220 – age × 0.7
- Temperature: A rise in body temperature to 37.2° C–37.5° C (99° F–99.6° F) (oral) is considered the temperature cut-off point for typical workers. If possible, a baseline temperature should be established for each individual response team member. A maximum increase of 0.8° C (1.5° F) in temperature is allowed. Body temperature should return to within 0.5% of baseline before the worker is allowed to return to work. Rectal temperature is the most accurate for determining actual body core temperature, but it is not practical for field use. Thermometers measuring the temperature of the blood in the tympanic membrane give a reliable indication of core temperature and a more accurate reading than oral measurements. These thermometers are available at reasonable prices and offer increased speed and accuracy in field temperature monitoring.

- Body weight: Fluid loss when wearing impermeable protective clothing may be as high as 3.5 L/hr. If these fluids are not replaced, a drop in body weight will be seen. Total body water loss (BWL) should not be allowed to exceed 1.5% of total body weight. Ideally, the hazmat responder should be weighed before and after heat exposure. A scale that is accurate to ±/- 0.25 pound should be available. This procedure may not be practical in emergency response situations and is usually conducted in remediation work.

ACCLIMATION

- Acclimation to hot environments and to the use of protective equipment in those environments helps prevent heat stress. Acclimation takes time and is an important factor in remediation work. It is not feasible for emergency operations.
- Acclimation periods may be feasible for long-duration events. The following schedule demonstrates acclimation time (14 days) required for adjustment to full-day work in extreme heat.

Acclimation Schedule

- *TIME TO ACCLIMATE WORK AND ENVIRONMENTAL DESCRIPTION*

  Day 1 to 3: Light work during the morning or late afternoon, not to exceed 2 hours.

  Day 4 to 6: Light work during the morning or late afternoon, not to exceed 3 hours.

  Day 6 to 8: Light work during the morning or late afternoon, not to exceed 4 hours.

  Day 8 to 10: Moderate work during the morning and afternoon, approximately 4 hours.

  Day 10 to12: Moderate work during the middle of the day, approximately 5 hours.

  Day 12 to 14 : Moderate work during the middle of the day, approximately 6 hours.

  After day 14 : Full days of moderate work.
- Shorter acclimation schedules (4 to 7 days) are available for less extreme environments.

SPECIAL CONSIDERATIONS

- Individual baseline temperature should be established over a 2-week period with averaging of daily temperature measurements. Obviously, this is a preplanning procedure.
- Many of the preceding procedures are designed for hazardous material remediation operations. These may be adapted for emergency response needs. Consult with your medical advisor.

Patient Transportation

INITIAL EMERGENCY DEPARTMENT CONTACT

- Early contact essential.
- Be sure to communicate the following information:
  - Number of patients.
  - Nature of accident.
  - Substance(s) involved.
  - Route of exposure.
  - Duration of exposure.
  - Associated trauma.
  - Victim examination findings and vital signs.
  - Initial signs and symptoms.
  - Treatment administered.
  - Signs and symptoms now.
  - Decontamination carried out?
  - Need for further decontamination?
  - Estimated time of arrival.

TRANSPORTATION CONSIDERATIONS

- Exposure potential exists if contaminated patients are transported.
- New ambulance units meeting KKK-A-1822 E standard are required to have a complete air exchange every 2 minutes. This standard has been in effect since the early 1990s (as KKK-A-1822 A 3.13.6 and later editions). Older units have a relatively poor air exchange rate, with resultant increased risk of secondary exposure to EMS personnel. Some ambulance manufacturers are now incorporating filters efficient enough to capture airborne biological contaminants down to 0.3 micron in size into their ventilation systems.
- Windows are bidirectional, allowing contamination to come back into the ambulance. Opening of rear windows may allow exhaust fumes (carbon monoxide) into the ambulance.
- Lining ambulance patient compartment in plastic may increase secondary inhalation hazard by limiting ventilation.

REDUCING EXPOSURE POTENTIAL

- Decontaminate before transport.
- Reverse isolation procedures such as transportation bags, plastic, blankets, and zip-front body bags may reduce EMS responders' exposure risk. CAUTION: If patient has not been adequately decontaminated, these reverse isolation procedures may increase the patient's chemical exposure risk.
- Provide adequate ambulance ventilation (intake and exhaust fans of proper size).
- Provide adequate EMS personnel protective equipment.
- Patients with toxic ingestion may vomit during transport. The vomitus may contain volatile compounds that may present an inhalation hazard. Vomitus should be immediately isolated in a sealed plastic bag.

AIR TRANSPORTATION

- Usually contraindicated unless rapid transport is necessary and patient is **COMPLETELY** decontaminated or was exposed to a chemical with no risk of secondary contamination. Vomitus may still pose a threat, and measures should be in place for immediate isolation of emesis contents.
- Helicopter landing area should be a safe distance from hot zone to avoid spreading the contamination.
- Flight crews must be advised of scene conditions to ensure a safe approach.
- Many flight services are apprehensive about transporting patients from a hazmat scene. If helicopter transport is necessary in your area, preincident plans should be made with the flight service. Explain decontamination procedures and demonstrate safe scene practices. This may resolve any potential problems.
- Flight services should not be ignored in hazmat response planning. They may be the only reasonable way to transport severely injured patients from rural areas. Helicopters may also be called to an unrecognized hazmat incident and be on the scene very quickly. Flight crews should receive adequate training in hazardous materials recognition and response.
- Helicopter transport of hazardous materials victims should be used when needed and when safety concerns allow.

Useful EMS/Hazardous Materials Equipment

STANDARD PROTECTIVE EQUIPMENT

- Body substance isolation equipment for "cold zone" operations.
- Eye protection.
- Mask.
- Gloves (latex underglove and chemical-resistant outer gloves).
- Fluid-resistant gowns.
- Fluid-resistant shoe cover.
- Rain gear.

SPECIALIZED PROTECTIVE EQUIPMENT

- For "warm" or "hot zone" operations.
- Self-contained breathing apparatus (SCBA).
- Air-purifying respirators (APRs) or powered air-purifying respirators (PAPRs).
- Chemical-resistant gloves (with exam type underglove).
- Chemical-resistant suits.
- Boots or shoe covers.
- **Use of this equipment requires extensive training beyond the scope of this text. Responders should not attempt to use protective equipment without proper preplanning, training, medical examination, and fit testing as required. Selection of equipment by an informed/knowledgeable individual using appropriate reference sources is essential.**
- Having equipment is not enough. The equipment must be compatible with the chemical. Chemical protective equipment usually does not provide protection against fire or heat.
- Repeated training and practice with the equipment is essential for safe and effective use.

USEFUL, QUICK INFORMATION RESOURCES

- *North American Emergency Response Guidebook* (NAERG).
- Material Safety Data Sheets (MSDS).
- National Institute of Occupational Safety and Health (NIOSH) *Pocket Guide to Chemical Hazards.*
- United States Coast Guard CHRIS manual.
- Chemical Manufacturers Association (CMA) CHEMTREC (1-800-424-9300) and MEDTREC programs.
- Emergency information number listed on the shipping papers.
- Regional poison center.
- Numerous other texts, periodicals, and computer programs are available.

MISCELLANEOUS SUPPORT EQUIPMENT

- Binoculars.
- Plastic bags and basins.

- Oxygen supplies for prolonged or multiple patient care situations.
- Patient transportation isolation system (e.g., transport bags, zip-front body bags).
- Disposable blankets and patient gowns.
- Disposable equipment (e.g., suction system, laryngoscopes, stethoscopes, blood pressure cuffs).
- Irrigation fluid and IV tubing.
- Morgan Therapeutic Eye Irrigation Lens.

MINIMUM SUGGESTED EQUIPMENT FOR EMS RESPONSE UNITS

- Binoculars..
- Body substance isolation equipment..
- *North American Emergency Response Guidebook.*
- Patient transport isolation system (e.g., transport bags, zip-front body bags).

SUGGESTED SPECIFIC PHYSIOLOGIC ANTAGONISTS (ANTIDOTES) FOR FIELD USE

- Activated charcoal.
- Atropine (multidose vials) (Mark I antidote kits).
- Calcium gluconate.
- Calcium gluconate gel.
- Cyanide antidote kit.
- Flumazenil.
- Methylene blue.
- Naloxone.
- Pralidoxime chloride (vial) (Mark I antidote kit).
- Use of these agents requires specific approval from local medical control.
- See guidelines for specific applications.

DECONTAMINATION EQUIPMENT

- Decontamination pools or premanufactured decontamination stretchers.
- Saw horses.
- Backboards.
- Soft brushes/sponges.
- Pump sprayers.
- Variable-spray nozzle and hose.
- Mild soap (mild liquid soap/baby shampoo).
- Towels.
- Barrier tape.
- Buckets.
- Items on fire apparatus (hose lines, salvage covers, ladders).

Postincident Concerns

HANDLING CONTAMINATED MATERIALS

- All articles that are possibly contaminated must be isolated for further decontamination, testing, and/or proper disposal according to federal, state, and local regulations.
- These items may include:
  - Patient clothes and personal possessions.
  - Any contaminated patient care equipment.
  - Responders' contaminated uniforms or protective equipment.

AMBULANCE CONCERNS

- Isolate unit until decontaminated.
- Decontamination of patient compartment.
- Mechanical and outside decontamination.
- CHEMTREC and local health department can assist with decision making.

MEDICAL RESPONDER CONCERNS

- Isolation of any possible contaminated clothing and personal possessions.
- All scene responders should shower and change clothes as soon as possible after incident response is terminated.
- Medical follow-up for EMS personnel as needed.
- Completion of all patient records.
- Completion of EMS personnel exposure record.

POST-INCIDENT ANALYSIS

- All responders should participate.
- Key questions to ask:
  - What caused incident?
  - Was proper notification made?
  - Were adequate personnel available?
  - Was adequate equipment available?
  - Were communication systems adequate?
  - Were communications adequate and appropriate?
  - What areas need improvement?

CRITICAL INCIDENT STRESS MANAGEMENT

- Factors that cause EMS response team stress:
  - Inability to intervene at scene because of inadequate equipment or training.
  - Multiple victims/triage decisions.
  - Concern about response team member safety.
  - Concern about possible exposure and delayed effects.
- Obtain professional critical incident stress debriefing team intervention as needed.

Hazardous Materials Team Member Medical Monitoring Program

MEDICAL SURVEILLANCE

- Required for every hazardous materials response team member.
- Requires specialized physician awareness of hazmat team operations and hazardous material toxicology.
- Identify physician to whom team members report.
- Identify physician to monitor all charts, preferably a medical toxicologist.
- Records must be kept for 30 years after termination of employment.

BASELINE PHYSICAL EXAMINATION

- Medical history.
- Occupational history.
- Exposure history.
- Hobbies.
- Physical examination.
- Laboratory testing as required.
- Examination and laboratory results reviewed by designated physician.
- Letter reporting findings to team member.
- Summary letter to employer.
- Fitness form:
  - Indicate fitness to wear respirator.
  - List any specific work restrictions.

ANNUAL EXAMINATION

- Medical history update.
- Occupational history update.
- Interval exposure history.
- Physical examination.
- Laboratory studies.
- Additional laboratory testing as required.
- Examination and laboratory results reviewed by designated physician.
- Letter reporting findings to team member.
- Summary letter to employer.
- Fitness form:
  - Indicate fitness to wear respirator.
  - List any specific work restrictions.

EXPOSURE-SPECIFIC EXAMINATION

- For exposed or possibly exposed individuals.
- Detailed history of exposure event.

- Symptoms at the time of exposure.
- Medical treatment.
- Current symptoms.
- Current treatment.
- Physical examination.
- Laboratory studies as indicated.
- Examination and laboratory results reviewed by designated physician.
- Letter stating findings to team member:
  - Address possible need for future medical monitoring.
  - Implications for team member.
- Summary letter to employer.

EXIT EXAMINATION

- Interval medical history.
- Interval occupational history.
- Repeat baseline physical examination.
- Repeat baseline laboratory studies.
- Keep all records for at least 30 years after employment termination.
- Examination and laboratory results reviewed by designated physician.
- Letter reporting exit findings to team member.
- Summary letter to employer.

LABORATORY STUDIES

- Complete blood count.
- Biochemistry profile, including:
  - Serum electrolytes.
  - Blood urea nitrogen (BUN).
  - Glucose.
  - Cholesterol, triglycerides.
  - Liver function.
  - Renal function.
  - Thyroid function.
- Additional biochemistry studies as required.
- Urinalysis.
- Poison-specific tests:
  - Lead.
  - Free erythrocyte protoporphyrin (FEP)/zinc protoporphyrin (ZPP).
  - Mercury.
  - Arsenic.
  - Cadmium.
  - Red blood cell cholinesterase.
  - Plasma cholinesterase.
  - Specific chemical screening based on area dangers.
  - NOTE: Paucity of poison-specific laboratory studies.
- Urine screening for drugs of abuse.

DIAGNOSTIC STUDIES

- ECG.
- Chest radiograph.
- Audiogram.

- Pulmonary function studies.
- Exercise treadmill examination.
- Additional studies as required by examining physician/toxicologist.

EXPOSURE DIARY

- Hazardous material team member should be encouraged to keep an exposure diary.
- Record all exposures:
  - Symptoms—immediate and delayed.
  - Treatment.
  - Outcome.

Section Six

REFERENCES

GUIDELINES

GUIDELINE 1

Books

CANUTEC: *Initial emergency response guide 1992,* Ottawa, Canada, 1992, Canada Communication Group.

CCINFO: *MSDS/CHEMINFO* (CD-ROM version), Hamilton, Ontario, Canada, 1993, Canadian Centre for Occupational Health and Safety.

DOT: *2000 Emergency response guidebook,* Office of Hazardous Materials Transportation, Research and Special Programs Administration, Washington, DC, 2000, US Department of Transportation.

Mackison FW, Stricoff RS, Partridge LJ Jr, editors: *Occupational health guidelines for chemical hazards,* NIOSH/OSHA, Washington, DC, 1981, US Government Printing Office.

NIOSH/OSHA/USCG/EPA: *Occupational safety and health guidance manual for hazardous waste site activities,* Washington, DC, 1985, DHHS (NIOSH) Publication No 85-115, US Government Printing Office.

Sittig M: *Handbook of toxic and hazardous chemicals and carcinogens,* ed 3, Park Ridge, NJ, 1992, Noyes Publications.

Smeby LC, editor: *Hazardous materials response handbook,* ed 3, Quincy, Mass, 1997, National Fire Protection Association.

Journals

Abrahms J: Nitroglycerin and long-acting nitrates in clinical practice, *Am J Med* 74:85-94, 1983.

Craig R, et al: Sixteen-year follow up of workers in an explosives factory, *J Soc Occup Med* 35:107-110, 1985.

Curry S: Methemoglobinemia, *Ann Emerg Med* 11:214-221, 1982.

Fraser P, Chilvers C, Goldblatt P: Census-based mortality study of fertilizer manufacturers, *Br J Ind Med* 39:323-329, 1982.

Goldhaber SZ: Cardiovascular effects of potential occupational hazards, *J Am Coll Cardiol* 2:1210-1215, 1983.

Kuhlberg A: Substance abuse: clinical identification and management, *Pediatr Clin North Am* 33:325-361, 1986.

Leftwich R, et al: Dinitrophenol poisoning: a diagnosis to consider in undiagnosed fever, *South Med J* 75:182-184, 1982.

Soares E, Tift J: Phenol poisoning: three fatal cases, *J Forensic Sci* 27:729-731, 1982.

Vlay S, Cohn P: Nitrate therapy in angina and congestive heart failure, *Cardiology* 72:322-328, 1985.

GUIDELINE 2

Books

Amdur MO, Doull J, Klaassen CD, editors: *Casarett and Doull's toxicology, the basic science of poisons,* ed 4, New York, 1991, Pergamon Press.

CANUTEC: *Initial emergency response guide 1992,* Ottawa, Canada, 1992, Canada Communication Group.

CCINFO: *MSDS/CHEMINFO* (CD-ROM version), Hamilton, Ontario, Canada, 1993, Canadian Centre for Occupational Health and Safety.

DOT: *CHRIS hazardous chemical data,* US Department of Transportation/United States Coast Guard, Washington, DC, 1984, US Government Printing Office.

DOT: *2000 Emergency response guidebook,* Office of Hazardous Materials Transportation, Research and Special Programs Administration, Washington, DC, 2000, US Department of Transportation.

DOT: Research and Special Programs Administration, US Department of Transportation, 49 CFR 173.300.

Haddad LM, et al: *Clinical management of poisoning and drug overdose,* ed 3, Philadelphia, 1997, Saunders.

Levy G: *Level II hazardous materials text,* Fort Collins, Colo, 1985, GML Consultants.

Mackison FW, Stricoff RS, Partridge LJ Jr, editors: *Occupational health guidelines for chemical hazards,* NIOSH/OSHA, Washington, DC, 1981, US Government Printing Office.

NIOSH: *NIOSH pocket guide to chemical hazards* (CD-ROM version), Cincinnati, 2000, DHHS (NIOSH), US Government Printing Office.

NIOSH/OSHA/USCG/EPA: *Occupational safety and health guidance manual for hazardous waste site activities,* Washington, DC, 1985, DHHS References(NIOSH) Publication No 85-115, US Government Printing Office.

Smeby LC, editor: *Hazardous materials response handbook,* ed 3, Quincy, Mass, 1997, National Fire Protection Association.

GUIDELINE 3

Books

Amdur MO, Doull J, Klaassen CD, editors: *Casarett and Doull's Toxicology, the basic science of poisons,* ed 4, New York, 1991, Pergamon Press.

CANUTEC: *Initial emergency response guide 1992,* Ottawa, Canada, 1992, Canada Communication Group.

CCINFO: *MSDS/CHEMINFO* (CD-ROM version), Hamilton, Ontario, Canada, 1993, Canadian Centre for Occupational Health and Safety.

DOT: *CHRIS hazardous chemical data,* US Department of Transportation/United States Coast Guard, Washington, DC, 1984, US Government Printing Office.

DOT: *2000 Emergency response guidebook,* Office of Hazardous Materials Transportation, Research and Special Programs Administration, Washington, DC, 2000, US Department of Transportation.

Gosselin RE, Smith RP, Hodge HC: *Clinical toxicology of commercial products,* ed 5, Baltimore, 1984, Williams & Wilkins.

Haddad LM, et al: *Clinical management of poisoning and drug overdose,* ed 3, Philadelphia, 1997, Saunders.

Levy G: *Level II hazardous materials text,* Fort Collins, Colo, 1985, GML Consultants.

Mackison FW, Stricoff RS, Partridge LJ Jr, editors: *Occupational health guidelines for chemical hazards,* NIOSH/OSHA, Washington, DC, 1981, US Government Printing Office.

NIOSH: *NIOSH pocket guide to chemical hazards* (CD-ROM version), Cincinnati, 2000, DHHS (NIOSH), US Government Printing Office.

NIOSH/OSHA/USCG/EPA: *Occupational safety and health guidance manual for hazardous waste site activities,* Washington, DC, 1985, DHHS (NIOSH) Publication No 85-115, US Government Printing Office.

Smeby LC, editor: *Hazardous materials response handbook,* ed 3, Quincy, Mass, 1997, National Fire Protection Association.

Tokle G, editor: *Hazardous materials response handbook,* ed 2, Quincy, Mass, 1993, National Fire Protection Association.

Journals

Arwood R, Hammond J, Ward G: Ammonia inhalation, *J Trauma* 25:444-446, 1985.

Binder J, Roberts R: Carbon monoxide intoxication in children, *Clin Toxicol* 16:287-295, 1980.

Cohen M, Guzzard LJ: Inhalation of products of combustion, *Ann Emerg Med* 12:628-632, 1983.

Craft A: Circumstances surrounding deaths from accidental poisoning 1974-1980, *Arch Disabled Child* 58:544-546, 1983.

Hoeffler J, Schweppe J, Greenberg S: Bronchiectasis following pulmonary ammonia burn, *Arch Pathol Lab Med* 106:686-687, 1982.

Klein J, Olson K: Caustic injury from household ammonia (letter), *J Pediatr* 108:328, 1986.

Klein J, Olson K, McKinney H: Caustic injury from household ammonia, *Am J Emerg Med* 3:320, 1985.

Winneke G: The neurotoxicity of dichloromethane, *Neurobehav Toxicol Teratol* 3:391-395, 1981.

Zimmerman S, Truxal B: Carbon monoxide poisoning, *Pediatrics* 68:125-124, 1981.

GUIDELINE 4

Books

Amdur MO, Doull J, Klaassen CD, editors: *Casarett and Doull's toxicology, the basic science of poisons,* ed 4, New York, 1991, Pergamon Press.

CANUTEC: *Initial emergency response guide 1992,* Ottawa, Canada, 1992, Canada Communication Group.

CCINFO: *MSDS/CHEMINFO* (CD-ROM version), Hamilton, Ontario, Canada, 1993, Canadian Centre for Occupational Health and Safety.

DOT: *CHRIS hazardous chemical data,* US Department of Transportation/United States Coast Guard, Washington, DC, 1984, US Government Printing Office.

DOT: *2000 Emergency response guidebook,* Office of Hazardous Materials Transportation, Research and Special Programs Administration, Washington, DC, 2000, US Department of Transportation.

Gosselin RE, Smith RP, Hodge HC: *Clinical toxicology of commercial products,* ed 5, Baltimore, 1984, Williams & Wilkins.

Haddad LM, et al: *Clinical management of poisoning and drug overdose,* ed 3, Philadelphia, 1997, Saunders.

Levy G: *Level II hazardous materials text,* Fort Collins, Colo, 1985, GML Consultants.

Mackison FW, Stricoff RS, Partridge LJ Jr, editors: *Occupational health guidelines for chemical hazards, NIOSH/OSHA,* Washington, DC, 1981, US Government Printing Office.

NIOSH: *NIOSH pocket guide to chemical hazards* (CD-ROM version), Cincinnati, 2000, DHHS (NIOSH), US Government Printing Office.

NIOSH/OSHA/USCG/EPA: *Occupational safety and health guidance manual for hazardous waste site activities,* Washington, DC, 1985, DHHS (NIOSH) Publication No 85-115, US Government Printing Office.

Snyder R, editor: *Ethel Browning's toxicity and metabolism of industrial solvents,* vol I, Hydrocarbons, New York, 1987, Elsevier Science Publishers.

Smeby LC, editor: *Hazardous materials response handbook,* ed 3, Quincy, Mass, 1997, National Fire Protection Association

Journals

Amitai I, et al: Pneumatocele in infants and children: report of 12 cases, *Clin Pediatr* 222:420-422, 1983.

Annobil S: Chest radiographic patterns following kerosene poisoning in Ghanaian children, *Clin Radiol* 34:643-646, 1983.

Aronow R, Spiegel RW: Implications of camphor poisoning, *Drug Intell Clin Pharm* 10:631-634, 1976.

Catchings TT, et al: Adult respiratory distress syndrome secondary to ethylene glycol ingestion, *Ann Emerg Med* 14:594-596, 1985.

Panson R, Winek C: Aspiration toxicity of ketones, *Clin Toxicol* 17:271-317, 1980.

GUIDELINE 5

Books

Amdur MO, Doull J, Klaassen CD, editors: *Casarett and Doull's toxicology, the basic science of poisons,* ed 4, New York, 1991, Pergamon Press.

CANUTEC: *Initial emergency response guide 1992,* Ottawa, Canada, 1992, Canada Communication Group.

CCINFO: *MSDS/CHEMINFO* (CD-ROM version), Hamilton, Ontario, Canada, 1993, Canadian Centre for Occupational Health and Safety.

DOT: *CHRIS hazardous chemical data,* US Department of Transportation/United States Coast Guard, Washington, DC, 1984, US Government Printing Office.

DOT: *2000 Emergency response guidebook,* Office of Hazardous Materials Transportation, Research and Special Programs Administration, Washington, DC, 2000, US Department of Transportation.

Gosselin RE, Smith RP, Hodge HC: *Clinical toxicology of commercial products,* ed 5, Baltimore, 1984, Williams & Wilkins.

Haddad LM, et al: *Clinical management of poisoning and drug overdose,* ed 3, Philadelphia, 1997, Saunders.

Levy G: *Level II hazardous materials text,* Fort Collins, Colo, 1985, GML Consultants.

Mackison FW, Stricoff RS, Partridge LJ Jr, editors: *Occupational health guidelines for chemical hazards,* NIOSH/OSHA, Washington, DC, 1981, US Government Printing Office.

Snyder R, editor: *Ethel Browning's toxicity and metabolism of industrial solvents,* vol I, Hydrocarbons, New York, 1987, Elsevier Science Publishers.

Smeby LC, editor: *Hazardous materials response handbook,* ed 3, Quincy, Mass, 1997, National Fire Protection Association.

Journals

Annobil S: Chest radiographic patterns following kerosene poisoning in Ghanaian children, *Clin Radiol* 34:643-646, 1983.

Meredith TJ, et al: Diagnosis and treatment of acute poisoning with volatile substances, *Hum Toxicol* 8:277-286, 1989.

Panson R, Winek C: Aspiration toxicity of ketones, *Clin Toxicol* 17:271-317, 1980.

Popendorf W: Vapor pressure and solvent vapor hazards, *Am Ind Hyg Assoc J* 45:719-726, 1984.

GUIDELINE 6

Books

CANUTEC: *Initial emergency response guide 1992,* Ottawa, Canada, 1992, Canada Communication Group.

CCINFO: *MSDS/CHEMINFO* (CD-ROM version), Hamilton, Ontario, Canada, 1993, Canadian Centre for Occupational Health and Safety.

DOT: *CHRIS hazardous chemical data,* US Department of Transportation/United States Coast Guard, Washington, DC, 1984, US Government Printing Office.

DOT: *2000 Emergency response guidebook,* Office of Hazardous Materials Transportation, Research and Special Programs Administration, Washington, DC, 2000, US Department of Transportation.

Gosselin RE, Smith RP, Hodge HC: *Clinical toxicology of commercial products,* ed 5, Baltimore, 1984, Williams & Wilkins.

Levy G: *Level II hazardous materials text,* Fort Collins, Colo, 1985, GML Consultants.

Mackison FW, Stricoff RS, Partridge LJ Jr, editors: *Occupational health guidelines for chemical hazards,* NIOSH/OSHA, Washington, DC, 1981, US Government Printing Office.

Smeby LC, editor: *Hazardous materials response handbook,* ed 3, Quincy, Mass, 1997, National Fire Protection Association.

Journals

Chernow B, et al: Iatrogenic hyperphosphatemia: a metabolic consideration in critical care medicine, *Crit Care Med* 9:772-774, 1981.

Chiarenza A, Gallone C: Match dermatitis. *Contact Dermatitis* 7:346-347, 1981.

Clausen J, Rastogi SC: Heavy metal pollution among auto workers. II. cadmium, chromium, copper, manganese and nickel, *Br J Ind Med* 34:216-220, 1977.

McCarron MM, Gaddis GP: Acute yellow phosphorus poisoning from pesticide pastes, *Clin Toxicol* 18: 693-711, 1981.

Pena M, et al: Contact urticaria and dermatitis from phosphorus sesquisulphide, *Contact Dermatitis* 13:126-127, 1985.

Stewart C: Chemical skin burns, *Am Fam Phys* 31:149-157, 1985.

Wason S, et al: Phosphorus trichloride toxicity: preliminary report, *Am J Med* 77:1039-1042, 1984.

GUIDELINE 7

Books

Amdur MO, Doull J, Klaassen CD, editors: *Casarett and Doull's toxicology, the basic science of poisons,* ed 4, New York, 1991, Pergamon Press.

CANUTEC: *Initial emergency response guide 1992,* Ottawa, Canada, 1992, Canada Communication Group.

CCINFO: *MSDS/CHEMINFO* (CD-ROM version), Hamilton, Ontario, Canada, 1993, Canadian Centre for Occupational Health and Safety.

DOT: *CHRIS hazardous chemical data,* US Department of Transportation/United States Coast Guard, Washington, DC, 1984, US Government Printing Office.

DOT: *2000 Emergency response guidebook,* Office of Hazardous Materials Transportation, Research and Special Programs Administration, Washington, DC, 2000, US Department of Transportation.

Gosselin RE, Smith RP, Hodge HC: *Clinical toxicology of commercial products,* ed 5, Baltimore, 1984, Williams & Wilkins.

Haddad LM, et al: *Clinical management of poisoning and drug overdose,* ed 3, Philadelphia, 997, Saunders.

Levy G: *Level II hazardous materials text,* Fort Collins, Colo, 1985, GML Consultants.

Mackison FW, Stricoff RS, Partridge LJ Jr, editors: *Occupational health guidelines for chemical hazards,* NIOSH/OSHA, Washington, DC, 1981, US Government Printing Office.

Sittig M: *Handbook of toxic and hazardous chemicals and carcinogens,* ed 3, Park Ridge, NJ, 1992, Noyes Publications.

Smeby LC, editor: *Hazardous materials response handbook,* ed 3, Quincy, Mass, 1997, National Fire Protection Association.

Journals

Goldhaber S Z: Cardiovascular effects of potential occupational hazards, J Am Coll Cardiol 2:1210-1215, 1983.

GUIDELINE 8

Books

Amdur MO, Doull J, Klaassen CD, editors: *Casarett and Doull's toxicology, the basic science of poisons,* ed 4, New York, 1991, Pergamon Press.

CANUTEC: *Initial emergency response guide 1992,* Ottawa, Canada, 1992, Canada Communication Group.

CCINFO: *MSDS/CHEMINFO* (CD-ROM version), Hamilton, Ontario, Canada, 1993, Canadian Centre for Occupational Health and Safety.

DOT: *CHRIS hazardous chemical data,* US Department of Transportation/United States Coast Guard, Washington, DC, 1984, US Government Printing Office.

DOT: *2000 Emergency response guidebook,* Office of Hazardous Materials Transportation, Research and Special Programs Administration, Washington, DC, 2000, US Department of Transportation.

Gosselin RE, Smith RP, Hodge HC: *Clinical toxicology of commercial products,* ed 5, Baltimore, 1984, Williams & Wilkins.

Levy G: *Level II hazardous materials text,* Fort Collins, Colo, 1985, GML Consultants.

Mackison FW, Stricoff RS, Partridge LJ Jr, editors: *Occupational health guidelines for chemical hazards,* NIOSH/OSHA, Washington, DC, 1981, US Government Printing Office.

NIOSH/OSHA/USCG/EPA: *Occupational safety and health guidance manual for hazardous waste site activities,* Washington, DC, 1985, DHHS (NIOSH) Publication No 85-115, U.S. Government Printing Office.

Smeby LC, editor: *Hazardous materials response handbook,* ed 3, Quincy, Mass, 1997, National Fire Protection Association.

GUIDELINE 9

Books

Amdur MO, Doull J, Klaassen CD, editors: *Casarett and Doull's toxicology, the basic science of poisons,* ed 4, New York, 1991, Pergamon Press.

CANUTEC: *Initial emergency response guide 1992,* Ottawa, Canada, 1992, Canada Communication Group.

CCINFO: *MSDS/CHEMINFO* (CD-ROM version), Hamilton, Ontario, Canada, 1993, Canadian Centre for Occupational Health and Safety.

DOT: *CHRIS hazardous chemical data,* US Department of Transportation/United States Coast Guard, Washington, DC, 1984, US Government Printing Office.

DOT: *2000 Emergency response guidebook,* Office of Hazardous Materials Transportation, Research and Special Programs Administration, Washington, DC, 2000, US Department of Transportation.

Gosselin RE, Smith RP, Hodge HC: *Clinical toxicology of commercial products,* ed 5, Baltimore, 1984, Williams & Wilkins.

Levy G: *Level II hazardous materials text,* Fort Collins, Colo, 1985, GML Consultants.

Mackison FW, Stricoff RS, Partridge LJ Jr, editors: *Occupational health guidelines for chemical hazards,* NIOSH/OSHA, Washington, DC, 1981, US Government Printing Office.

NIOSH: *NIOSH pocket guide to chemical hazards* (CD-ROM version), Cincinnati, 2000, DHHS (NIOSH), US Government Printing Office.

NIOSH/OSHA/USCG/EPA: *Occupational safety and health guidance manual for hazardous waste site activities,* Washington, DC, 1985, DHHS (NIOSH) Publication No 85-115, U.S. Government Printing Office.

Sittig M: *Handbook of toxic and hazardous chemicals and carcinogens,* ed 3, Park Ridge, NJ, 1992, Noyes Publications.

Smeby LC, editor: *Hazardous materials response handbook,* ed 3, Quincy, Mass, 1997, National Fire Protection Association.

Journals

Wegman DH, Eisen EA: Acute irritants, more than a nuisance (editorial), *Chest* 97:773-775, 1990.

Blackwood M: Health risks of smoking increased by exposure to workplace chemicals, *Occup Health Safety* 54:23-27, 1985.

Goldstein B, Melia R, Florey C: Indoor nitrogen oxide, *Bull N Y Acad Med* 57:873-882, 1981.

Goldstein E, Hackney J, Rokaw S: Photochemical air pollution: part I, *West J Med* 142:369-376, 1985.

Hu H, Christiani D: Reactive airways dysfunction after exposure to teargas (letter), *Lancet* 339:1535, 1992.

Morrow P: Toxicological data on NOx: an overview, *Toxicol Environ Health* 13:205-227, 1984.

Oxides of nitrogen and health (editorial), *Lancet* 10:81-82, 1981.

Ro YS, Lee CW: Tear gas dermatitis, allergic contact sensitization due to CS, *Int J Dermatol* 30:576-577, 1991.

Speizer F: Ozone and photochemical pollutants: status after 25 years, *West J Med* 142:377-379, 1985.

GUIDELINE 10

Books

Amdur MO, Doull J, Klaassen CD, editors: *Casarett and Doull's toxicology, the basic science of poisons,* ed 4, New York, 1991, Pergamon Press.

CANUTEC: *Initial emergency response guide 1992,* Ottawa, Canada, 1992, Canada Communication Group.

CCINFO: *MSDS/CHEMINFO* (CD-ROM version), Hamilton, Ontario, Canada, 1993, Canadian Centre for Occupational Health and Safety.

DOT: *CHRIS hazardous chemical data,* US Department of Transportation/United States Coast Guard, Washington, DC, 1984, US Government Printing Office.

DOT: *2000 Emergency response guidebook,* Office of Hazardous Materials Transportation, Research and Special Programs Administration, Washington, DC, 2000, US Department of Transportation.

Gosselin RE, Smith RP, Hodge HC: *Clinical toxicology of commercial products,* ed 5, Baltimore, 1984, Williams & Wilkins.

Levy G: *Level II hazardous materials text,* Fort Collins, Colo, 1985, GML Consultants.

Mackison FW, Stricoff RS, Partridge LJ Jr, editors: *Occupational health guidelines for chemical hazards,* NIOSH/OSHA, Washington, DC, 1981, US Government Printing Office.

NIOSH: *NIOSH pocket guide to chemical hazards* (CD-ROM version), Cincinnati, 2000, DHHS (NIOSH), US Government Printing Office.

NIOSH/OSHA/USCG/EPA: *Occupational safety and health guidance manual for hazardous waste site activities,* Washington, DC, 1985, DHHS (NIOSH) Publication No 85-115, U.S. Government Printing Office.

Sittig M: *Handbook of toxic and hazardous chemicals and carcinogens,* ed 3, Park Ridge, NJ, 1992, Noyes Publications.

Smeby LC, editor: *Hazardous materials response handbook,* ed 3, Quincy, Mass, 1997, National Fire Protection Association.

Journals

Dittrich K, Bayer M, Wanke L: A case of fatal strychnine poisoning, *J Emerg Med* 1:327-330, 1984.

Hutton G, Christians B: Sources, symptoms and signs of arsenic poisoning, *J Fam Pract* 17:423-426, 1983.

Johnson M: Initiation of organophosphate-induced delayed neuropathy, *Neurobehav Toxicol Teratol* 4:759-765, 1982.

Slimak M, Delos C: Environmental pathways of exposure to 129 priority pollutants, *J Toxicol Clin Toxicol* 84:39-63, 1983.

GUIDELINE 11

Books

CANUTEC: *Initial emergency response guide 1992,* Ottawa, Canada, 1992, Canada Communication Group.

DOT: *2000 Emergency response guidebook,* Office of Hazardous Materials Transportation, Research and Special Programs Administration, Washington, DC, 2000, US Department of Transportation.

Levy G: *Level II hazardous materials text,* Fort Collins, Colo, 1985, GML Consultants.

NIOSH/OSHA/USCG/EPA: *Occupational safety and health guidance manual for hazardous waste site activities,* Washington, DC, 1985, DHHS (NIOSH) Publication No 85-115, US Government Printing Office.

Smeby LC, editor: *Hazardous materials response handbook,* ed 3, Quincy, Mass, 1997, National Fire Protection Association.

Journals

CDC: Guidelines for counseling persons infected with human T-lymphotropic virus type-I (HTLV-I) and type II, *Ann Intern Med* 118:448-454, 1993.

Gerberding J: Is antiretroviral treatment after percutaneous HIV exposure justified? (editorial), *Ann Intern Med* 118:979-980, 1993.

Marcus R, CDC Cooperative Needlestick Surveillance Group: surveillance of health care workers exposed to blood from patients infected with the human immunodeficiency virus, *N Engl J Med* 319:1118-1123, 1988.

McCray E, CDC Cooperative Needlestick Surveillance Group: Occupational risk of the acquired immunodeficiency syndrome among health care workers, *N Engl J Med* 314:1127-1132, 1986.

OSHA: Occupational exposure to bloodborne pathogens; 29 CFR Part 1910.1030, Final rule, Dec 6, 1991.

Protection against viral hepatitis: recommendations of the Immunization Practices Advisory Committee (ACIP), *MMWR Morb Mortal Wkly Rep* 39(No. RR-2):1-26, 1990.

Tokars JI, et al: Surveillance of HIV Infection and zidovudine use among health care workers after occupational exposure to HIV-infected blood, *Ann Intern Med* 118:913-919, 1993.

GUIDELINE 12

Books

CANUTEC: *Initial emergency response guide 1992,* Ottawa, Canada, 1992, Canada Communication Group.

CCINFO: *MSDS/CHEMINFO* (CD-ROM version), Hamilton, Ontario, Canada, 1993, Canadian Centre for Occupational Health and Safety.

DOT: *CHRIS hazardous chemical data,* US Department of Transportation/United States Coast Guard, Washington, DC, 1984, US Government Printing Office.

DOT: *2000 Emergency response guidebook,* Office of Hazardous Materials Transportation, Research and Special Programs Administration, Washington, DC, 2000, US Department of Transportation.

Guideline for Public Sector Hazardous Materials Training Draft 2, Emmitsburg, Md, 1993, FEMA, National Emergency Training Center.

Levy G: *Level II hazardous materials text,* Fort Collins, Colo, 1985, GML Consultants.

Mackison FW, Stricoff RS, Partridge LJ Jr, editors: *Occupational health guidelines for chemical hazards,* NIOSH/OSHA, Washington, DC, 1981, US Government Printing Office.

NIOSH/OSHA/USCG/EPA: *Occupational safety and health guidance manual for hazardous waste site activities,* Washington, DC, 1985, DHHS (NIOSH) Publication No 85-115, U.S. Government Printing Office.

Noji EK, Kelen GD, editors: *Manual of toxicologic emergencies,* Chicago, Ill, 1989, Year Book Medical Publishers.

Smeby LC, editor: *Hazardous materials response handbook,* ed 3, Quincy, Mass, 1997, National Fire Protection Association.

Journals

Leonard RB, Ricks RC: Emergency department radiation accident protocol, *Ann Emerg Med* 9:462-470, 1980.

Richter LL, et al: A systems approach to the management of radiation accidents, *Ann Emerg Med* 9:303-309, 1980.

GUIDELINE 13

Books

Amdur MO, Doull J, Klaassen CD, editors: *Casarett and Doull's toxicology, the basic science of poisons,* ed 4, New York, 1991, Pergamon Press.

CANUTEC: *Initial emergency response guide 1992,* Ottawa, Canada, 1992, Canada Communication Group.

CCINFO: *MSDS/CHEMINFO* (CD-ROM version), Hamilton, Ontario, Canada, 1993, Canadian Centre for Occupational Health and Safety.

DOT: *CHRIS hazardous chemical data,* US Department of Transportation/United States Coast Guard, Washington, DC, 1984, US Government Printing Office.

DOT: *2000 Emergency response guidebook,* Office of Hazardous Materials Transportation, Research and Special Programs Administration, Washington, DC, 2000, US Department of Transportation.

Gosselin RE, Smith RP, Hodge HC: *Clinical toxicology of commercial products,* ed 5, Baltimore, 1984, Williams & Wilkins.

Levy G: *Level II hazardous materials text,* Fort Collins, Colo, 1985, GML Consultants.

Mackison FW, Stricoff RS, Partridge LJ Jr, editors: *Occupational health guidelines for chemical hazards,* NIOSH/OSHA, Washington, DC, 1981, US Government Printing Office.

NIOSH: *NIOSH pocket guide to chemical hazards* (CD-ROM version), Cincinnati, 2000, DHHS (NIOSH), US Government Printing Office.

NIOSH/OSHA/USCG/EPA: *Occupational safety and health guidance manual for hazardous waste site activities,* Washington, DC, 1985, DHHS (NIOSH) Publication No 85-115, US Government Printing Office.

Sittig M: *Handbook of toxic and hazardous chemicals and carcinogens,* ed 3, Park Ridge, NJ, 1992, Noyes Publications.

Smeby LC, editor: *Hazardous materials response handbook,* ed 3, Quincy, Mass, 1997, National Fire Protection Association.

JOURNALS

Gimmon Z, Durst A: Acid corrosive gastritis, *Am J Surg* 141:381-383, 1981.

LaDou J: Potential occupational health hazards in the microelectronics industry, *Scand J Work Environ Health* 9:42-46, 1983.

Leonard LG, Scheulen JJ, Munster AM: Chemical burns: effect of prompt first aid, *J Trauma* 22:420-424, 1982.

Milner J: The office treatment of minor skin burns, *Cutis* 29:185-186, 1982.

Pfister RR: Chemical corneal burns, *Int Ophthalmol Clin* 24:157-168, 1984.

GUIDELINE 14

Books

Amdur MO, Doull J, Klaassen CD, editors: *Casarett and Doull's toxicology, the basic science of poisons,* ed 4, New York, 1991, Pergamon Press.

CANUTEC: *Initial emergency response guide 1992,* Ottawa, Canada, 1992, Canada Communication Group.

CCINFO: *MSDS/CHEMINFO* (CD-ROM version), Hamilton, Ontario, Canada, 1993, Canadian Centre for Occupational Health and Safety.

DOT: *CHRIS hazardous chemical data,* US Department of Transportation/United States Coast Guard, Washington, DC, 1984, US Government Printing Office.

DOT: *2000 Emergency response guidebook,* Office of Hazardous Materials Transportation, Research and Special Programs Administration, Washington, DC, 2000, US Department of Transportation.

Gosselin RE, Smith RP, Hodge HC: *Clinical toxicology of commercial products,* ed 5, Baltimore, 1984, Williams & Wilkins.

Mackison FW, Stricoff RS, Partridge LJ Jr, editors: *Occupational health guidelines for chemical hazards,* NIOSH/OSHA, Washington, DC, 1981, US Government Printing Office.

NIOSH: *NIOSH pocket guide to chemical hazards* (CD-ROM version), Cincinnati, 2000, DHHS (NIOSH), US Government Printing Office.

Olson KR, editor: *Poisoning & drug overdose,* ed 3, East Norwalk, Conn, 1999, Appleton & Lange.

Sittig M: *Handbook of toxic and hazardous chemicals and carcinogens,* ed 3, Park Ridge, NJ, 1992, Noyes Publications.

Sullivan JB, Kriger GR, editors: *Clinical environmental health and hazardous materials toxicology,* Baltimore, 1997, Williams & Wilkins.

Journals

Brooks SM, Weiss MA, Bernstein IL: Reactive airways dysfunction syndrome after high level irritant exposure, *Chest* 88:376-384, 1985.

Gimmon Z, Durst A: Acid corrosive gastritis, *Am J Surg* 141:381-383, 1981.

Milner J: The office treatment of minor skin burns, *Cutis* 29:185-186, 1982.

Penner GE: Acid ingestion: toxicology and treatment, *Ann Emerg Med* 9:374-379, 1980.

Reisz GR, Gammon RS: Toxic pneumonitis from mixing household cleaners, *Chest* 89:49-52, 1986.

Schlesinger RB: Effects of inhaled acids on respiratory tract defense mechanisms, *Environ Health Perspect* 63:25-38, 1985.

Siebert S: Ocular trauma from lead-acid vehicle battery explosions, *Aust J Ophthalmol* 10:53-61, 1982.

Stewart C: Chemical skin burns, *Am Fam Phys* 31:149-157, 1985.

GUIDELINE 15

Books

Amdur MO, Doull J, Klaassen CD, editors: *Casarett and Doull's toxicology, the basic science of poisons,* ed 4, New York, 1991, Pergamon Press.

CANUTEC: *Initial emergency response guide 1992,* Ottawa, Canada, 1992, Canada Communication Group.

CCINFO: *MSDS/CHEMINFO* (CD-ROM version), Hamilton, Ontario, Canada, 1993, Canadian Centre for Occupational Health and Safety.

DOT: *CHRIS hazardous chemical data,* US Department of Transportation/United States Coast Guard, Washington, DC, 1984, US Government Printing Office.

DOT: *2000 emergency response guidebook,* Office of Hazardous Materials Transportation, Research and Special Programs Administration, Washington, DC, 2000, US Department of Transportation.

Gosselin RE, Smith RP, Hodge HC: *Clinical toxicology of commercial products,* ed 5, Baltimore, 1984, Williams & Wilkins.

Haddad LM, et al: *Clinical management of poisoning and drug overdose,* ed 3, Philadelphia, 1997, Saunders.

Mackison FW, Stricoff RS, Partridge LJ Jr, editors: *Occupational health guidelines for chemical hazards,* NIOSH/OSHA, Washington, DC, 1981, US Government Printing Office.

NIOSH: *NIOSH pocket guide to chemical hazards* (CD-ROM version), Cincinnati, 2000, DHHS (NIOSH), US Government Printing Office.

Olson KR, editor: *Poisoning & drug overdose,* ed 3, East Norwalk, Conn, 1999, Appleton & Lange.

Sullivan JB, Kriger GR, editors: *Clinical environmental health and hazardous materials toxicology,* Baltimore, 1997, Williams & Wilkins.

Journals

Gimmon Z, Durst A: Acid corrosive gastritis, *Am J Surg* 141:381-383, 1981.

Kern DG: Outbreak of the reactive airways dysfunction syndrome after a spill of glacial acetic acid, *Am Rev Respir Dis* 144:1058-1064, 1991.

LaDou J: Potential occupational health hazards in the microelectronics industry, *Scand J Work and Environ Health* 9:42-46, 1983.

Milner J: The office treatment of minor skin burns, *Cutis* 29:185-186, 1982.

Schlesinger R B: Effects of inhaled acids on respiratory tract defense mechanisms, *Environ Health Perspect* 63:25-38, 1985.

Siebert S: Ocular trauma from lead-acid vehicle battery explosions, *Aust J Ophthalmol* 10:53-61, 1982.

Stewart C: Chemical skin burns, *Am Fam Phys* 31:149-157, 1985.

GUIDELINE 16

Books

Amdur MO, Doull J, Klaassen CD, editors: *Casarett and Doull's toxicology, the basic science of poisons,* ed 4, New York, 1991, Pergamon Press.

CANUTEC: *Initial emergency response guide 1992,* Ottawa, Canada, 1992, Canada Communication Group.

CCINFO: *MSDS/CHEMINFO* (CD-ROM version), Hamilton, Ontario, Canada, 1993, Canadian Centre for Occupational Health and Safety.

DOT: *CHRIS hazardous chemical data.* US Department of Transportation/United States Coast Guard. Washington, DC, 1984, US Government Printing Office.

DOT: *2000 Emergency response guidebook,* Office of Hazardous Materials Transportation, Research and Special Programs Administration, Washington, DC, 2000, US Department of Transportation.

Goldfrank LR, et al: *Goldfrank's toxicologic emergencies,* ed 6, New York, 1998, McGraw-Hill Professional.

Gosselin RE, Smith RP, Hodge HC: *Clinical toxicology of commercial products,* ed 5, Baltimore, 1984, Williams & Wilkins.

Haddad LM, et al: *Clinical management of poisoning and drug overdose,* ed 3, Philadelphia, 1997, Saunders.

Mackison FW, Stricoff RS, Partridge LJ Jr, editors: *Occupational health guidelines for chemical hazards,* NIOSH/OSHA, Washington, DC, 1981, US Government Printing Office.

NIOSH: *NIOSH pocket guide to chemical hazards* (CD-ROM version), Cincinnati, 2000, DHHS (NIOSH), US Government Printing Office.

Olson KR, editor: *Poisoning & drug overdose,* ed 3, East Norwalk, Conn, 1999, Appleton & Lange.

Sullivan JB, Kriger GR, editors: *Clinical environmental health and hazardous materials toxicology,* Baltimore, 1997, Williams & Wilkins.

Journals

Baran R: Acute onycholysis from rust-removing agents, *Arch Derm* 116:382-383, 1980.

Bertolini JC: Hydrofluoric acid: a review of toxicity, *J Emerg Med* 10:163-168, 1992.

Braun J, Stoss J, Zorber A: Intoxication following the inhalation of hydrogen fluoride, *Arch Toxicol* 56:50-54, 1984.

Brown M: Fluoride exposure from hydrofluoric acid in a motor gasoline alkylation unit, *Am Ind Hyg Assoc J* 46:662-669, 1985.

Cappell MS, Simon T: Fulminant acute colitis following a self-administered hydrofluoric acid enema. *Am J Gastroenterol 88*:122-126, 1993.

Catton V: Prevention and treatment of hydrofluoric acid burns, *Occup Health* 35:227-231, 1983.

Chick LR, Borah G: Calcium carbonate gel therapy for hydrofluoric acid burns of the hand, *Plast Reconstr Surg* 86:935-940, Nov 1990.

Dunn BJ: Hydrofluoric acid dermal burns. An assessment of treatment efficacy using an experimental pig model. *J Occup Med* 34(9):902-909, Sept 1992.

Fitzpatrick K, Moylan J: Emergency care of chemical burns, *Postgrad Med* 78:189-194, 1985.

Mayer T, Gross P: Fatal systemic fluorosis due to hydrofluoric acid burns, *Ann Emerg Med* 14:149-153, 1985.

Menchel S, Dunn W: Hydrofluoric acid poisoning, *J Am J Forensic Med Pathol* 5:245-248, 1984.

Schenker M: Occupational lung diseases in the industrializing and industrialized world due to moderate industries and modern pollutants. *Tuber Lung Dis* 73:27-32, 1992.

Stremski ES, Grande GA, Ling LJ: Survival following hydrofluoric acid ingestion, *Ann Emerg Med* 21(11):1396-1399, 1992.

Trevino M, Herrmann G, Sprout W: Treatment of severe hydrofluoric acid exposures, *J Occup Med* 25:861-863, 1983.

Tepperman P: Fatality due to acute systemic fluoride poisoning following a hydrofluoric acid burn, *J Occup Med* 22:691-692, 1980.

Upfal M, Doyle C: Medical management of hydrofluoric acid exposure. *J Occup Med* 32:726-731, 1990.

Vance MV, et al: Digital hydrofluoric acid burns: treatment with intraarterial calcium infusion, *Ann Emerg Med* 15:890-896, 1986.

Velvart J: Arterial perfusion for hydrofluoric acid burns, *Hum Toxicol* 2:233-238, 1983.

White DA: Hydrofluoric acid—a chronic poisoning effect, *J Soc Occup Med* 30:12-14, 1980.

White J: Hydrofluoric acid burns, *Cutis* 34:241-244, 1984.

Wing JS, et al: Acute health effects in a community after a release of hydrofluoric acid, *Arch Environ Health* 46:155-160, 1991.

GUIDELINE 17

Books

Amdur MO, Doull J, Klaassen CD, editors: *Casarett and Doull's Toxicology, the basic science of poisons,* ed 4, New York, 1991, Pergamon Press.

CANUTEC: *Initial emergency response guide 1992,* Ottawa, Canada, 1992, Canada Communication Group.

CCINFO: *MSDS/CHEMINFO* (CD-ROM version), Hamilton, Ontario, Canada, 1993, Canadian *MSDS/CHEMINFO* Centre for Occupational Health and Safety.

DOT: *CHRIS hazardous chemical data.* US Department of Transportation/United States Coast Guard. Washington, DC, 1984, US Government Printing Office.

DOT: *2000 Emergency response guidebook,* Office of Hazardous Materials Transportation, Research and Special Programs Administration, Washington, DC, 2000, US Department of Transportation.

Goldfrank LR, et al: *Goldfrank's toxicologic emergencies,* ed 6, New York, 1998,McGraw-Hill Professional.

Gosselin RE, Smith RP, Hodge HC: *Clinical toxicology of commercial products,* ed 5, Baltimore, 1984, Williams & Wilkins.

Haddad LM, et al: *Clinical management of poisoning and drug overdose,* ed 3, Philadelphia, 1997, Saunders.

Mackison FW, Stricoff RS, Partridge LJ Jr, editors: *Occupational health guidelines for chemical hazards,* NIOSH/OSHA, Washington, DC, 1981, US Government Printing Office.

NIOSH: *NIOSH pocket guide to chemical hazards* (CD-ROM version), Cincinnati, 2000, DHHS (NIOSH), US Government Printing Office.

Journals

Campbell WA: Oxalic acid, epsom salt and the poison bottle, *Hum Toxicol* 1:187-193, 1982.

Clarke MJ: Poisoned by oxalic acid (letter), *Lancet* 335:233-234, 1990.

Farre M, et al: Fatal oxalic acid poisoning from sorrel soup (letter), *Lancet* 334:1524, 1989.

Fitzpatrick K, Moylan J: Emergency care of chemical burns, *Postgrad Med* 78:189-194, 1985.

GUIDELINE 18

Books

CANUTEC: *Initial emergency response guide 1992,* Ottawa, Canada, 1992, Canada Communication Group.

DOT: *2000 Emergency response guidebook,* Office of Hazardous Materials Transportation, Research and Special Programs Administration, Washington, DC, 2000, US Department of Transportation.

Sullivan JB, Kriger GR, editors: *Clinical environmental health and hazardous materials toxicology,* Baltimore, 1997, Williams & Wilkins.

Journals

Abrams J, El-Mallakh RS, Meyer R: Suicidal sodium azide ingestion, *Ann Emerg Med* 1378-1380, 1987.

Albertson TE, Reed S, Siefkin A: A case of fatal sodium azide ingestion, *Clin Toxicol* 24:339-351, 1986.

Gordon SM, et al: Epidemic hypotension in a dialysis center caused by sodium azide, *Kidney Int* 37:110-115, 1990.

Howard JD, et al: Death following accidental sodium azide ingestion, *J Forensic Sci* 35:193-196, 1990.

Judge KW, Ward NE: Fatal azide-induced cardiomyopathy presenting as acute myocardial infarction, *Am J Cardiol* 64:830-831, 1989.

Personal Communication (PLC), Ford Motor Company, 1993.

Smally AJ, et al: Alkaline chemical keratitis: eye injury from airbags, *Ann Emerg Med* 21:1400-1402, 1992.

GUIDELINE 19

Books

Amdur MO, Doull J, Klaassen CD, editors: *Casarett and Doull's toxicology, the basic science of poisons,* ed 4, New York, 1991, Pergamon Press.

CANUTEC: *Initial emergency response guide 1992,* Ottawa, Canada, 1992, Canada Communication Group.

CCINFO: *MSDS/CHEMINFO* (CD-ROM version), Hamilton, Ontario, Canada, 1993, Canadian Centre for Occupational Health and Safety.

DOT: *CHRIS hazardous chemical data.* US Department of Transportation/United States Coast Guard. Washington, DC, 1984, US Government Printing Office.

DOT: *2000 Emergency response guidebook,* Office of Hazardous Materials Transportation, Research and Special Programs Administration, Washington, DC, 2000, US Department of Transportation.

Ellenhorn MJ, Barceloux DG: *Medical toxicology diagnosis and treatment of human poisoning,* New York, 1988, Elsevier Science Publishing.

Gosselin RE, Smith RP, Hodge HC: *Clinical toxicology of commercial products,* ed 5, Baltimore, 1984, Williams & Wilkins.

Haddad LM, et al: *Clinical management of poisoning and drug overdose,* ed 3, Philadelphia, 1997, Saunders.

Mackison FW, Stricoff RS, Partridge LJ Jr, editors: *Occupational health guidelines for chemical hazards,* NIOSH/OSHA, Washington, DC, 1981, US Government Printing Office.

NIOSH: *NIOSH pocket guide to chemical hazards* (CD-ROM version), Cincinnati, 2000, DHHS (NIOSH), US Government Printing Office.

Noji EK, Kelen GD, editors: *Manual of toxicologic emergencies,* Chicago, Ill, 1989, Year Book Medical Publishers.

Olson KR, editor: *Poisoning & drug overdose,* ed 3, East Norwalk, Conn, 1999, Appleton & Lange.

Journals

Anderson KD, Rouse TM, Randolph JG: A controlled trial of corticosteroids in children with corrosive injury of the esophagus, *N Engl J Med* 323:637-640, 1990.

Anderson KD, Rouse TM, Randolph JG: Corticosteroids in children with corrosive injury of the esophagus, *N Engl J Med* 324:418-419, 1991.

Gelmetti C, Cecca E: Caustic ulcers caused by calcium hydroxide in 2 adolescent football players, *Contact Dermatitis* 27:19-20, 1992.

Gomez SR, et al: Respiratory health effects of alkali dust in residents near desiccated Old Wives Lake, *Arch Environ Health* 47:364-369, 1992.

Gumaste VV, Dave PB: Ingestion of corrosive substances by adults, *Am J Gastroenterol* 87:1-5, 1992.

Lovejoy FH: Corrosive injury of the esophagus in children, *N Engl J Med* 323:668-670, 1990.

Rozenbaum D, Baruchin AM, Dafna Z: Chemical burns of the eye with special reference to alkali burns, *Burns* 17:136-140, 1991.

Zargar SA, et al: Ingestion of strong corrosive alkalis: spectrum of injury to upper gastrointestinal tract and natural history, *Am J Gastroenterol* 87:337-341, 1992.

GUIDELINE 20

Books

Amdur MO, Doull J, Klaassen CD, editors: *Casarett and Doull's toxicology, the basic science of poisons,* ed 4, New York, 1991, Pergamon Press.

CANUTEC: *Initial emergency response guide 1992,* Ottawa, Canada, 1992, Canada Communication Group.

CCINFO: *MSDS/CHEMINFO* (CD-ROM version), Hamilton, Ontario, Canada, 1993, Canadian Centre for Occupational Health and Safety.

DOT: *2000 Emergency response guidebook,* Office of Hazardous Materials Transportation, Research and Special Programs Administration, Washington, DC, 2000, US Department of Transportation.

Gosselin RE, Smith RP, Hodge HC: *Clinical toxicology of commercial products,* ed 5, Baltimore, 1984, Williams & Wilkins.

HSDB: *Hazardous Substances Data Bank,* National Library of Medicine, Bethesda, Md, 1993.

NIOSH: *NIOSH pocket guide to chemical hazards* (CD-ROM version), Cincinnati, 2000, DHHS (NIOSH), US Government Printing Office.

Sullivan JB, Kriger GR, editors: *Clinical environmental health and hazardous materials toxicology,* Baltimore, 1997, Williams & Wilkins.

Journal

Leung HW, Paustenbach DJ: Organic acids and bases: review of toxicological studies, *Am J Ind Med* 18:717-735, 1990.

GUIDELINE 21

Books

Amdur MO, Doull J, Klaassen CD, editors: *Casarett and Doull's toxicology, the basic science of poisons,* ed 4, New York, 1991, Pergamon Press.

CANUTEC: *Initial emergency response guide 1992,* Ottawa, Canada, 1992, Canada Communication Group.

CCINFO: *MSDS/CHEMINFO* (CD-ROM version), Hamilton, Ontario, Canada, 1993, Canadian Centre for Occupational Health and Safety.

DOT: *CHRIS hazardous chemical data.* US Department of Transportation/United States Coast Guard. Washington, DC, 1984, US Government Printing Office.

DOT: *2000 Emergency response guidebook,* Office of Hazardous Materials Transportation, Research and Special Programs Administration, Washington, DC, 2000, US Department of Transportation.

Ellenhorn MJ, Barceloux DG: *Medical toxicology diagnosis and treatment of human poisoning,* New York, 1988, Elsevier Science Publishing.

Gosselin RE, Smith RP, Hodge HC: *Clinical toxicology of commercial products,* ed 5, Baltimore, 1984, Williams & Wilkins.

Haddad LM, et al: *Clinical management of poisoning and drug overdose,* ed 3, Philadelphia, 1997, Saunders.

Mackison F W, Stricoff RS, Partridge LJ Jr, editors: *Occupational health guidelines for chemical hazards,* NIOSH/OSHA, Washington, DC, 1981, US Government Printing Office.

NIOSH: *NIOSH pocket guide to chemical hazards* (CD-ROM version), Cincinnati, 2000, DHHS (NIOSH), US Government Printing Office.

Sullivan JB, Kriger GR, editors: *Clinical environmental health and hazardous materials toxicology,* Baltimore, 1997, Williams & Wilkins.

Journals

Anderson KD, Rouse TM, Randolph JG: A controlled trial of corticosteroids in children with corrosive injury of the esophagus, *N Engl J Med* 323:637-640, 1990.

Arwood R, Hammond J, Ward G: Ammonia inhalation, *J Trauma* 25:444-446, 1985.

Hoeffler H, Schweppe H, Greenberg S: Bronchiectasis following pulmonary ammonia burn, *Arch Pathol Lab Med* 106:686-687, 1982.

Klein J, Olson K: Caustic injury from household ammonia (letter), *J Pediatr* 108:328, 1986.

Klein J, Olson K, McKinney H: Caustic injury from household ammonia, *Am J Emerg Med* 3:320, 1985.

Leduc D, et al: Acute and long term respiratory damage following inhalation of ammonia, *Thorax* 47:755-757, 1992.

Moon ME, Robertson IF: Retrospective study of alkali burns of the eye, *Aust J Ophthalmol* 11:281-286, 1983.

O'Kane GJ: Inhalation of ammonia vapor, a report on the management of eight patients during the acute stages, *Anesthesia* 38:1208-1213, 1983.

Swotinsky RB, Chase KH: Health effects of exposure to ammonia: scant information, *Am J Ind Med* 17:515-521, 1990.

Tsujii M, et al: Mechanism of gastric mucosal damage induced by ammonia, *Gastroenterology* 102:1881-1888, 1992.

GUIDELINE 22

Books

CANUTEC: *Initial emergency response guide 1992,* Ottawa, Canada, 1992, Canada Communication Group.

CCINFO: *MSDS/CHEMINFO* (CD-ROM version), Hamilton, Ontario, Canada, 1993, Canadian Centre for Occupational Health and Safety.

DOT: *CHRIS hazardous chemical data.* US Department of Transportation/United States Coast Guard. Washington, DC, 1984, US Government Printing Office.

DOT: *2000 Emergency response guidebook,* Office of Hazardous Materials Transportation, Research and Special Programs Administration, Washington, DC, 2000, US Department of Transportation.

Ellenhorn MJ, Barceloux DG: *Medical toxicology diagnosis and treatment of human poisoning,* New York, 1988, Elsevier Science Publishing.

Gosselin RE, Smith RP, Hodge HC: *Clinical toxicology of commercial products,* ed 5, Baltimore, 1984, Williams & Wilkins.

Haddad LM, et al: *Clinical management of poisoning and drug overdose,* ed 3, Philadelphia, 1997, Saunders.

NIOSH: *NIOSH pocket guide to chemical hazards* (CD-ROM version), Cincinnati, 2000, DHHS (NIOSH), US Government Printing Office.

Sullivan JB, Kriger GR, editors: *Clinical environmental health and hazardous materials toxicology,* Baltimore, 1997, Williams & Wilkins.

Journals

Hoy RH: Accidental systemic exposure to sodium hypochlorite (Clorox) during hemodialysis, *Am J Hosp Pharm* 38:1512-1514, 1981.

Jakobsson SW, et al: Poisoning with sodium hypochlorite solution. Report of a fatal case, supplemented with an experimental and clinico-epidemiological study, *Am J Forensic Med Pathol* 12:320-327, 1991.

Morgan DL: Intravenous injection of household bleach, *Ann Emerg Med* 21:1394-1395, 1992.

GUIDELINE 23

Books

CANUTEC: *Initial emergency response guide 1992,* Ottawa, Canada, 1992, Canada Communication Group.

CCINFO: *MSDS/CHEMINFO* (CD-ROM version), Hamilton, Ontario, Canada, 1993, Canadian Centre for Occupational Health and Safety.

DOT: *2000 Emergency response guidebook,* Office of Hazardous Materials Transportation, Research and Special Programs Administration, Washington, DC, 2000, US Department of Transportation.

Gosselin RE, Smith RP, Hodge HC: *Clinical toxicology of commercial products,* ed 5, Baltimore, 1984, Williams & Wilkins.

Haddad LM, et al: *Clinical management of poisoning and drug overdose,* ed 3, Philadelphia, 1997, Saunders.

NIOSH: *NIOSH pocket guide to chemical hazards* (CD-ROM version), Cincinnati, 2000, DHHS (NIOSH), US Government Printing Office.

Sullivan JB, Kriger GR, editors: *Clinical environmental health and hazardous materials toxicology,* Baltimore, 1997, Williams & Wilkins.

Journals

Gent WL, et al: Factors in hydrazine formation from isoniazid by pediatric and adult tuberculosis patients, *Eur J Clin Pharmacol* 43:131-136, 1992.

Keller WC: Toxicity assessment of hydrazine fuels, *Aviat Space Environ Med* 59(11 Suppl):A100-A106, 1988.

Preece NE, Ghatineh S, Timbrell JA: Studies on the disposition and metabolism of hydrazine in rats in vivo, *Hum Exp Toxicol* 11:121-127, 1992.

Wald N, et al: Occupational exposure to hydrazine and subsequent risk of cancer, *Br J Ind Med* 41:31-34, 1984.

Wrangsjo K, Martensson A: Hydrazine contact dermatitis from gold plating, *Contact Dermatitis* 15:244-245, 1986.

GUIDELINE 24

Books

Amdur MO, Doull J, Klaassen CD, editors: *Casarett and Doull's toxicology, the basic science of poisons,* ed 4, New York, 1991, Pergamon Press.

Arena J M, et al: *Poisoning.* Springfield, Ill, 1986, Charles C Thomas.

CANUTEC: *Initial emergency response guide 1992,* Ottawa, Canada, 1992, Canada Communication Group.

CCINFO: *MSDS/CHEMINFO* (CD-ROM version), Hamilton, Ontario, Canada, 1993, Canadian Centre for Occupational Health and Safety.

DOT: *CHRIS hazardous chemical data.* US Department of Transportation/United States Coast Guard. Washington, DC, 1984, US Government Printing Office.

DOT: *2000 Emergency response guidebook,* Office of Hazardous Materials Transportation, Research and Special Programs Administration, Washington, DC, 2000, US Department of Transportation.

Gosselin RE, Smith RP, Hodge HC: *Clinical toxicology of commercial products,* ed 5, Baltimore, 1984, Williams & Wilkins.

Haddad LM, et al: *Clinical management of poisoning and drug overdose,* ed 3, Philadelphia, 1997, Saunders.

Hartman DE: *Neuropsychological toxicology, identification and assessment of human neurotoxic syndromes,* New York, 1988, Pergamon Press.

Mackison FW, Stricoff RS, Partridge LJ Jr, editors: *Occupational health guidelines for chemical hazards,* NIOSH/OSHA, Washington, DC, 1981, US Government Printing Office.

NIOSH: *NIOSH pocket guide to chemical hazards* (CD-ROM version), Cincinnati, 2000, DHHS (NIOSH), US Government Printing Office.

Snyder R, editor: *Ethel Browning's toxicity and metabolism of industrial solvents,* vol I, Hydrocarbons, New York, 1987, Elsevier Science Publishers.

Sullivan JB, Kriger GR, editors: *Clinical environmental health and hazardous materials toxicology,* Baltimore, 1997, Williams & Wilkins.

Journals

Angerer J, Wolf H: Occupational chronic exposure to organic solvents, XI. Alkylbenzene exposure of varnish workers: effects on hematopoietic system, *Int Arch Occup Environ Health* 56:307-321, 1985.

Donald JM, Hooper K, Hopenhayn-Rich C: Reproductive and developmental toxicity of toluene: a review, *Environ Health Perspect* 94: 237-244, 1991.

Dudek BR, et al: Structure-activity relationship of a series of sensory irritants, *J Toxicol Environ Health* 37:511-518, 1992.

Filley CM, Heaton RK, Rosenberg NL: White matter dementia in chronic toluene abuse, *Neurology* 40:532-534, 1990.

Foo SC, Jeyaratnam J, Koh D: Chronic neurobehavioural effects of toluene, *Br J Ind Med* 47:480-484, 1990.

Grasso P, et al: Neurophysiological and psychological disorders and occupational exposure to organic solvents, *Food Chem Toxicol* 22:819-852, 1984.

Hollo G, Varga M, Leigh RJ: Toluene and visual loss, *Neurology* 42:266, 1992.

Ikeda N, et al: The course of respiration and circulation in toluene-sniffing, *Forensic Sci Intl* 44:151-158, 1990.

Jie L, Quan-Guan J, Wei-Dong Z: Persistent ethanol drinking increases liver injury induced by trinitrotoluene exposure: an in-plant case-control study, *Hum Exp Toxicol* 10:405-409, 1991.

Knight AT, et al: Upholsterers' glue associated with myocarditis, hepatitis, acute renal failure and lymphoma, *Med J Aust* 154:360-362, 1991.

Lof A, Wallen M, Hjelm EW: Influence of paracetamol and acetylsalicylic acid on toxicokinetics of toluene, *Pharmacol Toxicol* 66:138-141, 1990.

Luo J-C J, Nelsen KG, Fischbein A: Persistent reactive airway dysfunction syndrome after exposure to toluene diisocyanate, *Br J Ind Med* 47:239-241, 1990.

Ng TP, Foo SC, Yoong T: Menstrual function in workers exposed to toluene, *Br J Ind Med* 49:799-803, 1992.

Ng TP, Foo SC, Yoong T: Risk of spontaneous abortion in workers exposed to toluene, *Br J Ind Med* 49:804-808, 1992.

Pryor G, et al: The hearing loss associated with exposure to toluene is not caused by a metabolite, *Brain Res Bull* 27:109-113, 1991.

Sevcik P, Hep A, Peslova M: Intravenous xylene poisoning, *Int Care Med* 18:377-378, 1992.

Spencer PS, Schaumburg HH: Organic solvent neurotoxicity. Facts and research needs, *Scand J Work Environ Health* 11(Suppl 1):53-60, 1985.

Svensson BG, et al: Deaths and tumours among rotogravure printers exposed to toluene, *Br J Ind Med* 47:372-379, 1990.

Svensson BG, et al: Neuroendocrine effects in printing workers exposed to toluene, *Br J Ind Med* 49:402-408, 1992.

Svensson BG et al: Hormone status in occupational toluene exposure, *Am J Ind Med* 22:99-107, 1992.

Tan EL, et al: Mutagenicity of trinitrotoluene and its metabolites formed during composting, *J Toxicol Environ Health* 36:165-175, 1992.

GUIDELINE 25

Books

Amdur MO, Doull J, Klaassen CD, editors: *Casarett and Doull's toxicology, the basic science of poisons,* ed 4, New York, 1991, Pergamon Press.

CANUTEC*: Initial emergency response guide 1992,* Ottawa, Canada, 1992, Canada Communication Group.

CCINFO: *MSDS/CHEMINFO* (CD-ROM version), Hamilton, Ontario, Canada, 1993, Canadian Centre for Occupational Health and Safety.

DOT: *CHRIS hazardous chemical data,* US Department of Transportation/United States Coast Guard, Washington, DC, 1984, US Government Printing Office.

DOT: *2000 Emergency response guidebook,* Office of Hazardous Materials Transportation, Research and Special Programs Administration, Washington, DC, 2000, US Department of Transportation.

Gosselin RE, Smith RP, Hodge HC: *Clinical toxicology of commercial products,* ed 5, Baltimore, 1984, Williams & Wilkins.

Haddad LM, et al: *Clinical management of poisoning and drug overdose,* ed 3, Philadelphia, 1997, Saunders.

Mackison FW, Stricoff RS, Partridge LJ Jr, editors: *Occupational health guidelines for chemical hazards,* NIOSH/OSHA, Washington, DC, 1981, US Government Printing Office.

NIOSH: *NIOSH pocket guide to chemical hazards* (CD-ROM version), Cincinnati, 2000, DHHS (NIOSH), US Government Printing Office.

Olson KR, editor: *Poisoning & drug overdose,* ed 3, East Norwalk, Conn, 1999, Appleton & Lange.

Snyder R, editor: *Ethel Browning's toxicity and metabolism of industrial solvents,* vol I, Hydrocarbons, New York, 1987, Elsevier Science Publishers.

Sullivan JB, Kriger GR, editors: *Clinical environmental health and hazardous materials toxicology,* Baltimore, 1997, Williams & Wilkins.

Journals

Angerer J, Wolf H: Occupational chronic exposure to organic solvents, XI. Alkylbenzene exposure of varnish workers: effects on hematopoietic system, *Int Arch Occup Environ Health* 56:307-321, 1985.

Collins JJ et al: A study of the hematologic effects of chronic low-level exposure to benzene, *J Occup Med* 33:619-626, 1991.

Dean B: Recent findings on the genetic toxicology of benzene, toluene, xylenes and phenols, *Mutat Res* 154:153-181, 1985.

Infante PF: Benzene toxicity: studying a subject to death, *Am J Ind Med* 52:599-604, 1987.

Johnson ES, Lucier G: Perspectives on risk assessment impact of recent reports on benzene, *Am J Ind Med* 21:749-757, 1992.

Mehlman MA: Benzene health effects: Unanswered questions still not addressed, *Am J Ind Med* 20:707-711, 1991.

Midzenski MA, et al: Acute high dose exposure to benzene in shipyard workers, *Am J Ind Med* 22:553-565, 1992.

Popp W: Investigations of the frequency of DNA strand breakage and cross-linking and of sister chromatid exchange frequency in the lymphocytes of female workers exposed to benzene and toluene, *Carcinogenesis* 13:57-61, 1992.

Spencer PS, Schaumburg HH: Organic solvent neurotoxicity. Facts and research needs, *Scand J Work Environ Health* 11(Suppl 1):53-60, 1985.

Wolff SP: Correlation between car ownership and leukaemia: Is non-occupational exposure to benzene from petrol and motor vehicle exhaust a causative factor in leukaemia and lymphoma? *Experientia* 48:301-304, 1992.

Yardley-Jones A et al: Analysis of chromosomal aberrations in workers exposed to low level benzene, *Br J Ind Med* 47:48-51, 1990.

GUIDELINE 26

Books

Amdur MO, Doull J, Klaassen CD, editors: *Casarett and Doull's toxicology, the basic science of poisons,* ed 4, New York, 1991, Pergamon Press.

CANUTEC: *Initial emergency response guide 1992,* Ottawa, Canada, 1992, Canada Communication Group.

CCINFO: *MSDS/CHEMINFO* (CD-ROM version), Hamilton, Ontario, Canada, 1993, Canadian Centre for Occupational Health and Safety.

DOT: *2000 Emergency response guidebook,* Office of Hazardous Materials Transportation, Research and Special Programs Administration, Washington, DC, 2000, US Department of Transportation.

Ellenhorn MJ, Barceloux DG: *Medical toxicology diagnosis and treatment of human poisoning,* New York, 1988, Elsevier Science Publishing.

Gosselin RE, Smith RP, Hodge HC: *Clinical toxicology of commercial products,* ed 5, Baltimore, 1984, Williams & Wilkins.

Hartman DE: *Neuropsychological toxicology, identification and assessment of human neurotoxic syndromes,* New York, 1988, Pergamon Press.

NIOSH: *NIOSH pocket guide to chemical hazards* (CD-ROM version), Cincinnati, 2000, DHHS (NIOSH), US Government Printing Office.

Sullivan JB, Kriger GR, editors: *Clinical environmental health and hazardous materials toxicology,* Baltimore, 1997, Williams & Wilkins.

Journals

Davis ME: Dichloroacetic acid and trichloroacetic acid increase chloroform toxicity, *J Toxicol Environ Health* 37:139-148, 1992.

Hearne FT, Pifer JW, Grose F: Absence of adverse mortality effects to methylene chloride: an update, *J Occup Med* 32:234-240, 1990.

Houck P, Nebel D, Milham S: Organic solvent encephalopathy: an old hazard revisited, *Am J Ind Med* 22:109-115, 1992.

Ingber A: Occupational allergic contact dermatitis from methyl chloroform (1,1,1-trichloroethane), *Contact Dermatitis* 25:193, 1991.

Kostrzewski P, Jakubowski M, Kolacinski Z: Kinetics of trichloroethylene elimination from venous blood after acute inhalation poisoning, *Clin Toxicol* 31:353-363, 1993.

Lindbohm ML, et al: Spontaneous abortions among women exposed to organic solvents, *Am J Ind Med* 17:449-463, 1990.

Manno M, Rugge M, Cocheo V: Double fatal inhalation of dichloromethane, *Hum Exp Toxicol* 11:540-545, 1992.

Mutti A, et al: Nephropathies and exposure to perchloroethylene in dry-cleaners, *Lancet* 340:189-193, 1992.

Olsen J, et al: Low birthweight, congenital malformations, and spontaneous abortions among dry-cleaning workers in Scandinavia, *Scand J Work Environ Health* 16:163-168, 1990.

Ruijten MWMM, Verberk MM, Salle HJA: Nerve function in workers with long term exposure to trichloroethane, *Br J Ind Med* 48:87-92, 1991.

Shusterman D, et al: Methylene chloride intoxication in a furniture refinisher, *J Occup Med* 32:451-454, 1990.

Seeber A, Kiesswetter E, Blaszkewicz M: Correlations between subjective disturbances due to acute exposure to organic solvents and internal dose, *Neurotoxicology* 13:265-270, 1992.

Silva-Filho AR, Pires MLN, Shiotsuki N: Anticonvulsant and convulsant effects of organic solvents, *Pharmacol Biochem Behav* 41:79-82, 1991.

Snyder RW, Mishel HS, Christensen GC: Pulmonary toxicity following exposure to methylene chloride and its combustion product, phosgene, *Chest* 101:860-861, 1992.

Snyder RW, Mishel HS, Christensen GC: Pulmonary toxicity following exposure to methylene chloride and its combustion product, phosgene (letter), *Chest* 102:1921, 1992.

Verschuuren HG, De Rooij CG: Health risk assessment of environmental exposure to 1,1,1-trichloroethane, *Regul Toxicol Pharmacol* 11:90-99, 1990.

Wrensch M, et al: Pregnancy outcomes in women potentially exposed to solvent-contaminated drinking water in San Jose, California, *Am J Epidemiol* 131:283-300, 1990.

Wodka RM, Jeong EWS: Myocardial injury following the intentional inhalation of typewriter correction fluid, *Mil Med* 156:204-205, 1991.

GUIDELINE 27

Books

Amdur MO, Doull J, Klaassen CD, editors: *Casarett and Doull's toxicology, the basic science of poisons,* ed 4, New York, 1991, Pergamon Press.

CANUTEC: *Initial emergency response guide 1992,* Ottawa, Canada, 1992, Canada Communication Group.

CCINFO: *MSDS/CHEMINFO* (CD-ROM version), Hamilton, Ontario, Canada, 1993, Canadian Centre for Occupational Health and Safety.

DOT: *2000 Emergency response guidebook,* Office of Hazardous Materials Transportation, Research and Special Programs Administration, Washington, DC, 2000, US Department of Transportation.

Gosselin RE, Smith RP, Hodge HC: *Clinical toxicology of commercial products,* ed 5, Baltimore, 1984, Williams & Wilkins.

Hartman DE: *Neuropsychological toxicology, identification and assessment of human neurotoxic syndromes,* New York, 1988, Pergamon Press.

NIOSH: *NIOSH pocket guide to chemical hazards* (CD-ROM version), Cincinnati, 2000, DHHS (NIOSH), US Government Printing Office.

Sullivan JB, Kriger GR, editors: *Clinical environmental health and hazardous materials toxicology,* Baltimore, 1997, Williams & Wilkins.

Journals

Antti-Poika M, Heikkila J, Saarinen L: Cardiac arrhythmias during occupational exposure to fluorinated hydrocarbons, *Br J Ind Med* 47:138-140, 1990.

Burris JF, Schwartz SL: Occupational exposure to freon: an association with severe hypertension? *JAMA* 267:569, 1992.

Egeland GM, et al: Fluorocarbon 113 exposure and cardiac dysrhythmias among aerospace workers, *Am J Ind Med* 22:851-857, 1992.

Holness DL, House RA: Health effects of halon 1301 exposure, *J Occup Med* 34:722-725, 1992.

Kaufman JD, et al: A study of the cardiac effects of bromochlorodifluoromethane (Halon 1211) exposure during exercise, *Am J Ind Med* 21:223-233, 1992.

Perbellini L, et al: Acute trichloroethylene poisoning by ingestion: clinical and pharmacokinetic aspects, *Intensive Care Med* 17:234-235, 1991.

GUIDELINE 28

Books

Amdur MO, Doull J, Klaassen CD, editors: *Casarett and Doull's toxicology, the basic science of poisons,* ed 4, New York, 1991, Pergamon Press.

CANUTEC: *Initial emergency response guide 1992,* Ottawa, Canada, 1992, Canada Communication Group.

CCINFO: *MSDS/CHEMINFO* (CD-ROM version), Hamilton, Ontario, Canada, 1993, Canadian Centre for Occupational Health and Safety.

DOT: *CHRIS hazardous chemical data.* US Department of Transportation/United States Coast Guard. Washington, DC, 1984, US Government Printing Office.

DOT: *2000 Emergency response guidebook,* Office of Hazardous Materials Transportation, Research and Special Programs Administration, Washington, DC, 2000, US Department of Transportation.

Gosselin RE, Smith RP, Hodge HC: *Clinical toxicology of commercial products,* ed 5, Baltimore, 1984, Williams & Wilkins.

Haddad LM, et al: *Clinical management of poisoning and drug overdose,* ed 3, Philadelphia, 1997, Saunders.

Mackison FW, Stricoff RS, Partridge LJ Jr, editors: *Occupational health guidelines for chemical hazards,* NIOSH/OSHA, Washington, DC, 1981, US Government Printing Office.

Meeks RG, Harrison SD, Bull RJ, editors: *Hepatotoxicology,* Boca Raton, Florida, 1991, CRC Press.

NIOSH: *NIOSH pocket guide to chemical hazards* (CD-ROM version), Cincinnati, 2000, DHHS (NIOSH), US Government Printing Office.

Journals

Fogel R, et al: Carbon tetrachloride poisoning treated with hemodialysis and total parenteral nutrition, *J Can Med Assoc* 128:560-561, 1983.

Hills B, Venable K: The interaction of ethyl alcohol and industrial chemicals, *Am J Ind Med* 3:321-333, 1982.

Kaminski NE, Stevens WD: The role of metabolism in carbon tetrachloride-mediated immunosuppression: in vitro studies, *Toxicology* 75:175-188, 1992.

Lindelof B, Almkvist O, Gothe CJ: Sleep disturbances and exposure to organic solvents, *Arch Environ Health* 42:104-106, 1992.

Mathieson PW, Williams G, MacSweeney JE: Survival after massive ingestion of carbon tetrachloride treated by intravenous infusion of acetylcysteine, *Hum Toxicol* 4:627-631, 1985.

Roberts SM, et al: Potentiation of carbon tetrachloride hepatotoxicity by phenylpropanolamine, *Toxicol Appl Pharmacol* 111:175-188, 1991.

Simko V, et al: Protective effect of oral acetylcysteine against the hepatorenal toxicity of carbon tetrachloride potentiated by ethyl alcohol, *Alcohol Clin Exp Res* 16:795-799, 1992.

Sjogren B, et al: Pulmonary reactions caused by welding-induced decomposed trichloroethylene, *Chest* 99:237-238, 1991.

GUIDELINE 29

Books

Amdur MO, Doull J, Klaassen CD, editors: *Casarett and Doull's toxicology, the basic science of poisons,* ed 4, New York, 1991, Pergamon Press.

CANUTEC: *Initial emergency response guide 1992,* Ottawa, Canada, 1992, Canada Communication Group.

CCINFO: *MSDS/CHEMINFO* (CD-ROM version), Hamilton, Ontario, Canada, 1993, Canadian Centre for Occupational Health and Safety.

DOT: *CHRIS hazardous chemical data,* US Department of Transportation/United States Coast Guard, Washington, DC, 1984, US Government Printing Office.

DOT: *2000 Emergency response guidebook,* Office of Hazardous Materials Transportation, Research and Special Programs Administration, Washington, DC, 2000, US Department of Transportation.

Gosselin RE, Smith RP, Hodge HC: *Clinical toxicology of commercial products,* ed 5, Baltimore, 1984, Williams & Wilkins.

Haddad LM, et al: *Clinical management of poisoning and drug overdose,* ed 3, Philadelphia, 1997, Saunders.

Hartman DE: *Neuropsychological toxicology, identification and assessment of human neurotoxic syndromes,* New York, 1988, Pergamon Press.

Mackison FW, Stricoff RS, Partridge LJ Jr, editors: *Occupational health guidelines for chemical hazards,* NIOSH/OSHA, Washington, DC, 1981, US Government Printing Office.

Meeks RG, Harrison SD, Bull RJ, editors: *Hepatotoxicology,* Boca Raton, Florida, 1991, CRC Press.

Merigan WH, Weiss B, editors: *Neurotoxicity of the visual system,* New York, 1980, Raven Press.

NIOSH: *NIOSH pocket guide to chemical hazards* (CD-ROM version), Cincinnati, 2000, DHHS (NIOSH), US Government Printing Office.

Sullivan JB, Kriger GR, editors: *Clinical environmental health and hazardous materials toxicology,* Baltimore, 1997, Williams & Wilkins.

Journals

Alexander C, McBay A, Hudson R: Isopropanol and isopropanol deaths—ten years experience, *J Forensic Sci* 27:541-548, 1982.

Enterline P: Importance of sequential exposure in the production of epichlorohydrin and isopropanol, *Ann N Y Acad Sci* 381:344-349, 1982.

Hawley P, Faldo J: "Pseudo" renal failure after isopropyl alcohol intoxication, *South Med J* 75:630-631, 1982.

Hoffman RS, et al: Osmol gaps revisited: normal values and limitations, *Clin Toxicol* 31:81-93, 1993.

Kelner M, Bailey D: Isopropanol ingestion: interpretation of blood concentrations and clinical findings, *J Toxicol Clin Toxicol* 20:497-507, 1983.

Kumar S: Adverse drug reactions in the newborn, *Ann Clin Lab Sci* 15:195-203, 1985.

Lacouture R, Wason S, Abrams A, Lovejoy F: Acute isopropyl alcohol intoxication: diagnosis and management, *Am J Med* 75:680-686, 1983.

Litovitz R: The alcohols: ethanol, methanol, isopropanol, ethylene glycol, *Pediatr Clin North Am* 33:311-323, 1986.

Natocicz M, et al: Pharmacokinetic analysis of a case of isopropanol intoxication, *Clin Chem* 19:265-271, 1985.

Olson E, McEnrue J, Greenbaum D M: Clinical aspects of drug intoxication: alcohols and miscellaneous agents, *Heart Lung* 12:127-130, 1983.

Rosansky SJ: Isopropyl alcohol poisoning treated with hemodialysis: kinetics of isopropyl alcohol and acetone removal, *J Toxicol Clin Toxicol* 19:265-271, 1982.

Smith MS: Solvent toxicity: isopropanol, methanol, and ethylene glycol, *Ear Nose Throat J* 62:126-135, 1983.

Taylor CD, Cowart CO, Ryan NT: Isopropanol intoxication: managing the coma, *Hosp Pract* 20:173-175, 1985.

Webster H, Shutack J, Norman M, Raphaely R: Diagnostic clinical osmometry in the unconscious infant, *Crit Care Med* 31:1076-1077, 1985.

GUIDELINE 30

Books

CANUTEC: *Initial emergency response guide 1992,* Ottawa, Canada, 1992, Canada Communication Group.

CCINFO: *MSDS/CHEMINFO* (CD-ROM version), Hamilton, Ontario, Canada, 1993, Canadian Centre for Occupational Health and Safety.

DOT: *CHRIS hazardous chemical data.* US Department of Transportation/United States Coast Guard. Washington, DC, 1984, US Government Printing Office.

DOT: *2000 Emergency response guidebook,* Office of Hazardous Materials Transportation, Research and Special Programs Administration, Washington, DC, 2000, US Department of Transportation.

Goldfrank LR, Flomenbaum NE, Lewin NA, Weisman RS, Howland MA: *Goldfrank's toxicologic emergencies,* ed 4, Norwalk, Conn, 1990, Appleton & Lange.

Gosselin RE, Smith RP, Hodge HC: *Clinical toxicology of commercial products,* ed 5, Baltimore, 1984, Williams & Wilkins.

Haddad LM, et al: *Clinical management of poisoning and drug overdose,* ed 3, Philadelphia, 1997, Saunders.

Mackison FW, Stricoff RS, Partridge LJ Jr, editors: *Occupational health guidelines for chemical hazards,* NIOSH/OSHA, Washington, DC, 1981, US Government Printing Office.

Meeks RG, Harrison SD, Bull RJ, editors: *Hepatotoxicology,* Boca Raton, Florida, 1991, CRC Press.

NIOSH: *NIOSH pocket guide to chemical hazards* (CD-ROM version), Cincinnati, 2000, DHHS (NIOSH), US Government Printing Office.

Sullivan JB, Kriger GR, editors: *Clinical environmental health and hazardous materials toxicology,* Baltimore, 1997, Williams & Wilkins.

Journals

Henson EV: The toxicology of some aliphatic alcohols, part 2, *J Occup Med* 2:497-502, 1960.

McCreery MJ, Hunt WA: Physico-chemical correlates of alcohol intoxication, *Neuropharmacology* 17:451-461, 1978.

GUIDELINE 31

Books

Amdur MO, Doull J, Klaassen CD, editors: *Casarett and Doull's toxicology, the basic science of poisons,* ed 4, New York, 1991, Pergamon Press.

Baselt RC, Cravey RH: *Disposition of toxic drugs and chemicals in man,* ed 3, Chicago, 1989, Year Book Medical Publishers.

CANUTEC: *Initial emergency response guide 1992,* Ottawa, Canada, 1992, Canada Communication Group.

CCINFO: *MSDS/CHEMINFO* (CD-ROM version), Hamilton, Ontario, Canada, 1993, Canadian Centre for Occupational Health and Safety.

DOT: *CHRIS hazardous chemical data.* US Department of Transportation/United States Coast Guard. Washington, DC, 1984, US Government Printing Office.

DOT: *2000 Emergency response guidebook,* Office of Hazardous Materials Transportation, Research and Special Programs Administration, Washington, DC, 2000, US Department of Transportation.

Goldfrank LR, et al: *Goldfrank's toxicologic emergencies,* ed 6, New York, 1998, McGraw-Hill Professional.

Gosselin RE, Smith RP, Hodge HC: *Clinical toxicology of commercial products,* ed 5, Baltimore, 1984, Williams & Wilkins.

Haddad LM, et al: *Clinical management of poisoning and drug overdose,* ed 3, Philadelphia, 1997, Saunders.

Levy G: *Level II hazardous materials test.* Fort Collins, Colo, 1985, GML Consultants.

Mackison FW, Stricoff RS, Partridge LJ Jr, editors: *Occupational health guidelines for chemical hazards,* NIOSH/OSHA, Washington, DC, 1981, US Government Printing Office.

Meeks RG, Harrison SD, Bull RJ, editors: *Hepatotoxicology,* Boca Raton, Florida, 1991, CRC Press.

Merigan WH, Weiss B, editors: *Neurotoxicity of the Visual System,* New York, 1980, Raven Press.

NIOSH: *NIOSH pocket guide to chemical hazards* (CD-ROM version), Cincinnati, 2000, DHHS (NIOSH), US Government Printing Office.

Olson KR, editor: *Poisoning & drug overdose,* ed 3, East Norwalk, Conn, 1999, Appleton & Lange.

Journals

Becker C: Methanol poisoning, *J Emerg Med* 1:51-58, 1983.

Burgess E MD: Prolonged hemodialysis in methanol intoxication, *Pharmacotherapy* 12:238-239, 1992.

Eckfeldt J, Kershaw M: Hyperamylasemia following methyl alcohol intoxication, *Arch Intern Med* 146:193-194, 1986.

Ekins BR, et al: Standardized treatment of severe methanol poisoning with ethanol and hemodialysis, *West J Med* 142:337-340, 1985.

Grufferman S, Alvarez J: Methanol poisoning complicated by myoglobinuric renal failure, Am *J Emerg Med* 3:24-26, 1985.

Jarvie DR, Simpson D: Simple screening tests for the emergency identification of methanol and ethylene glycol in poisoned patients, *Clin Chem* 36:1957-1961, 1990.

Kruse JA: Methanol poisoning, *Intensive Care Med* 18:391-397, 1992.

Liesivuori J, Savolainen H: Methanol and formic acid toxicity: biochemical mechanisms, *Pharmacol Toxicol* 69:157-163, 1991.

Litovitz T: The alcohols: ethanol, methanol, isopropanol, ethylene glycol, *Pediatr Clin North Am* 33:311-323, 1986.

Osterloch J, Pond S, Gradty S, Becker C: Serum formate concentrations in methanol intoxication as a criterion for hemodialysis, *Ann Intern Med* 104:200-203, 1986.

Scrimgeour E, Dethlefs R, Kevau I: Delayed recovery of vision after blindness caused by methanol poisoning, *Med J Aust* 13:481-483 1982.

Shahangian S, Robinson V, Jennison T: Formate concentrations in a case of menthol ingestion, *Clin Chem* 30:1413-1414,1984.

GUIDELINE 32

Books

Amdur MO, Doull J, Klaassen CD, editors: *Casarett and Doull's toxicology, the basic science of poisons,* ed 4, New York, 1991, Pergamon Press.

CANUTEC: *Initial emergency response guide 1992,* Ottawa, Canada, 1992, Canada Communication Group.

CCINFO: *MSDS/CHEMINFO* (CD-ROM version), Hamilton, Ontario, Canada, 1993, Canadian Centre for Occupational Health and Safety.

DOT: *CHRIS hazardous chemical data.* US Department of Transportation/United States Coast Guard. Washington, DC, 1984, US Government Printing Office.

DOT: *2000 Emergency response guidebook,* Office of Hazardous Materials Transportation, Research and Special Programs Administration, Washington, DC, 2000, US Department of Transportation.

Goldfrank LR, et al: *Goldfrank's toxicologic emergencies,* ed 6, New York, 1998,McGraw-Hill Professional.

Goodman AG, et al, editors: *Goodman and Gilman's the pharmacological basis of therapeutics,* ed 8, New York, 1990, Pergamon Press.

Gosselin RE, Smith RP, Hodge HC: *Clinical toxicology of commercial products,* ed 5, Baltimore, 1984, Williams & Wilkins.

Haddad LM, et al: *Clinical management of poisoning and drug overdose,* ed 3, Philadelphia, 1997, Saunders.

Mackison FW, Stricoff RS, Partridge LJ Jr, editors: *Occupational health guidelines for chemical hazards,* NIOSH/OSHA, Washington, DC, 1981, US Government Printing Office.

Meeks RG, Harrison SD, Bull RJ, editors: *Hepatotoxicology,* Boca Raton, Florida, 1991, CRC Press.

NIOSH: *NIOSH pocket guide to chemical hazards* (CD-ROM version), Cincinnati, 2000, DHHS (NIOSH), US Government Printing Office.

Journals

Curry S, Methemoglobinemia, *Ann Emerg Med* 11:214-221, 1982.

Harvey J, Keitt A: Studies of the efficacy and potential hazards of methylene blue therapy in aniline-induced methemoglobinaemia, *Br J Haemotol* 54:19-41, 1983.

Kearney TE, Manoguerra AS, Dunford JV: Chemically induced methemoglobinemia from aniline poisoning, *West J Med* 140:282-286, 1984.

NIOSH Alert: Request for assistance in preventing bladder cancer from exposure to o-toluidine and aniline, *MMWR Morb Mortal Wkly Rep* 40(21):353-354, 1991.

Popp W, et al: Incidence of bladder cancer in a cohort of workers exposed to 4-chloro-o-toluidine while synthesising chlordimeform, *Br J Ind Med* 49:529-531, 1992.

GUIDELINE 33

Books

Amdur MO, Doull J, Klaassen CD, editors: *Casarett and Doull's toxicology, the basic science of poisons,* ed 4, New York, 1991, Pergamon Press.

CANUTEC: *Initial emergency response guide 1992,* Ottawa, Canada, 1992, Canada Communication Group.

CCINFO: *MSDS/CHEMINFO* (CD-ROM version), Hamilton, Ontario, Canada, 1993, Canadian Centre for Occupational Health and Safety.

DOT: *CHRIS hazardous chemical data.* US Department of Transportation/United States Coast Guard. Washington, DC, 1984, US Government Printing Office.

DOT: *2000 Emergency response guidebook,* Office of Hazardous Materials Transportation, Research and Special Programs Administration, Washington, DC, 2000, US Department of Transportation.

Gosselin RE, Smith RP, Hodge HC: *Clinical toxicology of commercial products,* ed 5, Baltimore, 1984, Williams & Wilkins.

Haddad LM, et al: *Clinical management of poisoning and drug overdose,* ed 3, Philadelphia, 1997, Saunders.

Hartman DE: *Neuropsychological toxicology, identification and assessment of human neurotoxic syndromes,* New York, 1988, Pergamon Press.

Mackison FW, Stricoff RS, Partridge LJ Jr, editors: *Occupational health guidelines for chemical hazards,* NIOSH/OSHA, Washington, DC, 1981, US Government Printing Office.

Meeks RG, Harrison SD, Bull RJ, editors: *Hepatotoxicology,* Boca Raton, Florida, 1991, CRC Press.

NIOSH: *NIOSH pocket guide to chemical hazards* (CD-ROM version), Cincinnati, 2000, DHHS (NIOSH), US Government Printing Office.

Snyder R, editor: *Ethel Browning's toxicity and metabolism of industrial solvents,* vol I, Hydrocarbons, New York, 1987, Elsevier Science Publishers.

Sullivan JB, Kriger GR, editors: *Clinical environmental health and hazardous materials toxicology,* Baltimore, 1997, Williams & Wilkins.

Journals

Banner W, Walson PD: Systemic toxicity following gasoline aspiration, Am *J Emerg Med* 3:292-294, 1983.

Binns H, Gursel E, Wilson N: Gasoline contact burns, *JACEP* 7:404-405, 1978.

Driscoll TR, et al: Concentrations of individual serum or plasma bile acids in workers exposed to chlorinated aliphatic hydrocarbons, *Br J Ind Med* 49:700-705, 1992.

Layton TR, Grant KJ, Vilella ER: Gasoline injection, *Clin Toxicol* 23:409-412, 1984.

GUIDELINE 34

Books

Amdur MO, Doull J, Klaassen CD, editors: *Casarett and Doull's toxicology, the basic science of poisons,* ed 4, New York, 1991, Pergamon Press.

CANUTEC: *Initial emergency response guide 1992,* Ottawa, Canada, 1992, Canada Communication Group.

CCINFO: *MSDS/CHEMINFO* (CD-ROM version), Hamilton, Ontario, Canada, 1993, Canadian Centre for Occupational Health and Safety.

DOT: *CHRIS hazardous chemical data.* US Department of Transportation/United States Coast Guard, Washington, DC, 1984, US Government Printing Office.

DOT: *2000 Emergency response guidebook,* Office of Hazardous Materials Transportation, Research and Special Programs Administration, Washington, DC, 2000, US Department of Transportation.

Gosselin RE, Smith RP, Hodge HC: *Clinical toxicology of commercial products,* ed 5, Baltimore, 1984, Williams & Wilkins.

Haddad LM, et al: *Clinical management of poisoning and drug overdose,* ed 3, Philadelphia, 1997, Saunders.

Mackison FW, Stricoff RS, Partridge LJ Jr, editors: *Occupational health guidelines for chemical hazards,* NIOSH/OSHA, Washington, DC, 1981, US Government Printing Office.

Manahan SE: *Environmental chemistry,* ed 7, Chelsea, Mich, 1999, Lewis Publishers.

NIOSH: *NIOSH pocket guide to chemical hazards* (CD-ROM version), Cincinnati, 2000, DHHS (NIOSH), US Government Printing Office.

Journals

Brook MP, McCarron MM, Mueller JA: Pine oil cleaner ingestion, *Ann Emerg Med* 18:391-395, 1989.

Bruhn P, Arlien-Sorborig Gldensted C, Christensen E: Prognosis in chronic toxic encephalopathy: a two-year follow-up study in 26 house painters with occupational encephalopathy, *Acta Neurol Scand* 64:259-272, 1981.

Conde-Salazar L, et al: Contact dermatitis in an oil painter, *Contact Dermatitis* 8:209-210, 1982.

Hendy M, Beattie B, Burge P: Occupational asthma due to an emulsified oil mist, *Br J Ind Med* 42:51-54, 1985.

Klein F, Hackler R: Hemorrhagic cystitis associated with turpentine ingestion, *Urology* 16:187, 1980.

Romaguera C, et al: Turpentine sensitization, *Contact Dermatitis* 14:197, 1986.

GUIDELINE 35

Books

Amdur MO, Doull J, Klaassen CD, editors: *Casarett and Doull's toxicology, the basic science of poisons,* ed 4, New York, 1991, Pergamon Press.

CANUTEC: *Initial emergency response guide 1992,* Ottawa, Canada, 1992, Canada Communication Group.

CCINFO: *MSDS/CHEMINFO* (CD-ROM version), Hamilton, Ontario, Canada, 1993, Canadian Centre for Occupational Health and Safety.

DOT: *CHRIS hazardous chemical data,* US Department of Transportation/United States Coast Guard. Washington, DC, 1984, US Government Printing Office.

DOT: *2000 Emergency response guidebook,* Office of Hazardous Materials Transportation, Research and Special Programs Administration, Washington, DC, 2000, US Department of Transportation.

Gosselin RE, Smith RP, Hodge HC: *Clinical toxicology of commercial products,* ed 5, Baltimore, 1984, Williams & Wilkins.

Mackison FW, Stricoff RS, Partridge LJ Jr, editors: *Occupational health guidelines for chemical hazards,* NIOSH/OSHA, Washington, DC, 1981, US Government Printing Office.

Manahan SE: *Environmental chemistry,* ed 7, Chelsea, Mich, 1999, Lewis Publishers.

Meeks RG, Harrison SD, Bull RJ, editors: *Hepatotoxicology,* Boca Raton, Florida, 1991, CRC Press.

NIOSH: *NIOSH pocket guide to chemical hazards* (CD-ROM version), Cincinnati, 2000, DHHS (NIOSH), US Government Printing Office.

Snyder R, editor: *Ethel Browning's toxicity and metabolism of industrial solvents,* vol I, Hydrocarbons, New York, 1987, Elsevier Science Publishers.

Journals

Annobil S: Chest radiographic patterns following kerosene poisoning in Ghanaian children, *Clin Radiol* 34:643-646, 1983.

Banner W, Walson PD: Systemic toxicity following gasoline aspiration, *Am J Emerg Med* 3:292-294, 1983.

Fortenberry JD: Gasoline sniffing, *Am J Med* 79:740-744, 1985.

Panson R, Winek C: Aspiration toxicity of ketones, *Clin Toxicol* 17:271-317, 1980.

GUIDELINE 36

Books

Amdur MO, Doull J, Klaassen CD, editors: *Casarett and Doull's toxicology, the basic science of poisons,* ed 4, New York, 1991, Pergamon Press.

CANUTEC: *Initial emergency response guide 1992,* Ottawa, Canada, 1992, Canada Communication Group.

CCINFO: *MSDS/CHEMINFO* (CD-ROM version), Hamilton, Ontario, Canada, 1993, Canadian Centre for Occupational Health and Safety.

DOT: *CHRIS hazardous chemical data.* US Department of Transportation/United States Coast Guard. Washington, DC, 1984, US Government Printing Office.

DOT: *2000 Emergency response guidebook,* Office of Hazardous Materials Transportation, Research and Special Programs Administration, Washington, DC, 2000, US Department of Transportation.

Goldfrank LR, et al: *Goldfrank's toxicologic emergencies,* ed 6, New York, 1998,McGraw-Hill Professional.

Gosselin RE, Smith RP, Hodge HC: *Clinical toxicology of commercial products,* ed 5, Baltimore, 1984, Williams & Wilkins.

Haddad LM, et al: *Clinical management of poisoning and drug overdose,* ed 3, Philadelphia, 1997, Saunders.

Mackison FW, Stricoff RS, Partridge LJ Jr, editors: *Occupational health guidelines for chemical hazards,* NIOSH/OSHA, Washington, DC, 1981, US Government Printing Office.

NIOSH: *NIOSH pocket guide to chemical hazards* (CD-ROM version), Cincinnati, 2000, DHHS (NIOSH), US Government Printing Office.

Olson KR, editor: *Poisoning & drug overdose,* ed 3, East Norwalk, Conn, 1999, Appleton & Lange.

Journals

Geller R J, et al: Camphor toxicity: development of a triage strategy, *Vet Hum Toxicol* 26(Suppl 2):8-10, 1984.

Jimenez J, et al: Chronic camphor ingestion mimicking Reye's syndrome. *Gastroenterology* 84:394-398, 1983.

Siegel W, Wason S: Camphor toxicity, *Pediatr Clin North Am* 33:375-379, 1986

GUIDELINE 37

Books

Amdur MO, Doull J, Klaassen CD, editors: *Casarett and Doull's toxicology, the basic science of poisons,* ed 4, New York, 1991, Pergamon Press.

CANUTEC: *Initial emergency response guide 1992,* Ottawa, Canada, 1992, Canada Communication Group.

CCINFO: *MSDS/CHEMINFO* (CD-ROM version), Hamilton, Ontario, Canada, 1993, Canadian Centre for Occupational Health and Safety.

DOT: *2000 Emergency response guidebook,* Office of Hazardous Materials Transportation, Research and Special Programs Administration, Washington, DC, 2000, US Department of Transportation.

Finkel AJ, editor: *Hamilton and Hardy's industrial toxicology,* ed 4, Littleton, Mass, 1983, PSG Publishing.

Gosselin RE, Smith RP, Hodge HC: *Clinical toxicology of commercial products,* ed 5, Baltimore, 1984, Williams & Wilkins.

HSDB: *Hazardous substances data bank,* National Library of Medicine, Bethesda, Maryland, 1993.

Meeks RG, Harrison SD, Bull RJ, editors: *Hepatotoxicology,* Boca Raton, Florida, 1991, CRC Press.

NIOSH: *NIOSH pocket guide to chemical hazards* (CD-ROM version), Cincinnati, 2000, DHHS (NIOSH), US Government Printing Office.

Journals

Daniel JW: Toxicity and metabolism of phthalate esters, *Clin Toxicol* 13:257-268, 1978.

von Oettingen WF: The aliphatic acids and their esters: toxicity and potential dangers, *Arch Ind Health* 21:28-65, 1960.

GUIDELINE 38

Books

CANUTEC: *Initial emergency response guide 1992,* Ottawa, Canada, 1992, Canada Communication Group.

CCINFO: *MSDS/CHEMINFO* (CD-ROM version), Hamilton, Ontario, Canada, 1993, Canadian Centre for Occupational Health and Safety.

DOT: *CHRIS hazardous chemical data.* US Department of Transportation/United States Coast Guard, Washington, DC, 1984, US Government Printing Office.

DOT: *2000 Emergency response guidebook,* Office of Hazardous Materials Transportation, Research and Special Programs Administration, Washington, DC, 2000, US Department of Transportation.

Goodman AG, et al, editors: *Goodman and Gilman's the pharmacological basis of therapeutics,* ed 8, New York, 1990, Pergamon Press.

Gosselin RE, Smith RP, Hodge HC: *Clinical toxicology of commercial products,* ed 5, Baltimore, 1984, Williams & Wilkins.

Manahan SE: *Environmental chemistry,* ed 7, Chelsea, Mich, 1999, Lewis Publishers.

NIOSH: *NIOSH pocket guide to chemical hazards* (CD-ROM version), Cincinnati, 2000, DHHS (NIOSH), US Government Printing Office.

GUIDELINE 39

Books

CANUTEC: *Initial emergency response guide 1992,* Ottawa, Canada, 1992, Canada Communication Group.

CCINFO: *MSDS/CHEMINFO* (CD-ROM version), Hamilton, Ontario, Canada, 1993, Canadian Centre for Occupational Health and Safety.

DOT: *2000 Emergency response guidebook,* Office of Hazardous Materials Transportation, Research and Special Programs Administration, Washington, DC, 2000, US Department of Transportation.

Finkel AJ, editor: *Hamilton and Hardy's industrial toxicology,* ed 4, Littleton, Mass, 1983, PSG Publishing.

Gosselin RE, Smith RP, Hodge HC: *Clinical toxicology of commercial products,* ed 5, Baltimore, 1984, Williams & Wilkins.

NIOSH: *NIOSH pocket guide to chemical hazards* (CD-ROM version), Cincinnati, 2000, DHHS (NIOSH), US Government Printing Office.

Sullivan JB, Kriger GR, editors: *Clinical environmental health and hazardous materials toxicology,* Baltimore, 1997, Williams & Wilkins.

Journal

Young JD, Braun WH, Rampy LW: Pharmacokinetics of 1,4-dioxane in humans, *J Toxicol Environ Health* 3:507-520, 1977.

GUIDELINE 40

Books

Amdur MO, Doull J, Klaassen CD, editors: *Casarett and Doull's toxicology, the basic science of poisons,* ed 4, New York, 1991, Pergamon Press.

CANUTEC: *Initial emergency response guide 1992,* Ottawa, Canada, 1992, Canada Communication Group.

Casarett LJ, Doull J: *Toxicology, the basic science of poisons,* ed 3. Klaassen CD, Amdur MO, Doull J, editors, New York, 1986, Macmillan.

CCINFO: *MSDS/CHEMINFO* (CD-ROM version), Hamilton, Ontario, Canada, 1993, Canadian Centre for Occupational Health and Safety.

DOT: *CHRIS hazardous chemical data.* US Department of Transportation/United States Coast Guard,Washington, DC, 1984, US Government Printing Office.

DOT: *2000 Emergency response guidebook,* Office of Hazardous Materials Transportation,

Research and Special Programs Administration, Washington, DC, 2000, US Department of Transportation.

Goldfrank LR, et al: *Goldfrank's toxicologic emergencies,* ed 6, New York, 1998,McGraw-Hill Professional.

Gosselin RE, Smith RP, Hodge HC: *Clinical toxicology of commercial products,* ed 5, Baltimore, 1984, Williams & Wilkins.

Haddad LM, et al: *Clinical management of poisoning and drug overdose,* ed 3, Philadelphia, 1997, Saunders.

HSDB: *Hazardous substances data bank,* National Library of Medicine, Bethesda, Maryland, 1993.

Meeks RG, Harrison SD, Bull RJ, editors: *Hepatotoxicology,* Boca Raton, Florida, 1991, CRC Press.

NIOSH: *NIOSH pocket guide to chemical hazards* (CD-ROM version), Cincinnati, 2000, DHHS (NIOSH), US Government Printing Office.

Sullivan JB, Kriger GR, editors: *Clinical environmental health and hazardous materials toxicology,* Baltimore, 1997, Williams & Wilkins.

Journals

Bauer PH, et al: Transient non-cardiogenic pulmonary edema following massive ingestion of ethylene glycol butyl ether, *Intensive Care Med* 18:250-251, 1992.

Bolt HM, Golka K: Maternal exposure to ethylene glycol monomethyl ether acetate and hypospadia in offspring: a case report, *Br J Ind Med* 47:352-353, 1990.

Browning RG, Curry SC: Effect of glycol ethers on plasma osmolality, *Hum Exp Toxicol* 11:488-490, 1992.

Cook R, et al: A cross-sectional study of ethylene glycol monomethyl ether process employees, *Arch Environ Health* 37:346-351, 1982.

Dean BS, Krenzelok EP: Clinical evaluation of pediatric ethylene glycol monobutyl ether poisonings, *Clin Toxicol* 30:557-563, 1992.

Egbert A, et al: Alcoholics who drink mouthwash: the spectrum of non-beverage alcohol use, *J Stud Alcohol* 46:473-481, 1985.

Frommer J, Ayus C: Acute ethylene glycol intoxication, *Am J Nephrol* 1:1-5, 1982.

Ghanayem BI, Sanchez IM, Matthews HB: Development of tolerance to 2-butoxyethanol–induced hemolytic anemia and studies to elucidate the underlying mechanisms, *Toxicol Appl Pharmacol* 112:198-206, 1992.

Hall AH, Bronstein AC, Smolinske SC, et al: Propylene glycol plasma level (letter), *Pediatrics* 4:654, 1985.

Jacobsen D, et al: Anion and osmolal gaps in the diagnosis of methanol and ethylene glycol poisoning, *Acta Med Scand* 212:17-20, 1982.

Jacobsen D, Akesson I, Shefter E: Urinary calcium oxzalate monohydrate crystals in ethylene glycol poisoning, *Scand J Clin Lab Invest* 42:231-234, 1982.

Karlson-Stiber C, Perrson H: Ethylene glycol poisoning: experiences from an epidemic in Sweden, *Clin Toxicol* 30:565-574, 1992.

Kothman A, et al: Short-term hemodialysis in childhood ethylene glycol poisoning, *J Pediatr* 108:153-155, 1984.

Litovitz T: The alcohols: ethanol, methanol, isopropanol, ethylene glycol, *Pediatr Clin North Am* 33:311-323, 1986.

Lund M, et al: Effect of alcohols and selected solvents on serum osmolality measurements, *J Toxicol Clin Toxicol* 20:115-132, 1983.

Tanii H, Saito S, Hashimoto K: Structure-toxicity relationship of ethylene glycol ethers, *Arch Toxicol* 66:368-371, 1992.

Walker JT, Keller MS, Katz SM: Computed tomographic and sonographic findings in acute ethylene glycol poisoning, *J Ultrasound Med* 2(9):429-431, 1983.

Wess, JA: Reproductive toxicity of ethylene glycol monomethyl ether, ethylene glycol monoethyl ether and their acetates, *Scand J Work Environ Health* 18(Suppl 2):43-45, 1992.

GUIDELINE 41

Books

Amdur MO, Doull J, Klaassen CD, editors: *Casarett and Doull's toxicology, the basic science of poisons,* ed 4, New York, 1991, Pergamon Press.

Bardana EJ, Montanaro A, O'Hollaren MT: *Occupational asthma,* Philadelphia, 1992, Hanley & Belfus.

CANUTEC: *Initial emergency response guide 1992,* Ottawa, Canada, 1992, Canada Communication Group.

CCINFO: *MSDS/CHEMINFO* (CD-ROM version), Hamilton, Ontario, Canada, 1993, Canadian Centre for Occupational Health and Safety.

DOT: *CHRIS hazardous chemical data.* US Department of Transportation/United States Coast Guard. Washington, DC, 1984, US Government Printing Office.

DOT: *2000 Emergency response guidebook,* Office of Hazardous Materials Transportation, Research and Special Programs Administration, Washington, DC, 2000, US Department of Transportation.

Goldfrank LR, et al: *Goldfrank's toxicologic emergencies,* ed 6, New York, 1998, McGraw-Hill Professional.

NIOSH: *NIOSH pocket guide to chemical hazards* (CD-ROM version), Cincinnati, 2000, DHHS (NIOSH), US Government Printing Office.

Sullivan JB, Kriger GR, editors: *Clinical environmental health and hazardous materials toxicology,* Baltimore, 1997, Williams & Wilkins.

Journals

Alexandersson R, Kolmodin-Hedman B, Hedenstierna G: Exposure to formaldehyde: effects on pulmonary function, *Arch Environ Health* 37:279-284, 1982.

Bardana EJ Jr, Montanaro A: Formaldehyde: An analysis of its respiratory, cutaneous, and immunologic effects, *Ann Allergy* 66:441-452, 1991.

Bardana E, Montanaro A: Formaldehyde asthma (letter), *J Allergy Clin Immunol* 77:384-385, 1986.

Bender J, Reinhardt C, Mullin L: Formaldehyde toxicity (letter), *JAMA* 248:308-309, 1982.

Clark R: Formaldehyde in pathology departments, *J Clin Pathol* 36:839-846, 1983.

Feigal RJ, Messer HH: A critical look at glutaraldehyde, *Pediatr Dent* 12:69-71, 1990.

Formaldehyde and cancer (editorial), *Lancet* 2:26, 1983.

Imbus H: Clinical evaluation of patients with complaints related to formaldehyde exposure, *J Allergy Clin Immunol* 76:831-840, 1985.

Infante P, Schneiderman M: Formaldehyde, lung cancer, and bronchitis (letter), *Lancet* 1:436-438, 1986.

Kilburn KH, Warshaw RH: Neurobehavioral effects of formaldehyde and solvents on histology technicians: repeated testing across time, *Environ Res* 58:134-146, 1992.

Lawler P: Inhalation of formaldehyde vapour: a potential hazard of a method of sterilization of bacterial filters, *Anesthesia* 37:1102-1103, 1982.

Newhouse M: UFFI dust: nonspecific irritant only? (Letter), *Chest* 82:511-512, 1982.

Wilhelmsson B, Holmstrom M: Possible mechanisms of formaldehyde-induced discomfort in the upper airways, *Scand J Work Environ Health* 18:403-407, 1992.

GUIDELINE 42

Books

Amdur MO, Doull J, Klaassen CD, editors: *Casarett and Doull's toxicology, the basic science of poisons,* ed 4, New York, 1991, Pergamon Press.

CANUTEC: *Initial emergency response guide 1992,* Ottawa, Canada, 1992, Canada Communication Group.

CCINFO: *MSDS/CHEMINFO* (CD-ROM version), Hamilton, Ontario, Canada, 1993, Canadian Centre for Occupational Health and Safety.

DOT: *2000 Emergency response guidebook,* Office of Hazardous Materials Transportation, Research and Special Programs Administration, Washington, DC, 2000, US Department of Transportation.

Gosselin RE, Smith RP, Hodge HC: *Clinical toxicology of commercial products,* ed 5, Baltimore, 1984, Williams & Wilkins.

NIOSH: *NIOSH pocket guide to chemical hazards* (CD-ROM version), Cincinnati, 2000, DHHS (NIOSH), US Government Printing Office.

Sullivan JB, Kriger GR, editors: *Clinical environmental health and hazardous materials toxicology,* Baltimore, 1997, Williams & Wilkins.

Journals

Kechijian P: Nail polish removers: are they harmful? *Semin Dermatol* 10:26-28, 1991.

Kopelman PO, Kalfayan PY: Severe metabolic acidosis after ingestion of butanone, *Br J Ind Med* 42:155-161, 1985.

Mendell JR, et al: Neuropathy and methyl n-butyl ketone, *N Engl J Med* 290:1263-1264, 1974.

Raleigh RL, McGee WA: Effects of short, high-concentration exposures to acetone as determined by observation in the work area, *J Occup Med* 14:607-610, 1972.

Williams H: Skin lightening creams containing hydroquinone, *Br Med J* 305:903-904, 1992.

GUIDELINE 43

Books

CANUTEC: *Initial emergency response guide 1992,* Ottawa, Canada, 1992, Canada Communication Group.

CCINFO: *MSDS/CHEMINFO* (CD-ROM version), Hamilton, Ontario, Canada, 1993, Canadian Centre for Occupational Health and Safety.

DOT: *CHRIS hazardous chemical data.* US Department of Transportation/United States Coast Guard. Washington, DC, 1984, US Government Printing Office.

DOT: *2000 Emergency response guidebook,* Office of Hazardous Materials Transportation, Research and Special Programs Administration, Washington, DC, 2000, US Department of Transportation.

Gosselin RE, Smith RP, Hodge HC: *Clinical toxicology of commercial products,* ed 5, Baltimore, 1984, Williams & Wilkins.

Mackison FW, Stricoff RS, Partridge LJ Jr, editors: *Occupational health guidelines for chemical hazards,* NIOSH/OSHA, Washington, DC, 1981, US Government Printing Office.

NIOSH: *NIOSH pocket guide to chemical hazards* (CD-ROM version), Cincinnati, 2000, DHHS (NIOSH), US Government Printing Office.

Snyder R, editor: *Ethel Browning's toxicity and metabolism of industrial solvents,* vol I, Hydrocarbons, New York, 1987, Elsevier Science Publishers.

Journals

Gidron E, Leurer J: Naphthalene poisoning, *Lancet* 1:228-230, 1956.

Illness associated with exposure to naphthalene in moth balls—Indiana, *MMWR Morb Mortal Wkly Rep* 32(2):43-45, 1983.

Ojwang PJ, Ahmed-Jushuf IH, Abdullah MS: Naphthalene poisoning following ingestion of moth balls: case report, *East Afr Med J* 62:71-73, 1985.

Siegel E, Wason S: Mothball toxicity, *Pediatr Clin North Am* 33:369-374, 1986.

Tindall JP: Chloracne and chloracnegens, *J Am Acad Dermatol* 13:539-558, 1985.

GUIDELINE 44

Books

Amdur MO, Doull J, Klaassen CD, editors: *Casarett and Doull's toxicology, the basic science of poisons,* ed 4, New York, 1991, Pergamon Press.

CANUTEC: *Initial emergency response guide 1992,* Ottawa, Canada, 1992, Canada Communication Group.

CCINFO: *MSDS/CHEMINFO* (CD-ROM version), Hamilton, Ontario, Canada, 1993, Canadian Centre for Occupational Health and Safety.

DOT: *CHRIS hazardous chemical data.* US Department of Transportation/United States Coast Guard. Washington, DC, 1984, US Government Printing Office.

DOT: *2000 Emergency response guidebook,* Office of Hazardous Materials Transportation, Research and Special Programs Administration, Washington, DC, 2000, US Department of Transportation.

Gosselin RE, Smith RP, Hodge HC: *Clinical toxicology of commercial products,* ed 5, Baltimore, 1984, Williams & Wilkins.

Haddad LM, et al: *Clinical management of poisoning and drug overdose,* ed 3, Philadelphia, 1997, Saunders.

Mackison FW, Stricoff RS, Partridge LJ Jr, editors: *Occupational health guidelines for chemical hazards,* NIOSH/OSHA, Washington, DC, 1981, US Government Printing Office.

NIOSH: *NIOSH pocket guide to chemical hazards* (CD-ROM version), Cincinnati, 2000, DHHS (NIOSH), US Government Printing Office.

Journals

Briggs L, Clarke R, Watkins J: An adverse reaction to the administration of disoprofol (Diprivan), *Anaesthesia* 37:1099–1101, 1982.

Conning DM, Hayes MJ: The dermal toxicity of phenol: an investigation of the most effective first-aid measures, *Br J Ind Med* 27:155-159, 1970.

Contamination of potable water by phenol from a solar water tank liner—Georgia, *MMWR Morb Mortal Wkly Rep* 32(38):493-494, 1983.

Hunter DM, et al: Effects of isopropyl alcohol, ethanol, and polyethylene glycol/industrial methylated spirits in the treatment of acute phenol burns, *Ann Emerg Med* 21:1303-1307, 1992.

Kintz P, Tracqui A, Mangin P: Accidental death caused by the absorption of 2,4-dichlorophenol through the skin, *Arch Toxicol* 66:298-299, 1992.

Koopman C: Phenol toxicity during face peels, *Otolaryngol Head Neck Surg* 90:383-384, 1982.

Leads from the MMWR. Contamination of potable water by phenol from a solar water tank, *JAMA* 250:1957, 1983.

Pryor W: Free radical biology; xenobiotics, cancer and aging, *Ann N Y Acad Sci* 393:1-22, 1982.

Soares E, Tift J: Phenol poisoning: three fatal cases, *J Forensic Sci* 27:729-731, 1982.

GUIDELINE 45

Books

Amdur MO, Doull J, Klaassen CD, editors: *Casarett and Doull's toxicology, the basic science of poisons,* ed 4, New York, 1991, Pergamon Press.

CANUTEC: *Initial emergency response guide 1992,* Ottawa, Canada, 1992, Canada Communication Group.

CCINFO: *MSDS/CHEMINFO* (CD-ROM version), Hamilton, Ontario, Canada, 1993, Canadian Centre for Occupational Health and Safety.

DOT: *CHRIS hazardous chemical data.* US Department of Transportation/United States Coast Guard. Washington, DC, 1984, US Government Printing Office.

DOT: *2000 Emergency response guidebook,* Office of Hazardous Materials Transportation, Research and Special Programs Administration, Washington, DC, 2000, US Department of Transportation.

Gosselin RE, Smith RP, Hodge HC: *Clinical toxicology of commercial products,* ed 5, Baltimore, 1984, Williams & Wilkins.

NIOSH: *NIOSH pocket guide to chemical hazards* (CD-ROM version), Cincinnati, 2000, DHHS (NIOSH), US Government Printing Office.

Sullivan JB, Kriger GR, editors: *Clinical environmental health and hazardous materials toxicology,* Baltimore, 1997, Williams & Wilkins.

Journals

Degarmo P, Varnas V: Ethylene oxide: A hazard to health care workers, *Oreg Nurse* 48:11-13, 1983.

Deschamps D, et al: Persistent asthma after accidental exposure to ethylene oxide, *Br J Ind Med* 49:523-525, 1992.

Fujishiro K, Mori K, Inoue N: Chronic inhalation effects of ethylene oxide on porphyrin-heme metabolism, *Toxicology* 61:1-11, 1990.

Greenberg HL, Ott MG, Shore RE: Men assigned to ethylene oxide production or other ethylene oxide related chemical manufacturing: a mortality study, *Br J Ind Med* 47:221-230, 1990.

Kiesselbach N, et al: A multicentre mortality study of workers exposed to ethylene oxide, *Br J Ind Med* 47:182-188, 1990.

Kuzuhara S, et al: Ethylene oxide polyneuropathy, *Neurology* 33:377-380, 1983.

Steenland K, et al: Mortality among workers exposed to ethylene oxide, *N Engl J Med* 324:1402-1407, 1991.

Wong, O: Mortality among workers exposed to ethylene oxide (letter), *N Engl J Med* 325:1254, 1991.

GUIDELINE 46

Books

Amdur MO, Doull J, Klaassen CD, editors: *Casarett and Doull's toxicology, the basic science of poisons,* ed 4, New York, 1991, Pergamon Press.

Baselt RC, Cravey RH: *Disposition of toxic drugs and chemicals in man,* ed 3, Chicago, 1989, Year Book Medical Publishers.

CANUTEC: *Initial emergency response guide 1992,* Ottawa, Canada, 1992, Canada Communication Group.

CCINFO: *MSDS/CHEMINFO* (CD-ROM version), Hamilton, Ontario, Canada, 1993, Canadian Centre for Occupational Health and Safety.

DOT: *2000 Emergency response guidebook,* Office of Hazardous Materials Transportation, Research and Special Programs Administration, Washington, DC, 2000, US Department of Transportation.

Gosselin RE, Smith RP, Hodge HC: *Clinical toxicology of commercial products,* ed 5, Baltimore, 1984, Williams & Wilkins.

Haddad LM, et al: *Clinical management of poisoning and drug overdose,* ed 3, Philadelphia, 1997, Saunders.

Hartman DE: *Neuropsychological toxicology, identification and assessment of human neurotoxic syndromes,* New York, 1988, Pergamon Press.

Hutzinger O, Frei RW, Merian E, Pocchiari F, editors: *Chlorinated dioxins & related compounds, impact on the environment,* New York, 1982, Pergamon Press.

Jenson AV: *Guidebook for hazardous materials incidents,* Washington, DC, 1983, Department of Transportation.

Mackison FW, Stricoff RS, Partridge LJ Jr, editors: *Occupational health guidelines for chemical hazards,* NIOSH/OSHA, Washington, DC, 1981, US Government Printing Office.

NIOSH: *NIOSH pocket guide to chemical hazards* (CD-ROM version), Cincinnati, 2000, DHHS (NIOSH), US Government Printing Office.

NIOSH/OSHA/USCG/EPA: *Occupational safety and health guidance manual for hazardous waste site activities,* Washington, DC, 1985, DHHS (NIOSH) Publication No 85-115, US Government Printing Office.

Journals

Frank R, et al: Organochlorine residues in adipose tissues, blood, and milk from Ontario residents, 1976-1985, *Can J Public Health* 79:150-158, 1988.

Jappinen P, Pukkala E: Cancer incidence among pulp and paper workers exposed to organic chlorinated compounds formed during chlorine pulp bleaching, *Scand J Work Environ Health* 17:356-359, 1991.

Kimbrough RD: Human health effects of polychlorinated biphenyls (PCBs) and polybrominated biphenyls (PBBs), *Annu Rev Pharmacol Toxicol* 27:87-111, 1987.

Kriess K: Studies on populations exposed to polychlorinated biphenyls, *Environ Health Perspect* 60:193-199, 1985.

Kunita N, et al: Causal agents of Yusho, *Am J Ind Med* 5:45-58, 1984.

Ouw HK, Simpson GR, Siyali DS: Use and health effects of aroclor 1242, a polychlorinated biphenyl, in an electrical industry, *Arch Environ Health* 31:189, 1976.

Rogan WJ, Gladen, BC: Neurotoxicology of PCBs and related compounds, *Neurotoxicology* 13:27-36, 1992.

Wolff MS, et al: Disposition of polychlorinated biphenyl congeners in occupationally exposed persons, *Toxicol Appl Pharmacol* 62:294-306, 1982.

GUIDELINE 47

Books

Amdur MO, Doull J, Klaassen CD, editors: *Casarett and Doull's toxicology, the basic science of poisons,* ed 4, New York, 1991, Pergamon Press.

CANUTEC: *Initial emergency response guide 1992,* Ottawa, Canada, 1992, Canada Communication Group.

CCINFO: *MSDS/CHEMINFO* (CD-ROM version), Hamilton, Ontario, Canada, 1993, Canadian Centre for Occupational Health and Safety.

DOT: *CHRIS hazardous chemical data,* US Department of Transportation/United States Coast Guard. Washington, DC, 1984, US Government Printing Office.

DOT: *2000 Emergency response guidebook,* Office of Hazardous Materials Transportation, Research and Special Programs Administration, Washington, DC, 2000, US Department of Transportation.

Ellenhorn MJ, Barceloux DG: *Medical toxicology diagnosis and treatment of human poisoning,* New York, 1988, Elsevier Science Publishing Co.

Gosselin RE, Smith RP, Hodge HC: *Clinical toxicology of commercial products,* ed 5, Baltimore, 1984, Williams & Wilkins.

Haddad LM, et al: *Clinical management of poisoning and drug overdose,* ed 3, Philadelphia, 1997, Saunders.

Mackison FW, Stricoff RS, Partridge LJ Jr, editors: *Occupational health guidelines for chemical hazards,* NIOSH/OSHA, Washington, DC, 1981, US Government Printing Office.

NIOSH: *NIOSH pocket guide to chemical hazards* (CD-ROM version), Cincinnati, 2000, DHHS (NIOSH), US Government Printing Office.

Sullivan JB, Kriger GR, editors: *Clinical environmental health and hazardous materials toxicology,* Baltimore, 1997, Williams & Wilkins.

Journals

Abrahams J: Nitroglycerin and long acting nitrates in clinical practice, *Am J Med* 74:85-94, 1983.

Archer AW, Geyer R: Production of cyanide in a sodium nitrite poisoning case using an acid distillation screening test, *J Forensic Sci Soc* 22:333-334, 1982.

Becker DJ: Side effects of transdermal nitrate (letter), *Ann Intern Med* 104:590, 1986.

Curry S: Methemoglobinemia, *Ann Emerg Med* 11:214-221, 1982.

Fraser P, Chilvers C, Goldblatt P: Census-based mortality study of fertilizer manufacturers, *Br J Ind Med* 39:323-329, 1982.

Frishmann WH: Pharmacology of the nitrates in angina pectoris, *Am J Cardiol* 45:81-131, 1984.

Goldhaber S Z: Cardiovascular effects of potential occupational hazards, *J Am Coll Cardiol* 2:1210-1215, 1983.

Hajela R, et al: Fatal pulmonary edema due to nitric acid fume inhalation in three pulp-mill workers, *Chest* 97:487-489, 1990.

Kuhlberg A: Substance abuse: clinical identification and management, *Pediatr Clin North Am* 33:325-361, 1986.

Lin JK: Nitrosamines as potential environmental carcinogens in man, *Clin Biochem* 23:67-71, 1990.

Linden CH: Volatile substances of abuse, *Emerg Med Clin North Am* 8:559-578, 1990.

Maloney WJ, MacFarlane MT, Rimsza ME: Methemoglobinemia in an infant, *Ariz Med* 40(10):700-702, 1983.

Mansouri A: Review: methemoglobinemia, *Am J Med Sci* 5:200-209, 1985,

Mirvish SS: The etiology of gastric cancer: intragastric nitrosamide formation and other theories, *J Natl Cancer Inst* 71:629-647, 1983.

Saxena K, Kingston R: Acute poisoning: management protocol, *Postgrad Med* 71:67-77, 1982.

Vlay S, Cohn P: Nitrate therapy in angina and congestive heart failure, *Cardiology* 72:322-328, 1985.

GUIDELINE 48

Books

Amdur MO, Doull J, Klaassen CD, editors: *Casarett and Doull's toxicology, the basic science of poisons,* ed 4, New York, 1991, Pergamon Press.

CANUTEC: *Initial emergency response guide 1992,* Ottawa, Canada, 1992, Canada Communication Group.

CCINFO: *MSDS/CHEMINFO* (CD-ROM version), Hamilton, Ontario, Canada, 1993, Canadian Centre for Occupational Health and Safety.

DOT: *CHRIS hazardous chemical data.* US Department of Transportation/United States Coast Guard, Washington, DC, 1984, US Government Printing Office.

DOT: *2000 Emergency response guidebook,* Office of Hazardous Materials Transportation, Research and Special Programs Administration, Washington, DC, 2000, US Department of Transportation.

Gosselin RE, Smith RP, Hodge HC: *Clinical toxicology of commercial products,* ed 5, Baltimore, 1984, Williams & Wilkins.

Mackison FW, Stricoff RS, Partridge LJ Jr, editors: *Occupational health guidelines for chemical hazards,* NIOSH/OSHA, Washington, DC, 1981, US Government Printing Office.

NIOSH: *NIOSH pocket guide to chemical hazards* (CD-ROM version), Cincinnati, 2000, DHHS (NIOSH), US Government Printing Office.

Sullivan JB, Kriger GR, editors: *Clinical environmental health and hazardous materials toxicology,* Baltimore, 1997, Williams & Wilkins.

Journals

Goldstein E, Hackney JD, Rokaw SN: Photochemical air pollution. I, *West J Med* 142(3):369-376, 1985.

Goldstein BD, Melia RJ, Florey CD: Indoor nitrogen oxides, *Bull N Y Acad Med* 57(10):973-982, 1981.

Guidotti TL: The higher oxides of nitrogen: inhalation toxicology, *Environ Res* 15:443-472, 1987.

Lindall T: Health effects of nitrogen dioxide and oxidants, *Scand J Work Environ Health* 11(Suppl 3):10-28, 1985.

Lowry T, Schuman LM: "Silo-filler's disease"—a syndrome caused by nitrogen dioxide, *JAMA* 162:153-160, 1956.

Maugh TH: Acid rain's effects on people assessed [News], *Science* 226:1408-1410, 1984.

Morrow PE: Toxicology data on NOx: an overview, *Toxicol Environ Health* 13(2-3):205-227, 1984.

Moskowitz RL, Lyons HA, Cottle HR: Silo filler's disease, *Am J Med* 36:457-462, 1964.

Oxides of nitrogen and health (editorial), *Lancet* 1:81-82, 1981.

Roger LJ, et al: Pulmonary function, airway responsiveness and respiratory symptoms in asthmatics following exercise in NO_2, *Toxicol Ind Health* 6:155-171, 1990.

Speizer FE: Ozone and photochemical pollutants, status after 25 years, *West J Med* 142:377-379, 1985.

GUIDELINE 49

Books

Amdur MO, Doull J, Klaassen CD, editors: *Casarett and Doull's toxicology, the basic science of poisons,* ed 4, New York, 1991, Pergamon Press.

CANUTEC: *Initial emergency response guide 1992,* Ottawa, Canada, 1992, Canada Communication Group.

CCINFO: *MSDS/CHEMINFO* (CD-ROM version), Hamilton, Ontario, Canada, 1993, Canadian Centre for Occupational Health and Safety.

DOT: *CHRIS hazardous chemical data,* US Department of Transportation/United States Coast Guard. Washington, DC, 1984, US Government Printing Office.

DOT: *2000 Emergency response guidebook,* Office of Hazardous Materials Transportation, Research and Special Programs Administration, Washington, DC, 2000, US Department of Transportation.

Goldfrank LR, et al: *Goldfrank's toxicologic emergencies,* ed 6, New York, 1998,McGraw-Hill Professional.

Goodman AG, et al, editors: *Goodman and Gilman's the pharmacological basis of therapeutics,* ed 8, New York, 1990, Pergamon Press.

Gosselin RE, Smith RP, Hodge HC: *Clinical toxicology of commercial products,* ed 5, Baltimore, 1984, Williams & Wilkins.

Hartman DE: *Neuropsychological toxicology, identification and assessment of human neurotoxic syndromes,* New York, 1988, Pergamon Press.

HSDB: *Hazardous substances data bank,* National Library of Medicine, Bethesda, Md, 1993.

Kaloyanova FP, El Batawi MA: *Human toxicology of pesticides,* Boca Raton, Florida, 1991, CRC Press.

Mackison FW, Stricoff RS, Partridge LJ Jr, editors: *Occupational health guidelines for chemical hazards,* NIOSH/OSHA, Washington, DC, 1981, US Government Printing Office.

Merigan WH, Weiss B, editors: *Neurotoxicity of the visual system,* New York, 1980, Raven Press.

Morgan DP: *Recognition and management of pesticide poisonings,* ed 4, Washington, DC, United States Environmental Protection Agency, 1989, US Government Printing Office.

NIOSH: *NIOSH pocket guide to chemical hazards* (CD-ROM version), Cincinnati, 2000, DHHS (NIOSH), US Government Printing Office.

Sullivan JB, Kriger GR, editors: *Clinical environmental health and hazardous materials toxicology,* Baltimore, 1997, Williams & Wilkins.

Journals

Adamis Z, et al: Occupational exposure to organophosphorus insecticides and synthetic pyrethroid, *Int Arch Occup Environ Health* 56:299-305, 1985.

Amitai Y, et al: Atropine poisoning in children during the Persian Gulf crisis. A national survey in Israel, *JAMA* 268:630-632, 1992.

Andonova S, Tzvetkove T: Cytomorphological and clinical studies among workers employed in the production of chemical agents for plant protection, *Folia Medica* 1:47-51, 1982.

Baker P, Selvey D: Malathion-induced epidemic hysteria in an elementary school, *Vet Hum Toxicol* 34:156-160, 1992.

Barr A: Organophosphate insecticide poisoning (letter), *Anesthesia* 40:1017, 1985.

Beyer S: Regulation and its alternatives: some remarks on organophosphate pesticides, *Neurotoxicology* 4:99-104, 1983.

Clifford NJ, Nies AS: Organophosphate poisoning from wearing a laundered uniform previously contaminated with parathion, *JAMA* 262:3035-3036, 1989.

Delilkan AE, Manazie M, Ong G: Organophosphate poisoning: a Malaysian intensive care experience of one hundred cases, *Med J Malaysia* 39:229-233, 1984.

DeSilva HJ, Wijewickrema R, Senanayake N: Does pralidoxime affect outcome of management in acute organophosphorus poisoning? *Lancet* 339:1136-1138, 1992.

Duncan R, Griffith J: Monitoring study of urinary metabolites and selected symptomatology among Florida citrus workers, *J Toxicol Environ Health* 17:509-21, 1985.

Jay W, Marcus R, Jay M: Primary position upbeat nystagmus with organophosphate poisoning, *J Pediatr Ophthalmol Strabismus* 19:318-319, 1982.

Johnson M: Initiation of organophosphate-induced delayed neuropathy, *Neurobehav Toxicol Teratol* 4:759-765, 1982.

Kiss Z, Fazkas T: Organophosphates and torsades de pointes ventricular tachycardia, *J R Soc Med* 76:984, 1983.

Lokan R, James R: Rapid death by mevinphos poisoning while under observation, *Forensic Sci Int* 22:179-182, 1983.

McConnell R, et al: Monitoring organophosphate insecticide-exposed workers for cholinesterase depression: new technology for office or field use, *J Occup Med* 34:34-37, 1992.

Metcalf R L: Historical perspective of organophosphorus ester-induced delayed neurotoxicity, *Neurotoxicology* 3:269-284, 1982.

Mhtsushita T, et al: Allergic contact dermatitis from organophosphorus insecticides, *Ind Health* 23:145-153, 1985.

Mizutani T, Naito H, Oohashi N: Rectal ulcer with massive haemorrhage due to activated charcoal treatment in oral organophosphate poisoning, *Hum Exp Toxicol* 10:385-386, 1991.

Mortensen M: Management of acute childhood poisonings caused by selected insecticides and herbicides, *Pediatr Clin North Am* 33:421-444, 1986.

Muldoon SR, Hodgson MJ: Risk factors for nonoccupational organophosphate pesticide poisoning, *J Occup Med* 34:38-41, 1992.

Newcombe DS: Immune surveillance, organophosphorus exposure and lymphomagenesis, *Lancet* 339:539-541, 1992.

Organophosphorus esters and polyneuropathy (editorial), *Ann Intern Med* 104:264-266, 1986.

Padilla S, et al: Paraoxon toxicity is not potentiated by prior reduction in blood acetylcholinesterase, *Toxicol Appl Pharmacol* 117:110-115, 1992.

Paul V, et al: Evidence for a hazardous interaction between ethanol and the insecticide endosulfan in rats, *Pharmacol Toxicol* 70:268-270, 1992.

Peedicayil J, et al: The effect of organophosphorus compounds on serum pseudocholinesterase levels in a group of industrial workers, *Hum Exp Toxicol* 10:275-278, 1991.

Reeves J: Household insecticide–associated blood dyscrasias in children, *Am J Pediatr Hematol Oncol* 4:438-439, 1982.

Rosenstock L, et al: Chronic central nervous system effects of acute organophosphate pesticide intoxication, *Lancet* 338:223-227, 1991.

Schuman SH, Wagner SL: Pesticide intoxication and chronic CNS effects, *Lancet* 338:948-949, 1991.

GUIDELINE 50

Books

Amdur MO, Doull J, Klaassen CD, editors: *Casarett and Doull's toxicology, the basic science of poisons,* ed 4, New York, 1991, Pergamon Press.

CANUTEC: *Initial emergency response guide 1992,* Ottawa, Canada, 1992, Canada Communication Group.

CCINFO: *MSDS/CHEMINFO* (CD-ROM version), Hamilton, Ontario, Canada, 1993, Canadian Centre for Occupational Health and Safety.

Dot: *CHRIS hazardous chemical data,* US Department of Transportation/United States Coast Guard, Washington, DC, 1984, US Government Printing Office.

DOT: *2000 Emergency response guidebook,* Office of Hazardous Materials Transportation, Research and Special Programs Administration, Washington, DC, 2000, US Department of Transportation.

Goldfrank LR, et al: *Goldfrank's toxicologic emergencies,* ed 6, New York, 1998,McGraw-Hill Professional.

Goodman AG, et al, *Goodman and Gilman's the pharmacological basis of therapeutics,* ed 8, New York, 1990, Pergamon Press.

Gosselin RE, Smith RP, Hodge HC: *Clinical toxicology of commercial products,* ed 5, Baltimore, 1984, Williams & Wilkins.

Hartman DE: *Neuropsychological toxicology, identification and assessment of human neurotoxic syndromes,* New York, 1988, Pergamon Press.

Kaloyanova FP, El Batawi MA: *Human toxicology of pesticides,* Boca Raton, Florida, 1991, CRC Press.

Mackison FW, Stricoff RS, Partridge LJ Jr, editors: *Occupational health guidelines for chemical hazards,* NIOSH/OSHA, Washington, DC, 1981, US Government Printing Office.

Morgan DP: *Recognition and management of pesticide poisonings,* ed 4, Washington, DC, United States Environmental Protection Agency, 1989, US Government Printing Office.

NIOSH: *NIOSH pocket guide to chemical hazards* (CD-ROM version), Cincinnati, 2000, DHHS (NIOSH), US Government Printing Office.

Sullivan JB, Kriger GR, editors: *Clinical environmental health and hazardous materials toxicology,* Baltimore, 1997, Williams & Wilkins.

Journals

Basol MS, Eren S, Sadar M H: Comparative toxicity of some pesticides on human health and some aquatic species, *J Environ Sci Health (B)* 15:993-1004, 1980.

Branch R, Jacqz E: Subacute neurotoxicity following long-term exposure to carbaryl, *Am J Med* 80:741-745, 1982.

Gallo MA: 'Tis the season (editorial), *J Med Soc NJ* 80:329-330, 1983.

Gold RE, et al: Exposure of urban applicators to carbaryl, *Arch Environ Contam Toxicol* 11:63-67, 1982.

Leavitt JR, et al: Exposure of professional pesticide applicators to carbaryl, *Arch Environ Contam Toxicol* 11:57-62, 1982.

Mount ME, Dehme FW: Carbaryl: A literature review, *Residue Rev* 80:1-64, 1981.

Natoff IL, Reiff B: Effect of oximes on the acute toxicity of acetylcholinesterase carbamates, *Toxicol Appl Pharmacol* 25:569-575, 1973.

Recommended health-based limits in occupational exposure to pesticides, *WHO Tech Rep Ser* 677:1-110, 1982.

Shah P, Guthrie F: Percutaneous penetration of three insecticides in rats: a comparison of two methods for in vivo determination, *J Invest Dermatol* 80:291-293, 1983.

Zwiener RJ, Ginsburg CM: Organophosphate and carbamate poisoning in infants and children, *Pediatrics* 81:121-126, 1988.

GUIDELINE 51

Books

Amdur MO, Doull J, Klaassen CD, editors: *Casarett and Doull's toxicology, the basic science of poisons,* ed 4, New York, 1991, Pergamon Press.

CANUTEC: *Initial emergency response guide 1992,* Ottawa, Canada, 1992, Canada Communication Group.

CCINFO: *MSDS/CHEMINFO* (CD-ROM version), Hamilton, Ontario, Canada, 1993, Canadian Centre for Occupational Health and Safety.

DOT: *CHRIS hazardous chemical data,* US Department of Transportation/United States Coast Guard. Washington, DC, 1984, US Government Printing Office.

DOT: *2000 Emergency response guidebook,* Office of Hazardous Materials Transportation, Research and Special Programs Administration, Washington, DC, 2000, US Department of Transportation.

Goldfrank LR, et al: *Goldfrank's toxicologic emergencies,* ed 6, New York, NY, 1998, McGraw-Hill Professional.

Goodman AG, et al, editors: *Goodman and Gilman's the pharmacological basis of therapeutics,* ed 8, New York, 1990, Pergamon Press.

Gosselin RE, Smith RP, Hodge HC: *Clinical toxicology of commercial products,* ed 5, Baltimore, 1984, Williams & Wilkins.

Haddad LM, et al: *Clinical management of poisoning and drug overdose,* ed 3, Philadelphia, 1997, Saunders.

Kaloyanova FP, El Batawi MA: *Human toxicology of pesticides,* Boca Raton, Florida, 1991, CRC Press.

Mackison FW, Stricoff RS, Partridge LJ Jr, editors: *Occupational health guidelines for chemical hazards,* NIOSH/OSHA, Washington, DC, 1981, US Government Printing Office.

Morgan DP: *Recognition and management of pesticide poisonings,* ed 4, Washington, DC, United States Environmental Protection Agency, 1989, US Government Printing Office.

NIOSH: *NIOSH pocket guide to chemical hazards* (CD-ROM version), Cincinnati, 2000, DHHS (NIOSH), US Government Printing Office.

Journals

Chaturvedi A, Rao N, McCoy F: A multi-chemical death involving caffeine, nicotine and malathion, *Forensic Sci Intl* 23:265-275, 1983.

Duteil L, et al: Objective assessment of topical corticosteroids and non-steroidal anti-inflammatory drugs in methyl-nicotinate-induced skin inflammation, *Clin Exp Dermatol* 15:195-199, 1990.

Ghosh S, et al: Occupational health problems among tobacco processing workers: a preliminary study, *Arch Environ Health* 40:318-321, 1985.

Gothoni P: Hypersensitivity to the tremorogenic action of nicotine in rats withdrawn from ethanol, *Med Biol* 61:344-345, 1983.

Hsu W: Toxicity and drug interactions of levamisole, *J Am Vet Med Assn* 176:1166-1169, 1980.

Jeremy J, Mikhailidis D, Dandona P: Cigarette smoke extracts, but not nicotine, inhibit prostacyclin (PG12) synthesis in human, rabbit and rat vascular tissue, *Prostaglandins Leukot Med* 19:261-270, 1985.

Kuzlowski L, et al: Nicotine, a prescribable drug available without prescription (letter), *Lancet* 6:334, 1982.

Malizia E, et al: Acute intoxication with nicotine alkaloids and cannabinoids in children from ingestion of cigarettes, *Hum Toxicol* 2:315-316, 1983.

Manoguerra A, Freeman D: Acute poisoning from the ingestion of *Nicotiana glauca, J Toxicol Clin Toxicol* 19:861-864, 1982.

MMWR: Green tobacco sickness in tobacco harvesters—Kentucky—1992, *JAMA* 269(21):2722-2724, 1993.

Sasagawa S, et al: Effects of nicotine on the functions of human polymorphonuclear leukocytes in vitro, *J Leukocyte Biol* 37:493-502, 1985.

Saxena K, Scheman A: Suicide plan by nicotine poisoning: a review of nicotine toxicity, *Vet Hum Toxicol* 27:495-497, 1985.

Short DD, Blinder BB: Nicotine used as emetic by a patient with bulimia (Letter), *Am J Psychiatry* 142:272, 1985.

GUIDELINE 52

Books

Amdur MO, Doull J, Klaassen CD, editors: *Casarett and Doull's toxicology, the basic science of poisons,* ed 4, New York, 1991, Pergamon Press.

Bronstein AC, Sullivan JB: Herbicides, fungicides, biocides, and pyrethrins. In Sullivan JB, Krieger GR, editors: *Hazardous material toxicology,* Baltimore, 1991, Williams & Wilkins.

CANUTEC: *Initial emergency response guide 1992,* Ottawa, Canada, 1992, Canada Communication Group.

CCINFO: *MSDS/CHEMINFO* (CD-ROM version), Hamilton, Ontario, Canada, 1993, Canadian Centre for Occupational Health and Safety.

DOT: *CHRIS hazardous chemical data,* US Department of Transportation/United States Coast Guard. Washington, DC, 1984, US Government Printing Office.

DOT: *2000 Emergency response guidebook,* Office of Hazardous Materials Transportation, Research and Special Programs Administration, Washington, DC, 2000, US Department of Transportation.

Gosselin RE, Smith RP, Hodge HC: *Clinical toxicology of commercial products,* ed 5, Baltimore, 1984, Williams & Wilkins.

Kaloyanova FP, El Batawi MA: *Human toxicology of pesticides,* Boca Raton, Florida, 1991, CRC Press.

Mackison FW, Stricoff RS, Partridge LJ Jr, editors: *Occupational health guidelines for chemical hazards,* NIOSH/OSHA, Washington, DC, 1981, US Government Printing Office.

Morgan DP: *Recognition and management of pesticide poisonings,* ed 4, Washington, DC, United States Environmental Protection Agency, 1989, US Government Printing Office.

NIOSH: *NIOSH pocket guide to chemical hazards* (CD-ROM version), Cincinnati, 2000, DHHS (NIOSH), US Government Printing Office.

Sullivan JB, Kriger GR, editors: *Clinical environmental health and hazardous materials toxicology,* Baltimore, 1997, Williams & Wilkins.

Journals

Coats J: Mechanisms of toxic action of structure-activity relationships for organochlorine and synthetic pyrethroid insecticides, *Environ Health Perspect* 87:255-262, 1990.

Dorman DC, Beasley VR: Neurotoxicology of pyrethrin and the pyrethroid insecticides, *Vet Hum Toxicol* 33:238-243, 1991.

Lessenger JE: Five office workers inadvertently exposed to cypermethrin, *J Toxicol Environ Health* 35:261-267, 1992.

Patton DL, Walker JS: Pyrethrin poisoning from commercial strength flea and tick spray, *Am J Emerg Med* 6:232-235, 1988.

GUIDELINE 53

Books

Amdur MO, Doull J, Klaassen CD, editors: *Casarett and Doull's toxicology, the basic science of poisons,* ed 4, New York, 1991, Pergamon Press.

CANUTEC: *Initial emergency response guide 1992,* Ottawa, Canada, 1992, Canada Communication Group.

CCINFO: *MSDS/CHEMINFO* (CD-ROM version), Hamilton, Ontario, Canada, 1993, Canadian Centre for Occupational Health and Safety.

DOT: *CHRIS hazardous chemical data,* US Department of Transportation/United States Coast Guard. Washington, DC, 1984, US Government Printing Office.

DOT: *2000 Emergency response guidebook,* Office of Hazardous Materials Transportation,

Research and Special Programs Administration, Washington, DC, 2000, US Department of Transportation.

Gosselin RE, Smith RP, Hodge HC: *Clinical toxicology of commercial products,* ed 5, Baltimore, 1984, Williams & Wilkins.

Mackison FW, Stricoff RS, Partridge LJ Jr, editors: *Occupational health guidelines for chemical hazards,* NIOSH/OSHA, Washington, DC, 1981, US Government Printing Office.

Morgan DP: *Recognition and management of pesticide poisonings,* ed 4, Washington, DC, United States Environmental Protection Agency, 1989, US Government Printing Office.

NIOSH: *NIOSH pocket guide to chemical hazards* (CD-ROM version), Cincinnati, 2000, DHHS (NIOSH), US Government Printing Office.

Sullivan JB, Kriger GR, editors: *Clinical environmental health and hazardous materials toxicology,* Baltimore, 1997, Williams & Wilkins.

Journals

Gosalvez M: Carcinogenesis with the insecticide rotenone, *Life Sci* 21:809-816, 1983.

Khera K, Whalen C, Angers G: Teratogenicity study on pyrethrum and rotenone (natural origin) and ronnel in pregnant rats, *J Toxicol Environ Health* 10:111-119, 1982.

GUIDELINE 54

Books

Amdur MO, Doull J, Klaassen CD, editors: *Casarett and Doull's toxicology, the basic science of poisons,* ed 4, New York, 1991, Pergamon Press.

CANUTEC: *Initial emergency response guide 1992,* Ottawa, Canada, 1992, Canada Communication Group.

CCINFO: *MSDS/CHEMINFO* (CD-ROM version), Hamilton, Ontario, Canada, 1993, Canadian Centre for Occupational Health and Safety.

DOT: *CHRIS hazardous chemical data,* US Department of Transportation/United States Coast Guard. Washington, DC, 1984, US Government Printing Office.

DOT: *2000 Emergency response guidebook,* Office of Hazardous Materials Transportation, Research and Special Programs Administration, Washington, DC, 2000, US Department of Transportation.

Gosselin RE, Smith RP, Hodge HC: *Clinical toxicology of commercial products,* ed 5, Baltimore, 1984, Williams & Wilkins.

Hartman DE: *Neuropsychological toxicology, identification and assessment of human neurotoxic syndromes,* New York, 1988, Pergamon Press.

HSDB: *Hazardous substances data bank,* National Library of Medicine, Bethesda, Maryland, 1993.

Kaloyanova FP, El Batawi MA: *Human toxicology of pesticides,* Boca Raton, Florida, 1991, CRC Press.

Morgan DP: *Recognition and management of pesticide poisonings,* ed 4, Washington, DC, United States Environmental Protection Agency, 1989, US Government Printing Office.

NIOSH: *NIOSH pocket guide to chemical hazards* (CD-ROM version), Cincinnati, 2000, DHHS (NIOSH), US Government Printing Office.

Sullivan JB, Kriger GR, editors: *Clinical environmental health and hazardous materials toxicology,* Baltimore, 1997, Williams & Wilkins.

Journals

Chlordane and heptachlor, *IARC Monogr Eval Carcinog Risks Hum* 53:115-175, 1991.

Chlordane contamination of a public water supply—Pittsburgh, Pennsylvania, *MMWR Morb Mortal Wkly Rep* 30(46):571-572, 577-578, 1981.

Curley A, Garretson L: Acute chlordane poisoning, clinical and chemical studies, *Arch Environ Health* 18:211-215, 1969.

Garrettson L, Guzelian P, Blanke R: Subacute chlordane poisoning, *J Toxicol Clin Toxicol* 22:565-571, 1984.

Kuiz F, et al: A fatal chlordane poisoning, *J Toxicol Clin Toxicol* 20:167-174, 1983.

Marquardt ED: Suicide attempt with rectally administered chlordane, *Drug Intell Clin Pharm* 16:247-248, 1982.

McConnachie PR, Zahalsky AC: Immune alterations in humans exposed to the termiticide technical chlordane, *Arch Environ Health* 47:295-301, 1992.

Olanoff L, Bristow W, Cololough J: Acute chlordane intoxication, *J Toxicol Clin Toxicol* 20:291-306, 1983.

Webster RC, et al: Percutaneous absorption of (^{14}C)chlordane from soil, *J Toxicol Environ Health* 35:269-277, 1992.

Wright CG, Leidy RB: Chlordane and heptachlor in the ambient air of houses treated for termites, *Bull Environ Contam Toxicol* 28:617-623, 1982.

GUIDELINE 55

Books

Amdur MO, Doull J, Klaassen CD, editors: *Casarett and Doull's toxicology, the basic science of poisons,* ed 4, New York, 1991, Pergamon Press.

CANUTEC: *Initial emergency response guide 1992,* Ottawa, Canada, 1992, Canada Communication Group.

CCINFO: *MSDS/CHEMINFO* (CD-ROM version), Hamilton, Ontario, Canada, 1993, Canadian Centre for Occupational Health and Safety.

DOT: *CHRIS hazardous chemical data,* US Department of Transportation/United States Coast Guard. Washington, DC, 1984, US Government Printing Office.

DOT: *2000 Emergency response guidebook,* Office of Hazardous Materials Transportation, Research and Special Programs Administration, Washington, DC, 2000, US Department of Transportation.

Gosselin RE, Smith RP, Hodge HC: *Clinical toxicology of commercial products,* ed 5, Baltimore, 1984, Williams & Wilkins.

Hartman DE: *Neuropsychological toxicology, identification and assessment of human neurotoxic syndromes,* New York, 1988, Pergamon Press.

Kaloyanova FP, El Batawi MA: *Human toxicology of pesticides,* Boca Raton, Florida, 1991, CRC Press.

Manahan SE: *Environmental chemistry,* ed 7, Chelsea, Mich, 1999, Lewis Publishers.

Meeks RG, Harrison SD, Bull RJ, editors: *Hepatotoxicology,* Boca Raton, Florida, 1991, CRC Press.

Morgan DP: *Recognition and management of pesticide poisonings,* ed 4, Washington, DC, United States Environmental Protection Agency, 1989, US Government Printing Office.

NIOSH: *NIOSH pocket guide to chemical hazards* (CD-ROM version), Cincinnati, 2000, DHHS (NIOSH), US Government Printing Office.

Journals

Bulgur W, Kupfer D: Estrogenic action of DDT analogs, *Am J Ind Med* 4:163-173, 1983.

Coulston F: The dilemma of DDT (editorial), *Reg Toxicol Pharmacol* 5:329-331, 1985.

Coulston F: Reconsideration of the dilemma of DDT for the establishment of an acceptable daily intake, *Reg Toxicol Pharmacol* 5:332-383, 1985.

DDT and associated compounds, *IARC Monogr Eval Carcinog Risks Hum* 53:179-249, 1991.

Higginson J: DDT: epidemiological evidence, *Arch Sci Publ* 65:107-117, 1985.

Kreiss K, et al: Cross-sectional study of a community with exceptional exposure to DDT, *JAMA* 245:1926-1930, 1981.

Lessenger JE, Riley N: Neurotoxicities and behavioral changes in a 12-year-old male exposed to dicofol, an organochloride pesticide, *J Toxicol Environ Health* 33:255-261, 1991.

Misra U K, Nag D, Murti C R: A study of cognitive functions in DDT sprayers, *Ind Health* 22:199-206, 1984.

Misra U K, et al: Some observations on the macula of pesticide workers, *Hum Toxicol* 4:135-145, 1985.

Ohyama T, Takashi T, Ogawa H: Effects of dichlorodiphenyltrichloroethane and its analogues on rat liver mitochondria, *Biochem Pharmacol* 31:387-404, 1982.

Report of ICPEMC task group 5 on the differentiation between genotoxic and non-genotoxic carcinogens, *Mutat Res* 133:1-49, 1984.

Wang G: Evaluation of pesticides which pose carcinogenicity potential in animal testing. II. Consideration of human exposure conditions for regulatory decision making, *Reg Toxicol Pharmacol* 4:361-371, 1984.

Wong O, et al: Mortality of workers potentially exposed to organic and inorganic brominated chemicals, DBCP, TRIS, PBB, and DDT, *Br J Ind Med* 41:15-24, 1984.

GUIDELINE 56

Books

Amdur MO, Doull J, Klaassen CD, editors: *Casarett and Doull's toxicology, the basic science of poisons,* ed 4, New York, 1991, Pergamon Press.

CANUTEC: *Initial emergency response guide 1992,* Ottawa, Canada, 1992, Canada Communication Group.

CCINFO: *MSDS/CHEMINFO* (CD-ROM version), Hamilton, Ontario, Canada, 1993, Canadian Centre for Occupational Health and Safety.

DOT: *CHRIS hazardous chemical data,* US Department of Transportation/United States Coast Guard. Washington, DC, 1984, US Government Printing Office.

DOT: *2000 Emergency response guidebook,* Office of Hazardous Materials Transportation, Research and Special Programs Administration, Washington, DC, 2000, US Department of Transportation.

Gosselin RE, Smith RP, Hodge HC: *Clinical toxicology of commercial products,* ed 5, Baltimore, 1984, Williams & Wilkins.

Kaloyanova FP, El Batawi MA: *Human toxicology of pesticides,* Boca Raton, Florida, 1991, CRC Press.

Morgan DP: *Recognition and management of pesticide poisonings,* ed 4, Washington, DC, United States Environmental Protection Agency, 1989, US Government Printing Office.

NIOSH: *NIOSH pocket guide to chemical hazards* (CD-ROM version), Cincinnati, 2000, DHHS (NIOSH), US Government Printing Office.

Sullivan JB, Kriger GR, editors: *Clinical environmental health and hazardous materials toxicology,* Baltimore, 1997, Williams & Wilkins.

Journals

Ribbens PH: Mortality study of industrial workers exposed to aldrin, dieldrin and endrin, *Int Arch Occup Environ Health* 56:75-79, 1985.

Sandifer SH, et al: A case control study of persons with elevated blood levels of dieldrin, *Arch Environ Contam Toxicol* 10:35-45, 1981.

Waller K, et al: Seizures after eating a snack food contaminated with the pesticide endrin, *West J Med* 157:648-651, 1992.

GUIDELINE 57

Books

Amdur MO, Doull J, Klaassen CD, editors: *Casarett and Doull's toxicology, the basic science of poisons,* ed 4, New York, 1991, Pergamon Press.

CANUTEC: *Initial emergency response guide 1992,* Ottawa, Canada, 1992, Canada Communication Group.

CCINFO: *MSDS/CHEMINFO* (CD-ROM version), Hamilton, Ontario, Canada, 1993, Canadian Centre for Occupational Health and Safety.

DOT: *2000 Emergency response guidebook,* Office of Hazardous Materials Transportation, Research and Special Programs Administration, Washington, DC, 2000, US Department of Transportation.

Kaloyanova FP, El Batawi MA: *Human toxicology of pesticides,* Boca Raton, Florida, 1991, CRC Press.

Morgan DP: *Recognition and management of pesticide poisonings,* ed 4, Washington, DC, United States Environmental Protection Agency, 1989, US Government Printing Office.

NIOSH: *NIOSH pocket guide to chemical hazards* (CD-ROM version), Cincinnati, 2000, DHHS (NIOSH), US Government Printing Office.

Sullivan JB, Kriger GR, editors: *Clinical environmental health and hazardous materials toxicology,* Baltimore, 1997, Williams & Wilkins.

Journals

Fitzloff J, Pan J: Epoxidation of the lindane metabolite, beta-PCCH, by human-and rat-liver microsomes, *Xenobiotica* 14:599-604, 1984.

Gurevitch A: Scabies and lice, *Pediatr Clin North Am* 32:987-1018, 1985.

Jaeger U, et al: Acute oral poisoning with lindane-solvent mixtures, *Vet Hum Toxicol* 26:11-14, 1984.

Konje JC, et al: Insecticide poisoning in pregnancy, *J Reprod Med* 37:992-994, 1992.

Purres J: Safety of gamma benzene hexachloride (letter). *J Am Acad Dermatol* 7:407-408, 1982.

Rauch AE, et al: Lindane (Kwell)-induced aplastic anemia, *Arch Intern Med* 150:2393-2395, 1990.

Recommended health-based limits in occupational exposure to pesticides, *WHO Tech Rep Ser* 677:1-110, 1982.

Rugman FP, Cosstick R: Aplastic anaemia associated with organochlorine pesticide: case reports and review of evidence, *J Clin Pathol* 43:98-101, 1990.

Telch J, Jarvis D: Acute intoxication with lindane, *Can Med Assn J* 127:821, 1982.

Tenenbein M: Seizures after lindane therapy, *J Am Geriatr Soc* 39:394-395, 1991.

GUIDELINE 58

Books

Amdur MO, Doull J, Klaassen CD, editors: *Casarett and Doull's toxicology, the basic science of poisons,* ed 4, New York, 1991, Pergamon Press.

CANUTEC: *Initial emergency response guide 1992,* Ottawa, Canada, 1992, Canada Communication Group.

CCINFO: *MSDS/CHEMINFO* (CD-ROM version), Hamilton, Ontario, Canada, 1993, Canadian Centre for Occupational Health and Safety.

DOT: *2000 Emergency response guidebook,* Office of Hazardous Materials Transportation, Research and Special Programs Administration, Washington, DC, 2000, US Department of Transportation.

Gosselin RE, Smith RP, Hodge HC: *Clinical toxicology of commercial products,* ed 5, Baltimore, 1984, Williams & Wilkins.

Kaloyanova FP, El Batawi MA: *Human toxicology of pesticides,* Boca Raton, Florida, 1991, CRC Press.

Manahan SE: *Environmental chemistry,* ed 7, Chelsea, Mich, 1999, Lewis Publishers.

Morgan DP: *Recognition and management of pesticide poisonings,* ed 4, Washington, DC, United States Environmental Protection Agency, 1989, US Government Printing Office.

NIOSH: *NIOSH pocket guide to chemical hazards* (CD-ROM version), Cincinnati, 2000, DHHS (NIOSH), US Government Printing Office.

WHO. *Environmental health criteria 45, Camphechlor,* Geneva, 1984, World Health Organization.

Journals

Sobti R, Krishan A, Davies J: Cytokinetic and cytogenetic effect of agricultural chemicals on human lymphoid cells in vitro, *Arch Toxicol* 52:221-231, 1983.

Starmont RT, Conley BE: Pharmacologic properties of toxaphene, a chlorinated hydrocarbon insecticide, *JAMA* 149:1135-1137, 1952.

GUIDELINE 59

Books

Amdur MO, Doull J, Klaassen CD, editors: *Casarett and Doull's toxicology, the basic science of poisons,* ed 4, New York, 1991, Pergamon Press.

CANUTEC: *Initial emergency response guide 1992,* Ottawa, Canada, 1992, Canada Communication Group.

CCINFO: *MSDS/CHEMINFO* (CD-ROM version), Hamilton, Ontario, Canada, 1993, Canadian Centre for Occupational Health and Safety.

DOT: *2000 Emergency response guidebook,* Office of Hazardous Materials Transportation, Research and Special Programs Administration, Washington, DC, 2000, US Department of Transportation.

Gosselin RE, Smith RP, Hodge HC: *Clinical toxicology of commercial products,* ed 5, Baltimore, 1984, Williams & Wilkins.

Manahan SE: *Environmental chemistry,* ed 7, Chelsea, Mich, 1999, Lewis Publishers.

Morgan DP: *Recognition and management of pesticide poisonings,* ed 4, Washington, DC, United States Environmental Protection Agency, 1989, US Government Printing Office.

NIOSH: *NIOSH pocket guide to chemical hazards* (CD-ROM version), Cincinnati, 2000, DHHS (NIOSH), US Government Printing Office.

Sullivan JB, Kriger GR, editors: *Clinical environmental health and hazardous materials toxicology,* Baltimore, 1997, Williams & Wilkins.

Journals

Astray AL, Jakab GL: The effects of acrolein exposure on pulmonary antibacterial defenses, *Toxicol Appl Pharmacol* 67:49-54, 1983.

Beauchamp RO, et al: A critical review of the literature on acrolein toxicity, *CRC Crit Rev Toxicol* 14:309-380, 1985.

Hales CA, et al: Synthetic smoke with acrolein but not HCl produces pulmonary edema, *J Appl Physiol* 64:1121-1133, 1988.

GUIDELINE 60

Books

Amdur MO, Doull J, Klaassen CD, editors: *Casarett and Doull's toxicology, the basic science of poisons,* ed 4, New York, 1991, Pergamon Press.

Bronstein AC, Sullivan JB: Herbicides, fungicides, biocides, and pyrethrins. In Sullivan JB, Krieger GR, editors: *Hazardous material toxicology,* Baltimore, 1991, Williams & Wilkins.

CANUTEC: *Initial emergency response guide 1992,* Ottawa, Canada, 1992, Canada Communication Group.

CCINFO: *MSDS/CHEMINFO* (CD-ROM version), Hamilton, Ontario, Canada, 1993, Canadian Centre for Occupational Health and Safety.

DOT: *CHRIS hazardous chemical data,* US Department of Transportation/United States Coast Guard. Washington, DC, 1984, US Government Printing Office.

DOT: *2000 Emergency response guidebook,* Office of Hazardous Materials Transportation, Research and Special Programs Administration, Washington, DC, 2000, US Department of Transportation.

Gosselin RE, Smith RP, Hodge HC: *Clinical toxicology of commercial products,* ed 5, Baltimore, 1984, Williams & Wilkins.

Hartman DE: *Neuropsychological toxicology, identification and assessment of human neurotoxic syndromes,* New York, 1988, Pergamon Press.

Hutzinger O, Frei RW, Merian E, Pocchiari F, editors: *Chlorinated dioxins and related compounds, impact on the environment,* New York,1982, Pergamon Press.

Kaloyanova FP, El Batawi MA: *Human toxicology of pesticides,* Boca Raton, Florida, 1991, CRC Press.

Mackison FW, Stricoff RS, Partridge LJ Jr, editors: *Occupational health guidelines for chemical hazards,* NIOSH/OSHA, Washington, DC, 1981, US Government Printing Office.

Morgan DP: *Recognition and management of pesticide poisonings,* ed 4, Washington, DC, United States Environmental Protection Agency, 1989, US Government Printing Office.

NIOSH: *NIOSH pocket guide to chemical hazards* (CD-ROM version), Cincinnati, 2000, DHHS (NIOSH), US Government Printing Office.

Sullivan JB, Kriger GR, editors: *Clinical environmental health and hazardous materials toxicology,* Baltimore, 1997, Williams & Wilkins.

Journals

Arnold EK, Beasley VA: The pharmacokinetics of chlorinated phenoxy acid herbicides: a literature review, *Vet Hum Toxicol* 31:121-125, 1989.

Bailar JC: How dangerous is dioxin? *N Engl J Med* 324;260-262, 1991.

Blackburn A: Review of the effects of agent orange, *Military Med* 148:333-340, 1983.

Calesnick B: Dioxin and agent orange, *Am Fam Phys* 29:303-305, 1984.

Durakovic Z, et al: Poisoning with 2,4-dichlorophenoxyacetic acid treated by hemodialysis, *Arch Toxicol* 66:518-521, 1992.

Fagan K, Pollak J K: The effect of the phenoxyacetic acid herbicides 2,4,5-trichlorophenoxyacetic acid and 2,4-dichlorophenoxy-acetic acid as ascertained by direct experimentation, *Residue Rev* 92:29-58, 1984.

Fraser A, Isner A, Perry R: Toxicologic studies in a fatal overdose of 2,4-D, mecoprop and dicamba, *J Forensic Sci* 29:1237-1241, 1984.

Goldstein NP, Jones PH: Peripheral neuropathy after exposure to an ester of dichlorophenoxyacetic acid, *JAMA* 171: 1306-1309, 1959.

Gunby P: More questions, not answers emerge from agent orange studies, *JAMA* 249:2743-2746, 1983.

Hall RF: Herbicides: liberators or poisoners of humankind? *Vet Hum Toxicol* 25:92-95, 1983.

Heikki AE, Luoma T, Ylitalo P: Inhibition of human and rabbit platelet aggregation by chlorophenoxy acid herbicides, *Arch Toxicol* 65:140-144, 1991.

Increased rates of sister chromatid exchanges induced by the herbicide, 2,4-D, *J Heredity* 6:213-214, 1985.

Michalek JE, Wolff WH, Miner JC: Health status of Air Force veterans occupationally exposed to herbicides in Vietnam. I. Mortality, *JAMA* 264:1832-1836, 1990.

Osterloh J, Lotti M, Pond S M: Toxicologic studies in a fatal overdose of 2,4-D, and chlorpyrifos, *J Anal Toxicol* 7:125-129, 1983.

Stevens K: Agent orange toxicity: a quantitative perspective, *Hum Toxicol* 1:31-39, 1981.

Tamburro CH: Chronic liver injury in phenoxy herbicide-exposed Vietnam veterans, *Environ Research* 59:175-188, 1992.

Wolff WH, et al: Health status of Air Force veterans occupationally exposed to herbicides in Vietnam. I. physical health, *JAMA* 264:1824-1831, 1990.

GUIDELINE 61

Books

CANUTEC: *Initial emergency response guide 1992,* Ottawa, Canada, 1992, Canada Communication Group.

CCINFO: *MSDS/CHEMINFO* (CD-ROM version), Hamilton, Ontario, Canada, 1993, Canadian Centre for Occupational Health and Safety.

DOT: *CHRIS hazardous chemical data,* US Department of Transportation/United States Coast Guard. Washington, DC, 1984, US Government Printing Office.

DOT: *2000 Emergency response guidebook,* Office of Hazardous Materials Transportation, Research and Special Programs Administration, Washington, DC, 2000, US Department of Transportation.

Ellenhorn MJ, Barceloux DG: *Medical toxicology: diagnosis and treatment of human poisoning,* New York, 1988, Elsevier Science Publishing.

Gosselin RE, Smith RP, Hodge HC: *Clinical toxicology of commercial products,* ed 5, Baltimore, 1984, Williams & Wilkins.

Morgan DP: *Recognition and management of pesticide poisonings,* ed 4, Washington, DC, United States Environmental Protection Agency, 1989, US Government Printing Office.

NIOSH: *NIOSH pocket guide to chemical hazards* (CD-ROM version), Cincinnati, 2000, DHHS (NIOSH), US Government Printing Office.

Sullivan JB, Kriger GR, editors: *Clinical environmental health and hazardous materials toxicology,* Baltimore, 1997, Williams & Wilkins.

Journals

Brouwer EJ, et al: Biological effect monitoring of occupational exposure to 1,3-dichloropropene: effects on liver and renal function and on glutathione conjugation, *Br J Ind Med* 48:167-172, 1991.

Markovitz A, Crosby W: Chemical carcinogenesis, a soil fumigant, 1,3-dicloropropene, as possible cause of hematologic malignancies, *Arch Int Med* 144:1409-1411, 1984.

Osterloh JD, et al: Urinary excretion of the n-acetyl cysteine conjugate of cis-1,3-dichloropropene by exposed individuals, *Arch Environ Health* 39:271-275, 1984.

Osterloh JD, et al: Biological monitoring of dichloropropene: air concentrations, urinary metabolite, and renal enzyme excretion, *Arch Environ Health* 44:207-213, 1989.

Van Sittert NJ, et al: Biological effect monitoring of occupational exposure to 1,3-dichlorpropene: effects on liver and renal function and on glutathione conjugation: Correspondence and author's reply, *Br J Ind Med* 48:646-648, 1991.

GUIDELINE 62

Books

Amdur MO, Doull J, Klaassen CD, editors: *Casarett and Doull's toxicology, the basic science of poisons,* ed 4, New York, 1991, Pergamon Press.

CANUTEC: *Initial emergency response guide 1992,* Ottawa, Canada, 1992, Canada Communication Group.

CCINFO: *MSDS/CHEMINFO* (CD-ROM version), Hamilton, Ontario, Canada, 1993, Canadian Centre for Occupational Health and Safety.

DOT: *CHRIS hazardous chemical data,* US Department of Transportation/United States

Coast Guard. Washington, DC, 1984, US Government Printing Office.

DOT: *2000 Emergency response guidebook,* Office of Hazardous Materials Transportation, Research and Special Programs Administration, Washington, DC, 2000, US Department of Transportation.

Gosselin RE, Smith RP, Hodge HC: *Clinical toxicology of commercial products,* ed 5, Baltimore, 1984, Williams & Wilkins.

Kaloyanova FP, El Batawi MA: *Human toxicology of pesticides,* Boca Raton, Florida, 1991, CRC Press.

Morgan DP: *Recognition and management of pesticide poisonings,* ed 4, Washington, DC, United States Environmental Protection Agency, 1989, US Government Printing Office.

NIOSH: *NIOSH pocket guide to chemical hazards* (CD-ROM version), Cincinnati, 2000, DHHS (NIOSH), US Government Printing Office.

Sullivan JB, Kriger GR, editors: *Clinical environmental health and hazardous materials toxicology,* Baltimore, 1997, Williams & Wilkins.

Journals

Bidstrup PL, Payne DJH: Poisoning by dinitro-orthop-cresol: report of eight fatal cases occurring in Great Britain, *Br Med J* 2:16-19, 1951.

Leftwich R, et al: Dinitrophenol poisoning: a diagnosis to consider in undiagnosed fever, *S Med J* 75:182-184, 1982.

Smith W: An investigation of suspected dinoseb poisoning after the agricultural use of a herbicide, Practitioner 225:923-926, 1981.

GUIDELINE 63

Books

Amdur MO, Doull J, Klaassen CD, editors: *Casarett and Doull's toxicology, the basic science of poisons,* ed 4, New York, 1991, Pergamon Press.

CANUTEC: *Initial emergency response guide 1992,* Ottawa, Canada, 1992, Canada Communication Group.

CCINFO: *MSDS/CHEMINFO* (CD-ROM version), Hamilton, Ontario, Canada, 1993, Canadian Centre for Occupational Health and Safety.

DOT: *2000 Emergency response guidebook,* Office of Hazardous Materials Transportation, Research and Special Programs Administration, Washington, DC, 2000, US Department of Transportation.

HSDB: *Hazardous substances data bank,* National Library of Medicine, Bethesda, Md, 1993.

Kaloyanova FP, El Batawi MA: *Human toxicology of pesticides,* Boca Raton, Florida, 1991, CRC Press.

Morgan DP: *Recognition and management of pesticide poisonings,* ed 4, Washington, DC, United States Environmental Protection Agency, 1989, US Government Printing Office.

NIOSH: *NIOSH pocket guide to chemical hazards* (CD-ROM version), Cincinnati, 2000, DHHS (NIOSH), US Government Printing Office.

Sullivan JB, Kriger GR, editors: *Clinical environmental health and hazardous materials toxicology,* Baltimore, 1997, Williams & Wilkins.

Journals

Busby C, et al: Dermatitis among workers cleaning the Sacramento River after a chemical spill—California, 1991. *MMWR Morb Mortal Wkly Rep* 40(48):825-833, 1991.

Crippa M, et al: Dyshidrotic eczema and sensitization to dithiocarbamates in a florist, *Contact Dermatitis* 23: 203-204, 1990.

Peluso AN, et al: Multiple sensitization due to bis-dithiocarbamate and thiophthalimide pesticides, *Contact Dermatitis* 25:327, 1991.

Piraccini BM, et al: A case of allergic contact dermatitis due to the pesticide maneb, *Contact Dermatitis* 24:381-382, 1991.

GUIDELINE 64

Books

Amdur MO, Doull J, Klaassen CD, editors: *Casarett and Doull's toxicology, the basic science of poisons,* ed 4, New York, 1991, Pergamon Press.

CANUTEC: *Initial emergency response guide 1992,* Ottawa, Canada, 1992, Canada Communication Group.

CCINFO: *MSDS/CHEMINFO* (CD-ROM version), Hamilton, Ontario, Canada, 1993, Canadian Centre for Occupational Health and Safety.

DOT: *2000 Emergency response guidebook,* Office of Hazardous Materials Transportation, Research and Special Programs Administration, Washington, DC, 2000, US Department of Transportation.

Ellenhorn MJ, Barceloux DG: *Medical toxicology: diagnosis and treatment of human poisoning,* New York, 1988, Elsevier Science Publishing.

Gosselin RE, Smith RP, Hodge HC: *Clinical toxicology of commercial products,* ed 5, Baltimore, 1984, Williams & Wilkins.

Morgan DP: *Recognition and management of pesticide poisonings,* ed 4, Washington, DC, United States Environmental Protection Agency, 1989, US Government Printing Office.

Journals

Chung HM: Acute renal failure caused by acute monofluoroacetate poisoning, *Vet Hum Toxicol* 26(Suppl 2):29-32, 1984.

Dipalma J: Human toxicity from rat poisons, *Am Fam Phys* 24:186-189, 1981.

Quick MP, et al: Sodium monochloroacetate poisoning of greenfinches, *Forensic Sci Int* 54:1-8, 1992

Taitelman U, Roy A, Hoffer E: Fluoroacetamide poisoning in man: the role of ionized calcium, *Arch Toxicol Suppl* 6:228-231, 1983.

Trabes J, Rason N, Avrahami E: Computed tomography demonstration of brain damage due to acute sodium monofluoroacetate poisoning, *Clin Toxicol* 10:85-92, 1983.

GUIDELINE 65

Books

Amdur MO, Doull J, Klaassen CD, editors: *Casarett and Doull's toxicology, the basic science of poisons,* ed 4, New York, 1991, Pergamon Press.

CANUTEC: *Initial emergency response guide 1992,* Ottawa, Canada, 1992, Canada Communication Group.

CCINFO: *MSDS/CHEMINFO* (CD-ROM version), Hamilton, Ontario, Canada, 1993, Canadian Centre for Occupational Health and Safety.

DOT: *2000 Emergency response guidebook,* Office of Hazardous Materials Transportation, Research and Special Programs Administration, Washington, DC, 2000, US Department of Transportation.

Gosselin RE, Smith RP, Hodge HC: *Clinical toxicology of commercial products,* ed 5, Baltimore, 1984, Williams & Wilkins.

Morgan DP: *Recognition and management of pesticide poisonings,* ed 4 Washington, DC, United States Environmental Protection Agency, 1989, US Government Printing Office.

Sullivan JB, Kriger GR, editors: *Clinical environmental health and hazardous materials toxicology,* Baltimore, 1997, Williams & Wilkins.

Journals

Colosio C, et al: Occupational triphenyltin acetate poisoning: a case report, *Br J Ind Med* 48:136-139, 1991.

Grace CT, Ng SK, Cheong LL: Recurrent irritant contact dermatitis due to tributyltin oxide on work clothes, *Contact Dermatitis* 25: 250-271, 1991.

Kreyber S, et al: Trimethyltin poisoning: report of a case with postmortem examination, *Clin Neuropathol* 11:256-259, 1992.

Shelton D, et al: Occupational asthma induced by a carpet fungicide—tributyl tin oxide, *J Allergy Clin Immunol* 65:274-275, 1992.

GUIDELINE 66

Books

Amdur MO, Doull J, Klaassen CD, editors: *Casarett and Doull's toxicology, the basic science of poisons,* ed 4, New York, 1991, Pergamon Press.

Baselt RC, Cravey RH: *Disposition of toxic drugs and chemicals in man,* ed 3, Chicago, 1989, Year Book Medical Publishers.

CANUTEC: *Initial emergency response guide 1992,* Ottawa, Canada, 1992, Canada Communication Group.

CCINFO: *MSDS/CHEMINFO* (CD-ROM version), Hamilton, Ontario, Canada, 1993, Canadian Centre for Occupational Health and Safety.

DOT: *CHRIS hazardous chemical data,* US Department of Transportation/United States Coast Guard. Washington, DC, 1984, US Government Printing Office.

DOT: *2000 Emergency response guidebook,* Office of Hazardous Materials Transportation, Research and Special Programs Administration, Washington, DC, 2000, US Department of Transportation.

Gosselin RE, Smith RP, Hodge HC: *Clinical toxicology of commercial products,* ed 5, Baltimore, 1984, Williams & Wilkins.

Kaloyanova FP, El Batawi MA: *Human toxicology of pesticides,* Boca Raton, Florida, 1991, CRC Press.

Mackison FW, Stricoff RS, Partridge LJ Jr, editors: *Occupational health guidelines for chemical hazards,* NIOSH/OSHA, Washington, DC, 1981, US Government Printing Office.

Morgan DP: *Recognition and management of pesticide poisonings,* ed 4, Washington, DC, United States Environmental Protection Agency, 1989, US Government Printing Office.

NIOSH: *NIOSH pocket guide to chemical hazards* (CD-ROM version), Cincinnati, 2000, DHHS (NIOSH), US Government Printing Office.

Sullivan JB, Kriger GR, editors: *Clinical environmental health and hazardous materials toxicology,* Baltimore, 1997, Williams & Wilkins.

Journals

Barnard JW, et al: Lung protection against paraquat is calcium dependent, *J Appl Physiol* 72:498-504, 1992.

Bismuth C, et al: Prognosis and treatment of paraquat poisoning: a review of 28 cases, *J Clin Toxicol* 19:461-474, 1982.

Braithwaite RA: Emergency analysis of paraquat in biological fluids, *Hum Toxicol* 6:83-86, 1987.

Chan KW, Cheong IK: Paraquat poisoning: a clinical and epidemiological review of 30 cases, *Med J Malaysia* 37:227-230, 1982.

Conradi S, Olanoff L, Dawson W: Fatality due to paraquat intoxication: confirmation by postmortem tissue analysis, *Am J Clin Pathol* 80:771-776, 1983.

Hart TB: Paraquat-review of safety in agricultural and horticultural use, *Hum Toxicol* 6:13-18, 1987.

Howard J: The myth of paraquat inhalation as a route for human poisonings (letter), *J Toxicol Clin Toxicol* 20:191-193, 1983.

Imamura T, et al: Pseudomembranous colitis in a patient of paraquat intoxication, *Acta Pathol Jpn* 36:309-316, 1986.

Mofenson H, et al: Paraquat intoxication: report of a fatal case: discussion of pathophysiology and rational treatment, *J Toxicol Clin Toxicol* 19:321-334, 1982.

Ozonek S, et al: Successful treatment of paraquat poisoning: activated charcoal per os and "continuous hemoperfusion," *J Toxicol Clin Toxicol* 19:807-819, 1982.

Pond SM: Manifestations and management of paraquat poisoning, *Med J Aust* 152:256-259, 1990.

Pond SM, et al: Kinetics of toxic doses of paraquat and the effects of hemoperfusion in the dog, *Clin Toxicol* 31:229-246, 1993.

Proudfoot AT, et al: Paraquat poisoning: significance of plasma paraquat concentrations, *Lancet* 2:330-332, 1979.

Rivero C, et al: Paraquat poisoning in children: survival of three cases, *Vet Hum Toxicol* 34:164-165, 1992.

Sonoda Y, et al: Paraquat poisoning—a review of four cases, *Tokai J Exp Clin Med* 7(4):489-496, 1982.

Smith L, Cohen G, Adridge W: Morphological and biochemical correlates of chemical induced injury in the lung, *Arch Toxicol* 58:214-218, 1986.

Vale JA, Meredith TJ, Buckley BM: Paraquat poisoning: Clinical features and immediate general management, *Hum Toxicol* 6:41-47, 1987.

Vale J, Meredith T, Buckley B: Paraquat poisoning (letter), *Lancet* 21:14, 1986.

Vandenborgaerde J, Colardyn F, Rijksuniversiteit G: Untractable fecaliths and hypercalcemia, both associated with Fuller's earth therapy in a fatal case of paraquat poisoning, *J Toxicol Clin Toxicol* 19:1011-1012, 1982.

Webb DB, Leopold JD: Vasodilatation and rehydration in paraquat poisoning, *Hum Toxicol* 2:531-534, 1983.

GUIDELINE 67

Books

Amdur MO, Doull J, Klaassen CD, editors: *Casarett and Doull's toxicology, the basic science of poisons,* ed 4, New York, 1991, Pergamon Press.

CANUTEC: *Initial emergency response guide 1992,* Ottawa, Canada, 1992, Canada Communication Group.

CCINFO: *MSDS/CHEMINFO* (CD-ROM version), Hamilton, Ontario, Canada, 1993, Canadian Centre for Occupational Health and Safety.

DOT: *2000 Emergency response guidebook,* Office of Hazardous Materials Transportation, Research and Special Programs Administration, Washington, DC, 2000, US Department of Transportation.

Gosselin RE, Smith RP, Hodge HC: *Clinical toxicology of commercial products,* ed 5, Baltimore, 1984, Williams & Wilkins.

Kaloyanova FP, El Batawi MA: *Human toxicology of pesticides,* Boca Raton, Florida, 1991, CRC Press.

Manahan SE: *Environmental chemistry,* ed 7, Chelsea, Mich, 1999, Lewis Publishers.

Meeks RG, Harrison SD, Bull RJ, editors: *Hepatotoxicology,* Boca Raton, Florida, 1991, CRC Press.

Morgan DP: *Recognition and management of pesticide poisonings,* ed 4, Washington, DC, United States Environmental Protection Agency, 1989, US Government Printing Office.

NIOSH: *NIOSH pocket guide to chemical hazards* (CD-ROM version), Cincinnati, 2000, DHHS (NIOSH), US Government Printing Office.

Journals

McConnachie PR, Zahalsky AC: Immunological consequences of exposure to pentachlorophenol, *Arch Environ Health* 46:249-253, 1991.

Pentachlorophenol, *IARC Monogr Eval Carcinog Risks Hum* 53:371-402, 1991.

GUIDELINE 68

Books

Amdur MO, Doull J, Klaassen CD, editors: *Casarett and Doull's toxicology, the basic science of poisons,* ed 4, New York, 1991, Pergamon Press.

Gosselin RE, Smith RP, Hodge HC: *Clinical toxicology of commercial products,* ed 5, Baltimore, 1984, Williams & Wilkins.

Morgan DP: *Recognition and management of pesticide poisonings,* ed 4, Washington, DC, United States Environmental Protection Agency, 1989, US Government Printing Office.

Sullivan JB, Kriger GR, editors: *Clinical environmental health and hazardous materials toxicology,* Baltimore, 1997, Williams & Wilkins.

Journals

Menkes D, Temple W, Edwards I: Intentional self-poisoning with glyphosate-containing herbicides, *Hum Exper Toxicol* 10:103-107, 1991.

Smith EA, Oehme FW: The biological activity of plants and animals: a literature review, *Vet Hum Toxicol* 34:531-543, 1992.

Webster RC, et al: Glyphosate skin binding, absorption, residual tissue distribution, and skin decontamination, *Fundamental Appl Toxicol* 16:725-732, 1991.

GUIDELINE 69

Books

Amdur MO, Doull J, Klaassen CD, editors: *Casarett and Doull's toxicology, the basic science of poisons,* ed 4, New York, 1991, Pergamon Press.

CANUTEC: *Initial emergency response guide 1992,* Ottawa, Canada, 1992, Canada Communication Group.

CCINFO: *MSDS/CHEMINFO* (CD-ROM version), Hamilton, Ontario, Canada, 1993, Canadian Centre for Occupational Health and Safety.

DOT: *CHRIS hazardous chemical data,* US Department of Transportation/United States Coast Guard. Washington, DC, 1984, US Government Printing Office.

DOT: *2000 Emergency response guidebook,* Office of Hazardous Materials Transportation, Research and Special Programs Administration, Washington, DC, 2000, US Department of Transportation.

Goldfrank LR, et al: *Goldfrank's toxicologic emergencies,* ed 6, New York, NY, 1998, McGraw-Hill Professional.

Goodman AG, et al, editors: *Goodman and Gilman's the pharmacological basis of therapeutics,* ed 8, New York, 1990, Pergamon Press.

Gosselin RE, Smith RP, Hodge HC: *Clinical toxicology of commercial products,* ed 5, Baltimore, 1984, Williams & Wilkins.

Haddad LM, et al: *Clinical management of poisoning and drug overdose,* ed 3, Philadelphia, 1997, Saunders.

Mackison FW, Stricoff RS, Partridge LJ Jr, editors: *Occupational health guidelines for chemical hazards,* NIOSH/OSHA, Washington, DC, 1981, US Government Printing Office.

Morgan DP: *Recognition and management of pesticide poisonings,* ed 4, Washington, DC, United States Environmental Protection Agency, 1989, US Government Printing Office.

NIOSH: *NIOSH pocket guide to chemical hazards* (CD-ROM version), Cincinnati, 2000, DHHS (NIOSH), US Government Printing Office.

Journals

Alliot L, Bryant G, Guth PS: Measurement of strychnine by high-performance liquid chromatography, *J Chromatogr* 232:440-442, 1982.

Blain P, Nightingale S, Stoddart J: Strychnine poisoning: abnormal eye movements, *J Toxicol Clin Toxicol* 119:215-217, 1982.

Boyd R, et al: Strychnine poisoning: recovery from profound lactic acidosis, hyperthermia and rhabdomyolysis, *Am J Med* 74:507-512, 1983.

Decker WJ, et al: Two deaths resulting from apparent parenteral injection of strychnine, *Vet Hum Toxicol* 24:161-162, 1982.

Dittrich K, Bayer M, Wanke L: A case of fatal strychnine poisoning, *J Emerg Med* 1:327-330, 1984.

Lambert J, Byrick R, Hdammeke M: Management of acute strychnine poisoning, *Can Med J* 124:1268-1270, 1981.

Mack RB: St. Ronald's ballet—strychnine poisoning, *NC Med J* 45:554-555, 1984.

Martens PR, Vandevelde K: A near lethal case of combined strychnine and aconitine poisoning, *Clin Toxicol* 31:133-138, 1993.

Perper J: Fatal strychnine poisoning—a case report and review of literature, *J Forensic Sci* 30:1248-1255, 1985.

Smith BA: Strychnine poisoning, *J Emerg Med* 8:321-325, 1990.

GUIDELINE 70

Books

Bronstein AC, Sullivan JB: Herbicides, fungicides, biocides, and pyrethrins. In Sullivan JB, Krieger GR, editors: *Hazardous material toxicology,* Baltimore, 1991, Williams & Wilkins.

Goodman AG, et al, editors: *Goodman and Gilman's the pharmacological basis of therapeutics,* ed 8, New York, 1990, Pergamon Press.

Gosselin RE, Smith RP, Hodge HC: *Clinical toxicology of commercial products,* ed 5, Baltimore, 1984, Williams & Wilkins.

Haddad LM, et al: *Clinical management of poisoning and drug overdose,* ed 3, Philadelphia, 1997, Saunders.

Morgan DP: *Recognition and management of pesticide poisonings,* ed 4, Washington, DC, United States Environmental Protection Agency, 1989, US Government Printing Office.

Sullivan JB, Kriger GR, editors: *Clinical environmental health and hazardous materials toxicology,* Baltimore, 1997, Williams & Wilkins.

Journal

Humphreys F, Cox NH: Thiabendazole-induced erythema multiforme with lesions around melanocytic naevi, *Br J Dermatol* 118:855-856, 1988.

GUIDELINE 71

Books

Amdur MO, Doull J, Klaassen CD, editors: *Casarett and Doull's toxicology, the basic science of poisons,* ed 4, New York, 1991, Pergamon Press.

CANUTEC: *Initial emergency response guide 1992,* Ottawa, Canada, 1992, Canada Communication Group.

CCINFO: *MSDS/CHEMINFO* (CD-ROM version), Hamilton, Ontario, Canada, 1993, Canadian Centre for Occupational Health and Safety.

DOT: *CHRIS hazardous chemical data,* US Department of Transportation/United States Coast Guard. Washington, DC, 1984, US Government Printing Office.

DOT: *2000 Emergency response guidebook,* Office of Hazardous Materials Transportation, Research and Special Programs Administration, Washington, DC, 2000, US Department of Transportation.

Goodman AG, et al, editors: *Goodman and Gilman's the pharmacological basis of therapeutics,* ed 8, New York, 1990, Pergamon Press.

Gosselin RE, Smith RP, Hodge HC: *Clinical toxicology of commercial products,* ed 5, Baltimore, 1984, Williams & Wilkins.

Mackison FW, Stricoff RS, Partridge LJ Jr, editors: *Occupational health guidelines for chemical hazards,* NIOSH/OSHA, Washington, DC, 1981, US Government Printing Office.

Morgan DP: *Recognition and management of pesticide poisonings,* ed 4, Washington, DC, United States Environmental Protection Agency, 1989, US Government Printing Office.

NIOSH: *NIOSH pocket guide to chemical hazards* (CD-ROM version), Cincinnati, 2000, DHHS (NIOSH), US Government Printing Office.

Journals

Braithwaite GB: Vitamin K and brodifacoum, *Am J Vet Med Assoc* 181:531-534, 1982.

Butcher GP, et al: Difenacoum poisoning as a cause of haematuria, *Hum Exper Toxicol* 11:553-554, 1992.

Chelbowski R, et al: Clinical and pharmacokinetic effects of combined warfarin and 5-fluorouracil in advanced colon cancer, *Cancer Research* 42:5827-5830, 1982.

Hackett L, Llett K, Chester A: Plasma warfarin concentrations after a massive overdose, *Med J Aust* 142:642-643, 1985.

Hoffman RS, Smilkstein MJ, Goldfrank LR: Evaluation of coagulation factor abnormalities in long-acting anticoagulant overdose, *J Toxicol Clin Toxicol* 26:233-248, 1988.

Jolson HM, et al: Adverse reaction reporting of interaction between warfarin and fluoroquinolones, *Arch Intern Med* 151:1003-1004, 1991.

Jones EC, Growe GH, Naiman SC: Prolonged anticoagulation in rat poisoning, *JAMA* 252:3009, 1984.

Lipton RA, Klass EM: Human ingestion of a "superwarfarin" rodenticide resulting in a prolonged anticoagulation effect, *JAMA* 252:3004, 1984.

Renowden S, et al: Oral cholestyramine increases elimination of warfarin after overdose, *Br Med J* 291:513-514, 1985.

Saunderson H, Fernandez L: Confusion between warfarin and propranol leading to warfarin overdosage (letter), *Can Med Assn J* 124:366, 1981.

Toolis F, Robson R, Critchley J: Warfarin poisoning in patients with prosthetic heart valves, *Br Med J* 283:581-582, 1981.

GUIDELINE 72

Books

Amdur MO, Doull J, Klaassen CD, editors: *Casarett and Doull's toxicology, the basic science of poisons,* ed 4, New York, 1991, Pergamon Press.

Baselt RC, Cravey RH: *Disposition of toxic drugs and chemicals in man,* ed 3, Chicago, 1989, Year Book Medical Publishers.

CANUTEC: *Initial emergency response guide 1992,* Ottawa, Canada, 1992, Canada Communication Group.

CCINFO: *MSDS/CHEMINFO* (CD-ROM version), Hamilton, Ontario, Canada, 1993, Canadian Centre for Occupational Health and Safety.

DOT: *CHRIS hazardous chemical data,* US Department of Transportation/United States Coast Guard. Washington, DC, 1984, US Government Printing Office.

DOT: *2000 Emergency response guidebook,* Office of Hazardous Materials Transportation, Research and Special Programs Administration, Washington, DC, 2000, US Department of Transportation.

Gosselin RE, Smith RP, Hodge HC: *Clinical toxicology of commercial products,* ed 5, Baltimore, 1984, Williams & Wilkins.

Hartman DE: *Neuropsychological toxicology, identification and assessment of human neurotoxic syndromes,* New York, 1988, Pergamon Press.

Kaloyanova FP, El Batawi MA: *Human toxicology of pesticides,* Boca Raton, Florida, 1991, CRC Press.

Mackison FW, Stricoff RS, Partridge LJ Jr, editors: *Occupational health guidelines for chemical hazards,* NIOSH/OSHA, Washington, DC, 1981, US Government Printing Office.

NIOSH: *NIOSH pocket guide to chemical hazards* (CD-ROM version), Cincinnati, 2000, DHHS (NIOSH), US Government Printing Office.

Morgan DP: *Recognition and management of pesticide poisonings,* ed 4, Washington, DC, United States Environmental Protection Agency, 1989, US Government Printing Office.

Journals

Donofrio PD, et al: Acute arsenic intoxication presenting as Guillain-Barre–like syndrome, *Muscle Nerve* 10;114-120, 1987.

Effects of toxic chemicals on the reproductive system, council on scientific affairs, *JAMA* 253:3431-3437, 1985.

Enterline PE, Henderson VL, Marsh GM: Exposure to arsenic and respiratory cancer: a reanalysis, *Am J Epidemiol* 125:929-938, 1987.

Falk H, et al: Arsenic-related hepatic angiosarcoma, *Am J Ind Med* 2:43-50, 1981.

Gidseg G: Toxic effects of marine plywood, *JAMA* 253:920-921, 1985.

Hindmarsh JT, McCurdy RF: Clinical and environmental aspects of arsenic toxicity, *CRC Crit Rev Clin Lab Sci* 23:315-347, 1986.

Hughes G, Davis L: Variegate porphyria and heavy metal poisoning from ingestion of moonshine, *South Med J* 76:1027-1029, 1983.

Hutton J, Christians B: Sources, symptoms and signs of arsenic poisoning, *J Fam Pract* 17:423-426, 1983.

IARC Monographs on the evaluation of the carcinogenic risk of chemicals to man, vol 23, some metals and metallic compounds: arsenic and arsenic compounds, pp 39-141. Lyon, International Agency for Research on Cancer, 1980.

Lilis R, et al: Effects of low-level lead and arsenic exposure on copper smelter workers, *Arch Environ Health* 40:38-47, 1985.

Rezuke WN, et al: Arsenic intoxication presenting as a myelodysplastic syndrome: a case report, *Am J Hematol* 36:291-293, 1991.

Schenker M: Occupational lung diseases in the industrializing and industrialized world due to modern industries and modern pollutants, *Tuber Lung Dis* 73:27-32, 1992.

Slimak M, Delos C: Environmental pathways of exposure to 129 priority pollutants, *J Toxicol Clin Toxicol* 84:39-63, 1983.

Weiss W: Respiratory cancer risk in relation to arsenic exposure and smoking (letter), *Arch Environ Health* 38:189-191, 1983.

Welch K, et al: Arsenic exposure, smoking, and respiratory cancer in copper smelter workers, *Arch Environ Health* 37:325-335, 1982.

Zaloga G, et al: Unusual manifestations of arsenic intoxication, *Am J Med Sci* 289:210-214, 1985.

GUIDELINE 73

Books

Amdur MO, Doull J, Klaassen CD, editors: *Casarett and Doull's toxicology, the basic science of poisons,* ed 4, New York, 1991, Pergamon Press.

CANUTEC: *Initial emergency response guide 1992,* Ottawa, Canada, 1992, Canada Communication Group.

CCINFO: *MSDS/CHEMINFO* (CD-ROM version), Hamilton, Ontario, Canada, 1993, Canadian Centre for Occupational Health and Safety.

DOT: *CHRIS hazardous chemical data,* US Department of Transportation/United States Coast Guard. Washington, DC, 1984, US Government Printing Office.

DOT: *2000 Emergency response guidebook,* Office of Hazardous Materials Transportation, Research and Special Programs Administration, Washington, DC, 2000, US Department of Transportation.

Gosselin RE, Smith RP, Hodge HC: *Clinical toxicology of commercial products,* ed 5, Baltimore, 1984, Williams & Wilkins.

Mackison FW, Stricoff RS, Partridge LJ Jr, editors: *Occupational health guidelines for chemical hazards,* NIOSH/OSHA, Washington, DC, 1981, US Government Printing Office.

Morgan DP: *Recognition and management of pesticide poisonings,* ed 4, Washington, DC, United States Environmental Protection Agency, 1989, US Government Printing Office.

NIOSH: *NIOSH pocket guide to chemical hazards* (CD-ROM version), Cincinnati, 2000, DHHS (NIOSH), US Government Printing Office.

Sullivan JB, Kriger GR, editors: *Clinical environmental health and hazardous materials toxicology,* Baltimore, 1997, Williams & Wilkins.

Journals

Aposhian J, et al: Anti-lewisite activity and stability of o-dimercaptosuccinic acid and 2,3-

dimercapto-1-propanesulfonic acid, *Life Sci* 31:2149-2156, 1982.
California Emergency Medical Services Authority: The toxics epidemiology program: Hazardous materials exposure: arsine gas, *J Emerg Nurs* 16:300-302, 1990.
Cullen W, et al: The wood preservative chromated copper arsenate is a substrate for trimethylarsine biosynthesis, *Appl Environ Microbiol* 47:443-444, 1984.
LaDou J: Potential occupational health hazards in the microelectronics industry, *Scand J Work Environ Health* 9:42-46, 1983.
Peterson D, Bhattacharya M: Hematological responses to arsine exposure: quantitation of exposure response in mice, *Fundam Appl Toxicol* 5:499-505, 1985.
Pirl JN, et al: Death by arsenic: a comparative evaluation of exhumed body tissues in the presence of external contamination, *J Anal Toxicol* 7:216-219, 1983.
Ringenberg QS, et al: Hematologic effects of heavy metal poisoning, *S Med J* 81:1132-1139, 1988.
Sheehy JW, Jones JH: Assessment of arsenic exposures and controls in gallium arsenide production, *Am Ind Hyg Assoc* 54:61-69, 1993.
Srivastava P, Hay H, Knapp F: Effects of alkyl and aryl substitution on the myocardial specificity of radioiodinated phosphonium, arsonium, and ammonium cations. *J Med Chem* 28:901-904, 1985.
Watson AP, Griffin GD: Toxicity of vesicant agents scheduled for destruction by the chemical stockpile, *Environ Health Perspect* 98:259-280, 1992.

GUIDELINE 74

Books

Amdur MO, Doull J, Klaassen CD, editors: *Casarett and Doull's toxicology, the basic science of poisons,* ed 4, New York, 1991, Pergamon Press.
CANUTEC: *Initial emergency response guide 1992,* Ottawa, Canada, 1992, Canada Communication Group.
CCINFO: *MSDS/CHEMINFO* (CD-ROM version), Hamilton, Ontario, Canada, 1993, Canadian Centre for Occupational Health and Safety.
DOT: *CHRIS hazardous chemical data,* US Department of Transportation/United States Coast Guard. Washington, DC, 1984, US Government Printing Office.
DOT: *2000 Emergency response guidebook,* Office of Hazardous Materials Transportation, Research and Special Programs Administration, Washington, DC, 2000, US Department of Transportation.
Gosselin RE, Smith RP, Hodge HC: *Clinical toxicology of commercial products,* ed 5, Baltimore, 1984, Williams & Wilkins.
Hartman DE: *Neuropsychological toxicology, identification and assessment of human neurotoxic syndromes,* New York, 1988, Pergamon Press.
Mackison FW, Stricoff RS, Partridge LJ Jr, editors: *Occupational health guidelines for chemical hazards,* NIOSH/OSHA, Washington, DC, 1981, US Government Printing Office.
NIOSH: *NIOSH pocket guide to chemical hazards* (CD-ROM version), Cincinnati, 2000, DHHS (NIOSH), US Government Printing Office.
Sittig M: *Handbook of toxic and hazardous chemicals and carcinogens,* ed 3, Park Ridge, NJ, 1992, Noyes Publications.

Journals

Brenniman G, et al: High barium levels in public drinking water and its association with elevated blood pressure, *Arch Environ Health* 36:28-32, 1981.
Brooks SM: Lung disorders resulting from the inhalation of metals, *Clin Chest Med* 2:235-254, 1981.
Johnson CH, VanTassell VJ: Acute barium poisoning with respiratory failure and rhabdomyolysis, *Ann Emerg Med* 20: 1138-1142, 1991.
Layzer R: Periodic paralysis and the sodium potassium pump, *Ann Neurol* 11:547-552, 1982.
Phelan D, Hagley S, Gurin M: Is hypokalaemia the cause of paralysis in barium poisoning? *Br Med J* 189:882, 1984.
Stewart D, Hummel R: Acute poisoning by a barium chloride burn, *J Trauma* 24:768-770, 1984.
Wetherill S, Guarino M, Cox R: Acute renal failure associated with barium chloride poisoning, *Ann Intern Med* 95:187-188, 1981.

GUIDELINE 75

Books

Amdur MO, Doull J, Klaassen CD, editors: *Casarett and Doull's toxicology, the basic science of poisons,* ed 4, New York, 1991, Pergamon Press.
CANUTEC: *Initial emergency response guide 1992,* Ottawa, Canada, 1992, Canada Communication Group.
CCINFO: *MSDS/CHEMINFO* (CD-ROM version), Hamilton, Ontario, Canada, 1993, Canadian Centre for Occupational Health and Safety.
DOT: *CHRIS hazardous chemical data,* US Department of Transportation/United States Coast Guard. Washington, DC, 1984, US Government Printing Office.

DOT: *2000 Emergency response guidebook,* Office of Hazardous Materials Transportation, Research and Special Programs Administration, Washington, DC, 2000, US Department of Transportation.

Gosselin RE, Smith RP, Hodge HC: *Clinical toxicology of commercial products,* ed 5, Baltimore, 1984, Williams & Wilkins.

NIOSH: *NIOSH pocket guide to chemical hazards* (CD-ROM version), Cincinnati, 2000, DHHS (NIOSH), US Government Printing Office.

Sittig M: *Handbook of toxic and hazardous chemicals and carcinogens,* ed 3, Park Ridge, NJ, 1992, Noyes Publications.

Sullivan JB, Kriger GR, editors: *Clinical environmental health and hazardous materials toxicology,* Baltimore, 1997, Williams & Wilkins.

Journals

Benoko V, Vasileva EV: Hygienic and toxicological aspects of occupational and environmental exposure to beryllium, *J Hyg Epidemiol Microbiol Immunol* 27:403-417, 1983.

Critchley JA: Working with beryllium, *Occup Health* (Lond) 33:457-460, 1981.

Eisenbud M, Lisson J: Epidemiological aspects of beryllium induced nonmalignant lung disease: a 30-year update, *J Occup Med* 25:196-202, 1983.

Kriess K, et al: The pulmonary toxicity of beryllium, *Am Rev Respir Dis* 137:464-473, 1988.

Maceira J, Fukuyama K, Epstein W: Appearance of T-cell subpopulations during the time course of beryllium-induced granulomas, *J Invest Dermatol* 83:314-316, 1984.

Newman L, et al: Pathologic and immunologic alterations in early stages of beryllium disease: reexamination of disease definition in natural history, *Am Rev Respir Dis* 139:1479-1486, 1989.

Rom W, et al: Reversible beryllium sensitization in prospective study of beryllium workers, *Arch Environ Health* 38:302-307, 1983.

Saracci R: Beryllium epidemiological evidence, *IARC Sci Publ* 65:203-219, 1985.

Sky-Peck H: Trace metals and neoplasia, *Clin Physiol Biochem* 4:99-111, 1986.

Suskind RR: Percutaneous absorption and chemical carcinogenesis, *J Dermatol (Tokyo)* 10:97-107, 1983.

Vilaplana J, Romaguera C, Grimalt F: Occupational and non-occupational allergic contact dermatitis from beryllium. *Contact Dermatitis* 26:295-298, 1992.

Ward E, et al: A mortality study of workers at seven beryllium processing plants, *Am J Ind Med* 22:885-904, 1992.

Williams W, Williams WJ: Development of beryllium lymphocyte transformation tests in chronic beryllium disease, *Int Arch Allergy Appl Immunol* 67:175-180, 1982.

GUIDELINE 76

Books

Amdur MO, Doull J, Klaassen CD, editors: *Casarett and Doull's toxicology, the basic science of poisons,* ed 4, New York, 1991, Pergamon Press.

Baselt RC, Cravey RH: *Disposition of toxic drugs and chemicals in man,* ed 3, Chicago, 1989, Year Book Medical Publishers.

CANUTEC: *Initial emergency response guide 1992,* Ottawa, Canada, 1992, Canada Communication Group.

CCINFO: *MSDS/CHEMINFO* (CD-ROM version), Hamilton, Ontario, Canada, 1993, Canadian Centre for Occupational Health and Safety.

DOT: *CHRIS hazardous chemical data,* US Department of Transportation/United States Coast Guard, Washington, DC, 1984, US Government Printing Office.

DOT: *2000 Emergency response guidebook,* Office of Hazardous Materials Transportation, Research and Special Programs Administration, Washington, DC, 2000, US Department of Transportation.

Gosselin RE, Smith RP, Hodge HC: *Clinical toxicology of commercial products,* ed 5, Baltimore, 1984, Williams & Wilkins.

Hartman DE: *Neuropsychological toxicology, identification and assessment of human neurotoxic syndromes,* New York, 1988, Pergamon Press.

Mackison FW, Stricoff RS, Partridge LJ Jr, editors: *Occupational health guidelines for chemical hazards,* NIOSH/OSHA, Washington, DC, 1981, US Government Printing Office.

NIOSH: *NIOSH pocket guide to chemical hazards* (CD-ROM version), Cincinnati, 2000, DHHS (NIOSH), US Government Printing Office.

Sullivan JB, Kriger GR, editors: *Clinical environmental health and hazardous materials toxicology,* Baltimore, 1997, Williams & Wilkins.

Journals

Barnhart S, Rosenstock L: Cadmium chemical pneumonitis, *Chest* 86:789-791, 1984.

Becking G: Recent advances in the toxicity of heavy metal—an overview, *Fundam Appl Toxicol* 1:348-352, 1981.

Chan HM, Cherian MG: Protective roles of metallothionein and glutathione in hepatotoxicity of cadmium, *Toxicology* 72:281-290, 1992.

Cowan V: Cadmium: protection from its effects, *Occup Health* (Lond) 34:261-270,1982.

Ellis K, Cohn S, Smith T: Cadmium inhalation exposure estimates: their significance with respect to kidney and liver cadmium burden, *J Toxicol Environ Health* 15:173-187, 1985.

Engvall J, Perk J: Prevalence of hypertension among cadmium-exposed workers, *Arch Environ Health* 40:185-190, 1985.

Fleig I, et al: Chromosome investigations of workers exposed to cadmium in the manufacturing of cadmium stabilizers and pigments, *Ecotoxicol Environ Saf* 7:106-110, 1983.

Hughes E: Biological monitoring of cadmium workers (letter), *Lancet* 2:1467-1468, 1984.

Jones MM, Cherian MG: The search for chelate antagonists for chronic cadmium intoxication, *Toxicology* 62:1-25, 1990.

Kazantzis G, Armstrong BG: A mortality study of cadmium workers in the United Kingdom, *Scand J Work Environ Health* 8(Suppl 1): 157-160, 1982.

Klaassen C: Pharmacokinetics in metal toxicity, *Fundam Appl Toxicol* 1:353-357, 1981.

Landrigan P: Occupational and community exposures to toxic metals: lead, cadmium, mercury and arsenic, *West J Med* 137:531-539, 1982.

Liu YZ, et al: Effects of cadmium on cadmium smelter workers, *Scand J Work Environ Health* 11(Suppl 4):29-32, 1985.

Roels H, et al: Evolution of cadmium-induced renal dysfunction in workers removed from exposure, *Scand J Work Environ Health* 8:191-200, 1982.

Sorahan T, Adams R, Waterhouse J: Analysis of mortality and nephrosis among nickel-cadmium battery workers, *J Occup Med* 25:609-612, 1983.

Townshend R: Acute cadmium pneumonitis: a 17-year follow-up, *Br J Ind Med* 39:411-412, 1982.

Winneke G, Lilienthal H, Zimmermann U: Neurobehavioral effects of lead and cadmium, *Dev Toxicol Environ Sci* 11:85-96, 1983.

GUIDELINE 77

Books

Amdur MO, Doull J, Klaassen CD, editors: *Casarett and Doull's toxicology, the basic science of poisons,* ed 4, New York, 1991, Pergamon Press.

Baselt RC, Cravey RH: *Disposition of toxic drugs and chemicals in man,* ed 3, Chicago, 1989, Year Book Medical Publishers.

CANUTEC: *Initial emergency response guide 1992,* Ottawa, Canada, 1992, Canada Communication Group.

CCINFO: *MSDS/CHEMINFO* (CD-ROM version), Hamilton, Ontario, Canada, 1993, Canadian Centre for Occupational Health and Safety.

DOT: *2000 Emergency response guidebook,* Office of Hazardous Materials Transportation, Research and Special Programs Administration, Washington, DC, 2000, US Department of Transportation.

Gosselin RE, Smith RP, Hodge HC: *Clinical toxicology of commercial products,* ed 5, Baltimore, 1984, Williams & Wilkins.

NIOSH: *NIOSH pocket guide to chemical hazards* (CD-ROM version), Cincinnati, 2000, DHHS (NIOSH), US Government Printing Office.

Sittig M: *Handbook of toxic and hazardous chemicals and carcinogens,* ed 3, Park Ridge, NJ, 1992, Noyes Publications.

Journals

Alexandersson R: Blood and urine concentrations as estimators of cobalt exposure, *Arch Environ Health* 43:299-303, 1988.

Chaudhary S, et al: Health hazard of poorly regulated exposure during manufacture of cemented tungsten carbide and cobalt, *Br J Ind Med* 49:832-836, 1992.

Jarvis JQ: Cobalt cardiomyopathy: a report of two cases from mineral assay laboratories and a review of the literature, *J Occup Med* 34:620-626, 1992.

Nemery B, et al: Survey of cobalt exposure and respiratory health in diamond polishers, *Am Rev Resp Dis* 145:610-616, 1992.

Shirakawa T, et al: Occupational asthma from cobalt sensitivity in workers exposed to hard metal dust, *Chest* 95:29-37, 1989.

Singgih SI, et al: Occupational dermatoses in hospital cleaning personnel, *Contact Dermatitis* 14:14-19, 1986.

GUIDELINE 78

Books

Amdur MO, Doull J, Klaassen CD, editors: *Casarett and Doull's toxicology, the basic science of poisons,* ed 4, New York, 1991, Pergamon Press.

Baselt RC, Cravey RH: *Disposition of toxic drugs and chemicals in man,* ed 3, Chicago, 1989, Year Book Medical Publishers.

CANUTEC: *Initial emergency response guide 1992,* Ottawa, Canada, 1992, Canada Communication Group.

CCINFO: *MSDS/CHEMINFO* (CD-ROM version), Hamilton, Ontario, Canada, 1993, Canadian Centre for Occupational Health and Safety.

DOT: *CHRIS hazardous chemical data,* US Department of Transportation/United States Coast Guard. Washington, DC, 1984, US Government Printing Office.

DOT: *2000 Emergency response guidebook,* Office of Hazardous Materials Transportation, Research and Special Programs Administration, Washington, DC, 2000, US Department of Transportation.

Goodman AG, et al, editors: *Goodman and Gilman's the pharmacological basis of therapeutics,* ed 8, New York, 1990, Pergamon Press.

Gosselin RE, Smith RP, Hodge HC: *Clinical toxicology of commercial products,* ed 5, Baltimore, 1984, Williams & Wilkins.

Haddad LM, et al: *Clinical management of poisoning and drug overdose,* ed 3, Philadelphia, 1997, Saunders.

Mackison FW, Stricoff RS, Partridge LJ Jr, editors: *Occupational health guidelines for chemical hazards,* NIOSH/OSHA, Washington, DC, 1981, US Government Printing Office.

Morgan DP: *Recognition and management of pesticide poisonings,* ed 4, Washington, DC, United States Environmental Protection Agency, 1989, US Government Printing Office.

NIOSH: *NIOSH pocket guide to chemical hazards* (CD-ROM version), Cincinnati, 2000, DHHS (NIOSH), US Government Printing Office.

Journals

Bowman M, Lewis M: The copper hypothesis of schizophrenia: a review, *Neurosci Behav Rev* 6:321-328, 1982.

Chaudhary S: Environmental factors: extensive use of copper utensils and vegetarian diet in the causation of Indian childhood cirrhosis (letter), *Indian Pediatr* 20:529-531, 1983.

Eastwood J, et al: Heparin inactivation, acidosis and copper poisoning due to presumed acid contamination of water in a hemodialysis unit, *Clin Nephrol* 20:197-201, 1983.

Lamont DL: Duflou JA: Copper sulfate. Not a harmless chemical, *Am J Forensic Med Pathol* 9:226-227, 1988.

Mehta A, et al: Copper sulphate poisoning—its impact on kidneys, *J Indian Med Assoc* 83:108-110, 1985.

Song ZY, Lu YP, Gu XQ: Treatment of yellow phosphorus skin burns with silver nitrate instead of copper sulphate, *Scand J Work Environ Health* 11(Suppl 4):33, 1985.

Sterry W, Schmoll M: Contact urticaria and dermatitis from self-adhesive pads, *Contact Dermatitis* 13:284-285, 1985.

Van Der Wal JF: Exposure of welders to fumes, Cr, Ni, Cu and gases in Dutch industries, *Ann Occup Hyg* 29:377-389, 1985.

Williams D, Halstead B: Chelating agents in medicine, *J Toxicol Clin Toxicol* 19:1081-1115, 1982.

Yanagihara R: Heavy metals and essential minerals in motor neuron disease, *Adv Neurol* 36:233-247, 1982.

Yelin G, Taff ML, Sadowski GE: Copper toxicity following massive ingestion of coins, *Am J Forensic Med Pathol* 8:78-85, 1987.

GUIDELINE 79

Books

Amdur MO, Doull J, Klaassen CD, editors: *Casarett and Doull's toxicology, the basic science of poisons,* ed 4, New York, 1991, Pergamon Press.

Baselt RC, Cravey RH: *Disposition of toxic drugs and chemicals in man,* ed 3, Chicago, 1989, Year Book Medical Publishers.

CANUTEC: *Initial emergency response guide 1992,* Ottawa, Canada, 1992, Canada Communication Group.

CCINFO: *MSDS/CHEMINFO* (CD-ROM version), Hamilton, Ontario, Canada, 1993, Canadian Centre for Occupational Health and Safety.

DOT: *CHRIS hazardous chemical data,* US Department of Transportation/United States Coast Guard. Washington, DC, 1984, US Government Printing Office.

DOT: *2000 Emergency response guidebook,* Office of Hazardous Materials Transportation, Research and Special Programs Administration, Washington, DC, 2000, US Department of Transportation.

Goldfrank LR, et al: *Goldfrank's toxicologic emergencies,* ed 6, New York, NY, 1998, McGraw-Hill Professional.

Goodman AG, et al, editors: *Goodman and Gilman's the pharmacological basis of therapeutics,* ed 8, New York, 1990, Pergamon Press.

Gosselin RE, Smith RP, Hodge HC: *Clinical toxicology of commercial products,* ed 5, Baltimore, 1984, Williams & Wilkins.

Haddad LM, et al: *Clinical management of poisoning and drug overdose,* ed 3, Philadelphia, 1997, Saunders.

NIOSH: *NIOSH pocket guide to chemical hazards* (CD-ROM version), Cincinnati, 2000, DHHS (NIOSH), US Government Printing Office.

Journals

Czajka P: Effect of bicarbonate, phosphate, and saline lavage solutions on the dissolution of ferrous sulfate tablets, *J Toxicol Clin Toxicol* 22:447-453, 1984.

Henretig FM, Temple AR: Acute iron poisoning in children, *Emerg Med Clin North Am* 2:121-132, 1984.

Henretig F, Karl S, Weintraub W: Severe iron poisoning treated with enteral and intravenous deferoxamine, *Ann Emerg Med* 12:306-309, 1983.

Hill L, Kleinberg F: Effects of drugs and chemicals on the fetus and newborn, *Mayo Clin Proc* 59:707-716, 1984.

Jalihal S, Barlow A: Hemochromatosis following prolonged oral iron ingestion, *J Royal Soc Med* 77:690-692, 1984.

Lacouture PG, et al: Emergency assessment of severity in iron overdose by clinical and laboratory methods, *J Pediatr* 99:89-92, 1981.

Peck M, Rogers J, Rivenbark J: Use of high doses of deferoxamine (Desferal) in an adult patient with acute iron overdosage, *J Toxicol Clin Toxicol* 19:865-869, 1982.

Rhyburn W, Donn S, Wolf M: Iron overdose during pregnancy: successful therapy with deferoxamine, *Am J Ob Gyn* 247:717-718, 1983.

Rosenmund A, Haeberli A, Straub P: Blood coagulation and acute iron toxicity: reversible iron-induced inactivation of serine proteases in vitro, *J Lab Clin Med* 103:524-533, 1984.

Tenenbein M: Inefficiency of gastric emptying procedures, *J Emerg Med* 3:133-136, 1985.

Tenenbein M, et al: Pulmonary toxic effects of continuous desferrioxamine administration in acute iron poisoning, *Lancet* 339:699-701, 1992.

GUIDELINE 80

Books

Amdur MO, Doull J, Klaassen CD, editors: *Casarett and Doull's toxicology, the basic science of poisons,* ed 4, New York, 1991, Pergamon Press.

Baselt RC, Cravey RH: *Disposition of toxic drugs and chemicals in man,* ed 3, Chicago, 1989, Year Book Medical Publishers.

CANUTEC: *Initial emergency response guide 1992,* Ottawa, Canada, 1992, Canada Communication Group.

CCINFO: *MSDS/CHEMINFO* (CD-ROM version), Hamilton, Ontario, Canada, 1993, Canadian Centre for Occupational Health and Safety.

DOT: *CHRIS hazardous chemical data,* US Department of Transportation/United States Coast Guard. Washington, DC, 1984, US Government Printing Office.

DOT: *2000 Emergency response guidebook,* Office of Hazardous Materials Transportation, Research and Special Programs Administration, Washington, DC, 2000, US Department of Transportation.

Ellenhorn MJ, Barceloux DG: *Medical toxicology: diagnosis and treatment of human poisoning,* New York, 1988, Elsevier Science Publishing.

Gosselin RE, Smith RP, Hodge HC: *Clinical toxicology of commercial products,* ed 5, Baltimore, 1984, Williams & Wilkins.

Hartman DE: *Neuropsychological toxicology, identification and assessment of human neurotoxic syndromes,* New York, 1988, Pergamon Press.

NIOSH: *NIOSH pocket guide to chemical hazards* (CD-ROM version), Cincinnati, 2000, DHHS (NIOSH), US Government Printing Office.

Sullivan JB, Kriger GR, editors: *Clinical environmental health and hazardous materials toxicology,* Baltimore, 1997, Williams & Wilkins.

Journals

Araki S, et al: Radial and median nerve conduction velocities in workers exposed to lead, copper, and zinc: a follow-up study for 2 years, *Environ Res* 61:308-316, 1993.

Chisolm JJ: BAL, EDTA, DMSA, DMPS in the treatment of lead poisoning in children, *Clin Toxicol* 30:493-504, 1992.

Fischbein A, et al: Subjective symptoms in workers with low-level exposure to lead, *J Appl Toxicol* 2:289-293, 1982.

Fischbein A, et al: Lead poisoning in an art conservatory, *JAMA* 247:2007-2009, 1982.

Graham J, Maxton D, Twort C: Painter's palsy: A difficult case of lead poisoning, *Lancet* 21:1159-1160, 1981.

Graziano JH, Lolacono NJ, Meyer P: Dose-response study of oral 2, 3-dimercaptosuccinic acid in children with elevated blood lead concentrations, *J Pediatr* 113:751-757, 1988.

Krigman MR, Bouldin TW, Mushak P: Metal toxicity in the nervous system, *Monogr Pathol* 26:58-100, 1985.

Landrigan P, et al: Exposure to lead from the Mystic River Bridge: The dilemma of deleading, *N Engl J Med* 306:673-676, 1982.

Le Quesne P: Metal-induced diseases of the nervous system, *Br J Hosp Med* 28:534-538, 1982.

Lilis R, et al: Effects of low-level lead and arsenic exposure on copper smelter workers, *Arch Environ Health* 40:38-47, 1985.

Murata K, et al: Assessment of central, peripheral, and autonomic nervous system functions in lead workers: neuroelectrophysiological studies, *Environ Res* 61:323-336, 1993.

Seeber A, et al: Neurobehavioral effects of a long-term exposure to tetraalkyllead, *Neurotoxicol Teratol* 12:653-655, 1990.

Tripathi RK, et al: Lead exposure in outdoor firearm instructors, *Am J Pub Health* 81:753-755, 1991.

Turk DS, et al: Sensitivity of erythrocyte protoporphyrin as a screening test for lead poisoning, *N Engl J Med* 326:137-138, 1992.

Waldron H: Chasing the lead (editorial), *Br Med J* 291:366-367, 1985.

Walsh T, Tilson H: Neurobehavioral toxicology of the organoleads, *Neurotoxicol* 5:67-86, 1984.

Williams B, Hajtmanicik M, Abreu M: Cardiac effects of lead, *Fed Proc* 42:2989-2993, 1983.

Winneke G, Lilienthal H, Zimmermann U: Neurobehavioral effects of lead and cadmium, *Dev Toxicol Environ Sci* 11:85-96, 1983.

Zatlin G, Senaldi E, Bruckheim A: Adult lead poisoning, *Am Fam Phys* 32:137-143, 1985.

GUIDELINE 81

Books

Amdur MO, Doull J, Klaassen CD, editors: *Casarett and Doull's toxicology, the basic science of poisons,* ed 4, New York, 1991, Pergamon Press.

Baselt RC, Cravey RH: *Disposition of toxic drugs and chemicals in man,* ed 3, Chicago, 1989, Year Book Medical Publishers.

CANUTEC: *Initial emergency response guide 1992,* Ottawa, Canada, 1992, Canada Communication Group.

CCINFO: *MSDS/CHEMINFO* (CD-ROM version), Hamilton, Ontario, Canada, 1993, Canadian Centre for Occupational Health and Safety.

DOT: *2000 emergency response guidebook,* Office of Hazardous Materials Transportation, Research and Special Programs Administration, Washington, DC, 2000, US Department of Transportation.

Goldfrank LR, et al: *Goldfrank's toxicologic emergencies,* ed 6, New York, NY, 1998, McGraw-Hill Professional.

Goodman AG, et al, editors: *Goodman and Gilman's the pharmacological basis of therapeutics,* ed 8, New York, 1990, Pergamon Press.

Gosselin RE, Smith RP, Hodge HC: *Clinical toxicology of commercial products,* ed 5, Baltimore, 1984, Williams & Wilkins.

Hartman DE: *Neuropsychological toxicology, identification and assessment of human neurotoxic syndromes,* New York, 1988, Pergamon Press.

NIOSH: *NIOSH pocket guide to chemical hazards* (CD-ROM version), Cincinnati, 2000, DHHS (NIOSH), US Government Printing Office.

Journals

Belanger DR, Tierney MG, Dickenson G: Effect of sodium polystyrene sulfonate on lithium bioavailability, *Ann Emerg Med* 21:1312-1315, 1992.

Friedberg RC, Spyker DA, Herold DA: Massive overdoses with sustained-release lithium carbonate preparations: pharmacokinetic model based on two case studies, *Clin Chem* 37:1205-1209, 1991.

Jacobson SJ, et al: Prospective multicentre study of pregnancy outcome after lithium exposure during first trimester, *Lancet* 339:530-533, 1992.

McHenry CR, et al: Lithiumogenic disorders of the thyroid and parathyroid glands as surgical disease, *Surgery* 108:1001-1005, 1990.

Smith SW, Ling LJ, Halstenson CE: Whole-bowel irrigation as a treatment for acute lithium overdose, *Ann Emerg Med* 20:536-539, 1991.

Tomaszewski C, et al: Lithium absorption prevented by sodium polystyrene sulfonate in volunteers, *Ann Emerg Med* 21:1308-1311, 1992.

GUIDELINE 82

Books

Amdur MO, Doull J, Klaassen CD, editors: *Casarett and Doull's toxicology, the basic science of poisons,* ed 4, New York, 1991, Pergamon Press.

Baselt RC, Cravey RH: *Disposition of toxic drugs and chemicals in man,* ed 3, Chicago, 1989, Year Book Medical Publishers.

CANUTEC: *Initial emergency response guide 1992,* Ottawa, Canada, 1992, Canada Communication Group.

CCINFO: *MSDS/CHEMINFO* (CD-ROM version), Hamilton, Ontario, Canada, 1993, Canadian Centre for Occupational Health and Safety.

DOT: *2000 emergency response guidebook,* Office of Hazardous Materials Transportation, Research and Special Programs Administration, Washington, DC, 2000, US Department of Transportation.

Gilmore DA, Bronstein AC: Magnesium and manganese. In Sullivan JB, Krieger GR, editors: *Hazardous material toxicology,* Baltimore, 1991, Williams & Wilkins.

Goodman AG, et al, editors: *Goodman and Gilman's the pharmacological basis of therapeutics,* ed 8, New York, 1990, Pergamon Press.

Gosselin RE, Smith RP, Hodge HC: *Clinical toxicology of commercial products,* ed 5, Baltimore, 1984, Williams & Wilkins.

NIOSH: *NIOSH pocket guide to chemical hazards* (CD-ROM version), Cincinnati, 2000, DHHS (NIOSH), US Government Printing Office.

Sullivan JB, Kriger GR, editors: *Clinical environmental health and hazardous materials toxicology,* Baltimore, 1997, Williams & Wilkins.

Journals

Cotzias GC: Manganese versus magnesium: why are they so similar in vitro and so different in vivo? *Fed Proc* 20:98-103, 1961.

Massry SG: Pharmacology of magnesium, *Annu Rev Pharmacol Toxicol* 17:67-82, 1977.

Mueller EJ, Seger DC: Metal fume fever: a review, *J Emerg Med* 2:271-275,1985.

Whang R, Whang DD, Ryan MP: Refractory potassium repletion. A consequence of magnesium deficiency, *Arch Intern Med* 152:40-45, 1992.

GUIDELINE 83

Books

Amdur MO, Doull J, Klaassen CD, editors: *Casarett and Doull's toxicology, the basic science of poisons,* ed 4, New York, 1991, Pergamon Press.

Baselt RC, Cravey RH: *Disposition of toxic drugs and chemicals in man,* ed 3, Chicago, 1989, Year Book Medical Publishers.

CANUTEC: *Initial emergency response guide 1992,* Ottawa, Canada, 1992, Canada Communication Group.

CCINFO: *MSDS/CHEMINFO* (CD-ROM version), Hamilton, Ontario, Canada, 1993, Canadian Centre for Occupational Health and Safety.

DOT: *2000 Emergency response guidebook,* Office of Hazardous Materials Transportation, Research and Special Programs Administration, Washington, DC, 2000, US Department of Transportation.

Gilmore DA, Bronstein AC: Magnesium and manganese. In Sullivan JB, Krieger GR, editors: *Hazardous material toxicology,* Baltimore, 1991, Williams & Wilkins.

Hartman DE: *Neuropsychological toxicology, identification and assessment of human neurotoxic syndromes,* New York, 1988, Pergamon Press.

NIOSH: *NIOSH pocket guide to chemical hazards* (CD-ROM version), Cincinnati, 2000, DHHS (NIOSH), US Government Printing Office.

Sittig M: *Handbook of toxic and hazardous chemicals and carcinogens,* ed 3, Park Ridge, NJ, 1992, Noyes Publications.

Sullivan JB, Kriger GR, editors: *Clinical environmental health and hazardous materials toxicology,* Baltimore, 1997, Williams & Wilkins.

Journals

Cotzias GC: Manganese versus magnesium: why are they so similar in vitro and so different in vivo? *Fed Proc* 20:98-103, 1961.

Himel HJ, et al: Molten metal burn of the foot: a preventable injury, *J Emerg Med* 10:147-150, 1992.

Hua MS, Huang CC: Chronic occupational exposure to manganese and neurobehavioral function, *J Clin Exper Neuropsychol* 13(4): 495-507, 1991.

Kilburn CJ: Manganese malformations and motor disorders: findings in a manganese exposed population, *Neurotoxicology* 8:421-430, 1987.

Mena I: The role of manganese in human disease, *Ann Clin Lab Sci* 4:487-491, 1974.

Piscator M: Health hazards from inhalation of metal fumes, *Environ Res* 11:268-270, 1976.

Wennberg A, Hagman M, Johansson L: Preclinical neurophysiological signs of parkinsonism in occupational manganese exposure, *Neurotoxicology* 13:271-274. 1992.

GUIDELINE 84

Books

Amdur MO, Doull J, Klaassen CD, editors: *Casarett and Doull's toxicology, the basic science of poisons,* ed 4, New York, 1991, Pergamon Press.

Baselt RC, Cravey RH: *Disposition of toxic drugs and chemicals in man,* ed 3, Chicago, 1989, Year Book Medical Publishers.

CANUTEC: *Initial emergency response guide 1992,* Ottawa, Canada, 1992, Canada Communication Group.

CCINFO: *MSDS/CHEMINFO* (CD-ROM version), Hamilton, Ontario, Canada, 1993, Canadian Centre for Occupational Health and Safety.

DOT: *CHRIS hazardous chemical data,* US Department of Transportation/United States Coast Guard. Washington, DC, 1984, US Government Printing Office.

DOT: *2000 Emergency response guidebook,* Office of Hazardous Materials Transportation, Research and Special Programs Administration, Washington, DC, 2000, US Department of Transportation.

Goldfrank LR, et al: *Goldfrank's toxicologic emergencies,* ed 6, New York, NY, 1998, McGraw-Hill Professional.

Goodman AG, et al, editors: *Goodman and Gilman's the pharmacological basis of therapeutics,* ed 8, New York, 1990, Pergamon Press.

Gosselin RE, Smith RP, Hodge HC: *Clinical toxicology of commercial products,* ed 5, Baltimore, 1984, Williams & Wilkins.

Mackison FW, Stricoff RS, Partridge LJ Jr, editors: *Occupational health guidelines for chemical hazards,* NIOSH/OSHA, Washington, DC, 1981, US Government Printing Office.

NIOSH: *NIOSH pocket guide to chemical hazards* (CD-ROM version), Cincinnati, 2000, DHHS (NIOSH), US Government Printing Office.

Sullivan JB, Kriger GR, editors: *Clinical environmental health and hazardous materials toxicology,* Baltimore, 1997, Williams & Wilkins.

Journals

Agocs MM, et al: Mercury exposure from interior latex paint, *N Engl J Med* 323:1096-1101, 1990.

Albers J, et al: Asymptomatic sensorimotor polyneuropathy in workers exposed to elemental mercury, *Neurology* 32:1168-1174, 1982.

Clarkson TW: Mercury—an element of mystery, *N Engl J Med* 323:1137-1139, 1990.

Clarkson T, Nordberg G, Sager P: Reproductive and developmental toxicity of metals, *Scand J Work Environ Health* 11:145-154, 1985.

Hamada R, et al: Computed tomography in fetal methylmercury poisoning, *Clin Toxicol* 31:101-106, 1993.

Kanluen S, Gottlieb CA: A clinical pathologic study of four adult cases of acute mercury inhalation toxicity, *Arch Pathol Lab Med* 115:56-60, 1991.

Krigman MR, Bouldin TW, Mushak P: Metal toxicity in the nervous system, *Monogr Pathol* 26:58-100, 1985.

Langolf GD, et al: Measurements of neurological functions in the evaluations of exposure to neurotoxic agents, *Ann Occup Hyg* 24:293-296, 1981.

Lilis R, Miller A, Lerman Y: Acute mercury poisoning with severe chronic pulmonary manifestations, *Chest* 88:306-309, 1985.

Markowitz L, Schalimburg H: Successful treatment of inorganic mercury neurotoxicity with n-acetyl-penicillamine despite an adverse reaction, *Neurology* 30:1000-1001, 1980.

Ridlington J, Whanger P: Interactions of selenium and antioxidants with mercury, cadmium and silver, *Fundam Appl Toxicol* 1:368-375, 1981.

Ship II, Shapiro IM: Preventing mercury poisoning in dental practice, *Anesth Prog* 30:76-78, 1983.

Triebig G, Schaller K: Neurotoxic effects in mercury-exposed workers, *Neurobehav Toxicol Teratol* 4:717-720, 1982.

Williams D, Halstead B: Chelating agents in medicine, *J Toxicol Clin Toxicol* 19:1081-1115, 1982.

Wolff M, Osborne J, Hanson A: Mercury toxicity and dental amalgam, *Neurotoxicology* 4:201-204, 1983.

Zelman M, et al: Toxicity from vacuumed mercury: A household hazard. *Clin Pediatr* 30:121-123, 1991.

GUIDELINE 85

Books

Amdur MO, Doull J, Klaassen CD, editors: *Casarett and Doull's toxicology, the basic science of poisons,* ed 4, New York, 1991, Pergamon Press.

Bardana EJ, Montanaro A, O'Hollaren MT: *Occupational asthma,* Philadelphia, 1992, Hanley & Belfus.

Baselt RC, Cravey RH: *Disposition of toxic drugs and chemicals in man,* ed 3, Chicago, 1989, Year Book Medical Publishers.

CANUTEC: *Initial emergency response guide 1992,* Ottawa, Canada, 1992, Canada Communication Group.

CCINFO: *MSDS/CHEMINFO* (CD-ROM version), Hamilton, Ontario, Canada, 1993, Canadian Centre for Occupational Health and Safety.

DOT: *2000 Emergency response guidebook,* Office of Hazardous Materials Transportation, Research and Special Programs Administration, Washington, DC, 2000, US Department of Transportation.

Gosselin RE, Smith RP, Hodge HC: *Clinical toxicology of commercial products,* ed 5, Baltimore, 1984, Williams & Wilkins.

Hartman DE: *Neuropsychological toxicology, identification and assessment of human neurotoxic syndromes,* New York, 1988, Pergamon Press.

NIOSH: *NIOSH pocket guide to chemical hazards* (CD-ROM version), Cincinnati, 2000, DHHS (NIOSH), US Government Printing Office.

Sittig M: *Handbook of toxic and hazardous chemicals and carcinogens,* ed 3, Park Ridge, NJ, 1992, Noyes Publications.

Sullivan JB, Kriger GR, editors: *Clinical environmental health and hazardous materials toxicology,* Baltimore, 1997, Williams & Wilkins.

Journals

Basketter DA, et al: Nickel, cobalt and chromium in consumer products: A role in allergic contact dermatitis? *Contact Dermatitis* 28:15-25, 1993.

Kiec-Swierczynska M: Allergy to chromate, cobalt and nickel in Lodz 1977-1988, *Contact Dermatitis* 22:229-231, 1990.

Srivastava AK, et al: Blood chromium and nickel in relation to respiratory symptoms among industrial workers, *Vet Hum Toxicol* 34:232-234, 1992.

Sunderman FW Jr: The treatment of acute nickel carbonyl poisoning by sodium diethyldithiocarbamate, *Ann Clin Res* 3:182-185, 1971.

Sunderman FW Jr: A review of the metabolism and toxicology of nickel, *Ann Clin Lab Sci* 7:377-398, 1977.

Sunderman FW Jr, et al: Nickel absorption and kinetics in human volunteers, *Proc Soc Exp Biol Med* 191:5-11, 19889.

GUIDELINE 86
Books
Amdur MO, Doull J, Klaassen CD, editors: *Casarett and Doull's toxicology, the basic science of poisons,* ed 4, New York, 1991, Pergamon Press.

Baselt RC, Cravey RH: *Disposition of toxic drugs and chemicals in man,* ed 3, Chicago, 1989, Year Book Medical Publishers.

CANUTEC: *Initial emergency response guide 1992,* Ottawa, Canada, 1992, Canada Communication Group.

CCINFO: *MSDS/CHEMINFO* (CD-ROM version), Hamilton, Ontario, Canada, 1993, Canadian Centre for Occupational Health and Safety.

DOT: *2000 Emergency response guidebook,* Office of Hazardous Materials Transportation, Research and Special Programs Administration, Washington, DC, 2000, US Department of Transportation.

Gosselin RE, Smith RP, Hodge HC: *Clinical toxicology of commercial products,* ed 5, Baltimore, 1984, Williams & Wilkins.

Hartman DE: *Neuropsychological toxicology, identification and assessment of human neurotoxic syndromes,* New York, 1988, Pergamon Press.

NIOSH: *NIOSH pocket guide to chemical hazards* (CD-ROM version), Cincinnati, 2000, DHHS (NIOSH), US Government Printing Office.

Journals
Combs GF: Growing interest in selenium, *West J Med* 153:192-194, 1990.

Contempre B, et al: Effect of selenium supplementation in hypothyroid subjects of an iodine- and selenium-deficient area: the possible danger of indiscriminate supplementation of iodine-deficient subjects with selenium, *J Clin Endocrinol Metabol* 73:213-215, 1991.

Fan AM, Kizer KW: Selenium—nutritional, toxicologic, and clinical aspects, *West J Med* 153:160-167, Aug 1990.

Ransome JW, Scott NM, Knoblock EC: Selenium sulfide intoxication, *N Engl J Med* 264:384-385, 1961.

GUIDELINE 87
Books
Amdur MO, Doull J, Klaassen CD, editors: *Casarett and Doull's toxicology, the basic science of poisons,* ed 4, New York, 1991, Pergamon Press.

Baselt RC, Cravey RH: *Disposition of toxic drugs and chemicals in man,* ed 3, Chicago, 1989, Year Book Medical Publishers.

CANUTEC: *Initial emergency response guide 1992,* Ottawa, Canada, 1992, Canada Communication Group.

CCINFO: *MSDS/CHEMINFO* (CD-ROM version), Hamilton, Ontario, Canada, 1993, Canadian Centre for Occupational Health and Safety.

DOT: *CHRIS hazardous chemical data,* US Department of Transportation/United States Coast Guard. Washington, DC, 1984, US Government Printing Office.

DOT: *2000 Emergency response guidebook,* Office of Hazardous Materials Transportation, Research and Special Programs Administration, Washington, DC, 2000, US Department of Transportation.

Goodman AG, et al, editors: *Goodman and Gilman's the pharmacological basis of therapeutics,* ed 8, New York, 1990, Pergamon Press.

Gosselin RE, Smith RP, Hodge HC: *Clinical toxicology of commercial products,* ed 5, Baltimore, 1984, Williams & Wilkins.

Hartman DE: *Neuropsychological toxicology, identification and assessment of human neurotoxic syndromes,* New York, 1988, Pergamon Press.

Mackison FW, Stricoff RS, Partridge LJ Jr, editors: *Occupational health guidelines for chemical hazards,* NIOSH/OSHA, Washington, DC, 1981, US Government Printing Office.

NIOSH: *NIOSH pocket guide to chemical hazards* (CD-ROM version), Cincinnati, 2000, DHHS (NIOSH), US Government Printing Office.

Sullivan JB, Kriger GR, editors: *Clinical environmental health and hazardous materials toxicology,* Baltimore, 1997, Williams & Wilkins.

Journals
Andersen D: Clinical evidence and therapeutic indications in neurotoxicology: exemplified by thallotoxicosis, *ACTA Neurol Scand* 100:185- 192, 1984.

Burnett JW: Thallium poisoning, *Cutis* 46:112-113, 1990.

Chakrabarti AK, Ghosh K, Chaudhuri AK: Thallium poisoning—a case report, *J Trop Med Hyg* 88:291-293, 1985.

De Backer W, et al: Thallium intoxication treated with combined hemofusion-hemodialysis, *J Toxicol Clin Toxicol* 19:259-264, 1982.

De Groot G, Van Leusen R, Van Heijst AN: Thallium concentrations in body fluids and tissues in a fatal case of thallium poisoning, *Vet Hum Toxicol* 27:115-119, 1985

De Groot G, et al: An evaluation of the efficiency of charcoal hemoperfusion in the treatment of three cases of acute thallium poisoning, *Arch Toxicol* 57:61-66, 1985.

Dolgner R, et al: Repeated surveillance of exposure to thallium in a population living in the vicinity of a cement plant emitting dust containing thallium, *Int Arch Occup Environ Health* 52:79-94, 1983.

Heath A: A Letter on thallium concentrations in body fluids and tissues in a fatal case of thallium poisoning, *Vet Hum Toxicol* 27:4331, 1985.

Heath A, et al: Thallium poisoning—toxin elimination and therapy in three cases, *J Toxicol Clin Toxicol* 20:451-463, 1983.

Luckit J, et al: Thrombocytopenia associated with thallium poisoning, *Hum Exp Toxicol* 9:47-48, 1990.

Marcus RL: Investigation of a working population exposed to thallium, *J Soc Occup Med* 35:4-9, 1985.

Mayfield S, Morgan D, Roberts R: Acute thallium poisoning in a 3-year-old child, *Clin Pediatr* 12:461-462, 1984.

Nogue S, et al: Acute thallium poisoning: an evaluation of different forms of treatment, *J Toxicol Clin Toxicol* 19:1015-1021, 1982.

Saddique A, Peterson CD: Thallium poisoning: a review, *Vet Hum Toxicol* 25:16-22, 1983.

Sawant BN, et al: Thallium poisoning: a case report, *J Assoc Phys India* 29:783-785, 1981.

Vergauwe PL, Knockaert DC, Van Tittelboom TJ: Near fatal subacute thallium poisoning necessitating prolonged mechanical ventilation, *Am J Emerg Med* 8:548-550, 1990.

Yokoyama K, Araki S, Haruo A: Distribution of nerve conduction velocities in acute thallium poisoning, *Muscle Nerve* 13:117-120, 1990.

GUIDELINE 88

Books

Amdur MO, Doull J, Klaassen CD, editors: *Casarett and Doull's toxicology, the basic science of poisons,* ed 4, New York, 1991, Pergamon Press.

Baselt RC, Cravey RH: *Disposition of toxic drugs and chemicals in man,* ed 3, Chicago, 1989, Year Book Medical Publishers.

CANUTEC: *Initial emergency response guide 1992,* Ottawa, Canada, 1992, Canada Communication Group.

CCINFO: *MSDS/CHEMINFO* (CD-ROM version), Hamilton, Ontario, Canada, 1993, Canadian Centre for Occupational Health and Safety.

DOT: *2000 Emergency response guidebook,* Office of Hazardous Materials Transportation, Research and Special Programs Administration, Washington, DC, 2000, US Department of Transportation.

Gosselin RE, Smith RP, Hodge HC: *Clinical toxicology of commercial products,* ed 5, Baltimore, 1984, Williams & Wilkins.

Hartman DE: *Neuropsychological toxicology, identification and assessment of human neurotoxic syndromes,* New York, 1988, Pergamon Press.

NIOSH: *NIOSH pocket guide to chemical hazards* (CD-ROM version), Cincinnati, 2000, DHHS (NIOSH), US Government Printing Office.

Sullivan JB, Kriger GR, editors: *Clinical environmental health and hazardous materials toxicology,* Baltimore, 1997, Williams & Wilkins.

Journals

Ameille J, et al: Occupational hypersensitivity pneumonitis in a smelter exposed to zinc fumes, *Chest* 101:862-863, 1992.

Broun ER, et al: Excessive zinc ingestion. A reversible cause of sideroblastic anemia and bone marrow depression, *JAMA* 264:1441-1443, 1990.

Fosmire GJ: Zinc toxicity, *Am J Clin Nutr* 51:225-227, 1990.

Frambach DA, Bendel RE: Zinc supplementation and anemia (letter), *JAMA* 265:869, 1991.

Gyorffy EJ, Chan H: Copper deficiency and microcytic anemia resulting from prolonged ingestion of over-the-counter zinc, *Am J Gastroenterol* 87:1054-1055, 1992.

Malo JL, Cartier A, Dolovich J: Occupational asthma due to zinc, *Eur Respir J* 6:447-450, 1993.

Ringenberg QS, et al: Hematologic effects of heavy metal poisoning, *S Med J* 81:1132-1139, 1988.

GUIDELINE 89

Books

Amdur MO, Doull J, Klaassen CD, editors: *Casarett and Doull's toxicology, the basic science of poisons,* ed 4, New York, 1991, Pergamon Press.

CANUTEC: *Initial emergency response guide 1992,* Ottawa, Canada, 1992, Canada Communication Group.

CCINFO: *MSDS/CHEMINFO* (CD-ROM version), Hamilton, Ontario, Canada, 1993, Canadian Centre for Occupational Health and Safety.

DOT: *CHRIS hazardous chemical data,* US Department of Transportation/United States Coast Guard. Washington, DC, 1984, US Government Printing Office.

Goldfrank LR, et al: *Goldfrank's toxicologic emergencies,* ed 6, New York, NY, 1998, McGraw-Hill Professional.

Gosselin RE, Smith RP, Hodge HC: *Clinical toxicology of commercial products,* ed 5, Baltimore, 1984, Williams & Wilkins.

Hartman DE: *Neuropsychological toxicology, identification and assessment of human neurotoxic syndromes,* New York, 1988, Pergamon Press.

Mackison FW, Stricoff RS, Partridge LJ Jr, editors: *Occupational health guidelines for chemical hazards,* NIOSH/OSHA, Washington, DC, 1981, US Government Printing Office.

NIOSH: *NIOSH pocket guide to chemical hazards* (CD-ROM version), Cincinnati, 2000, DHHS (NIOSH), US Government Printing Office.

Sullivan JB, Kriger GR, editors: *Clinical environmental health and hazardous materials toxicology,* Baltimore, 1997, Williams & Wilkins.

Snyder R, editor: *Ethel Browning's toxicity and metabolism of industrial solvents, vol I, Hydrocarbons,* New York, 1987, Elsevier Science Publishers.

Journals

Becker CE: The role of cyanide in fires, *Vet Hum Toxicol* 27:487-490, 1985.

Benignus VA, Muller KE, Malott CM: Dose-effects functions for carboxyhemoglobin and behavior, *Neurotoxicol Teratol* 12:111-118, 1990.

Binder J, Roberts R: Carbon monoxide intoxication in children, *Clin Toxicol* 16:287-295, 1980.

Chang KH, et al: Delayed encephalopathy after acute carbon monoxide intoxication: MR imaging features and distribution of cerebral white matter lesions, *Radiology* 184:117-122, 1992.

Chu Chs: Burns updated in China. II. Special burn injury and burns of special areas, *J Trauma* 22:574-580, 1982.

Cobb N, Etzel RA: Unintentional carbon monoxide–related deaths in the United States, 1979 through 1988, *JAMA* 266:659-663,1991.

Cohen M, Guzzard LJ: Inhalation of products of combustion, *Ann Emerg Med* 12:628-632, 1983.

Craft A: Circumstances surrounding deaths from accidental poisoning 1974-80, *Arch Disabl Child* 58:544-546, 1983.

Cramer C: Fetal death due to accidental maternal carbon monoxide poisoning, *J Clin Toxicol* 19:297-301, 1982.

Davies D, Smith D: Electrocardiographic changes in healthy men during continuous low-level carbon monoxide poisoning, *Environ Res* 21:197-206, 1980.

Diller J: The availability of CO_2 detectors, *JAMA* 226:3286, 1991.

Elkharrat D, et al: Acute carbon monoxide intoxication and hyperbaric oxygen in pregnancy, *Intensive Care Med* 17: 289-292, 1991.

Fawcett TA, et al: Warehouse workers' headache. Carbon monoxide poisoning from propane-fueled forklifts, *J Occup Med* 34:12-15, 1992.

Green JL, et al: Index of suspicion, *Pediatr Rev* 13:295-297, 1992.

Gregor MA, et al: Unintentional deaths from carbon monoxide poisoning—Michigan, 1987-1989, *JAMA* 268:3419, 1992.

Hampson NB, Norkool DM: Carbon monoxide poisoning in children riding in the back of pickup trucks, *JAMA* 267:538-540, 1992.

Heckerling PS, et al: Screening hospital admissions from the emergency department for occult carbon monoxide poisoning, *Am J Emerg Med* 8:301-304, 1990.

Hennequin Y, et al: In-utero carbon monoxide poisoning and multiple fetal abnormalities (letter), *Lancet* 341:240, 1993.

Janes S, Lock B: Carbon monoxide poisoning in childhood (letter), *Br Med J* 291:1725, 1985.

Kanaya N, et al: The utility of MRI in acute stage of carbon monoxide poisoning, *Intensive Care Med* 18:371-372, 1992.

Kurppa K, et al: Chemical exposures at work and cardiovascular morbidity. Atherosclerosis, ischemic heart disease, hypertension, cardiomyopathy and arrhythmias, *Scand J Work Environ Health* 10:381-388, 1984.

Lycka B: Carbon monoxide poisoning (letter), *Can Med Assoc J* 133(10):952, 1985.

Martin L: Occult carbon monoxide poisoning (letter), *Arch Intern Med* 142:2345-2346, 1982.

Messier LD, Myers RAM: A neuropsychological screening battery for emergency assessment of carbon-monoxide-poisoned patients, *J Clin Psychol* 47:675-684, 1991.

Mihevic PM, Gliner JA, Horvath SM: Carbon monoxide exposure and information processing during perceptual-motor performance, *Int Arch Occup Environ Health* 51:355-363, 1983.

Moore SJ, Ho IK, Hume AS: Severe hypoxia produced by concomitant intoxication with sublethal doses of carbon monoxide and cyanide, *Toxicol Appl Pharmacol* 109:412-420, 1991.

Myers RAM, et al: Value of hyperbaric oxygen in suspected carbon monoxide poisoning, *JAMA* 248:2478-2480, 1981.

Rottman SJ: Carbon monoxide screening in the ED, *Am J Emerg Med* 9:204-205, 1991.

Rudge MAJ FW: Treatment of methylene chloride induced carbon monoxide poisoning with hyperbaric oxygenation, *Milit Med* 155: 570-572, 1990.

Sangalli BC, Bidanset JH: A review of carboxyhemoglobin formation: a major mechanism of carbon monoxide toxicity, *Vet Hum Toxicol* 32:449-453, 1990.

Sharma P, Penney DG: Effects of ethanol in acute carbon monoxide poisoning, *Toxicology* 62:213-226, 1990.

Stonesifer L, Bone R, Hiller F: Thrombotic thrombocytopenic purpura in carbon monoxide poisoning: report of a case, *Arch Intern Med* 140:104-105, 1980.

Torne R, et al: Skin lesions in carbon monoxide intoxication, *Dermatologica* 183:212-215, 1991.

Williams J, Lewis RW II, Kealey GP: Carbon monoxide poisoning and myocardial ischemia in patients with burns, *J Burn Care Rehabil* 13(2), Part 1: 210-213, 1992.

Winneke G: The neurotoxicity of dichloromethane, *Neurotoxicol Teratol* 3:391-395, 1981.

Zimmerman S, Truxal B: Carbon monoxide poisoning, *Pediatrics* 68:124-125, 1981.

GUIDELINE 90

Books

Amdur MO, Doull J, Klaassen CD, editors: *Casarett and Doull's toxicology, the basic science of poisons,* ed 4, New York, 1991, Pergamon Press.

Baselt RC, Cravey RH: *Disposition of toxic drugs and chemicals in man,* ed 3, Chicago, 1989, Year Book Medical Publishers.

CANUTEC: *Initial emergency response guide 1992,* Ottawa, Canada, 1992, Canada Communication Group.

CCINFO: *MSDS/CHEMINFO* (CD-ROM version), Hamilton, Ontario, Canada, 1993, Canadian Centre for Occupational Health and Safety.

DOT: *CHRIS hazardous chemical data,* US Department of Transportation/United States Coast Guard. Washington, DC, 1984, US Government Printing Office.

DOT: *2000 Emergency response guidebook,* Office of Hazardous Materials Transportation, Research and Special Programs Administration, Washington, DC, 2000, US Department of Transportation.

Goldfrank LR, et al: *Goldfrank's toxicologic emergencies,* ed 6, New York, NY, 1998, McGraw-Hill Professional.

Gosselin RE, Smith RP, Hodge HC: *Clinical toxicology of commercial products,* ed 5, Baltimore, 1984, Williams & Wilkins.

Hartman DE: *Neuropsychological toxicology, identification and assessment of human neurotoxic syndromes,* New York, 1988, Pergamon Press.

Mackison FW, Stricoff RS, Partridge LJ Jr, editors: *Occupational health guidelines for chemical hazards,* NIOSH/OSHA, Washington, DC, 1981, US Government Printing Office.

NIOSH: *NIOSH pocket guide to chemical hazards* (CD-ROM version), Cincinnati, 2000, DHHS (NIOSH), US Government Printing Office.

Sullivan JB, Kriger GR, editors: *Clinical environmental health and hazardous materials toxicology,* Baltimore, 1997, Williams & Wilkins.

Journals

Ballantyne B: Artifacts in the definition of toxicity of cyanides and cyanogens, *Fundam Appl Toxicol* 3:400-408, 1983.

Baskin SI, Horowitz AM, Nealley EW: The antidotal action of sodium nitrite and sodium thiosulfate against cyanide poisoning, *J Clin Pharmacol* 32:368-375, 1992.

Baud FJ, et al: Elevated blood cyanide concentrations in victims of smoke inhalation, *N Engl J Med* 325:1761-1766, 1991.

Becker CE: The role of cyanide in fires, *Vet Hum Toxicol* 27:487-490, 1985.

Curry SC, Patrick HC: Lack of evidence for a percent saturation gap in cyanide poisoning, *Ann Emerg Med* 20:523-531, 1991.

Fernandez De Corres L, Lajarazu D: Allergic contact dermatitis to cyanide, *Contact Dermatitis* 8:346, 1982.

Forsyth JC, et al: Hydroxocobalamin as a cyanide antidote: safety, efficacy and pharmacokinetics in heavily smoking normal volunteers, *Clin Toxicol* 31:277-294, 1993.

Freeman A: Optic neuropathy and chronic cyanide toxicity (letter), *Lancet* 22:441-442, 1986.

Greenberg SR: The morphology of cyanide poisoning, *Proc Inst Med Chic* 35:131-132, 1982.

Hart GB, et al: Treatment of smoke inhalation by hyperbaric oxygen, *J Emerg Med* 3:211-215, 1985.

Kohlmeier C: Protocols for the management of patients with acute hazardous materials exposure, *J Emerg Nurs* 11:249-252, 1985.

Kulig K: Cyanide antidotes and fire toxicology, *N Engl J Med* 325(25):1801-1802, 1991.

Lafin SM, et al: A need to revise the cyanide antidote package instructions, *J Emerg Med* 10:623-625, 1992.

Litovitz T, Larkin R, Myers R: Cyanide poisoning treated with hyperbaric oxygen, *Am J Emerg Med* 1:94-101, 1983.

Marbury T, et al: Combined antidotal and hemodialysis treatments for nitroprusside-induced cyanide toxicity, *J Clin Toxicol* 19:475-482, 1982.

Pickering W: Cyanide toxicity and the hazards of dicobalt edetate (letter), *Br Med J* 291:1644, 1985.

Rindone JP, Sloane EP: Cyanide toxicity from sodium nitroprusside: risks and management, *Ann Pharmacother* 26: 515-519, 1992.

Robin ED, McCauley R: Nitroprusside-related cyanide poisoning, time (long past due) for urgent, effective interventions, *Chest* 102:1842-1845, 1992.

Scharf BA, Fricke RF, Baskin SI: Comparison of methemoglobin formers in protection against the toxic effects of cyanide, *Gen Pharm* 23(1):19-25, 1992.

Ten Eyck R, et al: Stroma-free methemoglobin solution as an antidote for cyanide poisoning: a preliminary study, *Clin Toxicol* 21:343-358, 1983.

Vincent F: Pathologic changes after cyanide poisoning (letter), *Neurology* 36:137, 1986.

Wald P, Goldfrank L: Cyanide intoxication (letter), *JAMA* 254:2889, 1985.

Yeh MH, et al: Is measurement of venous oxygen saturation useful in the diagnosis of cyanide poisoning? *Am J Med* 93: 582-583, 1992.

GUIDELINE 91

Books

Amdur MO, Doull J, Klaassen CD, editors: *Casarett and Doull's toxicology, the basic science of poisons,* ed 4, New York, 1991, Pergamon Press.

CANUTEC: *Initial emergency response guide 1992,* Ottawa, Canada, 1992, Canada Communication Group.

CCINFO: *MSDS/CHEMINFO* (CD-ROM version), Hamilton, Ontario, Canada, 1993, Canadian Centre for Occupational Health and Safety.

DOT: *CHRIS hazardous chemical data,* US Department of Transportation/United States Coast Guard. Washington, DC, 1984, US Government Printing Office.

DOT: *2000 Emergency response guidebook,* Office of Hazardous Materials Transportation, Research and Special Programs Administration, Washington, DC, 2000, US Department of Transportation.

Gosselin RE, Smith RP, Hodge HC: *Clinical toxicology of commercial products,* ed 5, Baltimore, 1984, Williams & Wilkins.

Haddad LM, et al: *Clinical management of poisoning and drug overdose,* ed 3, Philadelphia, 1997, Saunders.

Hartman DE: *Neuropsychological toxicology, identification and assessment of human neurotoxic syndromes,* New York, 1988, Pergamon Press.

Mackison FW, Stricoff RS, Partridge LJ Jr, editors: *Occupational health guidelines for chemical hazards,* NIOSH/OSHA, Washington, DC, 1981, US Government Printing Office.

NIOSH: *NIOSH pocket guide to chemical hazards* (CD-ROM version), Cincinnati, 2000, DHHS (NIOSH), US Government Printing Office.

Sullivan JB, Kriger GR, editors: *Clinical environmental health and hazardous materials toxicology,* Baltimore, 1997, Williams & Wilkins.

Journals

Arnold I, et al: Health implication of occupational exposures to hydrogen sulfide, *J Occup Med* 27:373-376, 1985.

Beauchamp RD Jr, et al: A critical review of the literature on hydrogen sulfide toxicity, *CRC Crit Rev Toxicol* 13:25-97, 1984.

Donham K, et al: Acute exposure to gases from liquid manure, *J Occup Med* 24:142-145, 1982.

Erickson PJ, Rossing DR, Barlow JF: Forty-year-old man in coma with respiratory distress after falling into a hog pit, *S D J Med* 37:5-9, 1984.

Gann P, Roseman J: Hazards of metal processing (letter), *JAMA* 248:1580, 1982.

Hagley SR, South DL: Fatal inhalation of liquid manure gas, *Med J Aust* 2:459-460,1983.

Higashi T, et al: Cross-sectional study of respiratory symptoms and pulmonary functions in rayon textile workers with special reference to H_2S exposure, *Ind Health* 21:281-292, 1983.

Hudeau FM, Gnanaharan C, Davey K: Hydrogen sulphide poisoning: associated with pelt processing, *N Z Med J* 98:145-147, 1985.

Kangas J, Jappinen P, Savolainen H: Exposure to hydrogen sulfide: mercaptans and sulfur dioxide in pulp industry, *Am Ind Hyg Assn J* 45:787-790, 1984.

Ravizza AG, et al: The treatment of hydrogen sulfide intoxication: Oxygen versus nitrites, *Vet Hum Toxicol* 24:241-242, 1982.

Reiffenstein RJ, Hulbert WC, Roth SH: Toxicology of hydrogen sulfide, *Annu Rev Pharmacol Toxicol* 109-134, 1992.

Ronk R, White MK: Hydrogen sulfide and the probabilities of "inhalation" through a tympanic membrane defect, *J Occup Med* 27:337-340, 1985.

Smilkstein MJ, et al: Hyperbaric oxygen therapy for severe hydrogen sulfide poisoning, *J Emerg Med* 3:27-30, 1985.

Thom SR: Experimental use of hyperbaric oxygen therapy (editorial), *J Emerg Med* 3:65, 1985.

Tvedt B, et al: Delayed neuropsychiatric sequelae after acute hydrogen sulfide poisoning: Affection of motor function, memory, vision and hearing, *Acta Neurol Scand* 84:348-351, 1991.

Vannatta JB: Hydrogen sulfide poisoning. Report of four cases and brief review of the literature, *J Okla State Med Assoc* 75:29-32, 1982.

Whitcraft DD, Bailey TD, Hart GB: Hydrogen sulfide poisoning treated with hyperbaric oxygen, *J Emerg Med* 3:23-25, 1985.

GUIDELINE 92

Books

Amdur MO, Doull J, Klaassen CD, editors: *Casarett and Doull's toxicology, the basic science of poisons,* ed 4, New York, 1991, Pergamon Press.

CANUTEC: *Initial emergency response guide 1992,* Ottawa, Canada, 1992, Canada Communication Group.

CCINFO: *MSDS/CHEMINFO* (CD-ROM version), Hamilton, Ontario, Canada, 1993, Canadian Centre for Occupational Health and Safety.

DOT: *CHRIS hazardous chemical data,* US Department of Transportation/United States Coast Guard. Washington, DC, 1984, US Government Printing Office.

DOT: *2000 Emergency response guidebook,* Office of Hazardous Materials Transportation, Research and Special Programs Administration, Washington, DC, 2000, US Department of Transportation.

Gosselin RE, Smith RP, Hodge HC: *Clinical toxicology of commercial products,* ed 5, Baltimore, 1984, Williams & Wilkins.

Haddad LM, et al: *Clinical management of poisoning and drug overdose,* ed 2, Philadelphia, 1990, Saunders.

Mackison FW, Stricoff RS, Partridge LJ Jr, editors: *Occupational health guidelines for chemical hazards,* NIOSH/OSHA, Washington, DC, 1981, US Government Printing Office.

Manahan SE: *Environmental chemistry,* ed 5, Chelsea, Mich, 1991, Lewis Publishers.

NIOSH: *NIOSH pocket guide to chemical hazards* (CD-ROM version), Cincinnati, 2000, DHHS (NIOSH), US Government Printing Office.

Sullivan JB, Kriger GR, editors: *Clinical environmental health and hazardous materials toxicology,* Baltimore, 1997, Williams & Wilkins..

Journal

Byard RW, Wilson GW: Death scene gas analysis in suspected methane asphyxia, *Am J Forensic Med Pathol* 13:69-71, 1992.

GUIDELINE 93

Books

Amdur MO, Doull J, Klaassen CD, editors: *Casarett and Doull's toxicology, the basic science of poisons,* ed 4, New York, 1991, Pergamon Press.

Baselt RC, Cravey RH: *Disposition of toxic drugs and chemicals in man,* ed 3, Chicago, 1989, Year Book Medical Publishers.

CANUTEC: *Initial emergency response guide 1992,* Ottawa, Canada, 1992, Canada Communication Group.

CCINFO: *MSDS/CHEMINFO* (CD-ROM version), Hamilton, Ontario, Canada, 1993, Canadian Centre for Occupational Health and Safety.

DOT: *CHRIS hazardous chemical data,* US Department of Transportation/United States Coast Guard. Washington, DC, 1984, US Government Printing Office.

DOT: *2000 Emergency response guidebook,* Office of Hazardous Materials Transportation, Research and Special Programs Administration, Washington, DC, 2000, US Department of Transportation.

Gosselin RE, Smith RP, Hodge HC: *Clinical toxicology of commercial products,* ed 5, Baltimore, 1984, Williams & Wilkins.

Haddad LM, et al: *Clinical management of poisoning and drug overdose,* ed 3, Philadelphia, 1997, Saunders

Mackison FW, Stricoff RS, Partridge LJ Jr, editors: *Occupational health guidelines for chemical hazards,* NIOSH/OSHA, Washington, DC, 1981, US Government Printing Office.

Manahan SE: *Environmental chemistry,* ed 7, Chelsea, Mich, 1999, Lewis Publishers.

NIOSH: *NIOSH pocket guide to chemical hazards* (CD-ROM version), Cincinnati, 2000, DHHS (NIOSH), US Government Printing Office.

Sullivan JB, Kriger GR, editors: *Clinical environmental health and hazardous materials toxicology,* Baltimore, 1997, Williams & Wilkins.

Journals

Campbell L, Jones A, Wilson H: Evaluation of occupational exposure to carbon disulphide by blood, exhaled air, and urine analysis, *Am J Ind Med* 142-153, 1985.

Effects of toxic chemicals on the reproductive system, council on scientific affairs, *JAMA*, 253:3431-3437, 1985.

Grasso P, et al: Neurophysiological and psychological disorders and occupational exposure to organic solvents, *Food Chem Toxicol* 22:819-852, 1984.

Johnson B, et al: Effects on the peripheral nervous system of workers' exposure to carbon disulfide, *Neurotoxicology* 4:53-66, 1983.

Krstev S, Perunicic B, Farkic B: The effects of long-term occupational exposure to carbon disulphide on serum lipids, *Eur J Drug Metab Pharmacokinet* 17:237-240, 1992.

Kurppa K, et al: Chemical exposure at work and cardiovascular morbidity, atherosclerosis, ischemic heart disease, hypertension, cardiomyopathy and arrhythmias, *Am J Work Environ Health* 10:382-388, 1984.

Peters HA, et al: Extrapyramidal and other neurologic manifestations associated with carbon disulfide fumigant exposure, *Arch Neurol* 45:537-540, 1988.

Spencer PS, Schaumburg HH: Organic solvent neurotoxicity: facts and research needs, *Scand J Work Environ Health* 11(Suppl 1):53-60, 1985.

GUIDELINE 94

Books

Amdur MO, Doull J, Klaassen CD, editors: *Casarett and Doull's toxicology, the basic science of poisons,* ed 4, New York, 1991, Pergamon Press.

Bardana EJ, Montanaro A, O'Hollaren MT: *Occupational asthma,* Philadelphia, 1992, Hanley & Belfus.

CANUTEC: *Initial emergency response guide 1992,* Ottawa, Canada, 1992, Canada Communication Group.

CCINFO: *MSDS/CHEMINFO* (CD-ROM version), Hamilton, Ontario, Canada, 1993, Canadian Centre for Occupational Health and Safety.

DOT: *CHRIS hazardous chemical data,* US Department of Transportation/United States Coast Guard. Washington, DC, 1984, US Government Printing Office.

DOT: *2000 Emergency response guidebook,* Office of Hazardous Materials Transportation, Research and Special Programs Administration, Washington, DC, 2000, US Department of Transportation.

Gosselin RE, Smith RP, Hodge HC: *Clinical toxicology of commercial products,* ed 5, Baltimore, 1984, Williams & Wilkins.

Mackison FW, Stricoff RS, Partridge LJ Jr, editors: *Occupational health guidelines for chemical hazards,* NIOSH/OSHA, Washington, DC, 1981, US Government Printing Office.

Manahan SE: *Environmental chemistry,* ed 7, Chelsea, Mich, 1999, Lewis Publishers.

NIOSH: *NIOSH pocket guide to chemical hazards* (CD-ROM version), Cincinnati, 2000, DHHS (NIOSH), US Government Printing Office.

Sullivan JB, Kriger GR, editors: *Clinical environmental health and hazardous materials toxicology,* Baltimore, 1997, Williams & Wilkins.

Journals

Banks DE, Rando RJ, Barkman HW: Persistence of toluene diisocyanate–induced asthma despite negligible workplace exposures, *Chest* 97:121-125, 1990.

Baur X: New aspects of isocyanate asthma, *Lung* 168(Suppl):606-613, 1990.

Berode M: Detoxification of an aliphatic amine by N-acetylation: experimental and clinical studies, *Biochem Int* 24:947-950, 1991.

Erjefalt I, Persson CG: Increased sensitivity to toluene diisocyanate (TDI) in airways previously exposed to low doses of TDI, *Clin Exp Allergy* 22:854-862, 1992.

Fabbri LM, Mapp C: Bronchial hyperresponsiveness, airway inflammation and occupational asthma induced by toluene diisocyanate, *Clin Exp Allergy* 21(Suppl 1): 42-47, 1991.

Ferguson JS, Alarie Y: Long-term pulmonary impairment following a single exposure to methyl isocyanate, *Toxicol Appl Pharmacol* 107:253-268, 1991.

Jones RN, et al: Abnormal lung function in polyurethane foam producers. weak relationship to toluene diisocyanate exposures, *Am Rev Respir Dis* 146:871-877, 1992.

Karol MH, Jin R: Mechanisms of immunotoxicity to isocyanates, *Chem Res Toxicol* 4:503-509, 1991.

Koplan JP, Falk H, Green G: Public health lessons from the Bhopal chemical disaster, *JAMA* 264:2795-2796, 1990.

Lee HS, Phoon WH: Diurnal variation in peak expiratory flow rate among workers exposed to toluene diisocyanate in the polyurethane foam manufacturing industry, *Br J Ind Med* 49:423-427, 1992.

Mehta PS, et al: Bhopal tragedy's health effects: a review of methyl isocyanate toxicity, *JAMA* 264:2781-2787, 1990.

Moscato G, et al: Toluene diisocyanate–induced asthma: clinical findings and bronchial responsiveness studies in 113 exposed subjects with work-related respiratory symptoms, *J Occup Med* 87:720-725, 1991.

Saetta M, et al: Airway mucosal inflammation in occupational asthma induced by toluene diisocyanate, *Am Rev Respir Dis* 145:160-168, 1992.

Schenker M: Occupational lung diseases in the industrializing and industrialized world due to modern industries and modern pollutants, *Tuber Lung Dis* 73:27-32, 1992.

Sharma S, et al: Objective thoracic CT scan findings in a Bhopal gas disaster victim, *Resp Med* 85:539-541, 1991.

Sharma BK, Singh S, Mehta R: Fatal poisoning with methyl isothiocyanate, *Br Med J* 283:18-19, 1981.

GUIDELINE 95

Books

Baselt RC, Cravey RH: *Disposition of toxic drugs and chemicals in man,* ed 3, Chicago, 1989, Year Book Medical Publishers.

CANUTEC: *Initial emergency response guide 1992,* Ottawa, Canada, 1992, Canada Communication Group.

CCINFO: *MSDS/CHEMINFO* (CD-ROM version), Hamilton, Ontario, Canada, 1993, Canadian Centre for Occupational Health and Safety.

DOT: *CHRIS hazardous chemical data,* US Department of Transportation/United States Coast Guard. Washington, DC, 1984, US Government Printing Office.

DOT: *2000 Emergency response guidebook,* Office of Hazardous Materials Transportation, Research and Special Programs Administration, Washington, DC, 2000, US Department of Transportation.

Goldfrank LR, et al: *Goldfrank's toxicologic emergencies,* ed 6, New York, 1998, McGraw-Hill Professional.

Gosselin RE, Smith RP, Hodge HC: *Clinical toxicology of commercial products,* ed 5, Baltimore, 1984, Williams & Wilkins.

Mackison FW, Stricoff RS, Partridge LJ Jr, editors: *Occupational health guidelines for chemical hazards,* NIOSH/OSHA, Washington, DC, 1981, US Government Printing Office.

NIOSH: *NIOSH pocket guide to chemical hazards* (CD-ROM version), Cincinnati, 2000, DHHS (NIOSH), US Government Printing Office.

Sullivan JB, Kriger GR, editors: *Clinical environmental health and hazardous materials toxicology,* Baltimore, 1997, Williams & Wilkins.

Journals

Chavez CT, Hepler RS, Straatsma BR: Methyl bromide optic atrophy, *Am J Ophthalmol* 15:715-719, 1985.

Lossos IS, Abolnik I, Breuer R: Pneumomediastinum: a complication of exposure to bromine. *Br J Ind Med* 47:784, 1990.

Van Den Oever RU, Roosels D, LaHaye D: Actual hazard of methyl bromide fumigation in soil disinfection, *Br J Ind Med* 39:140-144, 1982.

Van Gelderen CEM, et al: The no-effect level of sodium bromide in healthy volunteers, *Hum Exp Toxicol* 12:9-14, 1993.

GUIDELINE 96

Books

CANUTEC: *Initial emergency response guide 1992,* Ottawa, Canada, 1992, Canada Communication Group.

CCINFO: *MSDS/CHEMINFO* (CD-ROM version), Hamilton, Ontario, Canada, 1993, Canadian Centre for Occupational Health and Safety.

DOT: *CHRIS hazardous chemical data,* US Department of Transportation/United States Coast Guard. Washington, DC, 1984, US Government Printing Office.

DOT: *2000 Emergency response guidebook,* Office of Hazardous Materials Transportation, Research and Special Programs Administration, Washington, DC, 2000, US Department of Transportation.

Goldfrank LR, et al: *Goldfrank's toxicologic emergencies,* ed 6, New York, NY, 1998, McGraw-Hill Professional.

Gosselin RE, Smith RP, Hodge HC: *Clinical toxicology of commercial products,* ed 5, Baltimore, 1984, Williams & Wilkins.

Haddad LM, et al: *Clinical management of poisoning and drug overdose,* ed 3, Philadelphia, 1997, Saunders.

NIOSH: *NIOSH pocket guide to chemical hazards* (CD-ROM version), Cincinnati, 2000, DHHS (NIOSH), US Government Printing Office.

Journals

Gradus D, et al: Acute bromate poisoning associated with renal failure and deafness presenting as hemolytic uremic syndrome, *Am J Nephrol* 4:188-191, 1984.

Kutom A, et al: Bromate intoxication: hairdressers' anuria, *Am J Kidney Dis* 15:84-85, Jan 1990.

Kuwahara T, et al: 2 cases of potassium bromate poisoning requiring long-term hemodialysis therapy for irreversible tubular damage, *Nephron* 36:278-280, 1984.

Lue JN, Johnson CE, Edwards DL: Bromate poisoning from ingestion of professional hair-care neutralizer, *Clin Pharmacol* 7:66-70, 1988.

Matsumoto I, Morizono T, Paparella M: Hearing loss following potassium bromate: two case reports, *Otolaryngol Head Neck Surg* 88:625-629, 1980.

Oh Sh Lee Hy, et al: Acute renal failure due to potassium bromate poisoning, *Yonsei Med J* 21:106-109, 1980.

Warsaw B, et al: Bromate poisoning from hair permanent preparations, *Pediatrics* 76:975-978, 1985.

GUIDELINE 97

Books

Amdur MO, Doull J, Klaassen CD, editors: *Casarett and Doull's toxicology, the basic science of poisons,* ed 4, New York, 1991, Pergamon Press.

CANUTEC: *Initial emergency response guide 1992,* Ottawa, Canada, 1992, Canada Communication Group.

CCINFO: *MSDS/CHEMINFO* (CD-ROM version), Hamilton, Ontario, Canada, 1993, Canadian Centre for Occupational Health and Safety.

DOT: *CHRIS hazardous chemical data,* US Department of Transportation/United States Coast Guard. Washington, DC, 1984, US Government Printing Office.

DOT: *2000 Emergency response guidebook,* Office of Hazardous Materials Transportation, Research and Special Programs Administration, Washington, DC, 2000, US Department of Transportation.

Goldfrank LR, et al: *Goldfrank's toxicologic emergencies,* ed 6, New York, NY, 1998, McGraw-Hill Professional.

Gosselin RE, Smith RP, Hodge HC: *Clinical toxicology of commercial products,* ed 5, Baltimore, 1984, Williams & Wilkins.

Haddad LM, et al: *Clinical management of poisoning and drug overdose,* ed 3, Philadelphia, 1997, Saunders.

NIOSH: *NIOSH pocket guide to chemical hazards* (CD-ROM version), Cincinnati, 2000, DHHS (NIOSH), US Government Printing Office.

Journals

Cunningham NE: Chlorate poisoning—two cases diagnosed at autopsy, *Med Sci Law* 22:281-282, 1982.

Lubbers JR, Bianchine JR: Effects of the acute rising dose administration of chlorine dioxide, chlorate and chlorite to normal healthy adult male volunteers, *J Environ Pathol Toxicol Oncol* 5:215-228, 1984.

Lubbers JR, Chauhan S, Bianchine JR: Controlled clinical evaluations of chlorine dioxide, chlorite and chlorate in man, *Fundam Appl Toxicol* 1:334-338, 1981.

Lubbers JR, et al: The effects of chronic administration of chlorine dioxide, chlorite and chlorate to normal healthy adult male volunteers, *J Environ Pathol Toxicol Oncol* 5:229-238, 1984.

Singleman E, Steffen C: Increased erythrocyte rigidity in chlorate poisoning (letter), *J Clin Pathol* 36:719, 1983.

Steffen C, Seitz R: Severe chlorate poisoning: report of a case, *Arch Toxicol* 48:291-298, 1981.

GUIDELINE 98

Books

Amdur MO, Doull J, Klaassen CD, editors: *Casarett and Doull's toxicology, the basic science of poisons,* ed 4, New York, 1991, Pergamon Press.

CANUTEC: *Initial emergency response guide 1992,* Ottawa, Canada, 1992, Canada Communication Group.

CCINFO: *MSDS/CHEMINFO* (CD-ROM version), Hamilton, Ontario, Canada, 1993, Canadian Centre for Occupational Health and Safety.

DOT: *CHRIS hazardous chemical data,* US Department of Transportation/United States Coast Guard. Washington, DC, 1984, US Government Printing Office.

DOT: *2000 Emergency response guidebook,* Office of Hazardous Materials Transportation, Research and Special Programs Administration, Washington, DC, 2000, US Department of Transportation.

Gosselin RE, Smith RP, Hodge HC: *Clinical toxicology of commercial products,* ed 5, Baltimore, 1984, Williams & Wilkins.

Mackison FW, Stricoff RS, Partridge LJ Jr, editors: *Occupational health guidelines for chemical hazards,* NIOSH/OSHA, Washington, DC, 1981, US Government Printing Office.

Manahan SE: *Environmental chemistry,* ed 7, Chelsea, Mich, 1999, Lewis Publishers.

NIOSH: *NIOSH pocket guide to chemical hazards* (CD-ROM version), Cincinnati, 2000, DHHS (NIOSH), US Government Printing Office.

Olson KR, editor: *Poisoning & drug overdose,* ed 3, East Norwalk, Conn, 1999, Appleton & Lange.

Sullivan JB, Kriger GR, editors: *Clinical environmental health and hazardous materials toxicology,* Baltimore, 1997, Williams & Wilkins.

Journals

CDC: Chlorine gas toxicity from mixture of bleach with other cleaning products—California, *MMWR* 40:619-629, 1991.

CDC: Chlorine gas toxicity from mixture of bleach with other cleaning products—California: erratum, *MMWR* 40:819, 1991.

Charan N, et al: Effects of accidental chlorine inhalation on pulmonary function, *West J Med* 143:333-336, 1985.

Daniel F, et al: Genotoxic properties of haloacetonitrites: drinking water by-products of chlorine disinfection, *Fundam Appl Toxicol* 6:447-453, 1986.

Donnelly SC, FitzGerald MX: Reactive airways dysfunction syndrome (RADS) due to chlorine gas exposure, *Irish J Med Sci* 159:275-277, 1990.

Edwards I, Temple W, Dobbinson T: Acute chlorine poisoning from a high school experiment, *N Z Med J* 96:720-721, 1983.

Hasan F, Gehshan A, Fuleihan F: Resolution of pulmonary dysfunction following acute chlorine exposures, *Arch Environ Health* 38:76-80, 1983.

Kennedy SM, et al: Lung health consequences of reported accidental chlorine gas exposures among pulpmill workers, *Am Rev Respir Dis* 143:74-79, 1991.

Leung A: Erythema multiforme following swimming in chlorinated pool (letter), *J Natl Med Assn* 77:13, 1985.

Lubbers JR, Chauhan S, Bianchine J: Controlled clinical evaluations of chlorine dioxide, chlorite and chlorate in man, *Fundam Appl Toxicol* 1:334-338, 1981.

Moore BB, Sherman M: Chronic reactive airway disease following acute chlorine gas exposure in an asymptomatic atopic patient, *Chest* 100:855-856, 1991.

Penny P: Swimming pool wheezing, *Br Med J* 13:461-462, 1983.

Phillip R, et al: Domestic chlorine poisoning (letter), *Lancet* 31:495, 1985.

Recommended health-based occupational exposure limits for respiratory irritants. Report of a WHO Study Group, *WHO Tech Rep Ser* 707:1-154, 1984.

Salisbury DA, et al: First-aid reports of acute chlorine gassing among pulpmill workers as predictors of lung health consequences, *Am J Ind Med* 20:71-81, 1991.

Schenker M: Occupational lung diseases in the industrializing and industrialized world due to modern industries and modern pollutants, *Tuber Lung Dis* 73:27-32, 1992.

Schwartz DA, Smith DD, Lakshminarayan S: The pulmonary sequelae associated with accidental inhalation of chlorine gas, *Chest* 97:820-825, 1990.

Vinsel, PJ: Treatment of acute chlorine gas inhalation with nebulized sodium bicarbonate, *J Emerg Med* 8:327-329, 1990.

GUIDELINE 99

Books

Amdur MO, Doull J, Klaassen CD, editors: *Casarett and Doull's toxicology, the basic science of poisons,* ed 4, New York, 1991, Pergamon Press.

CANUTEC: *Initial emergency response guide 1992,* Ottawa, Canada, 1992, Canada Communication Group.

CCINFO: *MSDS/CHEMINFO* (CD-ROM version), Hamilton, Ontario, Canada, 1993, Canadian Centre for Occupational Health and Safety.

DOT: *CHRIS hazardous chemical data,* US Department of Transportation/United States Coast Guard. Washington, DC, 1984, US Government Printing Office.

DOT: *2000 Emergency response guidebook,* Office of Hazardous Materials Transportation, Research and Special Programs Administration, Washington, DC, 2000, US Department of Transportation.

Finkel AJ, editor: *Hamilton and Hardy's industrial toxicology,* ed 4, Littleton, Mass, 1983, PSG Publishing.

Gosselin RE, Smith RP, Hodge HC: *Clinical toxicology of commercial products,* ed 5, Baltimore, 1984, Williams & Wilkins.

Haddad LM, et al: *Clinical management of poisoning and drug overdose,* ed 3, Philadelphia, 1997, Saunders.

Mackison FW, Stricoff RS, Partridge LJ Jr, editors: *Occupational health guidelines for chemical hazards,* NIOSH/OSHA, Washington, DC, 1981, US Government Printing Office.

Manahan SE: *Environmental chemistry,* ed 7, Chelsea, Mich, 1999, Lewis Publishers.

NIOSH: *NIOSH pocket guide to chemical hazards* (CD-ROM version), Cincinnati, 2000, DHHS (NIOSH), US Government Printing Office.

Journals

Andlaw R: Acute fluoride toxicity (letter), *Br Dent J* 153:285, 1982.

Beardsley T: Fluoridation: Reluctant ban in Scotland (News), *Nature* 304:308, 1983.

Grandjean P, Thomsen G: Reversibility of skeletal fluorosis, *Br J Ind Med* 40:456-461, 1983.

Grandjean P, et al: Cancer incidence and mortality in workers exposed to fluoride, *J Natl Cancer Inst* 84:1903-1909, 1992.

Heifetz S, Horowitz H: Amounts of fluoride in self-administered dental products: safety considerations for children, *Pediatrics* 77:867-882, 1986.

Hodge HC, Smith FA: Occupational fluoride exposure, *J Occup Med* 19:12-39,1977.

Jha M, et al: Excessive ingestion of fluoride and the significance of sialic acid: glycosaminoglycans in the serum of rabbit and human subjects, *J Toxicol Clin Toxicol* 19:1023-1030, 1982.

Ligh R: Fluoride therapy, *Hawaii Dent J* 16:8-11, 1985.

Maduska A: Fluoride renal toxicity in fetus and neonate (letter), *Am J Obstet Gynecol* 136:1080, 1980.

McIvor M, et al: Hyperkalemia and cardiac arrest from fluoride exposure during hemodialysis, *Am J Cardiol* 51:901-902, 1983.

Miller J, Roberts M, Nilsen R: Acute fluoride toxicity (letter), *Br Dent J* 153:211-212, 1982.

Plummer JL, Cousins MJ, Hall P: Volatile anaesthetic metabolism and acute toxicity, *Q Rev Drug Metab Drug Interact* 4:49-98, 1982.

Singer L, Ophaug R: Ionic and nonionic fluoride in plasma (or serum), *CRC Crit Rev Clin Lab Sci* 18:111-140, 1982.

Smith G: Fluoride, teeth and bone, *Med J Aust* 243:283-286, 1985.

Stephen K, et al: Acute fluoride toxicity (letter), *Br Dent J* 153:317, 1982.

Stocker P: Acute fluoride toxicity (letter), *Br Dent J* 154:67, 1983.

Upholt WM: Health risks and exposure, *Basic Life Sci* 21:37-44, 1982.

GUIDELINE 100

Books

Amdur MO, Doull J, Klaassen CD, editors: *Casarett and Doull's toxicology, the basic science of poisons,* ed 4, New York, 1991, Pergamon Press.

CANUTEC: *Initial emergency response guide 1992,* Ottawa, Canada, 1992, Canada Communication Group.

CCINFO: *MSDS/CHEMINFO* (CD-ROM version), Hamilton, Ontario, Canada, 1993, Canadian Centre for Occupational Health and Safety.

DOT: *2000 Emergency response guidebook,* Office of Hazardous Materials Transportation, Research and Special Programs Administration, Washington, DC, 2000, US Department of Transportation.

Goodman AG, et al, editors: *Goodman and Gilman's the pharmacological basis of therapeutics,* ed 8, New York, 1990, Pergamon Press.

Gosselin RE, Smith RP, Hodge HC: *Clinical toxicology of commercial products,* ed 5, Baltimore, 1984, Williams & Wilkins.

Manahan SE: *Environmental chemistry,* ed 7, Chelsea, Mich, 1999, Lewis Publishers.

NIOSH: *NIOSH pocket guide to chemical hazards* (CD-ROM version), Cincinnati, 2000, DHHS (NIOSH), US Government Printing Office.

Journals

Mu L, et al: Endemic goitre in central China caused by excessive iodine intake, *Lancet* 2:257, 1987.

Pennington JA: A review of iodine toxicity reports, *J Am Diet Assoc* 90:1571-1581,1990.

Ward JM, Ohshima M: The role of iodine in carcinogenesis, *Adv Exp Med Biol* 206:529, 1986.

GUIDELINE 101

Books

Amdur MO, Doull J, Klaassen CD, editors: *Casarett and Doull's toxicology, the basic science of poisons,* ed 4, New York, 1991, Pergamon Press.

CANUTEC: *Initial emergency response guide 1992,* Ottawa, Canada, 1992, Canada Communication Group.

CCINFO: *MSDS/CHEMINFO* (CD-ROM version), Hamilton, Ontario, Canada, 1993, Canadian Centre for Occupational Health and Safety.

DOT: *CHRIS hazardous chemical data,* US Department of Transportation/United States Coast Guard. Washington, DC, 1984, US Government Printing Office.

DOT: *2000 Emergency response guidebook,* Office of Hazardous Materials Transportation, Research and Special Programs Administration, Washington, DC, 2000, US Department of Transportation.

Goldfrank LR, et al: *Goldfrank's toxicologic emergencies,* ed 6, New York, NY, 1998, McGraw-Hill Professional.

Gosselin RE, Smith RP, Hodge HC: *Clinical toxicology of commercial products,* ed 5, Baltimore, 1984, Williams & Wilkins.

Mackison FW, Stricoff RS, Partridge LJ Jr, editors: *Occupational health guidelines for chemical hazards,* NIOSH/OSHA, Washington, DC, 1981, US Government Printing Office.

NIOSH: *NIOSH pocket guide to chemical hazards* (CD-ROM version), Cincinnati, 2000, DHHS (NIOSH), US Government Printing Office.

Noji EK, Kelen GD, editors: *Manual of toxicologic emergencies,* Chicago, 1989, Year Book Medical Publishers.

Sullivan JB, Kriger GR, editors: *Clinical environmental health and hazardous materials toxicology,* Baltimore, 1997, Williams & Wilkins.

Journals

Berkmen Y: Aspiration and inhalation pneumonias, *Sem Roentgenol* 15:73-84, 1980.

Bradley BL, Unger KM: Phosgene inhalation: a case report, *Tex Med* 78:51-53, 1982.

Dalderup LM: TLV of carbonylfluoride (letter), *J Soc Occup Med* 30:87, 1980.

Diller W: The methenamine misunderstanding in the therapy of phosgene poisoning, *Arch Toxicol* 46:199-206, 1980.

Misra NP, Manoria PC, Saxena K: Fatal pulmonary edema with phosgene poisoning, *J Assoc Phys India* 33:430-431, 1985.

Polednak A: Mortality among men occupationally exposed to phosgene in 1943-1945, *Environ Res* 22:357-367, 1980.

Snyder RW, Mishel HS, Christensen GC: Pulmonary toxicity following exposure to methylene chloride and its combustion product, phosgene, *Chest* 101:860-861, 1992.

Summer W, Haponik E: Inhalation of irritant gases, *Clin Chest Med* 2:273-287, 1981.

GUIDELINE 102

Books

Amdur MO, Doull J, Klaassen CD, editors: *Casarett and Doull's toxicology, the basic science of poisons,* ed 4, New York, 1991, Pergamon Press.

CANUTEC: *Initial emergency response guide 1992,* Ottawa, Canada, 1992, Canada Communication Group.

CCINFO: *MSDS/CHEMINFO* (CD-ROM version), Hamilton, Ontario, Canada, 1993, Canadian Centre for Occupational Health and Safety.

DOT: *2000 Emergency response guidebook,* Office of Hazardous Materials Transportation, Research and Special Programs Administration, Washington, DC, 2000, US Department of Transportation.

Gosselin RE, Smith RP, Hodge HC: *Clinical toxicology of commercial products,* ed 5, Baltimore, 1984, Williams & Wilkins.

Manahan SE: *Environmental chemistry,* ed 7, Chelsea, Mich, 1999, Lewis Publishers.

NIOSH: *NIOSH pocket guide to chemical hazards* (CD-ROM version), Cincinnati, 2000, DHHS (NIOSH), US Government Printing Office.

Sittig M: *Handbook of toxic and hazardous chemicals and carcinogens,* ed 3, Park Ridge, NJ, 1992, Noyes Publications.

Sullivan JB, Kriger GR, editors: *Clinical environmental health and hazardous materials toxicology,* Baltimore, 1997, Williams & Wilkins.

Journals

Bender AP, Williams AN, Parker DL: Experiences of a state-sponsored notification and screening program for asbestos workers, *Am J Ind Med* 23:161-169, 1993.

Chellini E, et al: Pleural malignant mesothelioma in Tuscany, Italy (1970-1988). II. Identification of occupational exposure to asbestos, *Am J Ind Med* 21:577-585, 1992.

Dujie Z, et al: Biphasic lung diffusing capacity: detection of early asbestos induced changes in lung function, *Br J Ind Med* 49:260-267, 1992.

Ehrlich R, et al: Long term radiological effects of short term exposure to amosite asbestos among factory workers, *Br J Ind Med* 49:268-275, 1992.

Hilt B, et al: Chest radiographs in subjects with asbestos-related abnormalities: comparison between ILO categorizations and clinical reading, *Am J Ind Med* 21:855-861, 1992.

Jarvholm B: Dose-responses in epidemiology—age and time aspects, *Am J Ind Med* 21: 101-106, 1992.

Kern DG, Hanley KT, Roggli VL: Malignant mesothelioma in the jewelry industry, *Am J Ind Med* 21:409-416, 1992.

Kilburn KH, Warshaw RH: Severity of pulmonary asbestosis as classified by international labour organisation profusion of irregular opacities in 8749 asbestos-exposed American workers: those who never smoked compared with those who ever smoked, *Arch Intern Med* 152:325-327, 1992.

Kishimoto T: Cancer due to asbestos exposure. *Chest* 101(1): 58-63, 1992.

Lundy P, Barer M: Asbestos-containing materials in New York City buildings, *Environ Res* 58:15-24, 1992.

Miller A, et al: Relationship of pulmonary function to radiographic interstitial fibrosis in 2,611 long-term asbestos insulators. An assessment of the international labour office profusion score, *Am Rev Respir Dis* 145:263-270, 1992

Morgan WKC: Asbestos and cancer: history and public policy, *Br J Ind Med* 49:451, 1992.

Ribak J, Selikoff IJ: Survival of asbestos insulation workers with mesothelioma, *Br J Ind Med* 49:732-735, 1992.

Rogers A: Prediction of mesothelioma, lung cancer, and asbestosis in former Wittenoom asbestos workers, *Br J Ind Med* 49:451-452, 1992.

Rom WN: Accelerated loss of lung function and alveolitis in a longitudinal study of non-smoking individuals with occupational exposure to asbestos, *Am J Ind Med* 21:835-844, 1992.

Sanden A, et al: The risk of lung cancer and mesothelioma after cessation of asbestos exposure: a prospective cohort study of shipyard workers, *Eur Respir J* 5:281-285, 1992.

GUIDELINE 103

Books

Amdur MO, Doull J, Klaassen CD, editors: *Casarett and Doull's toxicology, the basic science of poisons,* ed 4, New York, 1991, Pergamon Press.

CANUTEC: *Initial emergency response guide 1992,* Ottawa, Canada, 1992, Canada Communication Group.

CCINFO: *MSDS/CHEMINFO* (CD-ROM version), Hamilton, Ontario, Canada, 1993, Canadian Centre for Occupational Health and Safety.

DOT: *CHRIS hazardous chemical data.* US Department of Transportation/United States Coast Guard. Washington, DC, 1984, US Government Printing Office.

DOT: *2000 Emergency response guidebook,* Office of Hazardous Materials Transportation, Research and Special Programs Administration,

Washington, DC, 2000, US Department of Transportation.

Ellenhorn MJ, Barceloux DG: *Medical toxicology: diagnosis and treatment of human poisoning,* New York, 1988, Elsevier Science Publishing.

Gosselin RE, Smith RP, Hodge HC: *Clinical toxicology of commercial products,* ed 5, Baltimore, 1984, Williams & Wilkins.

NIOSH: *NIOSH pocket guide to chemical hazards* (CD-ROM version), Cincinnati, 2000, DHHS (NIOSH), US Government Printing Office.

Sittig M: *Handbook of toxic and hazardous chemicals and carcinogens,* ed 3, Park Ridge, NJ, 1992, Noyes Publications.

Journals

Ishii Y, et al: A fatal case of acute boric acid poisoning, *Clin Toxicol* 31:345-352, 1993.

Naeger L, Leibman K: Mechanisms of decaborane toxicity, *Toxicol Appl Pharmacol* 22:517-527, 1972.

Rousch G: The toxicology of the boranes, *J Occup Med* 1:46-52, 1959.

Schenker M: Occupational lung diseases in the industrializing and industrialized world due to modern industries and modern pollutants, *Tuber Lung Dis* 73:27-32, 1992.

Von Burg R: Boron, boric acid, borates and boron oxide, *J Appl Toxicol* 12:149-152, 1992.

GUIDELINE 104

Books

Amdur MO, Doull J, Klaassen CD, editors: *Casarett and Doull's toxicology, the basic science of poisons,* ed 4, New York, 1991, Pergamon Press.

CANUTEC: *Initial emergency response guide 1992,* Ottawa, Canada, 1992, Canada Communication Group.

CCINFO: *MSDS/CHEMINFO* (CD-ROM version), Hamilton, Ontario, Canada, 1993, Canadian Centre for Occupational Health and Safety.

DOT: *CHRIS hazardous chemical data.* US Department of Transportation/United States Coast Guard. Washington, DC, 1984, US Government Printing Office.

DOT: *2000 Emergency response guidebook,* Office of Hazardous Materials Transportation, Research and Special Programs Administration, Washington, DC, 2000, US Department of Transportation.

Haddad LM, et al: *Clinical management of poisoning and drug overdose,* ed 3, Philadelphia, 1997, Saunders.

Mackison FW, Stricoff RS, Partridge LJ Jr, editors*: Occupational health guidelines for chemical hazards, NIOSH/OSHA,* Washington, DC, 1981, US Government Printing Office.

Manahan SE: *Environmental chemistry,* ed 7, Chelsea, Mich, 1999, Lewis Publishers.

NIOSH: *NIOSH pocket guide to chemical hazards* (CD-ROM version), Cincinnati, 2000, DHHS (NIOSH), US Government Printing Office.

Sittig M: *Handbook of toxic and hazardous chemicals and carcinogens,* ed 3, Park Ridge, NJ, 1992, Noyes Publications.

Journals

Bates DV: Epidemiologic basis for photochemical oxidant standard, *Environ Health Perspect* 52:125-129, 1983.

Beckett WS: Ozone, air pollution, and respiratory health, *Yale J Biol Med* 64:167-175, 1991.

Bedi J, Drechsler-Parks D, Horvath S: Duration of increased pulmonary function sensitivity to an initial ozone exposure, *Am Ind Hyg Assn J* 46:731-734, 1985.

Calabrese EJ, Horton HM: The effects of vitamin E on ozone and nitrogen dioxide toxicity, *World Rev Nutr Diet* 46:124-147, 1985.

Hobbs CH, Mauderly JL: Risk assessment for diesel exhaust and ozone: the data from people and animals, *Clin Toxicol* 29:375-384, 1991.

Hoek G, et al: Acute effects of ambient ozone on pulmonary function of children in the Netherlands, *Am Rev Respir Dis* 147:111-117, 1993.

Kleeberger SR, Hudak BB: Acute ozone-induced change in airway permeability: role of infiltrating leukocytes, *J Appl Physiol* 72:59-69, 1990.

Kulle T, et al: Pulmonary function and bronchial reactivity in human subjects with exposure to ozone and respirable sulfuric acid aerosol, *Hum Rev Respir Dis* 126:996-1000, 1982.

Lindvall T: Recommendations for air quality standards for nitrogen dioxide and ozone, *Scand J Work Environ Health* 11(Suppl 3):3-9, 1985.

Lindvall T: Health effects of nitrogen dioxide and oxidants, *Scand J Work Environ Health* 11(Suppl 3):10-28, 1985.

Linn W, et al: Response to ozone in volunteers with chronic obstructive pulmonary disease, *Arch Environ Health* 38:278-283, 1983.

Mayer D, Branscheid D: Exposure of human lung fibroblasts to ozone: cell mortality and hyaluronan metabolism, *J Toxicol Environ Health* 35:235-246, 1992.

McDonnell W, et al: Pulmonary effects of ozone exposure during exercise: dose-response characteristics, *J Appl Physiol* 54:1345-1352, 1983.

Mochitate K, et al: Long-term effects of ozone and nitrogen dioxide on the metabolism and population of alveolar macrophages, *J Toxicol Environ Health* 35:247-260, 1992.

Ostro BD, et al: Air pollution and respiratory morbidity among adults in Southern California, *Am J Epidemiol* 137:691-700, 1993.

Peterson JE: Limitations of ambient air quality standards in evaluating indoor environments, *Am Ind Hyg Assoc J* 53:216-220, 1992.

Steinberg JJ, Gleeson JL, Gil D: The pathobiology of ozone-induced damage, *Arch Environ Health* 45:80-87, 1990.

Tashkin DP, et al: Respiratory symptoms of flight attendants during high-altitude flight: possible relation to cabin ozone exposure, *Int Arch Occup Environ Health* 52:117-137, 1983.

GUIDELINE 105

Books

Amdur MO, Doull J, Klaassen CD, editors: *Casarett and Doull's toxicology, the basic science of poisons,* ed 4, New York, 1991, Pergamon Press.

CANUTEC: *Initial emergency response guide 1992,* Ottawa, Canada, 1992, Canada Communication Group.

CCINFO: *MSDS/CHEMINFO* (CD-ROM version), Hamilton, Ontario, Canada, 1993, Canadian Centre for Occupational Health and Safety.

DOT: *2000 Emergency response guidebook,* Office of Hazardous Materials Transportation, Research and Special Programs Administration, Washington, DC, 2000, US Department of Transportation

Finkel AJ, editor: *Hamilton and Hardy's industrial toxicology,* ed 4, Littleton, Mass, 1983, PSG Publishing.

Gosselin RE, Smith RP, Hodge HC: *Clinical toxicology of commercial products,* ed 5, Baltimore, 1984, Williams & Wilkins.

Manahan SE: *Environmental chemistry,* ed 7, Chelsea, Mich, 1999, Lewis Publishers.

NIOSH: *NIOSH pocket guide to chemical hazards* (CD-ROM version), Cincinnati, 2000, DHHS (NIOSH), US Government Printing Office.

Sullivan JB, Kriger GR, editors: *Clinical environmental health and hazardous materials toxicology,* Baltimore, 1997, Williams & Wilkins.

Journals

Beaumont JJ, et al: Lung cancer mortality in workers exposed to sulfuric acid mist and other acid mists, *J Natl Cancer Inst* 79:911-921, 1987.

Boulet LP: Increases in airway responsiveness following acute exposure to respiratory irritants: reactive airway dysfunction syndrome or occupational asthma? *Chest* 94(3):476-481, 1988.

Knapp MJ, Bunn WB; Stave GM: Adult respiratory distress syndrome from sulfuric acid fume inhalation, *South Med J* 84:1031-1033, 1991.

Kraut A, Lilis R: Pulmonary effects of acute exposure to degradation products of sulphur hexafluoride during electrical cable repair work, *Br J Ind Med* 47:829-832, 1990.

Rabinovitch S, et al: Clinical and laboratory features of acute sulfur dioxide inhalation poisoning: two-year follow-up, *Am Rev Respir Dis* 139:556-558, 1989.

GUIDELINE 106

Books

Amdur MO, Doull J, Klaassen CD, editors: *Casarett and Doull's toxicology, the basic science of poisons,* ed 4, New York, 1991, Pergamon Press.

CANUTEC: *Initial emergency response guide 1992,* Ottawa, Canada, 1992, Canada Communication Group.

CCINFO: *MSDS/CHEMINFO* (CD-ROM version), Hamilton, Ontario, Canada, 1993, Canadian Centre for Occupational Health and Safety.

DOT: *CHRIS hazardous chemical data.* US Department of Transportation/United States Coast Guard. Washington, DC, 1984, US Government Printing Office.

DOT: *2000 Emergency response guidebook,* Office of Hazardous Materials Transportation, Research and Special Programs Administration, Washington, DC, 2000, US Department of Transportation.

Gosselin RE, Smith RP, Hodge HC: *Clinical toxicology of commercial products,* ed 5, Baltimore, 1984, Williams & Wilkins.

Haddad LM, et al: *Clinical management of poisoning and drug overdose,* ed 3, Philadelphia, 1997, Saunders.

Mackison FW, Stricoff RS, Partridge LJ Jr, editors*: Occupational health guidelines for chemical hazards, NIOSH/OSHA,* Washington, DC, 1981, US Government Printing Office.

Manahan SE: *Environmental chemistry,* ed 7, Chelsea, Mich, 1999, Lewis Publishers.

NIOSH: *NIOSH pocket guide to chemical hazards* (CD-ROM version), Cincinnati, 2000, DHHS (NIOSH), US Government Printing Office.

Journals

Bischoff A: Clinical and experimental work in neurotoxicity, *Dev Toxicol Environ Sci* 8:39-51, 1980.

Johnson MK: The mechanism of delayed neuropathy caused by some organophosphorus esters: using the understanding to improve safety, *J Environ Sci Health (B)* 15(6):823-841, 1980.

Maydew M, et al: Clinical signs and histopathologic changes of the spinal cord in pigs treated with tri-o-cresyl phosphate, *Neurotoxicology* 4:163-171, 1983.

Morgan AA, Hughes JP: An investigation into the value of cholinesterase estimations of workers in a plant manufacturing tri-aryl phosphate plasticizers, *J Soc Occup Med* 31:69-75, 1981.

Morgan J: The Jamaica ginger paralysis, *JAMA* 15:1864-1867, 1982.

Morgan JP, Tulloss TC: The jake walk blues, a toxicologic tragedy mirrored in American popular music, *Ann Intern Med* 85:804-808, 1976.

Thomas P: Selective vulnerability of the centrifugal and centripetal axions of primary sensory neurons, *Muscle Nerve* 5:1117-1121, 1982.

Vasilescu C: Neuropathy after organophosphorus compounds poisoning (letter), *J Neurol Neurosurg Psychiatry* 45:942, 1982.

Vasilescu C, Florescu A: Clinical and electrophysiological study of neuropathy after organophosphorus compounds poisoning, *Arch Toxicol* 43:305-315, 1980.

Wilson J: Toxic chemicals in the third world (letter), *Lancet* 21:446, 1981.

GUIDELINE 107

Books

CANUTEC: *Initial emergency response guide 1992,* Ottawa, Canada, 1992, Canada Communication Group.

CCINFO: *MSDS/CHEMINFO* (CD-ROM version), Hamilton, Ontario, Canada, 1993, Canadian Centre for Occupational Health and Safety.

DOT: *2000 Emergency response guidebook,* Office of Hazardous Materials Transportation, Research and Special Programs Administration, Washington, DC, 2000, US Department of Transportation.

Finkel AJ, editor: *Hamilton and Hardy's industrial toxicology,* ed 4, Littleton, Mass, 1983, PSG Publishing.

Manahan SE: *Environmental chemistry,* ed 7, Chelsea, Mich, 1999, Lewis Publishers.

Sullivan JB, Kriger GR, editors: *Clinical environmental health and hazardous materials toxicology,* Baltimore, 1997, Williams & Wilkins.

Journals

Omae K, et al: Acute and subacute inhalation toxicity of silane 1000 ppm in mice, *Arch Toxicol* 66:750-753, 1992.

Promisloff RA, et al: Reactive airway dysfunction syndrome in three police officers following a roadside chemical spill, *Chest* 98:928-929, 1990.

Thanabalasingham T, Beckett MW, Murray V: Hospital response to a chemical incident: report on casualties of an ethyldichlorosilane spill, *Br Med J* 302:101-102, 1991.

GUIDELINE 108

Books

Amdur MO, Doull J, Klaassen CD, editors: *Casarett and Doull's toxicology, the basic science of poisons,* ed 4, New York, 1991, Pergamon Press.

CANUTEC: *Initial emergency response guide 1992,* Ottawa, Canada, 1992, Canada Communication Group.

CCINFO: *MSDS/CHEMINFO* (CD-ROM version), Hamilton, Ontario, Canada, 1993, Canadian Centre for Occupational Health and Safety.

DOT: *2000 Emergency response guidebook,* Office of Hazardous Materials Transportation, Research and Special Programs Administration, Washington, DC, 2000, US Department of Transportation.

Finkel AJ, editor: *Hamilton and Hardy's industrial toxicology,* ed 4, Littleton, Mass, 1983, PSG Publishing.

Manahan SE: *Environmental chemistry,* ed 7, Chelsea, Mich, 1999, Lewis Publishers.

NIOSH: *NIOSH pocket guide to chemical hazards* (CD-ROM version), Cincinnati, 2000, DHHS (NIOSH), US Government Printing Office.

Sullivan JB, Kriger GR, editors: *Clinical environmental health and hazardous materials toxicology,* Baltimore, 1997, Williams & Wilkins.

Journals

Chhina RS, Thukral R, Chawla LS: Aluminum phosphide–induced gastroduodenitis (letter), *Gastrointest Endosc* 38:635-636. 1992.

Chugh SN, et al: Incidence and outcome of aluminium phosphide poisoning in a hospital study, *Indian J Med Res* 94:232-235, 1991.

Mistra UK, et al: Acute phosphine poisoning following ingestion of aluminum phosphides, *Hum Toxicol* 7:343-345, 1988.

Schenker M: Occupational lung diseases in the industrializing and industrialized world due to modern industries and modern pollutants. *Tuber Lung Dis* 73:27-32, 1992.

Wald P, Becker C: Toxic gases used in the microelectronics industry: state of the art reviews, *Occup Med* 1:105-117, 1986.

GUIDELINE 109

Books

Amdur MO, Doull J, Klaassen CD, editors: *Casarett and Doull's toxicology, the basic science of poisons,* ed 4, New York, 1991, Pergamon Press.

CANUTEC: *Initial emergency response guide 1992,* Ottawa, Canada, 1992, Canada Communication Group.

CCINFO: *MSDS/CHEMINFO* (CD-ROM version), Hamilton, Ontario, Canada, 1993, Canadian Centre for Occupational Health and Safety.

DOT: *CHRIS hazardous chemical data.* US Department of Transportation/United States Coast Guard. Washington, DC, 1984, US Government Printing Office.

DOT: *2000 Emergency response guidebook,* Office of Hazardous Materials Transportation, Research and Special Programs Administration, Washington, DC, 2000, US Department of Transportation.

Finkel AJ, editor: *Hamilton and Hardy's industrial toxicology,* ed 4, Littleton, Mass, 1983, PSG Publishing.

Gosselin RE, Smith RP, Hodge HC: *Clinical toxicology of commercial products,* ed 5, Baltimore, 1984, Williams & Wilkins.

Haddad LM, et al: *Clinical management of poisoning and drug overdose,* ed 3, Philadelphia, 1997, Saunders.

Jenson AV: *Guidebook for hazardous materials incidents,* Washington, DC, 1983, Department of Transportation.

Mackison FW, Stricoff RS, Partridge LJ Jr, editors*: Occupational health guidelines for chemical hazards, NIOSH/OSHA,* Washington, DC, 1981, US Government Printing Office.

NIOSH: *NIOSH pocket guide to chemical hazards* (CD-ROM version), Cincinnati, 2000, DHHS (NIOSH), US Government Printing Office.

Sullivan JB, Kriger GR, editors: *Clinical environmental health and hazardous materials toxicology,* Baltimore, 1997, Williams & Wilkins.

Journals

Chernow B, et al: Iatrogenic hyperphosphatemia: a metabolic consideration in critical care medicine, *Crit Care Med* 9:772-774, 1981.

Chiarenza A, Gallone C: Match dermatitis, *Contact Dermatitis* 7:346-347, 1981.

Eldad A, et al: Phosphorous pentachloride chemical burn—a slowly healing injury, *Burns* 18:340-341, 1992.

Felton J: Classical syndromes in occupation medicine phosphorus necrosis—a classical occupational disease, *Am J Ind Med* 3:77-120, 1982.

Pena M, et al: Contact urticaria and dermatitis from phosphorous sesquisulphide, *Contact Dermatitis* 13:126-127, 1985.

Rodeheaver GT: Initial treatment of chemical skin and eye burns, *Compr Ther* 8:37-43, 1982.

Song ZY, Lu YP, Gu XQ: Treatment of yellow phosphorus skin burns with silver nitrate instead of copper sulfate, *Scand J Work Environ Health* 11(Suppl 4):33, 1985.

Steele M, Ive F: Recurrent facial eczema in females due to "Strike Anywhere" matches, *Br J Derm* 106:477-479, 1982.

Stewart C: Chemical skin burns, *Am Fam Physician* 31:149-157, 1985.

Wason S, et al: Phosphorus trichloride toxicity: preliminary report, *Am J Med* 77:1039-1042, 1984.

GUIDELINE 110

Books

CANUTEC: *Initial emergency response guide 1992,* Ottawa, Canada, 1992, Canada Communication Group.

Casarett A: *Radiation biology,* Englewood Cliffs, NJ, 1968, Prentice-Hall.

CCINFO: *MSDS/CHEMINFO* (CD-ROM version), Hamilton, Ontario, Canada, 1993, Canadian Centre for Occupational Health and Safety.

DOT: *CHRIS hazardous chemical data,* US Department of Transportation/United States Coast Guard, Washington, DC, 1984, US Government Printing Office.

DOT: *2000 Emergency response guidebook,* Office of Hazardous Materials Transportation, Research and Special Programs Administration, Washington, DC, 2000, US Department of Transportation.

Guideline for public sector hazardous materials training draft 2, Emmitsburg, MD, 1993, FEMA, National Emergency Training Center.

Levy G: *Level II hazardous materials text,* Fort Collins, Colo, 1985, GML Consultants.

Mackison FW, Stricoff RS, Partridge LJ Jr, editors*: Occupational health guidelines for chemical hazards, NIOSH/OSHA,* Washington, DC, 1981, US Government Printing Office.

NIOSH/OSHA/USCG/EPA: *Occupational safety and health guidance manual for hazardous waste site activities,* Washington, DC, 1985, DHHS (NIOSH) Publication No 85-115, US Government Printing Office.

Noji EK, Kelen GD, editors: *Manual of toxicologic emergencies,* Chicago, 1989, Year Book Medical Publishers.

Smeby LC, editor: *Hazardous materials response handbook,* ed 3, Quincy, Mass, 1997, National Fire Protection Association.

US ARMY: *Field manual 8-285 treatment of chemical agent patients and conventional military chemical patients,* Washington, DC, 1995, Department of the Army.

US ARMY: *Field manual 8-9 NATO handbook on medical aspects of NBC defensive operations,* Washington, DC, 1996, Department of the Army.

US ARMY: *Textbook of military medicine, medical consequences of nuclear warfare,* Washington, DC, 1990, Department of the Army.

Journals

Leonard RB, Ricks RC: Emergency department radiation accident protocol, *Ann Emerg Med* 9:462-470, 1980.

Richter LL, et al: A systems approach to the management of radiation accidents, *Ann Emerg Med* 9:303-309, 1980.

GUIDELINE 111

Books

CANUTEC: *Initial emergency response guide 1992,* Ottawa, Canada, 1992, Canada Communication Group.

Casarett A: *Radiation biology,* Englewood Cliffs, NJ, 1968, Prentice-Hall.

CCINFO: *MSDS/CHEMINFO* (CD-ROM version), Hamilton, Ontario, Canada, 1993, Canadian Centre for Occupational Health and Safety.

DOT: *CHRIS hazardous chemical data,* US Department of Transportation/United States Coast Guard, Washington, DC, 1984, US Government Printing Office.

DOT: *2000 Emergency response guidebook,* Office of Hazardous Materials Transportation, Research and Special Programs Administration, Washington, DC, 2000, US Department of Transportation.

Guideline for public sector hazardous materials training draft 2, Emmitsburg, MD, 1993, FEMA, National Emergency Training Center.

Levy G: *Level II hazardous materials text,* Fort Collins, Colo, 1985, GML Consultants.

Mackison FW, Stricoff RS, Partridge LJ Jr, editors: *Occupational health guidelines for chemical hazards, NIOSH/OSHA,* Washington, DC, 1981, US Government Printing Office.

NIOSH/OSHA/USCG/EPA: *Occupational safety and health guidance manual for hazardous waste site activities,* Washington, DC, 1985, DHHS (NIOSH) Publication No 85-115, US Government Printing Office.

Noji EK, Kelen GD, editors: *Manual of toxicologic emergencies,* Chicago, 1989, Year Book Medical Publishers.

Smeby LC, editor: *Hazardous materials response handbook,* ed 3, Quincy, Mass, 1997, National Fire Protection Association.

US ARMY: *Field manual 8-285 treatment of chemical agent patients and conventional military chemical patients,* Washington, DC, 1995, Department of the Army.

US ARMY: *Field manual 8-9 NATO handbook on medical aspects of NBC defensive operations,* Washington, DC, 1996, Department of the Army.

US ARMY: *Textbook of military medicine, medical consequences of nuclear warfare,* Washington, DC, 1990, Department of the Army.

Journals

Leonard RB, Ricks RC: Emergency department radiation accident protocol, *Ann Emerg Med* 9:462-470, 1980.

Richter LL, et al: A systems approach to the management of radiation accidents, *Ann Emerg Med* 9:303-309, 1980.

GUIDELINE 112

Books

CANUTEC: *Initial emergency response guide 1992,* Ottawa, Canada, 1992, Canada Communication Group.

Casarett A: *Radiation biology,* Englewood Cliffs, NJ, 1968, Prentice-Hall.

CCINFO: *MSDS/CHEMINFO* (CD-ROM version), Hamilton, Ontario, Canada, 1993, Canadian Centre for Occupational Health and Safety.

DOT: *CHRIS hazardous chemical data,* US Department of Transportation/United States Coast Guard, Washington, DC, 1984, US Government Printing Office.

DOT: *2000 Emergency response guidebook,* Office of Hazardous Materials Transportation, Research and Special Programs Administration, Washington, DC, 2000, US Department of Transportation.

Guideline for public sector hazardous materials training draft 2, Emmitsburg, MD, 1993, FEMA, National Emergency Training Center.

Levy G: *Level II hazardous materials text,* Fort Collins, Colo, 1985, GML Consultants.

Mackison FW, Stricoff RS, Partridge LJ Jr, editors: *Occupational health guidelines for chemical hazards, NIOSH/OSHA,* Washington, DC, 1981, US Government Printing Office.

NIOSH/OSHA/USCG/EPA: *Occupational safety and health guidance manual for hazardous waste site activities,* Washington, DC, 1985, DHHS (NIOSH) Publication No 85-115, US Government Printing Office.

Noji EK, Kelen GD, editors: *Manual of toxicologic emergencies,* Chicago, 1989, Year Book Medical Publishers.

Smeby LC, editor: *Hazardous materials response handbook,* ed 3, Quincy, Mass, 1997, National Fire Protection Association.

US ARMY: *Field manual 8-285 treatment of chemical agent patients and conventional military chemical patients, Washington, DC,* 1995, Department of the Army.

US ARMY: *Field Manual 8-9 NATO handbook on medical aspects of NBC defensive operations,* Washington, DC, 1996, Department of the Army.

US ARMY: *Textbook of military medicine, medical consequences of nuclear warfare,* Washington, DC, 1990, Department of the Army.

Journals

Leonard RB, Ricks RC: Emergency department radiation accident protocol, *Ann Emerg Med* 9:462-470, 1980.

Richter LL, et al: A systems approach to the management of radiation accidents, *Ann Emerg Med* 9:303-309, 1980.

GUIDELINE 113

Books

Armstrong D, Cohen J: *Infectious diseases,* London, 1999, Harcourt.

Chin J, editor: *Control of communicable diseases manual,* ed 17, Washington, DC, 2000, American Public Health Association.

Eitzen E, Pavlin J, Cieslak T: *Medical management of biological casualties handbook.* Fort Detrick, Maryland, 1998, US Army Medical Research Institute of Infectious Diseases (USAMRIID).

Friedlander AM: *Textbook of military medicine: medical aspects of chemical and biological warfare,* Office of the Surgeon General Department of the Army, United States of America, 1997.

Osterholm MT, Schwartz J: *Living terrors. What America needs to know to survive the coming bioterrorist catastrophe,* New York, 2000, Delacorte Press.

Weinstein RS, Alibek K: *Biological and chemical terrorism: a guide for healthcare providers and first responders,* New York, 2003, Thieme.

Professional guide to diseases, Springhouse, Pa, 1998, Springhouse Corporation.

Journals

Centers for Disease Control and Prevention (CDC): Notice to readers: use of anthrax vaccine in response to terrorism: Supplemental recommendations of the Advisory Committee on Immunization Practices, *MMWR Morb Mortal Wkly Rep* 51(45):1024-1026, 2002. Available at: http://www.cdc.gov/mmwr/preview/mmwrhtml/mm5145a4.htm

Franz D, Jahrlling R, Friedlander PB, et al: Clinical recognition and management of patients exposed to biological warfare agents, *JAMA* 278:399-411, 1997.

Inglesby TV, Henderson DA, Bartlett JG, et al: Anthrax as a biological weapon. Medical and public health management, *JAMA* 281:1735-1745, 1991.

Inglesby T, O'Toole T, Henderson D, et al: Anthrax as a biological weapon, 2002: updated recommendations for management, *JAMA* 287:2236-2252, 2002.

Leggiadro RJ: The threat of biological terrorism: a public health and infection control reality. *Infect Control Hosp Epidemiol* 21:53-56, 2002.

Malone JD: Bioterrorism readiness audio conference, *Association for Professionals in Infection Control and Epidemiology,* 1999.

Moran GJ: Biological terrorism. 1. Are we prepared? *Emerg Med* 32:14-38, 2000.

GUIDELINE 114

Books

Centers for Disease Control and Prevention (CDC): *Botulism in the United States 1899-1996: handbook for epidemiologists, clinicians, and laboratory workers,* Atlanta, GA, CDC, 1998. Available at: http://www.cdc.gov/ncidod/dbmd/diseaseinfo/botulism.pdf

Chin J, editor: *Control of communicable diseases manual,* ed 17, Washington, DC: 2000, American Public Health Association.

Sidell FR, Patrick WC, Dashiell TR: *Jane's chem-bio handbook,* Alexandria, Va, 1998, Jane's Information Group.

Sifton DW, editor: *PDR guide to biological and chemical warfare response,* ed 1, Montvale, NJ, 2002, Thomson/Physician's Desk Reference.

Weinstein RS, Alibek K: *Biological and chemical terrorism: a guide for healthcare providers and first responders,* New York, 2003, Thieme.

Journals

Arnon S, et al: Botulinum toxin as a biological weapon: medical and public health management, *JAMA* 285:1059-1070, 2001.

Gill MD: Bacterial toxins: a table of lethal amounts, *Microbiol Rev* 46:86-94, 1982.

GUIDELINE 115

Books

Chin J, editor: *Control of communicable diseases manual,* ed 17, Washington, DC, 2000, American Public Health Association.

Eitzen E, Pavlin J, Cieslak T: *Medical management of biological casualties handbook.* Fort Detrick, Maryland, 1998, US Army Medical Research Institute of Infectious Diseases (USAMRIID).

Mandell GL, Bennett JE, Dolin R, editors: *Mandell, Douglas, and Bennett's Principles and practice of infectious diseases,* ed 5, New York, 2002, Churchill Livingstone.

Sifton DW, editor: *PDR guide to biological and chemical warfare response,* ed 1, Montvale, NJ, 2002, Thomson/Physician's Desk Reference.

Weinstein RS, Alibek K: *Biological and chemical terrorism: a guide for healthcare providers and first responders,* New York, 2003, Thieme.

Journals

Centers for Disease Control and Prevention, Division of Bacterial and Mycotic Diseases: Disease information: brucellosis [cited 2003 Oct 27]. Available at: http://www.cdc.gov/ncidod/dbmd/diseaseinfo/brucellosis_g.htm

GUIDELINE 116

Books

Chin J, editor: *Control of communicable diseases manual,* ed 17, Washington, DC, 2000, American Public Health Association.

Mandell GL, Bennett JE, Dolin R, editors: *Mandell, Douglas, and Bennett's Principles and practice of infectious diseases,* ed 5, New York, 2002, Churchill Livingstone.

Sifton DW, editor: *PDR guide to biological and chemical warfare response,* ed 1, Montvale, NJ, 2002, Thomson/Physician's Desk Reference.

Strickland GT, editor. Hunter's tropical medicine and emerging infectious diseases, ed 8, Philadelphia, 2002, Saunders.

Weinstein RS, Alibek K: *Biological and chemical terrorism: a guide for healthcare providers and first responders,* New York, 2003, Thieme.

Journals

Borio L, et al Hemorrhagic fever viruses as biological weapons: medical and public health management, JAMA 287:2391-2405, 2002.

Burney MI, et al: Nosocomial outbreak of viral hemorrhagic fever caused by Crimean hemorrhagic fever–Congo virus in Pakistan, January 1976, *Am J Trop Med Hyg* 29:941-947, 1980.

Suleiman MN, et al: Congo/Crimean haemorrhagic fever in Dubai. An outbreak at the Rashid Hospital, *Lancet* 2:939-941, 1980.

Van Eeden PJ, et al: A nosocomial outbreak of Crimean-Congo haemorrhagic fever at Tygerberg Hospital. Part I. Clinical features, *S Afr Med J* 68:711-717, 1985.

GUIDELINE 117

Books

Chin J, editor: *Control of communicable diseases manual,* ed 17, Washington, DC, 2000, American Public Health Association.

Mandell GL, Bennett JE, Dolin R, editors: *Mandell, Douglas, and Bennett's Principles and practice of infectious diseases,* ed 5, New York, 2002, Churchill Livingstone.

Sidell FR, Patrick WC, Dashiell TR: *Jane's chem-bio handbook,* Alexandria, Va, 1998, Jane's Information Group.

Sifton DW, editor: *PDR guide to biological and chemical warfare response,* ed 1, Montvale, NJ, 2002, Thomson/Physician's Desk Reference.

Strickland GT, editor. *Hunter's tropical medicine and emerging infectious diseases,* ed 8, Philadelphia, 2002, Saunders.

Weinstein RS, Alibek K: *Biological and chemical terrorism: a guide for healthcare providers and first responders,* New York, 2003, Thieme.

Journals

Centers for Disease Control and Prevention, Division of Bacterial and Mycotic Diseases: Disease information: *Escherichia coli* O157:H7 [cited 2003 Oct 27]. Available at: http://www.cdc.gov/ncidod/dbmd/diseaseinfo/escherichiacoli_t.htm

Centers for Disease Control and Prevention, Division of Bacterial and Mycotic Diseases: Disease information: salmonellosis [cited 2003 Oct 27]. Available at: http://www.cdc.gov/ncidod/dbmd/diseaseinfo/salmonellosis_t.htm

Centers for Disease Control and Prevention, Division of Bacterial and Mycotic Diseases: Disease information: shigellosis [cited 2003 Oct 27]. Available at: http://www.cdc.gov/ncidod/dbmd/diseaseinfo/shigellosis_t.htm

GUIDELINE 118

Books

Alibek K: *Biohazard,* New York, 1999, Random House.

Chin J, editor: *Control of communicable diseases manual,* ed 17, Washington, DC, 2000, American Public Health Association.

Eitzen E, Pavlin J, Cieslak T: *Medical management of biological casualties handbook.* Fort Detrick, Maryland, 1998, US Army Medical Research Institute of Infectious Diseases (USAMRIID).

Mandell GL, Bennett JE, Dolin R, editors: *Mandell, Douglas, and Bennett's Principles and practice of infectious diseases,* ed 5, New York, 2002, Churchill Livingstone.

Sidell FR, Patrick WC, Dashiell TR: *Jane's chem-bio handbook,* Alexandria, Va, 1998, Jane's Information Group

Sifton DW, editor: *PDR guide to biological and chemical warfare response,* ed 1, Montvale, NJ, 2002, Thomson/Physician's Desk Reference.

Strickland GT, editor. *Hunter's tropical medicine and emerging infectious diseases,* ed 8, Philadelphia, 2002, Saunders.

Weinstein RS, Alibek K: *Biological and chemical terrorism: a guide for healthcare providers and first responders,* New York, 2003, Thieme.

Journal

Russell P, et al: Comparison of efficacy of ciprofloxacin and doxycycline against experimental melioidosis and glanders, *J Antimicrob Chemother* 45:813-818, 2000.

GUIDELINE 119

Books

Chin J, editor: *Control of communicable diseases manual,* ed 17, Washington, DC, 2000, American Public Health Association.

Mandell GL, Bennett JE, Dolin R, editors: *Mandell, Douglas, and Bennett's Principles and practice of infectious diseases,* ed 5, New York, 2002, Churchill Livingstone.

Sifton DW, editor: *PDR guide to biological and chemical warfare response,* ed 1, Montvale, NJ, 2002, Thomson/Physician's Desk Reference.

Strickland GT, editor. *Hunter's tropical medicine and emerging infectious diseases,* ed 8, Philadelphia, 2002, Saunders.

Weinstein RS, Alibek K: *Biological and chemical terrorism: a guide for healthcare providers and first responders,* New York, 2003, Thieme.

Journals

Graziano KI, Tempest B: Hantavirus pulmonary syndrome: a zebra worth knowing, *Am Fam Physician* 66:1015-1020, 2002.

Padula PJ, et al: Hantavirus pulmonary syndrome outbreak in Argentina: molecular evidence for person-to-person transmission of Andes virus, *Virology* 241:323-330, 1998.

Toro J, et al: An outbreak of hantavirus pulmonary syndrome, Chile, 1997, *Emerg Infect Dis* 4:687-694, 1998.

Wells R, et al: Hantavirus transmission in the United States, *Emerg Infect Dis* 3:361-365, 1997.

Wells RM, et al: An unusual hantavirus outbreak in southern Argentina: person-to-person transmission? *Emerg Infect Dis* 3:171-174, 1997.

GUIDELINE 120

Books

Chin J, editor: *Control of communicable diseases manual,* ed 17, Washington, DC, 2000, American Public Health Association.

Mandell GL, Bennett JE, Dolin R, editors: *Mandell, Douglas, and Bennett's Principles and practice of infectious diseases,* ed 5, New York, 2002, Churchill Livingstone.

Sidell FR, Patrick WC, Dashiell TR: *Jane's chem-bio handbook,* Alexandria, Va, 1998, Jane's Information Group.

Sifton DW, editor: *PDR guide to biological and chemical warfare response,* ed 1, Montvale, NJ, 2002, Thomson/Physician's Desk Reference.

Strickland GT, editor. Hunter's tropical medicine and emerging infectious diseases, ed 8, Philadelphia, 2002, Saunders.

Weinstein RS, Alibek K: *Biological and chemical terrorism: a guide for healthcare providers and first responders,* New York, 2003, Thieme.

Journals

Centers for Disease Control and Prevention, Division of Bacterial and Mycotic Diseases: Disease information: melioidosis *(Burkholderia pseudomallei)* [cited 2003 Oct 27]. Available at: http://www.cdc.gov/ncidod/dbmd/diseaseinfo/melioidosis_t.htm

GUIDELINE 121

Books

Armstrong D, Cohen J: *Infectious diseases,* London, 1999, Harcourt.

Chin J, editor: *Control of communicable diseases manual,* ed 17, Washington, DC, 2000, American Public Health Association.

Eitzen E, Pavlin J, Cieslak T: *Medical management of biological casualties handbook.* Fort Detrick, Maryland, 1998, US Army Medical Research Institute of Infectious Diseases (USAMRIID).

Mandell GL, Bennett JE, Dolin R, editors: *Mandell, Douglas, and Bennett's Principles and practice of infectious diseases,* ed 5, New York, 2002, Churchill Livingstone.

McGovern TW, Friedlander AM: *Textbook of military medicine: medical aspects of chemical and biological warfare.* Office of the Surgeon General, Department of the Army, United States of America; 1997.

Osterholm MT, Schwartz J: *Living terrors. What America needs to know to survive the coming bioterrorist catastrophe.* New York, 2000, Delacorte Press.

Professional guide to diseases, Springhouse, Pa, 1998, Springhouse Corporation.

Sidell FR, Patrick WC, Dashiell TR: *Jane's chem-bio handbook,* Alexandria, Va, 1998, Jane's Information Group.

Journals

Franz DR, et al: Clinical recognition and management of patients exposed to biological warfare agents, *JAMA* 278:399-411, 1997.

Inglesby TV, et al: Plague as a biological weapon: medical and public health management, *JAMA* 283:2281-2290, 2000.

Leggiadro RJ: The threat of biological terrorism: a public health and infection control reality, *Infect Control Hosp Epidemiol* 21:53-56, 2000.

Moran GJ: Biological terrorism. 1. Are we prepared? *Emerg Med* 32:14-38, 2000.

GUIDELINE 122

Books

Mandell GL, Bennett JE, Dolin R, editors: *Mandell, Douglas, and Bennett's Principles and practice of infectious diseases,* ed 5, New York, 2002, Churchill Livingstone.

Chin J, editor: *Control of communicable diseases manual,* ed 17, Washington, DC, 2000, American Public Health Association.

Strickland GT, editor. *Hunter's tropical medicine and emerging infectious diseases,* ed 8, Philadelphia, 2002, Saunders.

Weinstein RS, Alibek K: *Biological and chemical terrorism: a guide for healthcare providers and first responders,* New York, 2003, Thieme.

Journal

Centers for Disease Control and Prevention, Division of Bacterial and Mycotic Diseases: Disease information: psittacosis [cited 2003 Oct 27]. Available at: http://www.cdc.gov/ncidod/dbmd/diseaseinfo/psittacosis_t.htm

GUIDELINE 123

Books

Chin J, editor: *Control of communicable diseases manual,* ed 17, Washington, DC, 2000, American Public Health Association.

Eitzen E, Pavlin J, Cieslak T: *Medical management of biological casualties handbook.* Fort Detrick, Maryland, 1998, US Army Medical Research Institute of Infectious Diseases (USAMRIID).

Mandell GL, Bennett JE, Dolin R, editors: *Mandell, Douglas, and Bennett's Principles and practice of infectious diseases,* ed 5, New York, 2002, Churchill Livingstone.

Sidell FR, Patrick WC, Dashiell TR: *Jane's chem-bio handbook,* Alexandria, Va, 1998, Jane's Information Group.

Sifton DW, editor: *PDR guide to biological and chemical warfare response,* ed 1, Montvale, NJ, 2002, Thomson/Physician's Desk Reference.

Strickland GT, editor. *Hunter's tropical medicine and emerging infectious diseases,* ed 8, Philadelphia, 2002, Saunders.

Weinstein RS, Alibek K: *Biological and chemical terrorism: a guide for healthcare providers and first responders,* New York, 2003, Thieme.

Journal

Centers for Disease Control and Prevention, Division of Viral and Rickettsial Diseases: Disease information: Q fever [cited 2003 Nov 1]. Available at: http://www.cdc.gov/ncidod/dvrd/qfever/index.htm

GUIDELINE 124

Books

Eitzen E, Pavlin J, Cieslak T: *Medical management of biological casualties handbook.* Fort Detrick, Maryland, 1998, US Army Medical Research Institute of Infectious Diseases (USAMRIID).

Sidell FR, Patrick WC, Dashiell TR: *Jane's chem-bio handbook,* Alexandria, Va, 1998, Jane's Information Group.

Sifton DW, editor: *PDR guide to biological and chemical warfare response,* ed 1, Montvale, NJ, 2002, Thomson/Physician's Desk Reference.

Weinstein RS, Alibek K: *Biological and chemical terrorism: a guide for healthcare providers and first responders,* New York, 2003, Thieme.

Journals

Balint GA: Ricin: the toxic protein of castor oil seeds, *Toxicology* 2:77-102, 1974.

Centers for Disease Control and Prevention, Emergency Preparedness and Response: Chemical agent information: facts about ricin [cited 2003 Nov 1]. Available at: http://www.bt.cdc.gov/agent/ricin/facts.asp

Olsnes S, et al: Mechanism of action of the toxic lectins abrin and ricin, *Nature* 249:627-631, 1974.

GUIDELINE 125

Books

Armstrong D, Cohen J: *Infectious diseases,* London, 1999, Harcourt.

Chin J, editor: *Control of communicable diseases manual,* ed 17, Washington, DC, 2000, American Public Health Association.

Eitzen E, Pavlin J, Cieslak T: *Medical management of biological casualties handbook.* Fort Detrick, Maryland, 1998, US Army Medical Research Institute of Infectious Diseases (USAMRIID).

McClain DJ: *Textbook of military medicine: medical aspects of chemical and biological warfare.* Office of the Surgeon General, Department of the Army, United States of America, 1997.

Osterholm MT, Schwartz J: *Living terrors. What America needs to know to survive the coming bioterrorist catastrophe,* New York, 2000, Delacorte Press.

Professional guide to diseases, Springhouse, Pa, 1998, Springhouse Corporation.

Sidell FR, Patrick WC, Dashiell TR: *Jane's chem-bio handbook,* Alexandria, Va, 1998, Jane's Information Group.

Sifton DW, editor: *PDR guide to biological and chemical warfare response,* ed 1, Montvale, NJ, 2002, Thomson/Physician's Desk Reference.

Weinstein RS, Alibek K: *Biological and chemical terrorism: a guide for healthcare providers and first responders,* New York, 2003, Thieme.

Journals

Franz DR, et al: Clinical recognition and management of patients exposed to biological warfare agents, *JAMA* 278:399-411, 1997.

Henderson DA, et al: Smallpox as a biological weapon: medical and public health management, *JAMA* 281:2127-2137, 1999.

Leggiadro RJ: The threat of biological terrorism: a public health and infection control reality, *Infect Control Hosp Epidemiol* 21:53-56, 2000.

Moran GJ: Biological terrorism. 1. Are we prepared? *Emerg Med* 32:14-38, 2000.

GUIDELINE 126

Books

Eitzen E, Pavlin J, Cieslak T: *Medical management of biological casualties handbook.* Fort Detrick, Maryland, 1998, US Army Medical Research Institute of Infectious Diseases (USAMRIID).

Sidell FR, Patrick WC, Dashiell TR: *Jane's chem-bio handbook,* Alexandria, Va, 1998, Jane's Information Group.

Sifton DW, editor: *PDR guide to biological and chemical warfare response,* ed 1, Montvale, NJ, 2002, Thomson/Physician's Desk Reference.

Weinstein RS, Alibek K: *Biological and chemical terrorism: a guide for healthcare providers and first responders,* New York, 2003, Thieme.

GUIDELINE 127

Books

Armstrong D, Cohen J: *Infectious diseases,* London, 1999, Harcourt.

Eitzen E, Pavlin J, Cieslak T: *Medical management of biological casualties handbook.* Fort Detrick, Maryland, 1998, US Army Medical Research Institute of Infectious Diseases (USAMRIID).

Mandell GL, Bennett JE, Dolin R, editors: *Mandell, Douglas, and Bennett's Principles and practice of infectious diseases,* ed 5, New York, 2002, Churchill Livingstone.

Sidell FR, Patrick WC, Dashiell TR: *Jane's chem-bio handbook,* Alexandria, Va, 1998, Jane's Information Group.

Sifton DW, editor: *PDR guide to biological and chemical warfare response,* ed 1, Montvale, NJ, 2002, Thomson/Physician's Desk Reference.

Weinstein RS, Alibek K: *Biological and chemical terrorism: a guide for healthcare providers and first responders,* New York, 2003, Thieme.

Journals

Day WC, Bernendt RF: Experimental tularemia in *Macaca mulatta:* relationship of aerosol particle size to the infectivity of airborne *Pasteurella tularensis, Infect Immun* 5:77-82, 1972.

Dennis DT, et al: Working Group on Civilian Biodefense. Tularemia as a biological weapon: medical and public health management, *JAMA* 285:2763-2773, 2001.

Enderlin G, et al: Streptomycin and alternative agents for the treatment of tularemia: review of the literature, *Clin Infect Dis* 19:42-47, 1994.

Francis E: Landmark article April 25, 1925: Tularemia. By Edward Francis, *JAMA* 250:3216-3224, 1983.

Gill V, Cunha BAL: Tularemia pneumonia, *Semin Respir Infect* 12:61-67, 1997.

Johansson A, et al: Ciprofloxacin for treatment of tularemia in children, *Pediatr Infect Dis J* 19:449-453, 2000.

Limaye AP, Hooper CJ: Treatment of tularemia with fluoroquinolones: two cases and review, *Clin Infect Dis* 29:922-924, 1999.

Martone WJ, et al: Tularemia pneumonia in Washington, DC. A report of three cases with possible common-source exposures, *JAMA* 242:2315-2317, 1979.

Penn RL, Kinasewitz GT: Factors associated with a poor outcome in tularemia, *Arch Intern Med* 147:265-268, 1987.

Rohrbach BW, Westerman E, Istre GR: Epidemiology and clinical characteristics of tularemia in Oklahoma, 1979 to 1985, *South Med J* 84:1091-1096, 1991.

Sanford JP: Landmark perspective: tularemia, *JAMA* 250:3225-3226, 1983.

Schrickeker RL, et al: Pathogenesis of tularemia in monkeys aerogenically exposed to *Francisella tularensis* 425, *Infect Immun* 5:734-744, 1972.

Spach DH, et al: Tick-borne diseases in the United States, *N Engl J Med* 329:936-947, 1993.

Teutsch SM, et al: Pneumonic tularemia on Martha's Vineyard, *N Engl J Med* 301:826-828, 1979.

GUIDELINE 128

Books

Eitzen E, Pavlin J, Cieslak T: *Medical management of biological casualties handbook.* Fort Detrick, Maryland, 1998, US Army Medical Research Institute of Infectious Diseases (USAMRIID).

Mandell GL, Bennett JE, Dolin R, editors: *Mandell, Douglas, and Bennett's Principles and practice of infectious diseases,* ed 5, New York, 2002, Churchill Livingstone.

Sifton DW, editor: *PDR guide to biological and chemical warfare response,* ed 1, Montvale, NJ, 2002, Thomson/Physician's Desk Reference.

Strickland GT, editor. *Hunter's tropical medicine and emerging infectious diseases,* ed 8, Philadelphia, 2002, Saunders.

Weinstein RS, Alibek K: *Biological and chemical terrorism: a guide for healthcare providers and first responders,* New York, 2003, Thieme.

GUIDELINE 129

Books

Eitzen E, Pavlin J, Cieslak T: *Medical management of biological casualties handbook.* Fort Detrick, Maryland, 1998, US Army Medical Research Institute of Infectious Diseases (USAMRIID).

Mandell GL, Bennett JE, Dolin R, editors: *Mandell, Douglas, and Bennett's Principles and practice of infectious diseases,* ed 5, New York, 2002, Churchill Livingstone.

Sidell FR, Patrick WC, Dashiell TR: *Jane's chem-bio handbook,* Alexandria, Va, 1998, Jane's Information Group.

Sifton DW, editor: *PDR guide to biological and chemical warfare response,* ed 1, Montvale, NJ, 2002, Thomson/Physician's Desk Reference.

Strickland GT, editor. *Hunter's tropical medicine and emerging infectious diseases,* ed 8, Philadelphia, 2002, Saunders.

Weinstein RS, Alibek K: *Biological and chemical terrorism: a guide for healthcare providers and first responders,* New York, 2003, Thieme.

Journal

Centers for Disease Control and Prevention, Division of Vector-Borne Infectious Diseases: Eastern equine encephalitis fact sheet [cited 2003 Nov 6]. Available at: http://www.cdc.gob/ncidod/dvbid/arbor/eeefact.htm

GUIDELINE 130

Books

Eitzen E, Pavlin J, Cieslak T: *Medical management of biological casualties handbook.* Fort Detrick, Maryland, 1998, US Army Medical Research Institute of Infectious Diseases (USAMRIID).

Mandell GL, Bennett JE, Dolin R, editors: *Mandell, Douglas, and Bennett's Principles and practice of infectious diseases,* ed 5, New York, 2002, Churchill Livingstone.

Sidell FR, Patrick WC, Dashiell TR: *Jane's chem-bio handbook,* Alexandria, Va, 1998, Jane's Information Group.

Sifton DW, editor: *PDR guide to biological and chemical warfare response,* ed 1, Montvale, NJ, 2002, Thomson/Physician's Desk Reference.

Strickland GT, editor. *Hunter's tropical medicine and emerging infectious diseases,* ed 8, Philadelphia, 2002, Saunders.

Weinstein RS, Alibek K: *Biological and chemical terrorism: a guide for healthcare providers and first responders,* New York, 2003, Thieme.

Journals

Borio L, et al: Working Group on Civilian Biodefense. Hemorrhagic fever viruses as biological weapons: medical and public health management, *JAMA* 287:2391-2405, 2002.

Centers for Disease Control and Prevention, Special Pathogens Branch: Viral hemorrhagic fevers [cited 2003 Nov 6]. Available at: http://www.cdc.gov/ncidod/dvrd/spb/mnpages/dispages/vhf.htm

GUIDELINE 131

Books

Mandell GL, Bennett JE, Dolin R, editors: *Mandell, Douglas, and Bennett's Principles and practice of infectious diseases,* ed 5, New York, 2002, Churchill Livingstone.

Sidell FR, Patrick WC, Dashiell TR: *Jane's chem-bio handbook,* Alexandria, Va, 1998, Jane's Information Group.

Sifton DW, editor: *PDR guide to biological and chemical warfare response,* ed 1, Montvale, NJ, 2002, Thomson/Physician's Desk Reference.

Weinstein RS, Alibek K: *Biological and chemical terrorism: a guide for healthcare providers and first responders,* New York, 2003, Thieme.

Journals

Centers for Disease Control and Prevention, Division of Parasitic Diseases: Disease information: cryptosporidiosis [cited 2003 Nov 7]. Available at: http://www.cdc.gov/ncidod/dpd/parasites/cryptosporidiosis/factsht_cryptosporidiosis.htm

Colley DG: Waterborne cryptosporidiosis threat addressed, *Emerg Infect Dis* 1:67-68, 1995.

Guerrant RL: Cryptosporidiosis: an emerging, highly infectious threat, *Emerg Infect Dis* 3:51-57, 1997.

GUIDELINE 132

Books

Amdur MO, Doull J, Klaassen CD, editors: *Casarett and Doull's toxicology, the basic science of poisons,* ed 4, New York, 1991, Pergamon Press.

Baselt RC, Cravey RH: *Disposition of toxic drugs and chemicals in man,* ed 3, Chicago, 1989, Year Book Medical Publishers.

CANUTEC: *Initial emergency response guide 1992,* Ottawa, Canada, 1992, Canada Communication Group.

CCINFO: *MSDS/CHEMINFO* (CD-ROM version), Hamilton, Ontario, Canada, 1993, Canadian Centre for Occupational Health and Safety.

Danon YL, et al, editors: *Chemical warfare medicine,* Jerusalem, 1994, Gefen.

DOT: *CHRIS hazardous chemical data.* US Department of Transportation/United States Coast Guard. Washington, DC, 1984, US Government Printing Office.

DOT: *2000 Emergency response guidebook,* Office of Hazardous Materials Transportation, Research and Special Programs Administration, Washington, DC, 2000, US Department of Transportation.

Goldfrank LR, et al: *Goldfrank's toxicologic emergencies,* ed 6, New York, 1998, McGraw-Hill.

Gosselin RE, Smith RP, Hodge HC: *Clinical toxicology of commercial products,* ed 5, Baltimore, 1984, Williams & Wilkins.

Hartman DE: *Neuropsychological toxicology, identification and assessment of human neurotoxic syndromes,* New York, 1988, Pergamon Press.

Mackison FW, Stricoff RS, Partridge LJ Jr, editors: *Occupational health guidelines for chemical hazards, NIOSH/OSHA,* Washington, DC, 1981, US Government Printing Office.

NIOSH: *NIOSH pocket guide to chemical hazards* (CD-ROM version), Cincinnati, 2000, DHHS (NIOSH), US Government Printing Office.

Sifton DW, editor: *PDR guide to biological and chemical warfare response,* Montvale, NJ, 2002, Thomson/Physician's Desk Reference.

Sullivan JB, Kriger GR, editors: *Clinical environmental health and hazardous materials toxicology,* Baltimore, 1997, Williams & Wilkins.

USAMRICD, Chemical Casualty Care Division: *Medical management of chemical casualties handbook, ed 3,* Aberdeen, MD, 1999, Department of the Army.

US ARMY: *Field manual 8-285 treatment of chemical agent patients' and conventional military chemical patients,* Washington, DC, 1995, Department of the Army.

US ARMY: *Field Manual 8-9 NATO handbook on medical aspects of NBC defensive operations,* Washington, DC, 1996, Department of the Army.

US ARMY: *Textbook of military medicine,* Washington, DC, 1990, Department of the Army.

Zajtchuk R, et al, editors: *Medical aspects of chemical and biological warfare*, Washington, DC, 1997, Department of the Army.

Journals

Ballantyne B: Artifacts in the definition of toxicity of cyanides and cyanogens, *Fundam Applied Toxicol* 3:400-408, 1983.

Baskin SI, Horowitz AM, Nealley EW: The antidotal action of sodium nitrite and sodium thiosulfate against cyanide poisoning, *J Clin Pharmacol* 32:368-375, 1992.

Baud FJ, et al: Elevated blood cyanide concentrations in victims of smoke inhalation, *N Engl J Med* 325:1761-1766, 1991.

Becker CE: The role of cyanide in fires, *Vet Hum Toxicol* 27:487-490, 1985.

Curry SC, Patrick HC: Lack of evidence for a percent saturation gap in cyanide poisoning, *Ann Emerg Med* 20:523-531, 1991.

Fernandez De Corres L, Lajarazu D: Allergic contact dermatitis to cyanide, *Contact Dermatitis* 8:346, 1982.

Forsyth JC, et al: Hydroxocobalamin as a cyanide antidote: safety, efficacy and pharmacokinetics in heavily smoking normal volunteers, *Clin Toxicol* 31:277-294, 1993.

Freeman A: Optic neuropathy and chronic cyanide toxicity (letter), *Lancet* 22:441-442, 1986.

Greenberg SR: The morphology of cyanide poisoning, *Proc Inst Med Chic* 35:131-132, 1982.

Hart GB, et al: Treatment of smoke inhalation by hyperbaric oxygen, *J Emerg Med* 3:211-215, 1985.

Kohlmeier C: Protocols for the management of patients with acute hazardous materials exposure, *J Emerg Nurs* 11:249-252, 1985.

Kulig K: Cyanide antidotes and fire toxicology, *N Engl J Med* 325:1801-1802, 1991.

Lafin SM, et al: A need to revise the cyanide antidote package instructions, *J Emerg Med* 10:623-625, 1992.

Litovitz T, Larkin R, Myers R: Cyanide poisoning treated with hyperbaric oxygen, *Am J Emerg Med* 1:94-101, 1983.

Marbury T, et al: Combined antidotal and hemodialysis treatments for nitroprusside-induced cyanide toxicity, *J Clin Toxicol* 19:475-482, 1982.

Pickering W: Cyanide toxicity and the hazards of dicobalt edetate (letter), *Br Med J* 291:1644, 1985.

Rindone JP, Sloane EP: Cyanide toxicity from sodium nitroprusside: risks and management, *Ann Pharmacotherapy* 26:515-519, 1992.

Robin ED, McCauley R: Nitroprusside-related cyanide poisoning, time (long past due) for urgent, effective interventions, *Chest* 102:1842-1845, 1992.

Scharf BA, Fricke RF, Baskin SI: Comparison of methemoglobin formers in protection against the toxic effects of cyanide, *Gen Pharmacol* 23:19-25, 1992.

Ten Eyck R, et al: Stroma-free methemoglobin solution as an antidote for cyanide poisoning: a preliminary study, *Clin Toxicol* 21:343-358, 1983.

Vincent F: Pathologic changes after cyanide poisoning (letter), *Neurology* 36:137, 1986.

Wald P, Goldfrank L: Cyanide intoxication (letter), *JAMA* 254:2889, 1985.

Yeh MH, et al: Is measurement of venous oxygen saturation useful in the diagnosis of cyanide poisoning? *Am J Med* 93:582-583, 1992.

GUIDELINE 133

Books

Amdur MO, Doull J, Klaassen CD, editors: *Casarett and Doull's toxicology, the basic science of poisons,* ed 4, New York, 1991, Pergamon Press.

CANUTEC: *Initial emergency response guide 1992,* Ottawa, Canada, 1992, Canada Communication Group.

CCINFO: *MSDS/CHEMINFO* (CD-ROM version), Hamilton, Ontario, Canada, 1993, Canadian Centre for Occupational Health and Safety.

Danon YL, et al, editors: *Chemical warfare medicine,* Jerusalem, 1994, Gefen.

DOT: *CHRIS hazardous chemical data.* US Department of Transportation/United States Coast Guard. Washington, DC, 1984, US Government Printing Office.

DOT: *2000 Emergency response guidebook,* Office of Hazardous Materials Transportation, Research and Special Programs Administration, Washington, DC, 2000, US Department of Transportation.

Gosselin RE, Smith RP, Hodge HC: *Clinical toxicology of commercial products,* ed 5, Baltimore, 1984, Williams & Wilkins.

Mackison FW, Stricoff RS, Partridge LJ Jr, editors*: Occupational health guidelines for chemical hazards, NIOSH/OSHA,* Washington, DC, 1981, US Government Printing Office.

Manahan SE: *Environmental chemistry,* ed 7, Chelsea, Mich, 1999, Lewis Publishers.

NIOSH: *NIOSH pocket guide to chemical hazards* (CD-ROM version), Cincinnati, 2000, DHHS (NIOSH), US Government Printing Office.

Olson KR, editor: *Poisoning & drug overdose*, ed 3, East Norwalk, Conn, 1999, Appleton & Lange.

Sifton, DW, editor: *PDR guide to biological and chemical warfare response,* Montvale, NJ, 2002, Thomson/Physician's Desk Reference.

Sullivan JB, Kriger GR, editors: *Clinical environmental health and hazardous materials toxicology,* Baltimore, 1997, Williams & Wilkins.

USAMRICD, Chemical Casualty Care Division: *Medical management of chemical casualties handbook,* ed 3, Aberdeen, MD, 1999, Department of the Army.

US ARMY: *Field manual 8-285 treatment of chemical agent patients and conventional military chemical patients, Washington, DC,* 1995, Department of the Army.

US ARMY: *Field Manual 8-9 NATO handbook on medical Aspects of NBC defensive operations,* Washington, DC, 1996, Department of the Army.

US ARMY: *Textbook of military medicine,* Washington, DC, 1990, Department of the Army.

Zajtchuk R, et al, editors: *Medical aspects of chemical and biological warfare,* Washington, DC, 1997, Department of the Army.

GUIDELINE 134

Books

Danon YL, et al, editors: *Chemical warfare medicine,* Jerusalem, 1994, Gefen.

Sifton, DW, editor: *PDR Guide to Biological and Chemical Warfare Response,* Montvale, NJ, 2002, Thomson/Physician's Desk Reference.

USAMRICD: Chemical Casualty Care Division: *Medical management of chemical casualties handbook, ed 3,* Aberdeen, MD, 1999, Department of the Army.

US ARMY: Conventional military chemical patients, Washington, DC, 1995, Department of the Army.

US ARMY: *Field Manual 8-9 NATO handbook on medical aspects of NBC defensive operations,* Washington, DC, 1996, Department of the Army.

US ARMY: *Textbook of military medicine,* Washington, DC, 1990, Department of the Army.

Zajtchuk R, et al, editors: *Medical aspects of chemical and biological warfare*, Washington, DC, 1997, Department of the Army.

GUIDELINE 135

Books

Amdur MO, Doull J, Klaassen CD, editors: *Casarett and Doull's toxicology, the basic science of poisons,* ed 4, New York, 1991, Pergamon Press.

CANUTEC: *Initial emergency response guide 1992,* Ottawa, Canada, 1992, Canada Communication Group.

CCINFO: *MSDS/CHEMINFO* (CD-ROM version), Hamilton, Ontario, Canada, 1993, Canadian Centre for Occupational Health and Safety.

Danon YL, et al, editors: *Chemical warfare medicine,* Jerusalem, 1994, Gefen.

DOT: *CHRIS hazardous chemical data.* US Department of Transportation/United States Coast Guard. Washington, DC, 1984, US Government Printing Office.

DOT: *2000 Emergency response guidebook,* Office of Hazardous Materials Transportation, Research and Special Programs Administration, Washington, DC, 2000, US Department of Transportation.

Goldfrank LR, et al: *Goldfrank's toxicologic emergencies,* ed 6, New York, 1998, McGraw-Hill Professional.

Goodman AG, et al, editors: *Goodman and Gilman's The pharmacological basis of therapeutics,* ed 8, New York, 1990, Pergamon Press.

Gosselin RE, Smith RP, Hodge HC: *Clinical toxicology of commercial products,* ed 5, Baltimore, 1984, Williams & Wilkins.

Hartman DE: *Neuropsychological toxicology, identification and assessment of human neurotoxic syndromes,* New York, 1988, Pergamon Press.

HSDB: *Hazardous substances data bank,* National Library of Medicine, Bethesda, MD, 1993.

Kaloyanova FP, El Batawi MA: *Human toxicology of pesticides,* Boca Raton, Florida, 1991, CRC Press.

Mackison FW, Stricoff RS, Partridge LJ Jr, editors: *Occupational health guidelines for chemical hazards, NIOSH/OSHA,* Washington, DC, 1981, US Government Printing Office.

Merigan WH, Weiss B, editors: *Neurotoxicity of the visual system,* New York, 1980, Raven Press.

Morgan DP: *Recognition and management of pesticide poisonings,* ed 4, Washington, DC, United States Environmental Protection Agency, 1989, US Government Printing Office.

NIOSH: *NIOSH pocket guide to chemical hazards* (CD-ROM version), Cincinnati, 2000, DHHS (NIOSH), US Government Printing Office.

Sifton, DW, editor: *PDR guide to biological and chemical warfare response,* Montvale, NJ, 2002, Thomson/Physician's Desk Reference.

Sullivan JB, Kriger GR, editors: *Clinical environmental health and hazardous materials toxicology,* Baltimore, 1997, Williams & Wilkins.

USAMRICD: Chemical Casualty Care Division: *Medical management of chemical casualties handbook,* ed 3, Aberdeen, MD, 1999, Department of the Army.

US ARMY: *Field manual 8-285 treatment of chemical agent patients and conventional military chemical patients,* Washington, DC, 1995, Department of the Army.

US ARMY: *Field manual 8-9 NATO handbook on medical aspects of NBC defensive operations,* Washington, DC, 1996, Department of the Army.

US ARMY: *Textbook of military medicine,* Washington, DC, 1990, Department of the Army.

Zajtchuk R, et al, editors: *Medical aspects of chemical and biological warfare,* Washington, DC, 1997, Department of the Army.

Journals

Adamis Z, et al: Occupational exposure to organophosphorus insecticides and synthetic pyrethroid, *Int Arch Occup Environ Health* 56:299-305, 1985.

Amitai Y, et al: Atropine poisoning in children during the Persian Gulf crisis. A national survey in Israel, *JAMA* 268:630-632, 1992.

Andonova S, Tzvetkove T: Cytomorphological and clinical studies among workers employed in the production of chemical agents for plant protection, *Folia Medica* 1:47-51, 1982.

Baker P, Selvey D: Malathion-induced epidemic hysteria in an elementary school, *Vet Hum Toxicol* 34:156-160, 1992.

Barr A: Organophosphate insecticide poisoning (letter), *Anesthesia* 40:1017, 1985.

Beyer S: Regulation and its alternatives: some remarks on organophosphate pesticides, *Neurotoxicology* 4:99-104, 1983.

Clifford NJ, Nies AS: Organophosphate poisoning from wearing a laundered uniform previously contaminated with parathion, *JAMA* 262:3035-3036, 1989.

Delilkan AE, Manazie M, Ong G: Organophosphate poisoning: a Malaysian intensive care experience of one hundred cases, *Med J Malaysia* 39:229-233, 1984.

DeSilva HJ, Wijewickrema R, Senanayake N: Does pralidoxime affect outcome of management in acute organophosphorus poisoning? *Lancet* 339:1136-1138, 1992.

Duncan R, Griffith J: Monitoring study of urinary metabolites and selected symptomatology among Florida citrus workers, *J Toxicol Environ Health* 17:509-521, 1985.

Jay W, Marcus R, Jay M: Primary position upbeat nystagmus with organophosphate poisoning, *J Pediatr Ophthalmol Strabismus* 19:318-319, 1982.

Johnson M: Initiation of organophosphate-induced delayed neuropathy, *Neurobehav Toxicol Teratol* 4:759-765, 1982.

Kiss Z, Fazkas T: Organophosphates and torsades de pointes ventricular tachycardia, *J R Soc Med* 76:984, 1983.

Lokan R, James R: Rapid death by mevinphos poisoning while under observation, *Forensic Sci Intl* 22:179-182, 1983.

McConnell R, et al: Monitoring organophosphate insecticide-exposed workers for cholinesterase depression: new technology for office or field use, *J Occup Med* 34:34-37, 1992.

Metcalf R L: Historical perspective of organophosphorus ester-induced delayed neurotoxicity, *Neurotoxicology* 3:269-284, 1982.

Mhtsushita T, et al: Allergic contact dermatitis from organophosphorus insecticides, *Ind Health* 23:145-153, 1985.

Mizutani T, Naito H, Oohashi N: Rectal ulcer with massive haemorrhage due to activated charcoal treatment in oral organophosphate poisoning, *Hum Exp Toxicol* 10:385-386, 1991.

Mortensen M: Management of acute childhood poisonings caused by selected insecticides and herbicides, *Pediatr Clin North Am* 33:421-444, 1986.

Muldoon SR, Hodgson MJ: Risk factors for nonoccupational organophosphate pesticide poisoning, *J Occup Med* 34:38-41, 1992.

Newcombe DS: Immune surveillance, organophosphorus exposure and lymphomagenesis, *Lancet* 339:539-541, 1992.

Organophosphorus esters and polyneuropathy (editorial), *Ann Intern Med* 104:264-266, 1986.

Padilla S, et al: Paraoxon toxicity is not potentiated by prior reduction in blood acetylcholinesterase, *Toxicol Appl Pharmacol* 117:110-115, 1992.

Paul V, et al: Evidence for a hazardous interaction between ethanol and the insecticide endosulfan in rats, *Pharmacol Toxicol* 70:268-270, 1992.

Peedicayil J, et al: The effect of organophosphorus compounds on serum pseudocholinesterase levels in a group of industrial workers, *Hum Exp Toxicol* 10:275-278, 1991.

Reeves J: Household insecticide–associated blood dyscrasias in children, *Am J Pediatr Hematol Oncol* 4:438-439, 1982.

Rosenstock L, et al: Chronic central nervous system effects of acute organophosphate pesticide intoxication, *Lancet* 338:223-227, 1991.

Schuman SH, Wagner SL: Pesticide intoxication and chronic CNS effects, *Lancet* 338:948-949, 1991.

GUIDELINE 136

Books

Amdur MO, Doull J, Klaassen CD, editors: *Casarett and Doull's toxicology, the basic science of poisons,* ed 4, New York, 1991, Pergamon Press.

CANUTEC: *Initial emergency response guide 1992,* Ottawa, Canada, 1992, Canada Communication Group.

CCINFO: *MSDS/CHEMINFO* (CD-ROM version), Hamilton, Ontario, Canada, 1993, Canadian Centre for Occupational Health and Safety.

Danon YL, et al, editors: *Chemical warfare medicine,* Jerusalem, 1994, Gefen.

DOT: *CHRIS hazardous chemical data*, US Department of Transportation/United States Coast Guard, Washington, DC, 1984, US Government Printing Office.

DOT: *2000 Emergency response guidebook,* Office of Hazardous Materials Transportation, Research and Special Programs Administration, Washington, DC, 2000, US Department of Transportation.

Gosselin RE, Smith RP, Hodge HC: *Clinical toxicology of commercial products,* ed 5, Baltimore, 1984, Williams & Wilkins.

Levy G: *Level II hazardous materials text,* Fort Collins, Colo, 1985, GML Consultants.

Mackison FW, Stricoff RS, Partridge LJ Jr, editors: *Occupational health guidelines for chemical hazards, NIOSH/OSHA,* Washington, DC, 1981, US Government Printing Office.

NIOSH: *NIOSH pocket guide to chemical hazards* (CD-ROM version), Cincinnati, 2000, DHHS (NIOSH), US Government Printing Office.

NIOSH/OSHA/USCG/EPA: *Occupational safety and health guidance manual for hazardous waste site activities,* Washington, DC, 1985, DHHS (NIOSH) Publication No 85-115, U.S. Government Printing Office.

Sifton, DW, editor: *PDR guide to biological and chemical warfare response,* Montvale, NJ, 2002, Thomson/Physician's Desk Reference.

Sittig M: *Handbook of toxic and hazardous chemicals and carcinogens,* ed 3, Park Ridge, NJ, 1992, Noyes Publications.

Smeby LC, editor: *Hazardous materials response handbook,* ed 3, Quincy, Mass, 1997, National Fire Protection Association.

USAMRICD, Chemical Casualty Care Division: *Medical management of chemical casualties handbook, ed 3,* Aberdeen, MD, 1999, Department of the Army.

US ARMY: *Field manual 8-285 treatment of chemical agent patients and conventional military chemical patients,* Washington, DC, 1995, Department of the Army.

US ARMY: *Field manual 8-9 NATO handbook on medical aspects of NBC defensive operations,* Washington, DC, 1996, Department of the Army.

US ARMY: *Textbook of military medicine,* Washington, DC, 1990, Department of the Army.

Zajtchuk R, et al, editors: *Medical aspects of chemical and biological warfare,* Washington, DC, 1997, Department of the Army.

Journals

Wegman DH, Eisen EA: Acute irritants, more than a nuisance (editorial), *Chest* 97: 773-775, 1990.

Blackwood M: Health risks of smoking increased by exposure to workplace chemicals, *Occup Health Saf* 54:23-27, 1985.

Goldstein B, Melia R, Florey C: Indoor nitrogen oxide, *Bull N Y Acad Med* 57:873-882, 1981.

Goldstein E, Hackney J, Rokaw S: Photochemical air pollution: part I, *West J Med* 142:369-376, 1985.

Hu H, Christiani D: Reactive airways dysfunction after exposure to teargas (letter), *Lancet* 339: 1535, 1992.

Morrow P: Toxicological data on NOx: an overview, *Toxicol Environ Health* 13:205-227, 1984.

Oxides of nitrogen and health (editorial), *Lancet* 10:81-82, 1981.

Ro YS, Lee CW: Tear gas dermatitis, allergic contact sensitization due to CS, *Int J Dermatol* 30:576-577, 1991.

Speizer F: Ozone and photochemical pollutants: status after 25 years, *West J Med* 142:377-379, 1985.

GUIDELINE 137

Books

USAMRICD, Chemical Casualty Care Division: *Medical management of chemical casualties handbook, ed 3,* Aberdeen, MD, 1999, Department of the Army.

US ARMY: *Field manual 8-285 treatment of chemical agent patients and conventional military chemical patients,* Washington, DC, 1995, Department of the Army.

US ARMY: *Field manual 8-9 NATO handbook on medical aspects of NBC defensive operations,* Washington, DC, 1996, Department of the Army.

US ARMY: *Textbook of military medicine,* Washington, DC, 1990, Department of the Army.

Zajtchuk R, et al, editors: *Medical aspects of chemical and biological warfare,* Washington, DC, 1997, Department of the Army.

GUIDELINE 138

Books

Amdur MO, Doull J, Klaassen CD, editors: *Casarett and Doull's toxicology, the basic science of poisons,* ed 4, New York, 1991, Pergamon Press.

CANUTEC: *Initial emergency response guide 1992,* Ottawa, Canada, 1992, Canada Communication Group.

CCINFO: *MSDS/CHEMINFO* (CD-ROM version), Hamilton, Ontario, Canada, 1993, Canadian Centre for Occupational Health and Safety.

DOT: *CHRIS hazardous chemical data.* US Department of Transportation/United States Coast Guard, Washington, DC, 1984, US Government Printing Office.

DOT: *2000 Emergency response guidebook,* Office of Hazardous Materials Transportation, Research and Special Programs Administration, Washington, DC, 2000, US Department of Transportation.

Gosselin RE, Smith RP, Hodge HC: *Clinical toxicology of commercial products,* ed 5, Baltimore, 1984, Williams & Wilkins.

Mackison FW, Stricoff RS, Partridge LJ Jr, editors*: Occupational health guidelines for chemical hazards, NIOSH/OSHA,* Washington, DC, 1981, US Government Printing Office.

Manahan SE: *Environmental chemistry,* ed 7, Chelsea, Mich, 1999, Lewis Publishers.

NIOSH: *NIOSH pocket guide to chemical hazards* (CD-ROM version), Cincinnati, 2000, DHHS (NIOSH), US Government Printing Office.

Olson KR, editor: *Poisoning & drug overdose,* ed 3, East Norwalk, Conn, 1999, Appleton & Lange.

Sifton, DW, editor: *PDR guide to biological and chemical warfare response*, Montvale, NJ, 2002, Thomson/Physician's Desk Reference.

Sullivan JB, Kriger GR, editors: *Clinical environmental health and hazardous materials toxicology,* Baltimore, 1997, Williams & Wilkins.

USAMRICD: Chemical Casualty Care Division: *Medical management of chemical casualties handbook, ed 3,* Aberdeen, MD, 1999, Department of the Army.

US ARMY: *Field manual 8-9 NATO handbook on medical aspects of NBC defensive operations,* Washington, DC, 1996, Department of the Army.

US ARMY: *Textbook of military medicine,* Washington, DC, 1990, Department of the Army.

Zajtchuk R, et al, editors: *Medical aspects of chemical and biological warfare,* Washington, DC, 1997, Department of the Army.

GUIDELINE 139

Books

Amdur MO, Doull J, Klaassen CD, editors: *Casarett and Doull's toxicology, the basic science of poisons,* ed 4, New York, 1991, Pergamon Press.

Baselt RC, Cravey RH: *Disposition of toxic drugs and chemicals in man,* ed 3, Chicago, 1989, Year Book Medical Publishers.

CANUTEC: *Initial emergency response guide 1992,* Ottawa, Canada, 1992, Canada Communication Group.

CCINFO: *MSDS/CHEMINFO* (CD-ROM version), Hamilton, Ontario, Canada, 1993, Canadian Centre for Occupational Health and Safety.

Danon YL, et al, editors: *Chemical warfare medicine,* Jerusalem, 1994, Gefen.

DOT: *CHRIS hazardous chemical data.* US Department of Transportation/United States Coast Guard. Washington, DC, 1984, US Government Printing Office.

DOT: *2000 Emergency response guidebook,* Office of Hazardous Materials Transportation, Research and Special Programs Administration, Washington, DC, 2000, US Department of Transportation.

Gosselin RE, Smith RP, Hodge HC: *Clinical toxicology of commercial products,* ed 5, Baltimore, 1984, Williams & Wilkins.

Hartman DE: *Neuropsychological toxicology, identification and assessment of human neurotoxic syndromes,* New York, 1988, Pergamon Press.

Kaloyanova FP, El Batawi MA: *Human toxicology of pesticides,* Boca Raton, Florida, 1991, CRC Press.

Mackison FW, Stricoff RS, Partridge LJ Jr, editors*: Occupational health guidelines for chemical hazards, NIOSH/OSHA,* Washington, DC, 1981, US Government Printing Office.

NIOSH: *NIOSH pocket guide to chemical hazards* (CD-ROM version), Cincinnati, 2000, DHHS (NIOSH), US Government Printing Office.

Sifton, DW, editor: *PDR guide to biological and chemical warfare response,* Montvale, NJ, 2002, Thomson/Physician's Desk Reference.

USAMRICD, Chemical Casualty Care Division: *Medical management of chemical casualties handbook,* ed 3, Aberdeen, MD, 1999, Department of the Army.

US ARMY: *Field manual 3-5 decontamination,* Washington, DC, 1993, Department of the Army.

US ARMY: *Field manual 8-285 treatment of chemical agent patients and conventional military chemical patients,* Washington, DC, 1995, Department of the Army.

US ARMY: *Field manual 8-9 NATO handbook on medical aspects of NBC defensive operations,* Washington, DC, 1996, Department of the Army.

US ARMY: *Textbook of military medicine,* Washington, DC, 1990, Department of the Army.

Zajtchuk R, et al, editors: *Medical aspects of chemical and biological warfare,* Washington, DC, 1997, Department of the Army.

GUIDELINE 140

Books

Sifton, DW, editor: *PDR guide to biological and chemical warfare response,* Montvale, NJ, 2002, Thomson/Physician's Desk Reference.

USAMRICD, Chemical Casualty Care Division: *Medical management of chemical casualties handbook,* ed 3, Aberdeen, MD, 1999, Department of the Army.

US ARMY: *Field manual 8-285 treatment of chemical agent patients and conventional military chemical patients, Washington, DC,* 1995, Department of the Army.

US ARMY: *Field manual 8-9 NATO handbook on medical aspects of NBC defensive operations,* Washington, DC, 1996, Department of the Army.

US ARMY: *Textbook of military medicine,* Washington, DC, 1990, Department of the Army.

Zajtchuk R, et al, editors: *Medical aspects of chemical and biological warfare,* Washington, DC, 1997, Department of the Army.

TREATMENT PROTOCOLS

INHALATION EXPOSURE

Books

Amdur MO, Doull J, Klaassen CD, editors: *Casarett and Doull's toxicology, the basic science of poisons,* ed 4, New York, 1991, Pergamon Press.

American Conference of Governmental and Industrial Hygienists: *1992-1993 Threshold limit values for chemical substances and physical agents and biological exposure indices,* Cincinnati, 1992, American Conference of Governmental Industrial Hygienists.

Bardana EJ, Montanaro A, O'Hollaren MT: *Occupational asthma,* Philadelphia, 1992, Hanley & Belfus.

Finkel AJ, editor: *Hamilton and Hardy's industrial toxicology,* ed 4, Littleton, Mass, 1983, PSG Publishing.

Sullivan JB, Kriger GR, editors: *Clinical environmental health and hazardous materials toxicology,* Baltimore, 1997, Williams & Wilkins.

DERMAL EXPOSURE

Books

Amdur MO, Doull J, Klaassen CD, editors: *Casarett and Doull's toxicology, the basic science of poisons,* ed 4, New York, 1991, Pergamon Press.

American Conference of Governmental and Industrial Hygienists: *1992-1993 Threshold limit values for chemical substances and physical agents and biological exposure indices,* Cincinnati, 1992, American Conference of Governmental Industrial Hygienists.

Bardana EJ, Montanaro A, O'Hollaren MT: *Occupational asthma,* Philadelphia, 1992, Hanley & Belfus.

Finkel AJ, editor: *Hamilton and Hardy's industrial toxicology,* ed 4, Littleton, Mass, 1983, PSG Publishing.

Sullivan JB, Kriger GR, editors: *Clinical environmental health and hazardous materials toxicology,* Baltimore, 1997, Williams & Wilkins.

INGESTION EXPOSURE

Books

Amdur MO, Doull J, Klaassen CD, editors: *Casarett and Doull's toxicology, the basic science of poisons,* ed 4, New York, 1991, Pergamon Press.

American Conference of Governmental and Industrial Hygienists: *1992-1993 Threshold limit values for chemical substances and physical agents and biological exposure indices,* Cincinnati, 1992, American Conference of Governmental Industrial Hygienists.

Goldfrank LR, et al: *Goldfrank's toxicologic emergencies,* ed 6, New York, 1998, McGraw-Hill Professional.

Rosen P, Barkin RM, et al, editors: *Emergency medicine, concepts and clinical practice,* ed 3, St Louis, 1992, Mosby.

Sullivan JB, Kriger GR, editors: *Clinical environmental health and hazardous materials toxicology,* Baltimore, 1997, Williams & Wilkins.

CARDIAC

Books

Amdur MO, Doull J, Klaassen CD, editors: *Casarett and Doull's toxicology, the basic science of poisons,* ed 4, New York, 1991, Pergamon Press.

Rosen P, Barkin RM, et al, editors: *Emergency medicine, concepts and clinical practice,* ed 3, St Louis, 1992, Mosby.

Wilson JD, et al, editors: *Harrison's principles of internal medicine,* ed 12, New York, 1991, McGraw-Hill.

Journals

Emergency Cardiac Care Committee and Subcommittees, American Heart Association: Guidelines for cardiopulmonary resuscitation and emergency cardiac care, III: adult ACLS, *JAMA* 268:2199-2241, 1992.

Emergency Cardiac Care Committee and Subcommittees, American Heart Association: Guidelines for cardiopulmonary resuscitation and emergency cardiac care, VI: pediatric ACLS, *JAMA* 268: 2262-2275, 1992.

CHEMICAL BURNS

Books

Abbott J, Gifford M, Rosen P: *Protocols for prehospital emergency medical care,* ed 2, Baltimore, 1984, Williams & Wilkins.

Caroline NL: *Emergency care in the streets,* Boston, 1983, Little, Brown and Company.

Gosselin RE, Smith RP, Hodge HC: *Clinical toxicology of commercial products,* ed 5, Baltimore, 1984, Williams & Wilkins.

Potter DL, et al, editors: *Nurses reference library, emergencies,* Springhouse, Pa, 1982, Intermed Communications.

Rosen P, Barkin RM, et al, editors: *Emergency medicine, concepts and clinical practice,* ed 3, St Louis, 1992, Mosby.

Stewart CE: *Environmental emergencies,* Baltimore, 1990, Williams & Wilkins.

Walraven G, et al: *Manual of advanced prehospital care,* ed 2, Bowie, MD, 1984, Robert J. Brady.

Journals

Bertolini JC: Hydrofluoric acid: a review of toxicity, *J Emerg Med* 10:163-168, 1992.

Stewart C: Chemical skin burns, *Am Fam Physician* 31:149-157, 1985.

Stremski ES, Grande GA, Ling LJ: Survival following hydrofluoric acid ingestion, *Ann Emerg Med* 21:1396-1399, 1992.

Wing JS, et al: Acute health effects in a community after a release of hydrofluoric acid, *Arch Environ Health* 46:155-160, 1991.

DECONTAMINATION

Books

CANUTEC: *Initial emergency response guide 1992,* Ottawa, Canada, 1992, Canada Communication Group.

Danon YL, et al, editors: *Chemical warfare medicine,* Jerusalem, 1994, Gefen.

DOT: *2000 Emergency response guidebook,* Office of Hazardous Materials Transportation, Research and Special Programs Administration,

Washington, DC, 2000, US Department of Transportation.

NIOSH/OSHA/USCG/EPA: *Occupational safety and health guidance manual for hazardous waste site activities,* Washington, DC, 1985, DHHS (NIOSH) Publication No 85-115, US Government Printing Office.

Olson KR, editor: *Poisoning & drug overdose,* ed 3, East Norwalk, Conn, 1999, Appleton & Lange.

Smeby LC, editor: *Hazardous materials response handbook,* ed 3, Quincy, Mass, 1997, National Fire Protection Association.

USAMRICD, Chemical Casualty Care Division: *Medical management of chemical casualties handbook, ed 3,* Aberdeen, MD, 1999, Department of the Army.

US ARMY: *Field manual 3-5 decontamination,* Washington, DC, 1993, Department of the Army.

US ARMY: *Field manual 8-9 NATO handbook on medical aspects of NBC defensive operations,* Washington, DC, 1996, Department of the Army.

EYE IRRIGATION

Books

Goldfrank LR, et al: *Goldfrank's toxicologic emergencies,* ed 6, New York, 1998, McGraw-Hill Professional.

Gosselin RE, Smith RP, Hodge HC: *Clinical toxicology of commercial products,* ed 5, Baltimore, 1984, Williams & Wilkins.

Olson KR, editor: *Poisoning & drug overdose,* ed 3, East Norwalk, Conn, 1999, Appleton & Lange.

Rosen P, Barkin RM, et al, editors: *Emergency medicine, concepts and clinical practice,* ed 3, St Louis, 1992, Mosby.

FROSTBITE

Books

Caroline NL: *Emergency medical treatment,* Boston, 1982, Little, Brown and Company.

Rosen P, Barkin RM, et al, editors: *Emergency medicine, concepts and clinical practice,* ed 3, St Louis, 1992, Mosby.

Stewart CE: *Environmental emergencies,* Baltimore, 1990, Williams & Wilkins.

Walraven G, et al: *Manual of advanced prehospital care,* ed 2, Bowie, MD, 1984, Robert J. Brady.

HEAT STRESS

Books

American Conference of Governmental and Industrial Hygienists: *1992-1993 Threshold limit values for chemical substances and physical agents and biological exposure indices,* Cincinnati, 1992, American Conference of Governmental Industrial Hygienists.

FEMA: *Emergency incident rehabilitation,* Washington, DC, 1992, Publication No FA-114, USFA Publications.

NIOSH: *Hot environments,* Cincinnati, 1980, DHHS (NIOSH) Publication No 80-132, US Government Printing Office.

NIOSH/OSHA/USCG/EPA: *Occupational safety and health guidance manual for hazardous waste site activities,* Washington, DC, 1985, DHHS (NIOSH) Publication No 85-115, US Government Printing Office.

Rosen P, Barkin RM, et al, editors: *Emergency medicine, concepts and clinical practice,* ed 3, St Louis, 1992, Mosby.

Stewart CE: Environmental emergencies, Baltimore, 1990, Williams & Wilkins.

Smeby LC, editor: *Hazardous materials response handbook,* ed 3, Quincy, Mass, 1997, National Fire Protection Association.

HYPOTHERMIA

Books

American Conference of Governmental and Industrial Hygienists: *1992-1993 Threshold limit values for chemical substances and physical agents and biological exposure indices,* Cincinnati, 1992, American Conference of Governmental Industrial Hygienists.

FEMA: *Emergency incident rehabilitation,* Washington, DC, 1992, Publication No FA-114, USFA Publications.

Goldfrank LR, et al: *Goldfrank's toxicologic emergencies,* ed 6, New York, 1998, McGraw-Hill Professional.

NIOSH/OSHA/USCG/EPA: *Occupational safety and health guidance manual for hazardous waste site activities,* Washington, DC, 1985, DHHS (NIOSH) Publication No 85-115, US Government Printing Office.

Rosen P, Barkin RM, et al, editors: *Emergency medicine, concepts and clinical practice,* ed 3, St Louis, 1992, Mosby.

Stewart CE: *Environmental emergencies,* Baltimore, 1990, Williams & Wilkins.

PATIENT EVALUATION

Books

Amdur MO, Doull J, Klaassen CD, editors: *Casarett and Doull's toxicology, the basic science of poisons,* ed 4, New York, 1991, Pergamon Press.

American Conference of Governmental and Industrial Hygienists: *1992-1993 Threshold limit values for chemical substances and physical agents and biological exposure indices,* Cincinnati, 1992, American Conference of Governmental Industrial Hygienists.

Goldfrank LR, et al: *Goldfrank's toxicologic emergencies,* ed 6, New York, 1998, McGraw-Hill Professional.

Gosselin RE, Smith RP, Hodge HC: *Clinical toxicology of commercial products,* ed 5, Baltimore, 1984, Williams & Wilkins.

NIOSH/OSHA/USCG/EPA: *Occupational safety and health guidance manual for hazardous waste site activities,* Washington, DC, 1985, DHHS (NIOSH) Publication No 85-115, US Government Printing Office.

Olson KR, editor: *Poisoning & drug overdose,* ed 3, East Norwalk, Conn, 1999, Appleton & Lange.

Rosen P, Barkin RM, et al, editors: *Emergency medicine, concepts and clinical practice,* ed 3, St Louis, 1992, Mosby.

PULMONARY EDEMA

Books

Abbott J, Gifford M, Rosen P: *Protocols for prehospital emergency medical care,* ed 2, Baltimore, 1984, Williams & Wilkins.

Amdur MO, Doull J, Klaassen CD, editors: *Casarett and Doull's toxicology, the basic science of poisons,* ed 4, New York, 1991, Pergamon Press.

Goldfrank LR, et al: *Goldfrank's toxicologic emergencies,* ed 6, New York, 1998, McGraw-Hill Professional.

Gosselin RE, Smith RP, Hodge HC: *Clinical toxicology of commercial products,* ed 5, Baltimore, 1984, Williams & Wilkins.

Olson KR, editor: *Poisoning & drug overdose,* ed 3, East Norwalk, Conn, 1999, Appleton & Lange.

Rosen P, Barkin RM, et al, editors: *Emergency medicine, concepts and clinical practice,* ed 3, St Louis, 1992, Mosby.

Walraven G, et al: *Manual of advanced prehospital care,* ed 2, Bowie, MD, 1984, Robert J. Brady.

Wilson JD, et al, editors: *Harrison's principles of internal medicine,* ed 12, New York, 1991, McGraw-Hill.

SEIZURES

Books

Abbott J, Gifford M, Rosen P: *Protocols for prehospital emergency medical care,* ed 2, Baltimore, 1984, Williams & Wilkins.

Goldfrank LR, et al: *Goldfrank's toxicologic emergencies,* ed 6, New York, 1998, McGraw-Hill Professional.

Goodman AG, et al, editors: *Goodman and Gilman's the pharmacological basis of therapeutics,* ed 8, New York, 1990, Pergamon Press.

Gosselin RE, Smith RP, Hodge HC: *Clinical toxicology of commercial products,* ed 5, Baltimore, 1984, Williams & Wilkins.

Olson KR, editor: *Poisoning & drug overdose,* ed 3, East Norwalk, Conn, 1999, Appleton & Lange.

Rosen P, Barkin RM, et al, editors: *Emergency medicine, concepts and clinical practice,* ed 3, St Louis, 1992, Mosby.

Walraven G, et al: *Manual of advanced prehospital care,* ed 2, Bowie, MD, 1984, Robert J. Brady.

Wilson JD, et al, editors: *Harrison's principles of internal medicine,* ed 12, New York, 1991, McGraw-Hill.

SHOCK

Books

Abbott J, Gifford M, Rosen P: *Protocols for prehospital emergency medical care,* ed 2, Baltimore, 1984, Williams & Wilkins.

Goldfrank LR, et al: *Goldfrank's toxicologic emergencies,* ed 6, New York, 1998, McGraw-Hill Professional.

Goodman AG, et al, editors: *Goodman and Gilman's the pharmacological basis of therapeutics,* ed 8, New York, 1990, Pergamon Press.

Gosselin RE, Smith RP, Hodge HC: *Clinical toxicology of commercial products,* ed 5, Baltimore, 1984, Williams & Wilkins.

Olson KR, editor: *Poisoning & drug overdose,* ed 3, East Norwalk, Conn, 1999, Appleton & Lange.

Rosen P, Barkin RM, et al, editors: *Emergency medicine, concepts and clinical practice,* ed 3, St Louis, 1992, Mosby.

Walraven G, et al: *Manual of advanced prehospital care,* ed 2, Bowie, MD, 1984, Robert J. Brady.

Wilson JD, et al, editors: *Harrison's principles of internal medicine,* ed 12, New York, 1991, McGraw-Hill.

DRUG PROTOCOLS

ADENOSINE

Books

Goodman AG, et al, editors: *Goodman and Gilman's the pharmacological basis of therapeutics,* ed 8, New York, 1990, Pergamon Press.

Loeb S, et al, editors: *Nurse's handbook of drug therapy,* Springhouse, Pa, 1993, Springhouse Corporation.

McEvoy GK, editor: *American Hospital Formulary Service (AHFS) drug information 1993,* Bethesda, MD, 1993, American Society of Hospital Pharmacists.

Journals

Emergency Cardiac Care Committee and Subcommittees, American Heart Association: Guidelines for cardiopulmonary resuscitation and emergency cardiac care, III: adult ACLS, *JAMA* 268:2199-2241, 1992.

Emergency Cardiac Care Committee and Subcommittees, American Heart Association: Guidelines for cardiopulmonary resuscitation and emergency cardiac care, VI: pediatric ACLS, *JAMA* 268:2262-2275, 1992.

LIDOCAINE

Books

Abbott J, Gifford M, Rosen P: *Protocols for prehospital emergency medical care,* ed 2, Baltimore, 1984, Williams & Wilkins.

Barber JM, Budassi SA: *Mosby's manual of emergency care, practices and procedures,* St Louis, 1979, Mosby.

Goodman AG, et al, editors: *Goodman and Gilman's the pharmacological basis of therapeutics,* ed 8, New York, 1990, Pergamon Press.

Loeb S, et al, editors: *Nurse's handbook of drug therapy,* Springhouse, Pa, 1993, Springhouse Corporation.

Madigan KG: *Prehospital emergency drugs,* St Louis, 1990, Mosby.

McEvoy GK, editor: *American Hospital Formulary Service (AHFS) drug information 1993,* Bethesda, MD, 1993, American Society of Hospital Pharmacists.

Journals

Emergency Cardiac Care Committee and Subcommittees, American Heart Association: Guidelines for cardiopulmonary resuscitation and emergency cardiac care, III: adult ACLS, *JAMA* 268:2199-2241, 1992.

Emergency Cardiac Care Committee and Subcommittees, American Heart Association: Guidelines for cardiopulmonary resuscitation and emergency cardiac care, VI: pediatric ACLS, *JAMA* 268:2262-2275, 1992.

MAGNESIUM SULFATE

Books

Goodman AG, et al, editors: *Goodman and Gilman's the pharmacological basis of therapeutics,* ed 8, New York, 1990, Pergamon Press.

Loeb S, et al, editors: *Nurse's handbook of drug therapy,* Springhouse, Pa, 1993, Springhouse Corporation.

McEvoy GK, editor: *American Hospital Formulary Service (AHFS) drug information 1993,* Bethesda, MD, 1993, American Society of Hospital Pharmacists.

Journals

Emergency Cardiac Care Committee and Subcommittees, American Heart Association: Guidelines for cardiopulmonary resuscitation and emergency cardiac care, III: adult ACLS, *JAMA* 268:2199-2241, 1992.

Emergency Cardiac Care Committee and Subcommittees, American Heart Association: Guidelines for cardiopulmonary resuscitation and emergency cardiac care, VI: pediatric ACLS, *JAMA* 268:2262-2275, 1992.

PROCAINAMIDE

Books

Goodman AG, et al, editors: *Goodman and Gilman's the pharmacological basis of therapeutics,* ed 8, New York, 1990, Pergamon Press.

Loeb S, et al, editors: *Nurse's handbook of drug therapy,* Springhouse, Pa, 1993, Springhouse Corporation.

Madigan KG: *Prehospital emergency drugs,* St Louis, 1990, Mosby.

McEvoy GK, editor: *American Hospital Formulary Service (AHFS) drug information 1993,* Bethesda, MD, 1993, American Society of Hospital Pharmacists.

Journals

Emergency Cardiac Care Committee and Subcommittees, American Heart Association: Guidelines for cardiopulmonary resuscitation and emergency cardiac care, III: adult ACLS, *JAMA* 268:2199-2241, 1992.

Emergency Cardiac Care Committee and Subcommittees, American Heart Association: Guidelines for cardiopulmonary resuscitation and emergency cardiac care, VI: pediatric ACLS, *JAMA* 268:2262-2275, 1992.

ANTIBIOTICS

Books

Alibek K: *Biohazard*, New York, 1999, Random House.

Armstrong D, Cohen J: *Infectious diseases*, London, 1999, Harcourt Publishers, Ltd.

Chin J, ed: *Control of communicable diseases manual,* ed 17, Washington, DC, 2000, American Public Health Association.

Eitzen E, Pavlin J, Cieslak T: *Medical management of biological casualties handbook.* U.S. Army Medical Research Institute of Infectious Diseases (USAMRIID). Fort Detrick, Md, 1998.

Friedlander AM: *Textbook of military medicine: medical aspects of chemical and biological warfare.* Office of the Surgeon General

Department of the Army, United States of America; 1997, pp 467-475.

Mandell GL, Bennett JE, Dolin R, eds: *Mandell, Douglas, and Bennett's principles and practice of infectious disease,* ed 5, Philadelphia, 2000, Churchill Livingstone.

McGovern TW, Friedlander AM: *Textbook of military medicine: medical aspects of chemical and biological warfare.* Office of the Surgeon General Department of the Army, United States of America, 1997, pp 479-499.

Osterholm MT, Schwartz J: *Living terrors. What America needs to know to survive the coming bioterrorist catastrophe*, New York, 2000, Delacorte Press.

Professional guide to diseases. Springhouse, Pa, 1998, Springhouse Corporation.

Sidell FR, Patrick WC, Dashiell TR: *Jane's chem-bio handbook,* Alexandria, Va, 1998, Jane's Information Group.

Sifton DW, ed: *PDR guide to biological and chemical warfare response,* Montvale, NJ, 2002, Thomson/Physician's Desk Reference.

Strickland GT, ed: *Hunter's tropical medicine and emerging infectious diseases,* ed 8, Philadelphia, 2000, WB Saunders.

Weinstein RS, Alibek K: *Biological and chemical terrorism: a guide for healthcare providers and first responders*, New York, 2003, Thieme.

Journals

Centers for Disease Control and Prevention (CDC). Notice to readers: use of anthrax vaccine in response to terrorism: supplemental recommendations of the Advisory Committee on Immunization Practices. *Morb Mortal Wkly Rep* 2002. 51(45);1024-1026. Available at: http://www.cdc.gov/mmwr/preview/mmwrhtml/mm5145a4.htm

Centers for Disease Control and Prevention, Division of Bacterial and Mycotic Diseases. Disease Information: Brucellosis [cited 2003 Oct 27] Available at: http://www.cdc.gov/ncidod/dbmd/diseaseinfo/brucellosis_g.htm

Centers for Disease Control and Prevention, Division of Bacterial and Mycotic Diseases. Disease Information: Escherichia coli O157:H7 [cited 2003 Oct 27] Available at: http://www.cdc.gov/ncidod/dbmd/diseaseinfo/escherichiacoli_t.htm

Centers for Disease Control and Prevention, Division of Bacterial and Mycotic Diseases. Disease Information: Melioidosis *(Burkholderia pseudomallei)* [cited 2003 Oct 27] Available at: http://www.cdc.gov/ncidod/dbmd/diseaseinfo/melioidosis_g.htm

Centers for Disease Control and Prevention, Division of Bacterial and Mycotic Diseases. Disease Information: Psittacosis [cited 2003 Oct 27] Available at: http://www.cdc.gov/ncidod/dbmd/diseaseinfo/psittacosis_t.htm

Centers for Disease Control and Prevention, Division of Viral and Rickettsial Diseases. Disease Information: Q Fever [cited 2003 Nov 1] Available at: http://www.cdc.gov/ncidod/dvrd/qfever/index.htm

Centers for Disease Control and Prevention, Division of Bacterial and Mycotic Diseases. Disease Information: Salmonellosis [cited 2003 Oct 27] Available at: http://www.cdc.gov/ncidod/dbmd/diseaseinfo/salmonellosis_t.htm

Centers for Disease Control and Prevention, Division of Bacterial and Mycotic Diseases. Disease Information: Shigellosis [cited 2003 Oct 27] Available at: http://www.cdc.gov/ncidod/dbmd/diseaseinfo/shigellosis_t.htm

Day WC, Bernendt RF: Experimental tularemia in *Macaca mulatta:* relationship of aerosol particle size to the infectivity of airborne *Pasteurella tularensis*, *Infection Immunity* 5(1):77-82, 1972.

Dennis DT, Inglesby TV, Henderson DA, et al: Working Group on Civilian Biodefense. Tularemia as a biological weapon: medical and public health management, *JAMA* 285(21):2763-2773, 2001.

Enderlin G, Morales L, Jacobs RF, Cross JT: Streptomycin and alternative agents for the treatment of tularemia: review of the literature, *Clin Infect Dis* 19(1):42-47, 1994.

Francis E: Landmark article April 25, 1925: Tularemia, by Edward Francis, *JAMA* 250(23):3216-3224, 1983.

Franz DR, Jahrlling PB, Friedlander AM, et al: Clinical recognition and management of patients exposed to biological warfare agents, *JAMA* 278(5):399-411, 1997.

Gill V, Cunha BA: Tularemia pneumonia, *Semin Resp Infect* 12(1):61-67, 1997.

Inglesby TV, Henderson DA, Bartlett JG, et al: Anthrax as a biological weapon. Medical and public health management, *JAMA* 281(18):1735-1745, 1999.

Inglesby T, O'Toole T, Henderson D, et al: Anthrax as a biological weapon, 2002: Updated recommendations for management, *JAMA* 287:2236-2252, 2002.

Johansson A, Berglund L, Gothefors L, et al: Ciprofloxacin for treatment of tularemia in children, *Pediatr Infect Dis J* 19(5):449-453, 2000.

Leggiadro RJ: The threat of biological terrorism: a public health and infection control reality, *Infect Control Hosp Epidemiol* 21(1):53-56, 2000.

Limaye AP, Hooper CJ: Treatment of tularemia with fluoroquinolones: two cases and review, *Clin Infect Dis* 29(4):922-924, 1999.

Malone JD: Bioterrorism Readiness Audioconference, APIC, 1999.

Martone WJ, Marshall LW, Kaufmann AF, et al: Tularemia pneumonia in Washington, DC. A report of three cases with possible common-source exposures *JAMA* 242(21):2315-2317, 1979.

Moran GJ: Biological terrorism. 1. Are we prepared? *Emerg Med* 32(2):14-38, 2000.

Penn RL, Kinasewitz GT: Factors associated with a poor outcome in tularemia. *Arch Intern Med* 147(2):265-268, 1987.

Rohrbach BW, Westerman E, Istre GR: Epidemiology and clinical characteristics of tularemia in Oklahoma, 1979 to 1985, *South Med J* 84(9):1091-1096, 1991.

Russell P, Eley SM, Ellis J, et al: Comparison of efficacy of ciprofloxacin and doxycycline against experimental melioidosis and glanders, *J. Antimicrob Chemother* 45(6): 813-818, 2000.

Sanford JP: Landmark perspective: tularemia, *JAMA* 250(23):3225-3226, 1983.

Schricker RL, Eigelsbach HT, Miten JQ, Hall WC: Pathogenesis of tularemia in monkeys aerogenically exposed to *Francisella tularensis* 425, *Infect Immun* 5(5):734-744, 1972.

Spach DH, Liles WC, Campbell GL, et al: Tick-borne diseases in the United States, *N Engl J Med* 329(13):936-947, 1993.

Teutsch SM, Martone WJ, Brink EW, et al: Pneumonic tularemia on Martha's Vineyard, *N Engl J Med* 301(15):826-828, 1979.

DIAZEPAM

Books

Abbott J, Gifford M, Rosen P: *Protocols for prehospital emergency medical care,* ed 2, Baltimore, 1984, Williams & Wilkins.

Barber JM, Budassi SA: *Mosby's manual of emergency care, practices and procedures,* St Louis, 1979, Mosby.

Goodman AG, et al, editors: *Goodman and Gilman's the pharmacological basis of therapeutics,* ed 8, New York, 1990, Pergamon Press.

Loeb S, et al, editors: *Nurse's handbook of drug therapy,* Springhouse, Pa, 1993, Springhouse Corporation.

Madigan KG: *Prehospital emergency drugs,* St Louis, 1990, Mosby.

McEvoy GK, editor: *American Hospital Formulary Service (AHFS) drug information 1993,* Bethesda, MD, 1993, American Society of Hospital Pharmacists.

LORAZEPAM

Books

Goodman AG, et al, editors: *Goodman and Gilman's the pharmacological basis of therapeutics,* ed 8, New York, 1990, Pergamon Press.

Loeb S, et al, editors: *Nurse's handbook of drug therapy,* Springhouse, Pa, 1993, Springhouse Corporation.

McEvoy GK, editor: *American Hospital Formulary Service (AHFS) drug information 1993,* Bethesda, MD, 1993, American Society of Hospital Pharmacists.

DOBUTAMINE

Books

Goodman AG, et al, editors: *Goodman and Gilman's the pharmacological basis of therapeutics,* ed 8, New York, 1990, Pergamon Press.

Loeb S, et al, editors: *Nurse's handbook of drug therapy,* Springhouse, Pa, 1993, Springhouse Corporation.

Madigan KG: *Prehospital emergency drugs,* St Louis, 1990, Mosby.

McEvoy GK, editor: *American Hospital Formulary Service (AHFS) drug information 1993,* Bethesda, MD, 1993, American Society of Hospital Pharmacists.

Journals

Emergency Cardiac Care Committee and Subcommittees, American Heart Association: Guidelines for cardiopulmonary resuscitation and emergency cardiac care, III: adult ACLS, *JAMA* 268:2199-2241, 1992.

Emergency Cardiac Care Committee and Subcommittees, American Heart Association: Guidelines for cardiopulmonary resuscitation and emergency cardiac care, VI: pediatric ACLS, *JAMA* 268:2262-2275, 1992.

DOPAMINE

Books

Abbott J, Gifford M, Rosen P: *Protocols for prehospital emergency medical care,* ed 2, Baltimore, 1984, Williams & Wilkins.

Barber JM, Budassi SA: *Mosby's manual of emergency care, practices and procedures,* St Louis, 1979, Mosby.

Goodman AG, et al, editors: *Goodman and Gilman's the pharmacological basis of therapeutics,* ed 8, New York, 1990, Pergamon Press.

Loeb S, et al, editors: *Nurse's handbook of drug therapy,* Springhouse, Pa, 1993, Springhouse Corporation.

Madigan KG: *Prehospital emergency drugs,* St Louis, 1990, Mosby.

McEvoy GK, editor: *American Hospital Formulary Service (AHFS) drug information 1993,* Bethesda, MD, 1993, American Society of Hospital Pharmacists.

Journals

Emergency Cardiac Care Committee and Subcommittees, American Heart Association: Guidelines for cardiopulmonary resuscitation and emergency cardiac care, III: adult ACLS, *JAMA* 268:2199-2241, 1992.

Emergency Cardiac Care Committee and Subcommittees, American Heart Association: Guidelines for cardiopulmonary resuscitation and emergency cardiac care, VI: pediatric ACLS, *JAMA* 268:2262-2275, 1992.

EPINEPHRINE

Books

Abbott J, Gifford M, Rosen P: *Protocols for prehospital emergency medical care,* ed 2, Baltimore, 1984, Williams & Wilkins.

Barber JM, Budassi SA: *Mosby's manual of emergency care, practices and procedures,* St Louis, 1979, Mosby.

Goodman AG, et al, editors: *Goodman and Gilman's the pharmacological basis of therapeutics,* ed 8, New York, 1990, Pergamon Press.

Loeb S, et al, editors: *Nurse's handbook of drug therapy,* Springhouse, Pa, 1993, Springhouse Corporation.

Madigan KG: *Prehospital emergency drugs,* St Louis, 1990, Mosby.

McEvoy GK, editor: *American Hospital Formulary Service (AHFS) drug information 1993,* Bethesda, MD, 1993, American Society of Hospital Pharmacists.

Journals

Emergency Cardiac Care Committee and Subcommittees, American Heart Association: Guidelines for cardiopulmonary resuscitation and emergency cardiac care, III: adult ACLS, *JAMA* 268:2199-2241, 1992.

Emergency Cardiac Care Committee and Subcommittees, American Heart Association: Guidelines for cardiopulmonary resuscitation and emergency cardiac care, VI: pediatric ACLS, *JAMA* 268:2262-2275, 1992.

ISOPROTERENOL

Books

Abbott J, Gifford M, Rosen P: *Protocols for prehospital emergency medical care,* ed 2, Baltimore, 1984, Williams & Wilkins.

Barber JM, Budassi SA: *Mosby's manual of emergency care, practices and procedures,* St Louis, 1979, Mosby.

Goodman AG, et al, editors: *Goodman and Gilman's the pharmacological basis of therapeutics,* ed 8, New York, 1990, Pergamon Press.

Loeb S, et al, editors: *Nurse's handbook of drug therapy,* Springhouse, Pa, 1993, Springhouse Corporation.

Madigan KG: *Prehospital emergency drugs,* St Louis, 1990, Mosby.

McEvoy GK, editor: *American Hospital Formulary Service (AHFS) drug information 1993,* Bethesda, MD, 1993, American Society of Hospital Pharmacists.

Journals

Emergency Cardiac Care Committee and Subcommittees, American Heart Association: Guidelines for cardiopulmonary resuscitation and emergency cardiac care, III: adult ACLS, *JAMA* 268:2199-2241, 1992.

Emergency Cardiac Care Committee and Subcommittees, American Heart Association: Guidelines for cardiopulmonary resuscitation and emergency cardiac care, VI: pediatric ACLS, *JAMA* 268:2262-2275, 1992.

NOREPINEPHRINE

Books

Abbott J, Gifford M, Rosen P: *Protocols for prehospital emergency medical care,* ed 2, Baltimore, 1984, Williams & Wilkins.

Barber JM, Budassi SA: *Mosby's manual of emergency care, practices and procedures,* St Louis, 1979, Mosby.

Goodman AG, et al, editors: *Goodman and Gilman's the pharmacological basis of therapeutics,* ed 8, New York, 1990, Pergamon Press.

Loeb S, et al, editors: *Nurse's handbook of drug therapy,* Springhouse, Pa, 1993, Springhouse Corporation.

McEvoy GK, editor: *American Hospital Formulary Service (AHFS) drug information 1993,* Bethesda, MD, 1993, American Society of Hospital Pharmacists.

Journals

Emergency Cardiac Care Committee and Subcommittees, American Heart Association: Guidelines for cardiopulmonary resuscitation and emergency cardiac care, III: adult ACLS, *JAMA* 268:2199-2241, 1992.

Emergency Cardiac Care Committee and Subcommittees, American Heart Association: Guidelines for cardiopulmonary resuscitation and emergency cardiac care, VI: pediatric ACLS, *JAMA* 268:2262-2275, 1992.

DEFEROXAMINE

Books

Goldfrank LR, et al: *Goldfrank's toxicologic emergencies,* ed 6, New York, 1998, McGraw-Hill Professional.

Goodman AG, et al, editors: *Goodman and Gilman's the pharmacological basis of therapeutics,* ed 8, New York, 1990, Pergamon Press.

Gosselin RE, Smith RP, Hodge HC: *Clinical toxicology of commercial products,* ed 5, Baltimore, 1984, Williams & Wilkins.

McEvoy GK, editor: *American Hospital Formulary Service (AHFS) drug information 1993,* Bethesda, MD, 1993, American Society of Hospital Pharmacists.

DIMERCAPROL

Books

Goldfrank LR, et al: *Goldfrank's toxicologic emergencies,* ed 6, New York, 1998, McGraw-Hill Professional.

Goodman AG, et al, editors: *Goodman and Gilman's the pharmacological basis of therapeutics,* ed 8, New York, 1990, Pergamon Press.

Gosselin RE, Smith RP, Hodge HC: *Clinical toxicology of commercial products,* ed 5, Baltimore, 1984, Williams & Wilkins.

McEvoy GK, editor: *American Hospital Formulary Service (AHFS) drug information 1993,* Bethesda, MD, 1993, American Society of Hospital Pharmacists.

Sullivan JB, Kriger GR, editors: *Clinical environmental health and hazardous materials toxicology,* Baltimore, 1997, Williams & Wilkins.

EDETATE CALCIUM DISODIUM

Books

Goldfrank LR, et al: *Goldfrank's toxicologic emergencies,* ed 6, New York, 1998, McGraw-Hill Professional.

Goodman AG, et al, editors: *Goodman and Gilman's the pharmacological basis of therapeutics,* ed 8, New York, 1990, Pergamon Press.

Gosselin RE, Smith RP, Hodge HC: *Clinical toxicology of commercial products,* ed 5, Baltimore, 1984, Williams & Wilkins.

McEvoy GK, editor: *American Hospital Formulary Service (AHFS) drug information 1993,* Bethesda, MD, 1993, American Society of Hospital Pharmacists.

Sullivan JB, Kriger GR, editors: *Clinical environmental health and hazardous materials toxicology,* Baltimore, 1997, Williams & Wilkins.

PENICILLAMINE

Books

Goldfrank LR, et al: *Goldfrank's toxicologic emergencies,* ed 6, New York, 1998, McGraw-Hill Professional.

Goodman AG, et al, editors: *Goodman and Gilman's the pharmacological basis of therapeutics,* ed 8, New York, 1990, Pergamon Press.

Gosselin RE, Smith RP, Hodge HC: *Clinical toxicology of commercial products,* ed 5, Baltimore, 1984, Williams & Wilkins.

McEvoy GK, editor: *American Hospital Formulary Service (AHFS) drug information 1993,* Bethesda, MD, 1993, American Society of Hospital Pharmacists.

Olson KR, editor: *Poisoning & drug overdose,* ed 3, East Norwalk, Conn, 1999, Appleton & Lange.

Sullivan JB, Kriger GR, editors: *Clinical environmental health and hazardous materials toxicology,* Baltimore, 1997, Williams & Wilkins.

SUCCIMER

Books

McEvoy GK, editor: *American Hospital Formulary Service (AHFS) drug information 1993,* Bethesda, MD, 1993, American Society of Hospital Pharmacists.

Sullivan JB, Kriger GR, editors: *Clinical environmental health and hazardous materials toxicology,* Baltimore, 1997, Williams & Wilkins.

50% DEXTROSE

Books

Abbott J, Gifford M, Rosen P: *Protocols for prehospital emergency medical care,* ed 2, Baltimore, 1984, Williams & Wilkins.

Barber JM, Budassi SA: *Mosby's manual of emergency care, practices and procedures,* St Louis, 1979, Mosby.

Goodman AG, et al, editors: *Goodman and Gilman's the pharmacological basis of therapeutics,* ed 8, New York, 1990, Pergamon Press.

Loeb S, et al, editors: *Nurse's handbook of drug therapy,* Springhouse, Pa, 1993, Springhouse Corporation.

Madigan KG: *Prehospital emergency drugs,* St Louis, 1990, Mosby.

McEvoy GK, editor: *American Hospital Formulary Service (AHFS) drug information 1993,* Bethesda, MD, 1993, American Society of Hospital Pharmacists.

Journals

Emergency Cardiac Care Committee and Subcommittees, American Heart Association:

Guidelines for cardiopulmonary resuscitation and emergency cardiac care, III: adult ACLS, *JAMA* 268:2199-2241, 1992.

Emergency Cardiac Care Committee and Subcommittees, American Heart Association: Guidelines for cardiopulmonary resuscitation and emergency cardiac care, VI: pediatric ACLS, *JAMA* 268:2262-2275, 1992.

FUROSEMIDE

Books

Abbott J, Gifford M, Rosen P: *Protocols for prehospital emergency medical care,* ed 2, Baltimore, 1984, Williams & Wilkins.

Barber JM, Budassi SA: *Mosby's manual of emergency care, practices and procedures,* St Louis, 1979, Mosby.

Goodman AG, et al, editors: *Goodman and Gilman's the pharmacological basis of therapeutics,* ed 8, New York, 1990, Pergamon Press.

Loeb S, et al, editors: *Nurse's handbook of drug therapy,* Springhouse, Pa, 1993, Springhouse Corporation.

Madigan KG: *Prehospital emergency drugs,* St Louis, 1990, Mosby.

McEvoy GK, editor: *American Hospital Formulary Service (AHFS) drug information 1993,* Bethesda, MD, 1993, American Society of Hospital Pharmacists.

Journals

Emergency Cardiac Care Committee and Subcommittees, American Heart Association: Guidelines for cardiopulmonary resuscitation and emergency cardiac care, III: adult ACLS, *JAMA* 268:2199-2241, 1992.

Emergency Cardiac Care Committee and Subcommittees, American Heart Association: Guidelines for cardiopulmonary resuscitation and emergency cardiac care, VI: pediatric ACLS, *JAMA* 268:2262-2275, 1992.

HOMATROPINE HYDROBROMIDE (ISOPTO) 2% OPHTHALMIC SOLUTION

Books

Danon YL, et al, editors: *Chemical warfare medicine,* Jerusalem, 1994, Gefen.

Sifton, DW, editor: *PDR guide to biological and chemical warfare response,* Montvale, NJ, 2002, Thomson/Physician Desk Reference.

USAMRICD: Chemical Casualty Care Division: *Medical management of chemical casualties handbook, ed 3,* Aberdeen, MD, 1999, Department of the Army.

US ARMY: *Field manual 8-285 treatment of chemical agent patients and conventional military chemical patients,* Washington, DC, 1995, Department of the Army.

US ARMY: *Field Manual 8-9 NATO handbook on medical Aspects of NBC defensive operations,* Washington, DC, 1996, Department of the Army.

US ARMY: *Textbook of military medicine,* Washington, DC, 1990, Department of the Army.

Zajtchuk R, et al, editors: *Medical aspects of chemical and biological warfare,* Washington, DC, 1997, Department of the Army.

MORPHINE SULFATE

Books

Abbott J, Gifford M, Rosen P: *Protocols for prehospital emergency medical care,* ed 2, Baltimore, 1984, Williams & Wilkins.

Barber JM, Budassi SA: *Mosby's manual of emergency care, practices and procedures,* St Louis, 1979, Mosby.

Goodman AG, et al, editors: *Goodman and Gilman's the pharmacological basis of therapeutics,* ed 8, New York, 1990, Pergamon Press.

Loeb S, et al, editors: *Nurse's handbook of drug therapy,* Springhouse, Pa, 1993, Springhouse Corporation.

Madigan KG: *Prehospital emergency drugs,* St Louis, 1990, Mosby.

McEvoy GK, editor: *American Hospital Formulary Service (AHFS) drug information 1993,* Bethesda, MD, 1993, American Society of Hospital Pharmacists.

Journals

Emergency Cardiac Care Committee and Subcommittees, American Heart Association: Guidelines for cardiopulmonary resuscitation and emergency cardiac care, III: adult ACLS, *JAMA* 268:2199-2241, 1992.

Emergency Cardiac Care Committee and Subcommittees, American Heart Association: Guidelines for cardiopulmonary resuscitation and emergency cardiac care, VI: pediatric ACLS, *JAMA* 268:2262-2275, 1992.

PROPARACAINE HYDROCHLORIDE

Books

Goodman AG, et al, editors: *Goodman and Gilman's the pharmacological basis of therapeutics,* ed 8, New York, 1990, Pergamon Press.

McEvoy GK, editor: *American Hospital Formulary Service (AHFS) drug information 1993,* Bethesda, MD, 1993, American Society of Hospital Pharmacists.

Olson KR, editor: *Poisoning & drug overdose,* ed 3, East Norwalk, Conn, 1999, Appleton & Lange.

Rosen P, Barkin RM, et al, editors: *Emergency medicine, concepts and clinical practice,* ed 3, St Louis, 1992, Mosby.

SODIUM BICARBONATE

Books

Abbott J, Gifford M, Rosen P: *Protocols for prehospital emergency medical care,* ed 2, Baltimore, 1984, Williams & Wilkins.

Barber JM, Budassi SA: *Mosby's manual of emergency care, practices and procedures,* St Louis, 1979, Mosby.

Goodman AG, et al, editors: *Goodman and Gilman's the pharmacological basis of therapeutics,* ed 8, New York, 1990, Pergamon Press.

Loeb S, et al, editors: *Nurse's handbook of drug therapy,* Springhouse, Pa, 1993, Springhouse Corporation.

Madigan KG: *Prehospital emergency drugs,* St Louis, 1990, Mosby.

McEvoy GK, editor: *American Hospital Formulary Service (AHFS) drug information 1993,* Bethesda, MD, 1993, American Society of Hospital Pharmacists.

Journals

Emergency Cardiac Care Committee and Subcommittees, American Heart Association: Guidelines for cardiopulmonary resuscitation and emergency cardiac care, III: adult ACLS, *JAMA* 268:2199-2241, 1992.

Emergency Cardiac Care Committee and Subcommittees, American Heart Association: Guidelines for cardiopulmonary resuscitation and emergency cardiac care, VI: pediatric ACLS, *JAMA* 268:2262-2275, 1992.

ALBUTEROL

Books

Goodman AG, et al, editors: *Goodman and Gilman's the pharmacological basis of therapeutics,* ed 8, New York, 1990, Pergamon Press.

Loeb S, et al, editors: *Nurse's handbook of drug therapy,* Springhouse, Pa, 1993, Springhouse Corporation.

Madigan KG: *Prehospital emergency drugs,* St Louis, 1990, Mosby.

McEvoy GK, editor: *American Hospital Formulary Service (AHFS) drug information 1993,* Bethesda, MD, 1993, American Society of Hospital Pharmacists.

AMINOPHYLLINE

Books

Abbott J, Gifford M, Rosen P: *Protocols for prehospital emergency medical care,* ed 2, Baltimore, 1984, Williams & Wilkins.

Barber JM, Budassi SA: *Mosby's manual of emergency care, practices and procedures,* St Louis, 1979, Mosby.

Goodman AG, et al, editors: *Goodman and Gilman's the pharmacological basis of therapeutics,* ed 8, New York, 1990, Pergamon Press.

Loeb S, et al, editors: *Nurse's handbook of drug therapy,* Springhouse, Pa, 1993, Springhouse Corporation.

Madigan KG: *Prehospital emergency drugs,* St Louis, 1990, Mosby.

McEvoy GK, editor: *American Hospital Formulary Service (AHFS) drug information 1993,* Bethesda, MD, 1993, American Society of Hospital Pharmacists.

METAPROTERENOL SULFATE

Books

Goodman AG, et al, editors: *Goodman and Gilman's the pharmacological basis of therapeutics,* ed 8, New York, 1990, Pergamon Press.

Gosselin RE, Smith RP, Hodge HC: *Clinical toxicology of commercial products,* ed 5, Baltimore, 1984, Williams & Wilkins.

Loeb S, et al, editors: *Nurse's handbook of drug therapy,* Springhouse, Pa, 1993, Springhouse Corporation.

Madigan KG: *Prehospital emergency drugs,* St Louis, 1990, Mosby.

McEvoy GK, editor: *American Hospital Formulary Service (AHFS) drug information 1993,* Bethesda, MD, 1993, American Society of Hospital Pharmacists.

OXYGEN

Books

Abbott J, Gifford M, Rosen P: *Protocols for prehospital emergency medical care,* ed 2, Baltimore, 1984, Williams & Wilkins.

Barber JM, Budassi SA: *Mosby's manual of emergency care, practices and procedures,* St Louis, 1979, Mosby.

Goodman AG, et al, editors: *Goodman and Gilman's the pharmacological basis of therapeutics,* ed 8, New York, 1990, Pergamon Press.

Madigan KG: *Prehospital emergency drugs,* St Louis, 1990, Mosby.

Journals

Emergency Cardiac Care Committee and Subcommittees, American Heart Association: Guidelines for cardiopulmonary resuscitation and emergency cardiac care, III: adult ACLS, *JAMA* 268:2199-2241, 1992.

Emergency Cardiac Care Committee and Subcommittees, American Heart Association: Guidelines for cardiopulmonary resuscitation and emergency cardiac care, VI: pediatric ACLS, *JAMA* 268:2262-2275, 1992.

ACTIVATED CHARCOAL

Books

Goldfrank LR, et al: *Goldfrank's toxicologic emergencies,* ed 6, New York, 1998, McGraw-Hill Professional.

Goodman AG, et al, editors: *Goodman and Gilman's the pharmacological basis of therapeutics,* ed 8, New York, 1990, Pergamon Press.

Gosselin RE, Smith RP, Hodge HC: *Clinical toxicology of commercial products,* ed 5, Baltimore, 1984, Williams & Wilkins.

Loeb S, et al, editors: *Nurse's handbook of drug therapy,* Springhouse, Pa, 1993, Springhouse Corporation.

McEvoy GK, editor: *American Hospital Formulary Service (AHFS) drug information 1993,* Bethesda, MD, 1993, American Society of Hospital Pharmacists.

Journals

Bernstein G, et al: Failure of gastric emptying and charcoal administration in fatal sustained-release theophylline overdose: pharmacobezoar formation, *Ann Emerg Med* 21:1388-1390, 1992.

Mariani PJ, Pook N: Gastrointestinal tract perforation with charcoal peritoneum complicating orogastric intubation and lavage, *Ann Emerg Med* 22:606-609, 1993.

Mofenson HC, et al: Gastrointestinal dialysis with activated charcoal and cathartic in the treatment of adolescent intoxications, *Clin Pediatr* 24:678-684, 1985.

Sporer KA, Manning JJ: Massive ingestion of sustained-release verapamil with a concretion and bowel infarction, *Ann Emerg Med* 22:603-605, 1993.

Tenenbein M: Multiple doses of activated charcoal: time for reappraisal? *Ann Emerg Med* 20:529-531, 1991.

ATROPINE SULFATE

Books

Amdur MO, Doull J, Klaassen CD, editors: *Casarett and Doull's toxicology, the basic science of poisons,* ed 4, New York, 1991, Pergamon Press.

Goodman AG, et al, editors: *Goodman and Gilman's the pharmacological basis of therapeutics,* ed 8, New York, 1990, Pergamon Press.

Gosselin RE, Smith RP, Hodge HC: *Clinical toxicology of commercial products,* ed 5, Baltimore, 1984, Williams & Wilkins.

Loeb S, et al, editors: *Nurse's handbook of drug therapy,* Springhouse, Pa, 1993, Springhouse Corporation.

Madigan KG: *Prehospital emergency drugs,* St Louis, 1990, Mosby.

McEvoy GK, editor: *American Hospital Formulary Service (AHFS) drug information 1993,* Bethesda, MD, 1993, American Society of Hospital Pharmacists.

Journals

Emergency Cardiac Care Committee and Subcommittees, American Heart Association: Guidelines for cardiopulmonary resuscitation and emergency cardiac care, III: adult ACLS, *JAMA* 268:2199-2241, 1992.

Emergency Cardiac Care Committee and Subcommittees, American Heart Association: Guidelines for cardiopulmonary resuscitation and emergency cardiac care, VI: pediatric ACLS, *JAMA* 268:2262-2275, 1992.

CALCIUM GLUCONATE

Books

Goodman AG, et al, editors: *Goodman and Gilman's the pharmacological basis of therapeutics,* ed 8, New York, 1990, Pergamon Press.

Loeb S, et al, editors: *Nurse's handbook of drug therapy,* Springhouse, Pa, 1993, Springhouse Corporation.

McEvoy GK, editor: *American Hospital Formulary Service (AHFS) drug information 1993,* Bethesda, MD, 1993, American Society of Hospital Pharmacists.

Journals

Bracken WM, et al: Comparative effectiveness of topical treatment for hydrofluoric acid burns, *J Occup Med* 27:733-739, 1985.

Emergency Cardiac Care Committee and Subcommittees, American Heart Association: Guidelines for cardiopulmonary resuscitation and emergency cardiac care, III: adult ACLS, *JAMA* 268:2199-2241, 1992.

Emergency Cardiac Care Committee and Subcommittees, American Heart Association: Guidelines for cardiopulmonary resuscitation and emergency cardiac care, VI: pediatric ACLS, *JAMA* 268:2262-2275, 1992.

Trevino MA, Herrman GH, Spront WL: Treatment of severe hydrofluoric acid exposure, *J Occup Med* 25:861-863, 1983.

CYANIDE ANTIDOTE KIT

Books

Amdur MO, Doull J, Klaassen CD, editors: *Casarett and Doull's toxicology, the basic science of poisons,* ed 4, New York, 1991, Pergamon Press.

Goodman AG, et al, editors: *Goodman and Gilman's the pharmacological basis of therapeutics,* ed 8, New York, 1990, Pergamon Press.

Gosselin RE, Smith RP, Hodge HC: *Clinical toxicology of commercial products,* ed 5, Baltimore, 1984, Williams & Wilkins.

Haddad LM, et al: *Clinical management of poisoning and drug overdose,* ed 3, Philadelphia, 1997, Saunders.

McEvoy GK, editor: *American Hospital Formulary Service (AHFS) drug information 1993,* Bethesda, MD, 1993, American Society of Hospital Pharmacists.

Sullivan JB, Kriger GR, editors: *Clinical environmental health and hazardous materials toxicology,* Baltimore, 1997, Williams & Wilkins.

ETHANOL

Books

Goldfrank LR, et al: *Goldfrank's toxicologic emergencies,* ed 6, New York, 1998, McGraw-Hill Professional.

Goodman AG, et al, editors: *Goodman and Gilman's the pharmacological basis of therapeutics,* ed 8, New York, 1990, Pergamon Press.

Haddad LM, et al: *Clinical management of poisoning and drug overdose,* ed 3, Philadelphia, 1997, Saunders.

McEvoy GK, editor: *American Hospital Formulary Service (AHFS) drug information 1993,* Bethesda, MD, 1993, American Society of Hospital Pharmacists.

Olson KR, editor: *Poisoning & drug overdose,* ed 3, East Norwalk, Conn, 1999, Appleton & Lange.

Journals

Galvan LA, Watts MT: Generation of an osmolality gap–ethanol nomogram from routine laboratory data, *Ann Emerg Med* 21:1342-1348, 1992.

Hoffman RS, et al: Osmol gaps revisited: normal values and limitations, *Clin Toxicol* 31:81-93, 1993.

FLUMAZENIL

Books

Goodman AG, et al, editors: *Goodman and Gilman's the pharmacological basis of therapeutics,* ed 8, New York, 1990, Pergamon Press.

McEvoy GK, editor: *American Hospital Formulary Service (AHFS) drug information 1993,* Bethesda, MD, 1993, American Society of Hospital Pharmacists.

Journals

Flumazenil, *Med Lett Drugs Ther* 34:66-68, 1992.

Votey SR, et al: Flumazenil: a new benzodiazepine antagonist, *Ann Emerg Med* 20:181-188, 1991.

FOMEPIZOLE

Book

Olson KR, ed: Poisoning & drug overdose, ed 3, East Norwalk, Conn, 1999, Appleton & Lange.

MARK I ANTIDOTE KIT

Books

Danon YL, et al, editors: *Chemical warfare medicine,* Jerusalem, 1994, Gefen.

Sifton, DW, editor: *PDR Guide to biological and chemical warfare response,* Montvale, NJ, 2002, Thomson/Physician Desk Reference.

USAMRICD, Chemical Casualty Care Division: *Medical management of chemical casualties handbook,* ed 3, Aberdeen, MD, 1999, Department of the Army.

US ARMY: *Field manual 8-285 treatment of chemical agent patients and conventional military chemical patients,* Washington, DC, 1995, Department of the Army.

US ARMY: *Field manual 8-9 NATO handbook on medical aspects of NBC defensive operations,* Washington, DC, 1996, Department of the Army.

US ARMY: *Textbook of military medicine,* Washington, DC, 1990, Department of the Army.

Zajtchuk R, et al, editors: *Medical aspects of chemical and biological warfare,* Washington, DC, 1997, Department of the Army.

METHYLENE BLUE 1%

Books

Goldfrank LR, et al: *Goldfrank's toxicologic emergencies,* ed 6, New York, 1998, McGraw-Hill Professional.

Goodman AG, et al, editors: *Goodman and Gilman's the pharmacological basis of therapeutics,* ed 8, New York, 1990, Pergamon Press.

Gosselin RE, Smith RP, Hodge HC: *Clinical toxicology of commercial products,* ed 5, Baltimore, 1984, Williams & Wilkins.

McEvoy GK, editor: *American Hospital Formulary Service (AHFS) drug information 1993,* Bethesda, MD, 1993, American Society of Hospital Pharmacists.

Sullivan JB, Kriger GR, editors: *Clinical environmental health and hazardous materials toxicology,* Baltimore, 1997, Williams & Wilkins.

NALOXONE

Books

Abbott J, Gifford M, Rosen P: *Protocols for prehospital emergency medical care,* ed 2, Baltimore, 1984, Williams & Wilkins.

Barber JM, Budassi SA: *Mosby's manual of emergency care, practices and procedures,* St Louis, 1979, Mosby.

Goldfrank LR, et al: *Goldfrank's toxicologic emergencies,* ed 6, New York, 1998, McGraw-Hill Professional.

Goodman AG, et al, editors: *Goodman and Gilman's the pharmacological basis of therapeutics,* ed 8, New York, 1990, Pergamon Press.

Loeb S, et al, editors: *Nurse's handbook of drug therapy,* Springhouse, Pa, 1993, Springhouse Corporation.

Madigan KG: *Prehospital emergency drugs,* St Louis, 1990, Mosby.

McEvoy GK, editor: *American Hospital Formulary Service (AHFS) drug information 1993,* Bethesda, MD, 1993, American Society of Hospital Pharmacists.

Journals

Emergency Cardiac Care Committee and Subcommittees, American Heart Association: Guidelines for cardiopulmonary resuscitation and emergency cardiac care, III: adult ACLS, *JAMA* 268:2199-2241, 1992.

Emergency Cardiac Care Committee and Subcommittees, American Heart Association: Guidelines for cardiopulmonary resuscitation and emergency cardiac care, VI: pediatric ACLS, *JAMA* 268:2262-2275, 1992.

PRALIDOXIME CHLORIDE

Books

Goldfrank LR, et al: *Goldfrank's toxicologic emergencies,* ed 6, New York, 1998, McGraw-Hill Professional.

Goodman AG, et al, editors: *Goodman and Gilman's the pharmacological basis of therapeutics,* ed 8, New York, 1990, Pergamon Press.

Gosselin RE, Smith RP, Hodge HC: *Clinical toxicology of commercial products,* ed 5, Baltimore, 1984, Williams & Wilkins.

Loeb S, et al, editors: *Nurse's handbook of drug therapy,* Springhouse, Pa, 1993, Springhouse Corporation.

McEvoy GK, editor: *American Hospital Formulary Service (AHFS) drug information 1993,* Bethesda, MD, 1993, American Society of Hospital Pharmacists.

Sullivan JB, Kriger GR, editors: *Clinical environmental health and hazardous materials toxicology,* Baltimore, 1997, Williams & Wilkins.

OPERATIONAL PROCEDURES

PREPLANNING CONCERNS

Books

Hazardous material emergency planning guide. In Smeby LC, editor: *Hazardous materials response handbook,* ed 3, Quincy, Mass, 1997, National Fire Protection Association.

Keffer WJ: So you want to start a haz mat team! In Tokle G, editor: *Hazardous materials response handbook,* ed 2, suppl 2, Quincy, Mass, 1993, National Fire Protection Association, pp 485-500.

NIOSH/OSHA/USCG/EPA: *Occupational safety and health guidance manual for hazardous waste site activities,* Washington, DC, 1985, DHHS (NIOSH) Publication No 85-115, US Government Printing Office.

Olson KR, editor: *Poisoning & drug overdose,* ed 3, East Norwalk, Conn, 1999, Appleton & Lange.

Smeby LC, editor: *Hazardous materials response handbook,* ed 3, Quincy, Mass, 1997, National Fire Protection Association.

SCENE OPERATIONS AND RESPONSE

Books

EMS sector standard operating procedures. In Smeby LC, editor: *Hazardous materials response handbook,* ed 3, Quincy, Mass, 1997, National Fire Protection Association.

Keffer WJ: So you want to start a haz mat team! In Tokle G, editor: *Hazardous materials response handbook,* ed 2, suppl 2, Quincy, Mass, 1993, National Fire Protection Association, pp 485-500.

NIOSH/OSHA/USCG/EPA: *Occupational safety and health guidance manual for hazardous waste site activities,* Washington, DC, 1985, DHHS (NIOSH) Publication No 85-115, US Government Printing Office.

Summit County hazardous materials standard operating procedures. In Smeby LC, editor: *Hazardous materials response handbook,* ed 3, Quincy, Mass, 1997, National Fire Protection Association.

Smeby LC, editor: *Hazardous materials response handbook,* ed 3, Quincy, Mass, 1997, National Fire Protection Association.

CHEMICAL EXPOSURE AND TRIAGE

Books

NIOSH/OSHA/USCG/EPA: *Occupational safety and health guidance manual for hazardous waste site activities,* Washington, DC, 1985, DHHS (NIOSH) Publication No 85-115, US Government Printing Office.

Olson KR, editor: *Poisoning & drug overdose,* ed 3, East Norwalk, Conn, 1999, Appleton & Lange.

Smeby LC, editor: *Hazardous materials response handbook,* ed 3, Quincy, Mass, 1997, National Fire Protection Association.

HAZARDOUS MATERIALS RESPONSE TEAM MEDICAL SUPPORT

Books

EMS sector standard operating procedures. In Smeby LC, editor: *Hazardous materials response handbook,* ed 3, Quincy, Mass, 1997, National Fire Protection Association.

Keffer WJ: So you want to start a haz mat team! In Tokle G, editor: *Hazardous materials response handbook,* ed 2, suppl 2, Quincy, Mass, 1993, National Fire Protection Association, pp 485-500.

NFPA: NFPA 471, Recommended practice for responding to hazardous materials incidents, Quincy, MA, 2002, National Fire Protection Association.

NIOSH/OSHA/USCG/EPA: *Occupational safety and health guidance manual for hazardous waste site activities,* Washington, DC, 1985, DHHS (NIOSH) Publication No 85-115, US Government Printing Office.

OSHA: CFR 1910.120, Hazardous waste operations and emergency response, Final Rule, March 6, 1989.

Summit County hazardous materials standard operating procedures. In Smeby LC, editor: *Hazardous materials response handbook,* ed 3, Quincy, Mass, 1997, National Fire Protection Association.

Smeby LC, editor: *Hazardous materials response handbook,* ed 3, Quincy, Mass, 1997, National Fire Protection Association.

PATIENT TRANSPORTATION

Books

Olson KR, editor: *Poisoning & drug overdose,* ed 3, East Norwalk, Conn, 1999, Appleton & Lange.

Smeby LC, editor: *Hazardous materials response handbook,* ed 3, Quincy, Mass, 1997, National Fire Protection Association.

Journals

Bronstein AC, et al: *Measurements of ambulance ventilation rates: impact on chemical exposure,* AACT/AAPCC/ABMT/CAPCC, Annual Meeting, Toronto, Ontario, Canada, Oct 1-4, 1991.

EMS/HAZARDOUS MATERIALS EQUIPMENT

Books

NIOSH/OSHA/USCG/EPA: *Occupational safety and health guidance manual for hazardous waste site activities,* Washington, DC, 1985, DHHS (NIOSH) Publication No 85-115, US Government Printing Office.

Smeby LC, editor: *Hazardous materials response handbook,* ed 3, Quincy, Mass, 1997, National Fire Protection Association.

POSTINCIDENT CONCERNS

Books

NIOSH/OSHA/USCG/EPA: *Occupational safety and health guidance manual for hazardous waste site activities,* Washington, DC, 1985, DHHS (NIOSH) Publication No 85-115, US Government Printing Office.

Smeby LC, editor: *Hazardous materials response handbook,* ed 3, Quincy, Mass, 1997, National Fire Protection Association.

HAZARDOUS MATERIALS TEAM MEMBER MEDICAL MONITORING PROGRAM

Books

American Conference of Governmental and Industrial Hygienists: *1992-1993 Threshold limit values for chemical substances and physical agents and biological exposure indices,* Cincinnati, 1992, American Conference of Governmental Industrial Hygienists.

Keffer WJ: So you want to start a haz mat team! In Tokle G, editor: *Hazardous materials response handbook,* ed 2, suppl 2, Quincy, Mass, 1993, National Fire Protection Association, pp 485-500.

NIOSH/OSHA/USCG/EPA: *Occupational safety and health guidance manual for hazardous waste site activities,* Washington, DC, 1985, DHHS (NIOSH) Publication No 85-115, US Government Printing Office.

OSHA: 29 CFR 1910.120, Hazardous waste operations and emergency response, Final Rule, March 6, 1989.

Smeby LC, editor: *Hazardous materials response handbook,* ed 3, Quincy, Mass, 1997, National Fire Protection Association.

ABBREVIATIONS AND ACRONYMS

The following is a list of common abbreviation used in this text:

ABC Airway, Breathing, Circulation
ABCDE Airway, Breathing, Circulation/C-spine, Decontamination needs, Evaluation for systemic toxicity
ABGs arterial blood gases
AF atrial fibrillation
ACGIH American Conference of Governmental Industrial Hygienists
ACLS advanced cardiac life support
AG anion gap
ALS advanced life support
alt alanine aminotransferase (formerly serum glutamic-pyruvic transaminase [SGPT])
AML acute myelogenous leukemia
APR air-purifying respirator
ARDS acute respiratory distress syndrome
AST aspartate aminotransferase (formerly serum glutamic-pyruvic transaminase [SGOT])
ATP adenosine triphosphate
AV atrioventricular
BAL British Anti-Lewisite (dimercaprol)
BLEVE boiling liquid expanding vapor explosion
BLS basic life support
BP blood pressure
BSA body surface area
BUN blood urea nitrogen
BWL body water loss
CBC complete blood count
CHF congestive heart failure
CN cyanide
CNMHB cyanmethemoglobin
CPR cardiopulmonary resuscitation
Cyclic AMP
adenosine 3′,5′-cyclic monophosphate
C ° Centigrade degrees
CHF congestive heart failure
CNS central nervous system
COPD chronic obstructive pulmonary disease
DMAP 4-dimethylaminophenol
DMSA 2,3-dimercaptosuccinic acid
DOT Department of Transportation
D_5W 5% dextrose in water
ECG electrocardiogram
EDTA ethylenediaminetetraacetic acid
EMG electromyography
EMS Emergency Medical Services
EPA Environmental Protection Agency
ERG Emergency Response Guidebook
F ° Fahrenheit degrees
FDA Food and Drug Administration
FEMA U.S. Federal Emergency Management Agency
FEP free erythrocyte protoporphyrin
FEV_1 forced expiratory volume in 1 second
G6PD glucose-6-phospate dehydrogenase
g gram
GFR glomerular filtration rate
GI gastrointestinal
HAZMAT Hazardous Materials
HB hemoglobin
HF hydrofluoric (acid)
HBO hyperbaric oxygen
HIV human immunodeficiency virus
IA intraarterial
ICS Incident Command System
ID identification number
IM intramuscular
IO intraosseous
IV intravenous
KCl potassium chloride
kg kilogram
kPa kilopascal
L liter
LDH lactic dehydrogenase
LEPC local emergency planning committee
LR lactated Ringer's solution
LOC level of consciousness
LPG liquefied propane gas
ml milliliter
MSDS material safety data sheets
NAC *N*-acetylcysteine
NAP *N*-acetyl-penicillamine
NIOSH National Institute for Occupational Safety and Health
NFPA National Fire Protection Association
NA North American identification number
NCV nerve conduction velocity
n.o.s. not otherwise specified
NS normal saline solution
OG osmolar gap
OP organophosphate

ORMS other regulated materials
OSHA Occupational Safety and Health Administration
Pa water vapor pressure
PAPR powered air-purifying respirator
PBBs polybrominated biphenyls
PEEP positive end-expiratory pressure
PCBs polychlorinated biphenyls
PCDFs polychlorinated dibenzofurans
PEG polyethylene glycol
PIN product identification number
PPE personal protective equipment
ppm parts per million
psi pounds per square inch
PVC premature ventricular contraction
RADS reactive airways dysfunction syndrome/radiation absorbed dose
RCRA Resource Conservation and Recovery Act
SARA Superfund Amendments and Reauthorization Act of 1986 (PL 99-499)
SQ subcutaneous
SCBA self-contained breathing apparatus
SLUDGE *s*alivation, *l*acrimation, *u*rination, *d*efecation, *g*astrointestinal pain, and *e*mesis
SQ subcutaneous
T_{db} dry bulb temperature
TCDD dioxin (2,3,7,8-tetrachlorodibenzo-*p*-dioxin)
TDI toluene diisocyanate
TIBC total iron-binding capacity
TKO to keep open
TOCP tri-ortho-cresyl phosphate
UN United Nations
USCG United States Coast Guard
USP United States Pharmacopeia
VF ventricular fibrillation
VT ventricular tachycardia
WBGT wet bulb globe temperature
ZZP zinc protoporphyrin